HANDBOOK OF COSMETIC DERMATOLOGY

VOLUME 1

FOUNDATIONS AND TECHNIQUES IN AESTHETIC SKIN SCIENCE

Dr. Shreya Das

ALLIED HEALTH PRESS

Handbook of Cosmetic Dermatology Volume 1

Foundations and Techniques in Aesthetic Skin Science

Author: **Dr. Shreya Das**

Allied Health Press
4164 Lakeshore Road
Burlington ON L7L 1A4
Canada
www.alliedhealthpress.com
Email: orders@arclereducation.com

ISBN: 978-1-77956-828-1

Allied Health Press publishes wide variety of books and eBooks. For more information about Allied Health Press and its products, visit our website at www.alliedhealthpress.com

ABOUT THE AUTHOR

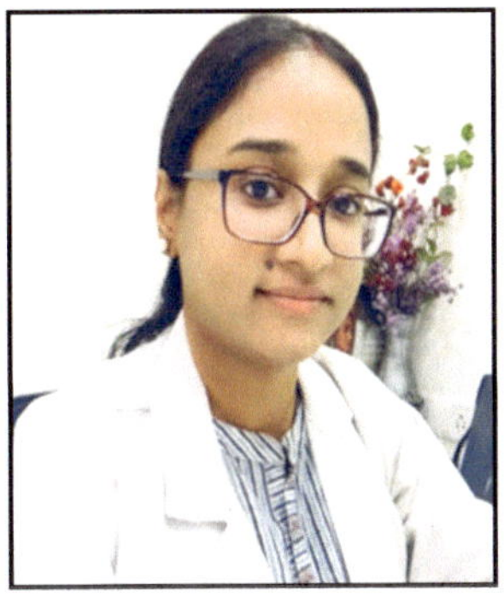

Dr. Shreya Das is an Oral and Maxillofacial Surgeon with specialized training and clinical experience in facial cosmetic surgery and aesthetic medicine. A university gold medalist, she completed her MDS in Oral and Maxillofacial Surgery and has since worked across reputed hospitals and wellness organizations. With a strong interest in facial aesthetics, her work bridges surgical precision and minimally invasive cosmetic procedures. She is passionate about advancing evidence-based practices in facial cosmetic and reconstructive surgery and contributing to the education of clinicians in this evolving field.

Brief Table of Contents

Getting Started with This Book

Chapter Openers

A list of Chapter Outline is presented providing a brief Introduction to what will be covered in the chapter.

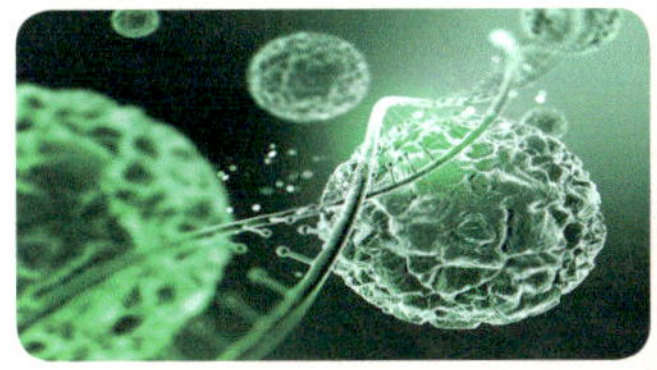

Introduction

Often referred to as the science of life, biology is a broad field of study aimed at comprehending the several kinds of life on Earth, from tiny creatures to sophisticated multicellular entities. Comprising several subfields, including molecular biology, ecology, and evolutionary biology, each of which advances our knowledge of living systems, this field clarifies the mechanisms controlling life events, including development, reproduction, and interaction with the surroundings, which is the central goal of biology. Moreover, biology fills in the void between the natural sciences and medicine by offering a necessary understanding of health, illness, and the interactions between organisms and their environments. Dealing with urgent global issues such as climate change, biodiversity loss, and new diseases depends on an awareness of these complex biological interactions, therefore highlighting the critical part biology plays in modern civilization. Fundamentally, biology explores and tests ideas about the living world using the scientific method. Through methodical observation and experimentation,

LEARNING OBJECTIVES

After studying this chapter, you will be able to:

1. Discuss the scientific method in biology;
2. Explain the cell theory;
3. Discuss the genetics and heredity;
4. Evolution and natural selection;
5. Focus on ecology and ecosystems;
6. Learn about human biology;
7. Evaluate the plant biology;
8. Explain the microbiology;
9. Focus on current trends in biology.

1.1. The Scientific Method in Biology

Learning Outcome

1. Describe the steps of the scientific method;
2. Focus on hypothesis formation;
3. Learn about experimental design.

Learning Outcomes

The beginning of each section of every chapter contains a set of Learning Outcomes that inform students of concepts they should understand. These outcomes help students understand what they should be able to do if they have mastered the material in that section.

Test Your Knowledge

Throughout each chapter, Test Your Knowledge cues you to note which topics have been covered and to self-test your understanding of the material presented.

Test Your Knowledge

1. Explain why correlation does not imply causation in scientific experiments.
2. How does the scientific method help reduce the influence of personal opinions in research?

Chapter Summary

The Summary Section appear at the end of each chapter and summarize main concepts covered throughout the chapter. These points provide key concepts in an engaging and meaningful way.

Summary

The investigation of biological principles highlights the importance of a comprehensive view of life by reflecting the intricate interactions that occur within living systems. The complexity of biology goes beyond individual species or systems, as this essay highlights; it also includes the interactions that mold ecosystems and affect biodiversity. Researchers can conduct in-depth analyses of metabolomic data using sophisticated technologies like MetaboAnalyst, which offer insights into the molecular mechanisms underlying these interactions. As demonstrated by the developments in MetaboAnalyst, for example, the integration of diverse omics data promotes a thorough understanding of metabolic pathways and helps identify important biological markers necessary for research on development and disease (Chong et al., 2018). Additionally, the phenomenon of ecological invasions is a key component of biological research and a vital field of study. The introduction of non-native species into unfamiliar habitats has significant ramifications and calls for multidisciplinary management strategies. Examining the origins and effects of these biological incursions, invasion science has become a crucial field that highlights the need to comprehend ecological dynamics and community interactions. As interest in biological invasions increases, new findings are emerging that put conventional ecological theories and practices to the test. The importance of incorporating various scientific viewpoints is shown by this developing discipline, which also highlights how invasive species shape ecosystems and advances our knowledge of ecological resilience (David et al., 2013). When taken as a whole, these discoveries from invasion science and metabolomics highlight the value of multidisciplinary biology research. Fostering cross-disciplinary collaboration and utilizing technological breakthroughs to improve our comprehension of intricate biological interactions are crucial as we look to the future of biological research. In addition to deepening our understanding of the complexities of life, this method lays the groundwork for tackling urgent environmental issues. Future studies can ensure the continued relevance of biology in a world that is constantly changing by acknowledging the interconnection of biological systems and opening the door to creative solutions that support sustainability and biodiversity conservation. We might imagine a thorough comprehension of life that serves both academia and society at large through ongoing investigation and integration of scientific knowledge.

Knowledge Assessment

The chapter includes material designed to review and reinforce each content. It includes Critical Thinking Questions to help test of your understanding of information presented in the chapter and Short answer Questions to review your understanding of the key concepts presented in the chapter.

Critical Thinking Questions

1. **Who is known as the "Father of Modern Biology"?**
   a. Aristotle
   b. Charles Darwin
   c. Gregor Mendel
   d. Louis Pasteur
2. **What is the basic unit of life?**
   a. Atom
   b. Molecule
   c. Cell
   d. Organism
3. **Which branch of biology studies the interaction of organisms with their environment?**
   a. Genetics
   b. Ecology
   c. Physiology
   d. Botany
4. **Which macromolecule is the main source of energy for living organisms?**
   a. Proteins
   b. Lipids
   c. Carbohydrates
   d. Nucleic acids
5. **DNA is primarily responsible for which function in living organisms?**
   a. Energy production
   b. Protein synthesis
   c. Storing genetic information
   d. Regulating body temperature

Short Answer Questions

1. What is biology, and why is it important to study biology?
2. What are the three main domains of life, and how are they different from one another?
3. Define homeostasis and give an example of how it works in living organisms.
4. What is the cell theory, and why is it fundamental to biology?
5. How do autotrophs and heterotrophs differ in the way they obtain energy?
6. What is the scientific method, and how is it applied in biological research?
7. Discuss how biology helps address global challenges such as climate change, disease, and food security.
8. Explain the levels of biological organization from the smallest unit to the largest. Provide examples at each level.
9. Describe the relationship between structure and function in biology, giving specific examples from cells or organs.
10. How has the discovery of genetics shaped our understanding of inheritance and variation among organisms?

Supplementary Materials

Key Terms: A list of key terms is given for quick reference

KEY TERMS FROM THIS CHAPTER

Annotation enrichment analysis
Cell theory
Ecosystems
Microbiology
Plant biology
Biological structure
Cellular structure
Genetics
Natural selection
Cell
Ecology
Human biology
Organism

Further Resources: Recommendations for additional readings, websites, and multimedia resources.

References

1. Argelaguet, R., Velten, B., Arnol, D., Dietrich, S., Zenz, T., Marioni, J. C., Buettner, F., et al. (2018). Multi-omics factor analysis—A framework for unsupervised integration of multi-omics data sets. *Molecular Systems Biology, 14*. https://doi.org/10.15252/msb.20178124.
2. Bacher, S., Blackburn, T. M., Essl, F., & Genovesi, P. (2017). *Socio-Economic Impact Classification of Alien Taxa (SEICAT)*. https://core.ac.uk/download/286567949.pdf (accessed on 8th March 2025).
3. Barnett, R., Brace, S., Cucchi, T., & Dobney, K. (2013). *Divergent Evolutionary Processes Associated with Colonization of Offshore Islands*. https://core.ac.uk/download/20664364.pdf (accessed on 8th March 2025).

Detailed Table of Contents

CHAPTER 5

Chemical Peels: Superficial to Deep 139

CHAPTER 6

Collagen Induction Therapy 173

CHAPTER 9

Mesotherapy 273

CHAPTER 10

Cryolipolysis and Body Contouring Technologies 307

CHAPTER 11

Botulinum Toxin: Types, Indications, Techniques 339

LIST OF FIGURES

PREFACE

Cosmetic dermatology exists uniquely at the intersection of medical science and cosmetic optimization. It involves not only the functional health of the skin as the body's largest organ, but also the human imperative of appearance optimization. Advancements in cellular biology, molecular pathways, and cutaneous immunology have created a platform for therapies that move beyond repair to deliver visible rejuvenation. From an understanding of the epidermal and dermal microarchitecture to the management of signal cascades governing collagen production, the specialty combines systematic inquiry with therapeutic imagination.

Over the past few decades, requests for minimally invasive treatments and personalized topical regimens have grown exponentially, driven as much by technological developments as by cultural shifts in attitudes toward self-care. Providers must balance evidence-based practice with patient expectations, safety and efficacy, and outcomes that satisfy personal goals. Whether halting the natural order of intrinsic aging or defending against dermal damage from ultraviolet radiation, treatments will be required to blend an extensive understanding of skin physiology with an informed assessment of risk factors, side-effect profiles, and long-term outcomes.

This book, *Handbook of Cosmetic Dermatology: Volume 1,* has been written to serve as a comprehensive guide, providing a complete reference for allied health professionals, scientists, and clinicians. It compiles basic principles, treatment approaches, and emerging technologies in one book. By providing core concepts with practical guidance, this handbook aims to ensure high-quality care and inform decision-making in diverse practice settings.

Chapter 1 provides an exhaustive account of skin anatomy and physiology, from the structural components of the epidermis, dermis, and subcutaneous tissue, as well as their interactions with vascular, nervous, and immune networks.

Chapter 2 describes intrinsic aging and photoaging, comparing the molecular pathways that drive chronological alterations with those triggered by ultraviolet radiation and outlining the associated clinical manifestations.

Chapter 3 covers the application of cosmeceuticals and topical products, evaluating active ingredients such as retinoids, peptides, and antioxidants, and formulating options for peak penetration and stability.

Chapter 4 covers photoprotection and sunscreens, including the physics of ultraviolet light, filter types, and application methods to achieve maximal patient compliance and cutoff wavelengths.

Chapter 5 discusses chemical peels, ranging from superficial alpha-hydroxy peels to deep phenol peeling, including indications, protocols, and post-procedure care.

Chapter 6 provides an in-depth review of collagen induction therapy (CIT), including microneedling devices, radiofrequency (RF) devices, and adjunctive growth factor applications.

Chapter 7 provides an overview of laser and light therapy, including chromophore targets, wavelength selection, and safety considerations for varying skin types. Chapter 8 brings non-ablative skin rejuvenation and fractional lasers up to date, comparing treatment endpoints, downtime considerations, and maintenance techniques.

Chapter 9 addresses mesotherapy techniques, outlining injection technique, solution composition, and contraindications.

Chapter 10 examines cryolipolysis and body contour devices, presenting the biophysical basis of adipocyte apoptosis, patient selection criteria, and combination approaches.

Chapter 11 provides coverage of the use of botulinum toxin (BT) types A and B, including neurotoxin pharmacology, calculation of dosing, landmarks for injection, and safety considerations regarding side effects.

Chapter 12 covers the use of dermal fillers, categorizing products such as hyaluronic acid, calcium hydroxylapatite (CaHA), and poly-L-lactic acid (PLLA) and detailing injection techniques for various anatomical regions.

This book is intended for dermatologists, plastic surgeons, aesthetic practitioners, nurse specialists, and postgraduate trainees who require a comprehensive foundation in cosmetic dermatology. It will also be helpful to basic scientists who are researching translational uses and industry specialists who formulate products. Merging theory and clinical pearls, this book is suitable for both new clinicians and established experts in the delivery of patient-centered care, underpinned by the best current evidence.

SKIN ANATOMY AND PHYSIOLOGY

1

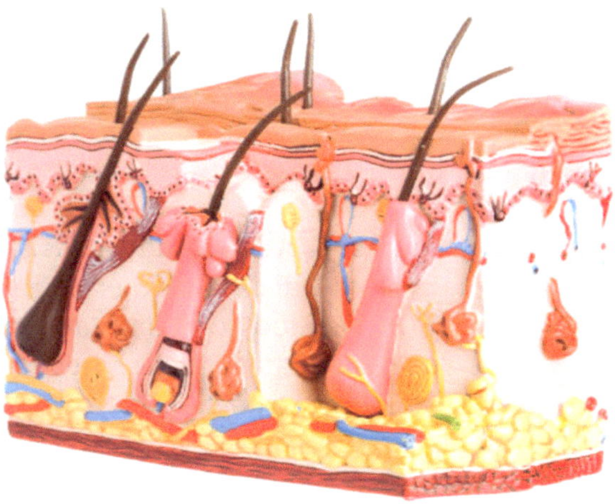

LEARNING OBJECTIVES

After studying this chapter, you will be able to:

1. Understand the structure of the skin
2. Explain the types of skin
3. Describe skin functions
4. Discuss skin cells and their roles
5. Define skin appendages
6. Focus on skin health and disorders

Introduction

The skin, the largest body organ of the human body, is required for defense and homeostasis against damage from the external world. Being the body's initial defense, it possesses various functions like barrier formation, reception of sensory stimuli, and temperature maintenance. It is crucial to understand the complex organization and physiology of the skin so that its interaction with various internal and external factors can be understood. Skin consists of three principal layers: epidermis, dermis, and hypodermis. All three layers contribute uniquely to the function and durability of skin, which has a remarkable capacity to acclimatize to changes in the surrounding external environment. This introduction will investigate skin's intricate anatomy and how its specialized cell and tissue arrangements enable it to perform essential functions with effectiveness, setting the stage for an integrated investigation into skin anatomy and physiology. Besides its protective function, the skin is also vital in many physiological processes. It plays a vital role in sensation and communication with the environment, possessing an assortment of nerve endings that respond to touch, temperature, and pain. Besides sensation, the skin plays a vital role in the immune system by offering immune cells that identify and combat infections. Besides, the skin is also involved in maintaining body temperature and fluid balance by its mechanisms of vasodilation and sweating. Such a multi-stage system clearly indicates the importance of the intrinsic function of the skin not just as a covering but also as an active participant in systemic homeostasis. Thus, careful consideration of skin anatomy and physiology has to be kept in mind for these functions, which clearly emphasize the importance of skin health for general health. Advancements in modern technology employed to study skin physiology have provided us with more insight into its structure and functioning, leading to new medical applications. Technologies such as hyperspectral imaging (HSI) are transforming the landscape of information regarding skin composition and illness by creating rich spectroscopic data on skin tissue. This enables researchers to extract valuable diagnostic information regarding conditions that affect the skin and related systems. Besides, non-invasive tools like transcranial electrical stimulation (tES) are able to potentially modulate subcutaneous tissue and skin responses very effectively. These developments offer researchers and practitioners a more nuanced understanding of the delicate interfacing of the skin with numerous physiological processes, complementing therapeutic intervention further. As we progress deeper into the intricate maze of dermatology's skin physiology and anatomy, these new technologies can be invaluable to both clinical use and fundamental research in dermatology and general health (Lu et al., 2014; Adam et al., 2015).

Definition of Skin and Its Importance

The human body's largest organ, skin, is a vital barrier to the outside world, critical to homeostasis and protection of the tissue beneath. Composed of three main layers, the epidermis, dermis, and subcutaneous tissue, the layers contribute distinct functions that are necessary for overall well-being. The epidermis provides a first line of defense against pathogens and toxins. Beneath this, the dermis has structural support and holds vital components such as blood vessels, nerves, and connective tissues. Not only does this active communication between the layers make the skin's protective functions stronger, but it also enables sensory perception to occur, which is of utmost importance for detecting environmental stimuli. Anatomy and physiology of skin are fundamental knowledge, as they emphasize its role in disease and health, illustrating how healthy skin is the body's general well-being. In addition to protection and sensation, the skin plays a crucial role in thermoregulation, which allows the body to maintain its internal temperature constant. With the mechanisms of perspiration and vasodilation, the skin effectively regulates heat loss through sweat evaporation and increased blood flow, respectively. This process of thermoregulation is not only crucial when exercising, but also because of environmental fluctuations. For instance, in high or low temperatures, the skin rapidly adapts to maintain the body's core temperature. Any interference in these regulatory processes can lead to situations such as hyperthermia or hypothermia, reflecting the skin's role in ensuring physiological stability. Hence, appreciating the skin's role is not restricted to this organ's primary function, highlighting its complexity in regulating homeostasis in a changing environment. Also, skin is responsible for playing a basic role in numerous metabolic activities, including vitamin D formation, essential for the immune system and healthy bones. Skin cells transform a precursor molecule that they absorb from ultraviolet light into vitamin D3, which is then activated by the kidneys and liver. This aspect of skin physiology demonstrates how skin is engaged in enabling essential nutrient production, further emphasizing its various roles in health. In addition, recent advances in wearable chemical sensors aim to push the role of skin in health monitoring, pointing to a growing interface between technology and biology. While wearable sensors are capable of monitoring hydration and detecting chemical changes, the capability of skin to monitor health continuously can bring revolutionized individualized medicine (Amay et al., 2016). Therefore, understanding the definition and function of skin transcends mere anatomy; it observes skin's key roles in protection, regulation, metabolism, and technological assimilation in health sciences (Figure 1.1).

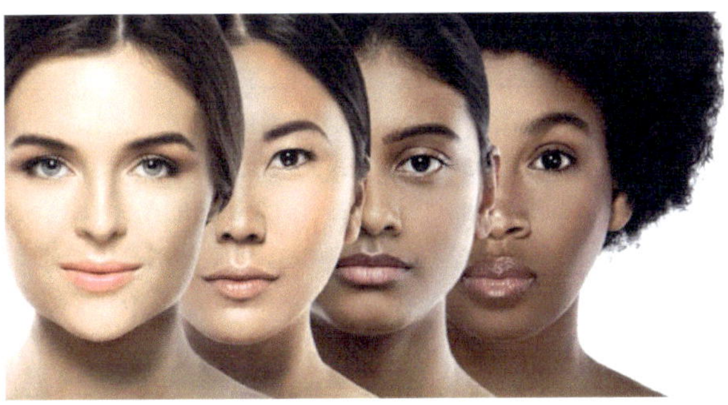

Figure 1.1. Representation of diverse skin types and tones, illustrating the range of human skin variation relevant to dermatological and cosmetic considerations.

Source: https://www.myerleepharmacy.com/wp-content/uploads/2019/07/skin-types.jpg.

Overview of Skin Functions

Skin is the body's first line of defense, with important protective functions to shield internal structures from the outside threat of danger. The barrier function is of great importance to maintaining homeostasis as it prevents invasion by pathogens, harmful chemicals, and water loss. The most external layer of skin is the epidermis and consists predominantly of keratinocytes that produce keratin, a hard protein that safeguards the skin against abrasion and environmental stress. In addition, melanocytes found in the epidermis are responsible for pigmentation of the skin to guard against ultraviolet (UV) radiation. The intrinsic ability of the skin to regenerate and repair itself further highlights its protective function, so that there is rapid recovery from minor injury. By these mechanisms, the skin is not only protective but also integral to health and wellness overall. This gives a focal emphasis to the interdependent relationship of skin physiology and body defense (Lotfollahi, 2024). In addition to its roles as protection, the skin is essential in thermoregulation, which is vital to the mechanism of stable body temperature maintenance. The skin regulates heat by mechanisms such as vasodilation and sweating; as temperature rises in the body, vessels in the dermis widen and heat is lost. Sweating serves a dual purpose, cooling the body via evaporation and hydrating the skin. At low temperatures, vasoconstriction reduces blood supply to the skin surface, conserving heat. The skin's thermoregulatory process also affects metabolic processes as well as overall energy expenditure. Thus, the skin is not merely a protective outer covering but an active participant in physiological functions, unveiling its complexity. The multilateral role of the skin also clarifies its function beyond obvious protection (Jörg, 2024). Lastly, the skin plays a vital sensory role, being equipped with various receptors that respond to physical stimuli, thus enabling the sense of touch, warmth, coldness, and pain. This sensory function is delegated to certain nerve endings that are located in the dermal layer and that advise the nervous system to deliver useful information about the outside world. The ability to perceive these stimuli is vital for survival since it enables instantaneous responses to harmful stimuli or changes in the environment. Besides, the function of the skin in sensory perception contributes to emotional and social relationships, as touch influences mood and behavior. Therefore, sensory functions of the skin transcend basic defensive mechanisms, demonstrating its importance in shaping human experiences and relationships (Lotfollahi, 2024).

1.1. Structure of the Skin

Learning Outcome

1. Describe the epidermis, the outermost layer
2. Define dermis, the middle layer
3. Explain the hypodermis, the innermost layer

Skin is a complex organ that reveals a multi-faceted composition made up of three principal layers: the epidermis, dermis, and hypodermis. The most superficial layer, the epidermis, is a barrier against environmental aggressors, harmful microbes, and water loss. The epidermis is composed mainly of keratinocytes, which produce keratin, a key protein discovered to help strengthen the skin and make it waterproof. Furthermore, melanocytes are present in the epidermis and are responsible for the secretion of melanin, the pigment that gives skin its color and protects it from UV radiation. The constant cycle of keratinocyte growth and shedding is critical to maintaining the integrity of the skin, influencing everything from wound healing to how the skin looks. The complexity of the outer layer is the setting for understanding the ways in which skin health can be influenced by internal factors, as well as external environmental factors. Beneath the epidermis lies the dermis, which is much thicker and gives structural and functional support to the epidermal layer. Made up of connective tissues, elastin, and collagen, the dermis lends the skin elasticity and strength. This layer is rich in vascularity, lymphatization, and innervation, making it possible for the provision of nutrients, removal of waste, and sensory perception. Further, the dermis contains varied skin appendages like hair follicles, sebaceous glands, and sweat glands, each of which plays a crucial role in thermoregulation, hydration, and protection. The intricate vascular bed of the dermis ensures the supply of the skin with nutrients, recognizing its value not as a barrier alone but also as an active participant in systemic homeostasis. Understanding how the dermis functions is crucial, particularly in considering dermatologic conditions arising which happen due to this layer's dysfunction. Fixing the skin to deeper tissues, the subcutaneous tissue, or hypodermis, consists primarily of loose connective tissue and adipose tissue. The layer has several functions, including cushioning the deeper structures such as muscles and bones, insulation, and storing energy. The inclusion of adipose tissue in the hypodermis regulates body temperature by providing insulation, alongside acting as an energy store during caloric deficit. Moreover, the hypodermis is also responsible for the overall mobility of the skin in that it permits it to glide freely on top of deeper anatomical structures. Understanding the structure and function of the hypodermis is essential in comprehending the interaction of the skin with other body systems, as well as how different health issues can impact skin integrity and function, particularly in terms of diseases that can impede these layers, such as psoriasis (Torres et al., 2023) and how immunizations affect skin physiology (Kamaleldin et al., 2022) (Figure 1.2).

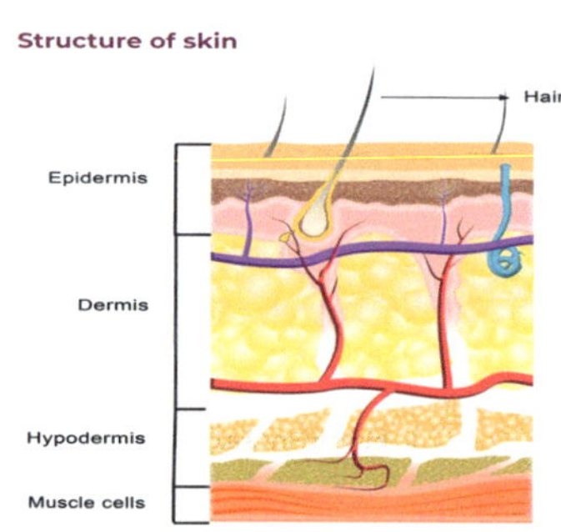

Figure 1.2. Skin structure.

Source: https://learnfatafat.com/wp-content/uploads/2020/02/Structure-of-skin-human.jpg.

1.1.1. Epidermis: The Outermost Layer

The outermost layer of skin, the epidermis, is a vital protective barrier between the body and environmental stressors and pathogens. The stratum is primarily composed of keratinocytes and plays a major role in preserving the integrity of the skin. The epidermis is stratified in several discrete layers, culminating in the outermost stratum corneum, consisting of dead keratinized cells that provide strength and waterproofing to the skin. This anatomy of the skin protects deeper tissues but also participates in the perception of stimuli and immune response, illustrating the epidermis and its multifunctional character in skin physiology. As the body's first line of defense against infection, the integrity of the epidermis is key to overall dermatological health and influences conditions such as psoriasis and dermatitis, highlighting the necessity for additional knowledge and epidermal-related pathologies' treatment (Lotfollahi, 2024). Aside from its defense functions, the epidermis is also engaged in osmoregulation so that normal hydration levels in the skin are sustained. The outermost stratum corneum is especially important in this context since it is the main barrier to transepidermal water loss (TEWL). The complex structure of this layer, in which corneocytes are embedded in a matrix of lipids, allows the retention of moisture while excluding harmful substances from outside that would otherwise penetrate into the skin. The health of the stratum corneum is significant to skin health and appearance and has therefore been a target for dermatologic interventions. Increasing environmental stress on skin barrier integrity has made preservation and restoration measures aimed at the stratum corneum increasingly important. This action acknowledges that the wellness of the epidermis is not just imperative aesthetically but also for the longevity of the skin's health (Tharakan & Lonczak, 2024). Furthermore, aging also has significant effects on the functional and structural properties of the epidermis. As a human being ages, the rate of keratinocyte turnover decreases, leading to thinner skin in the epidermis that provides poor defense against environmental aggressions. This alteration is the cause behind the manifestations of aging skin, such as greater dryness, reduced elasticity, and greater vulnerability to injury and disease. Effects of aging on the epidermis also extend to its barrier function, with decreased lipid synthesis eroding its ability to retain water. Knowledge of physiological changes due to aging is important for intervention programs designed to preserve skin integrity in the elderly. Studying treatments and products that were developed to enhance epidermal resilience, e.g., topical products to tighten up the stratum corneum, could potentially uncover a pathway toward ameliorating the adverse effects of skin aging, ultimately improving quality of life (Lotfollahi, 2024) (Figure 1.3).

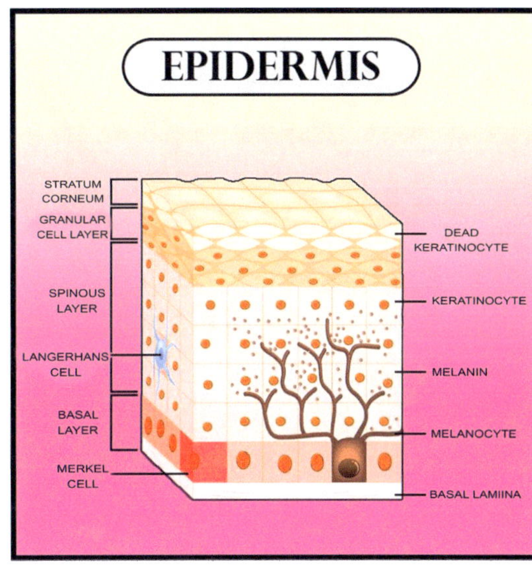

Figure 1.3. Epidermis.

Source: https://www.vedantu.com/question-sets/4dc2c2dd-fa76-46b4-8c4c-9477607083ae5509742480639124723.png.

1.1.2. Dermis: The Middle Layer

The dermis, the second layer of the skin, is a fundamental constituent of the structure and function of the integumentary system. The dermis is situated between the outer epidermis and inner subcutaneous tissue, lending strength and elasticity to the skin because of its high level of connective tissue. This layer is predominantly composed of elastin and collagen fibers, which lend mechanical strength and flexibility so that the skin is able to withstand stresses and strains. Apart from this, the dermis also houses important structures such as blood vessels, lymph vessels, nerve endings, and glands, all of which contribute significantly to the physiological activities of the skin. The intricate arrangement of the aforementioned elements is not only responsible for thermoregulation but also has a major role in sensory perception, emphasizing the role of the dermis in homeostasis in the body. Upon closer examination, the dermal elements are observed to play a dual structural and functional role. In the dermis, there are two main layers, the papillary and the reticular layers. The papillary layer, characterized by loose and thin connective tissue, interdigitates with the epidermis, a function that allows for increased oxygen and nutrient exchange. It is rich in sensory nerve endings, capillaries, and skin appendages, a function that also adds to sensation and nutrient delivery. The reticular layer, making up most of the dermis, is made of dense connective tissue that provides tensile strength. The arrangement of collagen fibers in this layer controls the skin's general firmness and elasticity, showing how the dermis not only organizes the epidermis but also controls the outside look and how long the skin will last, an area of concentration in most areas of science, including medicine and cosmetology (Igarashi et al., 2005).

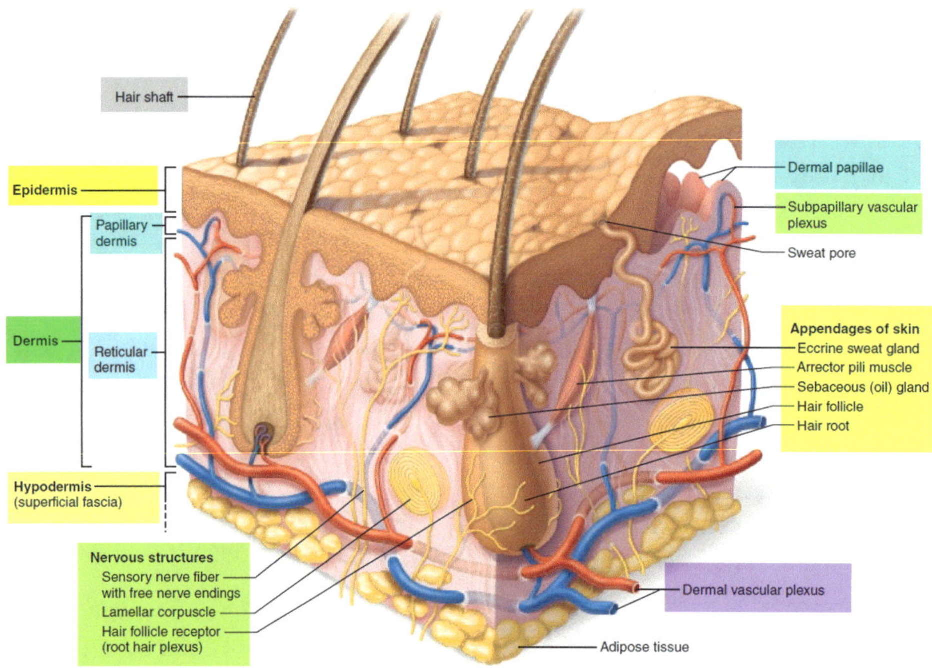

Figure 1.4. Dermis layers.

Source: https://healthjade.net/wp-content/uploads/2017/10/dermis-layers.jpg.

In learning about the dermis's contribution to skin physiology, the significance of its health becomes apparent in achieving full skin integrity and function. Damage to the dermis from injury, aging, or environmental stress can lead to complications like loss of elasticity, hindered healing, and even chronic skin conditions. Therefore, understanding the underlying mechanics of the dermis and its response to stressors is vital for developing effective skincare and therapeutic interventions. Moreover, advancements in cosmetic technology often target this layer, aiming to promote collagen production or enhance moisture retention to improve skin appearance and health. Therefore, the dermis not only exists as a structural entity but also as an active and complex component of skin anatomy and physiology and deserves further study and investigation in the scientific community (Cozart et al., 2017) (Figure 1.4).

1.1.3. Hypodermis: The Innermost Layer

The hypodermis, or the subcutaneous tissue, is an important feature of skin physiology and anatomy as the innermost tissue that holds the skin to the deeper tissues, essentially muscle and bone. It is primarily made up of loose connective tissue and fat tissue, which insulates and shock-absorbs and thus protects the body against exterior pressures. The hypodermis is an important reservoir of energy, containing fat that can be tapped when the caloric intake is minimal. As a transition zone between dermis and deeper tissues, the hypodermis makes it possible for the skin to slide freely, to extend and return to its original state without damage, and to play a significant role in the overall integrity and function of the skin as a protective barrier. Furthermore, the hypodermis contains significant vasculature, lymphatic vessels, and nerve endings, which indicate its role in thermoregulation and sensation. The hypodermal blood vessels play a significant role in temperature regulation of the body by regulating blood flow to the skin surface. In hot conditions, vasodilation is effective in increasing blood flow and heat dissipation. In cold temperatures, vasoconstriction is active in minimizing the loss of heat. The sensory nerves located in the hypodermis are responsible for the sense of pressure and vibration, as well as providing valuable feedback to the central nervous system regarding the external environment. The hypodermis thus serves not only to strengthen more peripheral layers of the skin but also contains numerous diverse physiological functions required for homeostasis. The hypodermis also ages, diets, and gets sick, and these changes can greatly influence the look as well as the overall well-being of an individual. With aging, the amount of adipose tissue within the hypodermis decreases, which leads to wrinkling and sagging of the skin typical of advanced age. Weight changes can also modify the thickness of the hypodermis, affecting both cosmetic issues and physiological well-being. This layer also plays a role in the pathogenesis of many dermatological conditions and treatments, as knowledge of its structure and functioning is necessary for successful interventions. From studies, improvements in techniques for assessing and reconstructing skin layers, including the hypodermis, can enhance insight into skin disease and help in more effective therapeutic approaches (Hofmann et al., 2023). Enhanced information on the function of subcutaneous tissues can result in dermatologic breakthroughs (Serra et al., 2022) (Figure 1.5).

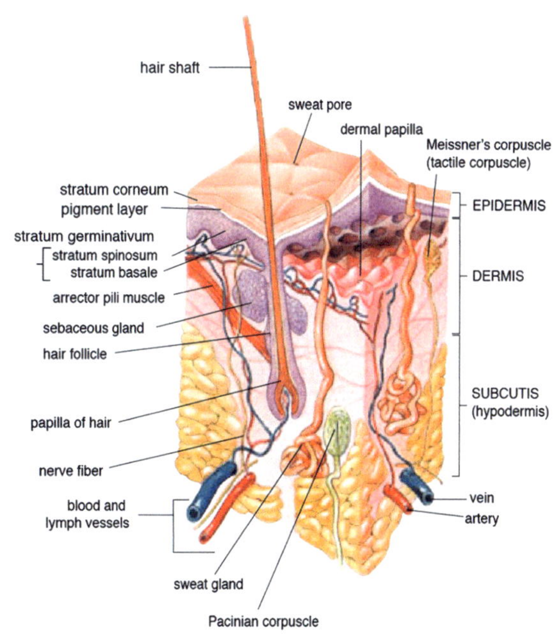

Figure 1.5. Hypodermis.

Source: https://upload.wikimedia.org/wikipedia/commons/thumb/2/27/Skin.png/800px-Skin.png

Test Your Knowledge

1. What are the three main layers of the skin?
2. What is the function of the dermis layer in the skin?

1.2. Types of Skin

Learning Outcome

1. Differentiate between thick skin and thin skin
2. Discuss variations in skin color
3. Understand various skin types

Understanding of the different skin types is basic to comprehending the overall anatomy and physiology of this organ. The human skin can be classified into four categories in general: normal, oily, dry, and combination skin. Normal skin possesses an optimal balance of oil and moisture with even texture and few blemishes. Oily skin results from overproduction of sebum, which typically gives the skin a shiny appearance and greater predisposition to obtain acne through clogged pores. Dry skin typically is rough in texture and tight or itchy due to underproduction of oil. Combination skin contains characteristics of more than one category, with oily patches on some areas and dry patches on others, requiring care in skincare regimens. A knowledge of these differences aids successful treatment and formulation of skincare in the clinic and cosmetic practice. Skin type is not merely about appearance, since it carries important implications for skin well-being and disease prevention. For instance, all skin types have unique physiological features that influence the manner in which the skin barrier functions and reacts to external aggression. Oily skin is generally more resilient against environmental trauma due to its lipid-filled barrier, yet it may be susceptible to specific dermatological states like acne. Dry skin, on the other hand, is more sensitive to irritants and allergens, and this makes moisturizing and maintenance of its barrier particularly crucial. According to recent findings, variations in skin type are observed among various populations, indicating the role of genes, lifestyle, and even location in the skin (Fan et al., 2025). Such diverse influences necessitate unique skincare and therapeutic approaches based on skin type and need. Furthermore, it is noteworthy to mention that skin types are dynamic and can change due to several intrinsic and extrinsic reasons like age, hormonal changes, and environmental influences. For example, studies have established that skin lipid profiles could dramatically alter with progressing age, thus possibly drastically altering the dynamics of skin type classification (Fan et al., 2025). Research on the facial stratum corneum lipid profiles, particularly in young women, shows significant variations with age and thus underscores the requirement for adaptive skincare routines over a period. These findings indicate that skin health is a continuous process, and it is necessary to have knowledge of the interaction between skin type and environmental conditions, thereby enhancing our ability to develop effective interventions against skin diseases and support overall skin health (Lotfollahi, 2024).

1.2.1. Thick Skin vs. Thin Skin

The distinction between thick skin and thin skin is important in the anatomy and physiology of the skin because the two serve different functions and have deep structural differences. Thick skin is predominantly found on the palms of the hands and soles of the feet, with a considerably thicker epidermis made up of all five layers of keratinocytes. This greater thickness provides a robust wall against mechanical wear and tear and external stress, and this is very important for these frictional areas. Thin skin, however, covers the majority of the body surface and consists only of four epidermal layers without the stratum lucidum. This reduction in layers allows for more flexibility and sensing, but accommodating the extensive diversity in skin functions in the various body regions while maintaining protection and thermoregulation (Almet et al., 2023). The structural physiological effect of thick and thin skin surpasses merely structure since it also encompasses variation in cellular composition and functioning. Thick skin contains a high density of keratinocytes that are also critical to the barrier since these cells are responsible for the formation of keratin, a protein that enhances the endurance of the skin against environmental damage. Similarly critical to desiccation resistance in areas that are under chronic abrasion is the stratum corneum thickness, a sheet composed of dead keratinized cells. Thin skin, on the other hand, has more advanced cell types, including melanocytes and Merkel cells, to contribute to pigmentation and sensory functions, respectively. These variations testify to the skin's adaptive development as a result of mechanical and environmental stresses by different parts of the body (Heng et al., 2021). Cellular and molecular studies of thick and thin skin are also expanding our understanding of skin disease and potential treatment. As emerging technologies, such as single-cell RNA sequencing, allow us to analyze populations of skin cells in fine detail, we are able to observe how various types of skin respond to damage, inflammation, or disease. Such a distinction is important as some skin disorders, like psoriasis or eczema, may manifest differently depending on whether they appear in thick or thin skin. Understanding such varied responses at the cellular level can pave the way for specific interventions and, therefore, enhance patient care in dermatology, finally emphasizing the importance of understanding the role of skin type heterogeneity in clinical practice (Axel et al., 2023) (Figure 1.6).

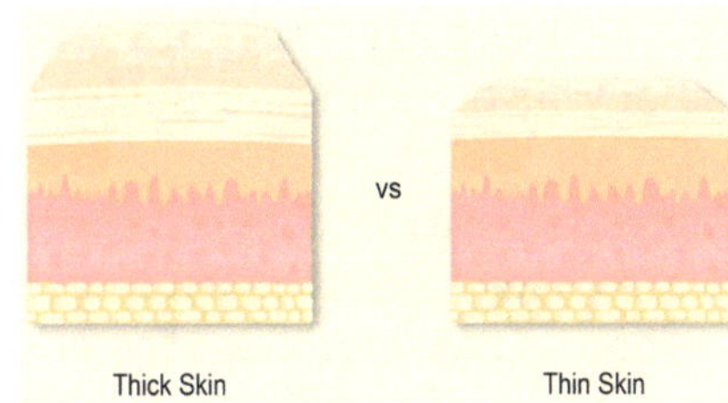

Figure 1.6. Thick skin vs. thin skin.

Source: https://knyamed.com/cdn/shop/articles/Difference_Between_Thick_And_Thin_Skin_Anatomy.jpg?v=1704287379.

1.2.2. Variations in Skin Color

Variations in skin pigmentation are primarily a function of the quantity and type of melanin, a pigment produced by melanocytes. Melanin occurs in two primary forms: eumelanin, brown or black, and pheomelanin, yellow or red. The ratio of these pigments determines a spectrum of skin colors among populations influenced by genetic factors and natural selection pressures to environmental factors. Of special interest, regions of enhanced UV radiation exposure tend to produce darker-skinned populations with protective capabilities against dangerous UV radiation. Such a melanoprotective role stresses an adaptive physiological adaptation to environmental stress, highlighting the intricate relationship between sun exposure and skin color variation in human populations. Moreover, separate from genetic determinants, environmental conditions and extrinsic factors also play a role in skin color variation. For instance, geography plays a role in that populations dwelling in equatorial regions will have more darkly pigmented skin compared to populations in higher latitudes, where lighter skin is the norm. This is normally explained in terms of the need for enough Vitamin D synthesis in low UV environments, where more light skin can make greater sunlight absorption possible. Climate and seasonal change can influence skin color as well; people can become tanned from heightened sun exposure, reflecting an interactive response between the physiology of the skin and environmental influences. This too shows how skin color is not as much a static as to dynamic factor but a state that can change based on external stimuli. Recent research has significantly enhanced our understanding of variations in skin color, notably from an evolutionary point and one of genetic plasticity. The literature points to the importance of phenotypic plasticity, where organisms express variations in physical features, including skin color, in response to changes in the environment. For instance, the adaptive traits of certain lizards, such as the Italian wall lizard, illustrate how environmental stresses can induce rapid evolutionary color changes as they relate to survival strategies. Increased activity in melanocortins, which regulate pigmentation, illustrates the molecular mechanisms for these adaptations.

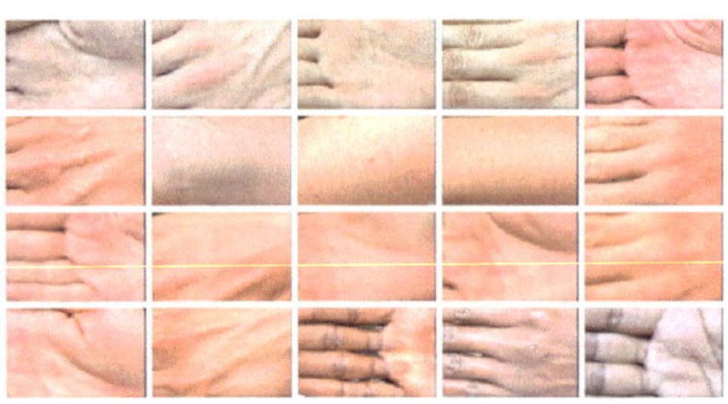

Figure 1.7. A representation of different human skin color variations.

Source: https://www.researchgate.net/profile/Gilles-Coppin/publication/50842378/figure/fig3/AS:305700325609483@1449896045445/A-representation-of-different-human-skin-color-variations.png.

This ongoing dialogue between the environment and genetics warrants that variability in skin color is due to complex interactions that create both physiology and evolutionary trajectories, consistent with the broader context of skin anatomy and human adaptation and health (Fulgione et al., 2023; Elizabeth et al., 2025) (Figure 1.7).

1.2.3. Skin Types: Oily, Dry, Combination

Understanding skin types is at the core of both dermatology and skincare since it plays a major role in determining the approach mode of treatment and product formulation. Skin can broadly be categorized into three broad types: oily, dry, and combination. Oily skin is caused by excess production of sebum from the sebaceous glands, leading to an oily appearance and greater susceptibility to acne and blemishes. This condition is typically accompanied by hyperactivity of the sebaceous glands, which is typically caused by hormonal changes or genetic predisposition. In contrast, dry skin is associated with inadequate sebum secretion, resulting in a dull, rough appearance that can further be accentuated by environmental factors such as low humidity. Detection of such differences is the foundation of the development of effective skincare routines that cater to the unique needs of each skin type, enhancing skin health and appearance (Aggarwal et al., 2022). Combination skin is especially challenging since it has elements of oily and dry skin types, which require special care. Typically, those with combination skin will experience oiliness across the T-zone (nose, forehead, and chin) but dryness or normal skin elsewhere on the face, such as the cheeks. This contrast in skin type and oil production demands a specific choice of products that will harmonize and maintain skin well-being. Combination skin care typically demands the use of light moisturizers and intense treatments targeting special concerns within different zones. Under guidance, one can find the best solution for combination skin. Furthermore, understanding the physiologic differences in skin types can avoid typical issues, such as over-drying the oily areas or irritating the dry areas, ultimately resulting in comprehensive skin harmony and functionality (Smolarz et al., 2021). The significance of consideration of these skin types extends beyond external beauty; it is highly associated with inner layers and complex mechanisms of skin anatomy and physiology. The relationship between skin type and health is illustrated in the skin's microbiome, which varies according to the oil and moisture conditions on the skin's surface. People with oily skin might have dissimilar microbial communities compared to dry skin types and this can have repercussions on the skin defense system and response to treatment. Furthermore, the awareness of these differences allows for more targeted research into the skin diseases of various skin types, such as acne on oily skin or eczema on dry skin. Therefore, evaluating skin types with the Anatomy and Physiology model not only improves our knowledge of skin health but also guides patient-specific therapeutic interventions (Aggarwal et al., 2022) (Figure 1.8).

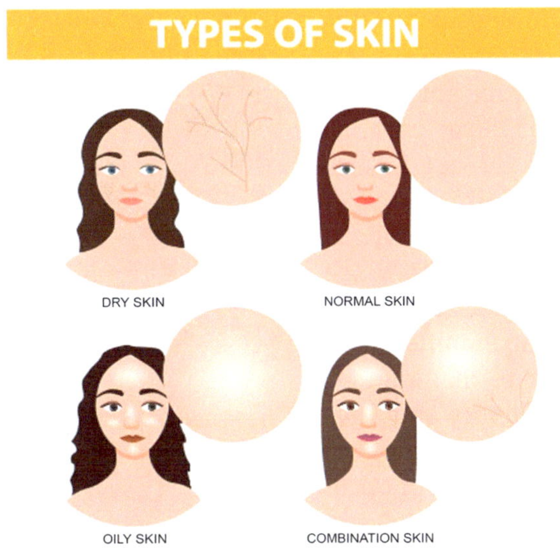

Figure 1.8. Types of skin.

Source: https://skinkraft.com/cdn/shop/articles/Evidence-Based_ae4d0bef-f9d6-48b8-99dc-4cf8a29e332e_1024x1024.jpg?v=1634809078.

Test Your Knowledge

1. Where is thick skin found on the human body?
2. What are the four main types of skin based on oil production?
3. What pigment is primarily responsible for variations in human skin color?

1.3. Skin Functions

Learning Outcome

1. Explain how skin protects against environmental hazards
2. Discuss about regulation of body temperature
3. Understand how skin serves a fundamental role in sensation and communication

The skin offers a complete range of functions required for the maintenance of overall health and homeostasis. Most importantly, it serves as a physical barrier that protects internal organs and systems from pathogens, environmental toxins, and physical trauma. This barrier function is essential not just to exclude infections but also to minimize loss of fluid and regulate temperature. The epidermal layer of the skin consists of keratinocytes, which secrete keratin, a protein that strengthens the barrier function. The skin is also supplied with other immune cells that work to maintain its protective nature, helping to identify and fight off invading foreign bodies. Immune responses of this sort are essential in the prevention of the development of infection and inflammatory dermatoses, highlighting the skin's position as a frontline protector in the body's defense system. In addition to its barrier role, the skin plays a critical role in sensory perception. Because of the presence of diverse sensory receptors, the skin is capable of sensing changes in the environment such as temperature, pressure, and pain, providing critical feedback for survival. These sensory functions are facilitated through specialized nerve endings in the dermal layer, which send signals to the central nervous system to enable perception and response to stimuli. This ability not only warns humans of potential danger but also contributes to everyday life, such as the enjoyment of contact and changes in temperature. As such, the skin does not just cover the body; it plays an active role in molding interactions with the environment, governing behaviors and reactions on the basis of touch. Further, the skin plays a crucial role in thermoregulation and metabolic function. By means such as sweat secretion and vasodilation, the skin absorbs heat, keeping the body temperature constant, which is vital for enzymatic reactions and general metabolic well-being. In addition, the skin is also a site for vitamin D formation, which is a fundamental component of calcium metabolism and bone accretion. This is catalyzed by exposure to ultraviolet light, thus highlighting the skin's role in facilitating vital biochemical processes. The complexity of such functions further highlights the importance of healthy skin since imbalances precipitated by disruptions can have cascading effects on physiological processes in the whole body. With the research advances towards reconstructing skin models, its multifaceted functions can be more clearly outlined with therapeutic significance to dermatological health (Abaci et al., 2017; Kastl et al., 2019) (Figure 1.9).

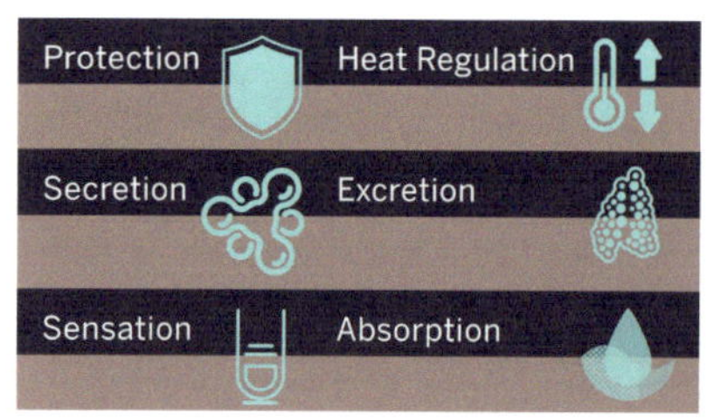

Figure 1.9. Functions of skin.

Source: https://images.squarespace-cdn.com/content/v1/5c376e29f8370a0c087f5ca5/1571764832988-TBQMFZYACJCC39EVU8OA/Functions-of-Skin.jpg.

1.3.1. Protection Against Environmental Hazards

The skin is also the body's front line in its defense against many environmental insults, including toxic substances, UV radiation, and infectious agents. The epidermis, which contains multiple layers, acts as a physical barrier to keep toxins out of the body and protect it against mechanical injury. The keratinocytes in the skin also secrete keratin, an important protein that supports the physical barrier function of the skin and allows it to regulate moisture. The inbuilt capability of the skin to regenerate perpetually enables it to repair minor damage and recover from environmental insults with ease. However, chronic exposure to environmental stressors has the potential to overwhelm such protective covering, compromising integrity and increasing susceptibility to skin disease. Understanding these mechanisms is clear on the significance of healthy skin and its requirement for proper protection against destructive elements of the environment, particularly in light of the dynamicity of contaminants to which human beings are subjected daily (Laura et al., 2023). In addition to its physical defense, skin also possesses inherent immune reactions that double the protective measure against environmental threats. The integrity of immune cells such as Langerhans cells (LCs) in the epidermis is important in pathogen recognition and neutralization. The dendritic cells engulf the antigens of invading microbes and initiate immunity by conversing with lymphocytes. The microbiome of the skin also supplements this protective function by competing with potentially harmful pathogens for resources and space. This complex interaction not only prevents infection but also reduces inflammation, ultimately maintaining skin homeostasis. This multi-component approach shows how skin immunity is a subset of the body's overall defense mechanism against invaders, emphasizing the significance of researching the enhancement of dermal immunity through environmental exposure management and skin hygiene practices (Christine, 2015). For optimal protection of skin against external insult, individuals can utilize various preventive measures promoting healthy skin. Methods including routine application of broad-spectrum sunscreen can avert UV-induced sun damage, reducing skin cancers and photodamage risks. The utilization of products containing antioxidants and moisturizers also avoids oxidative stress and maintains hydrated skin, maintaining its resistance. Reducing documented environmental toxins, such as certain chemicals in products or air contamination, is critical for preserving skin integrity. Implementing a detailed skincare protocol alongside safeguarding equipment, especially under conditions that are hazardous, can aid the skin's resistance to potential harm. With changing environmental dangers, continuous education and sensitivity are crucial in promoting practices that enhance the protective skills of the skin as well as overall health and contentment (Laura et al., 2023; Christine, 2015) (Figure 1.10).

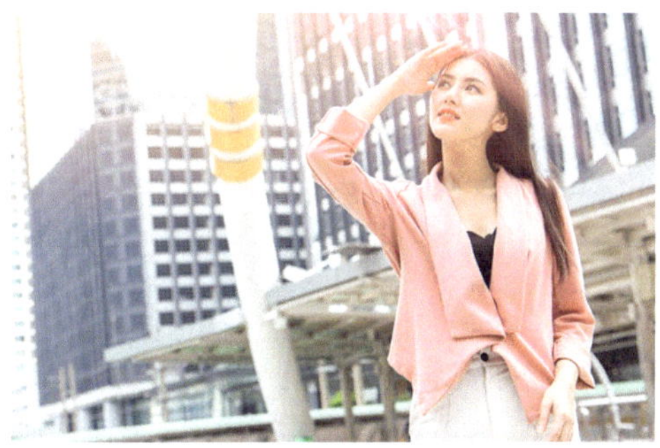

Figure 1.10. Protection against environmental hazards.

Source: https://www.megawecare.com.bd/wp-content/uploads/2021/11/The-secret-of-protecting-skin-from-harmful-effects-of-the-environment.jpg.

1.3.2. Regulation of Body Temperature

Body temperature control is a significant skin function closely tied to homeostasis in general. The skin is also the largest organ of the body and maintains the body in thermal balance through its dynamic interaction with the external environment. Physiologically, temperature control is maintained through such mechanisms as the vasoconstriction and vasodilation of blood vessels and the operation of sweat glands. When body temperature rises, dermal blood vessels become dilated, and hence, there is increased flow of blood and loss of heat through convection and radiation. Under cold environments, however, vasoconstriction occurs to counteract heat loss and preserve core body temperature. Such mechanisms underscore the complex anatomy of the skin, in which vascular and neural components communicate with one another to regulate thermal sensations and responses to environmental temperatures. Also, the integrated function of skin in thermoregulation is affected by a spectrum of pathophysiological processes that compromise circulation and integrity of the skin. For instance, disease conditions like hypoperfusion and vasopermeability can be detrimental to effective regulation of body temperature by the skin, leading to complications like hypothermia or hyperthermia. Disruptions in the vasculature of the skin can compromise the capacity of the skin to retain heat in cold weather as well as to dissipate heat in warmer temperatures. Additionally, structural damage to the integrity of the skin barrier can disrupt sweat gland health, diminishing evaporative cooling processes required for thermoregulation. Hence, uncontrolled temperature can create a cascade process leading to skin failure, a process recognized as part of systemic health and quality of life, as expressed in existing clinical language regarding the integumentary system's physiology (Jeffrey et al., 2022). Lastly, anatomical alterations brought about by aging make temperature regulation in the body even more complicated, since older individuals typically experience decreased thermoregulatory performance. With advancing age, elasticity and integrity of the skin are compromised, internal tissue blood flow falls, and sweat gland activity is decreased, all contributing quite significantly to the overall thermoregulatory capacity. These age-related changes can add to susceptibility to ambient temperature variations and thus enhance the risk of temperature disorders such as heat stroke or frostbite. These vulnerabilities highlight the relevance of knowledge about skin thermoregulation, especially in older populations, who can have cumulative risk factors secondary to comorbidities. When health care providers take into account thermoregulatory processes, treatment plans must include anticipated skin failures and other age-related deficits for the best patient outcomes (Habib et al., 2015) (Figure 1.11).

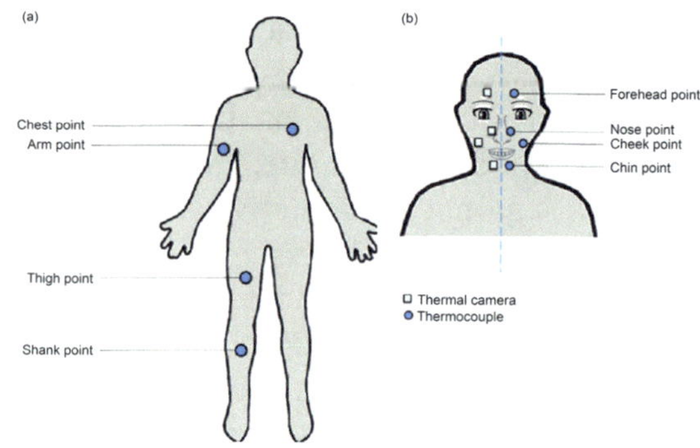

Figure 1.11. Measurement point of body skin temperature (a); and face skin temperature (b).

Source: https://www.researchgate.net/profile/Rachmawan-Budiarto/publication/349336761/figure/fig1/AS:991707051094016@1613452794169/Measurement-point-of-body-skin-temperature-a-and-face-skin-temperature-b-6.png.

1.3.3. Sensation and Communication

The skin has a fundamental role in sense and communication by serving as a vital interface between the external world and the body. The sensory receptors within the skin detect varied stimuli such as temperature, pain, and touch to relay information regarding the body's condition to the brain. The sensory information is processed through complex neural pathways that engage the central nervous system to facilitate adequate physiological responses. For instance, when skin receptors are activated by painful stimulation, they send signals to the brain, which responds by initiating a reflex withdrawal response. Such intricate interaction illustrates the interconnectedness of sensation and physiological response, showing how human survival is dependent on the sensory processes of the skin. These processes emphasize the importance of healthy skin in the ease of communication between the organism and the environment for both physiological and psychological health. Further, the role of the skin in sensation is not merely a matter of touch; it is also deeply embedded in emotional and social communication. The ability to convey emotions through skin reactions, e.g., blushing when embarrassed or sweating with fear, illustrates the skin's double purpose as protective covering and expressive channel. Its expressiveness is facilitated by the integumentary system's complex anatomy, comprising a multitude of nerve endings and receptors for reacting to internal and external stimuli. Delafield-Butt et al. (2013) observe that this mastery of sensory communication is not merely intellectual but is also present in emotional contexts where sensitivity and intentionality are central. In this sense, the skin not only conveys information about the state of one's body but also generates social interaction, thus being a fundamental component in interpersonal communication. Further research on the physiology of sensation demonstrates that connective tissue within the skin is also involved in pain sensation and mechanisms of chronic pain. Increased stiffness within the connective tissues, typically secondary to a state of disease, may further increase pain sensitivity and limit the skin's capacity to communicate. Reis et al. (2011) discuss how extracellular structures engage with fibroblasts in the subcutaneous layer and affect everything from collagen synthesis to the overall mechanosensitivity of the skin. The way that connective tissue stiffness affects pain sensation is significant in that it underlines the importance of understanding the skin's structural components within the broader picture, as they are paramount not only to sensation, but to outcomes related to health in the case of chronic pain disorders. Therefore, the integrity of both sensory receptors and connective tissue is necessary for the skin to function in its proper sense of sensation and communication and eventually one's quality of life.

Test Your Knowledge

1. What are the three main functions of the skin?
2. How does the skin help regulate body temperature?
3. Why is the skin considered part of the immune system?

1.4. Skin Cells and Their Roles

Learning Outcome

1. Discuss keratinocytes
2. Define melanocytes
3. Understand Langerhans cells

Human skin is a heterogeneous organ made up of numerous cell types, each playing a role in the general skin function and health. The epidermal cells that are most abundant in the epidermis are known as keratinocytes, and they are responsible for the synthesis of keratin, a protein that forms a protective barrier against external stressors such as pathogens and UV radiation. These cells differentiate when they migrate from the basal layer to the surface of the skin, where they are finally shed. Wound repair and replacement of skin rely on this ongoing turnover of keratinocytes. Keratinocytes also play a role in the immune response by releasing cytokines that recruit immune cells to sites of injury or infection, indicating their dual role in barrier function and immune surveillance. Other than the keratinocytes, melanocytes present in the basal layer of the epidermis contribute significantly to skin physiology by secreting melanin. The melanin is crucial for protecting skin cells against the harmful action of UV radiation. Melanin will absorb UV light and thus avert the potential for DNA damage resulting in skin cancer. Of significance, variation in the number and activity of melanocytes between individuals leads to variation in skin color and, therefore their susceptibility to skin diseases due to UV irradiation. Furthermore, there is also interaction between melanocytes and keratinocytes critical for the maintenance of skin homeostasis; e.g., keratinocytes can stimulate the production of melanin following UV exposure, indicating an intricate regulatory process essential for the protection and survival of the skin (Marcinkowska, 2020). Other skin cell types, such as LCs and fibroblasts, also augment the activity of the skin. LCs are epidermal dendritic cells that help protect against immunity by capturing and presenting antigens to T cells, thus initiating adaptive immune responses. Such an activity is crucial to detect and neutralize possible insults to the integrity of the skin. Fibroblasts are present in the dermis and hold the credit for the synthesis of collagen and elastin that provide structure and flexibility to the skin. They also contribute to wound healing and tissue remodeling by reacting to the signals from wounds by proliferating and synthesizing extracellular matrix components (Ralitsa et al., 2018). These populations of skin cells collectively create an active environment that sustains skin's protective, regulatory, and aesthetic functions, proving the complexity and importance of skin anatomy and physiology.

1.4.1. Keratinocytes: The Primary Cell Type

Keratinocytes, the predominant cell of the epidermis, form the core of skin anatomy and physiology. These cells originate from the basal layer of the epidermis, from which they proliferate and differentiate as they migrate towards the skin surface. The primary function of keratinocytes is to form a barrier against external injury in the form of pathogens and physical damage and also regulate moisture retention. This differentiation process is vital for the establishment of the skin's barrier function as keratinocytes secrete keratin, a fibrous protein that confers strength. The functioning and health of keratinocytes are also crucial not just to provide a strong skin barrier but also in wound healing as well as inflammation responses, which underlines their core role in overall skin homeostasis (Al-Dhubaibi et al., 2025). The regulation of keratinocyte differentiation may be a complex process that involves various intrinsic and extrinsic factors. Cytokines and growth factors, secreted by neighboring cells, have been shown to control the activity of keratinocytes, influencing their proliferation as well as differentiation status. For instance, it has been revealed that the influence of certain growth factors can stimulate keratinocyte migration and enhance the healing of damaged skin. Significantly, dysregulation of such mechanisms can lead to a number of dermatologic conditions, like psoriasis and atopic dermatitis, where the integrity of keratinocyte function is disturbed. Also, recent research shows the role of nutritional components, like myricetin, in regulating the activity of keratinocytes and enhancing the integrity of the skin barrier. By activating specific ion channels, e.g., the TRPV4 channel, myricetin has been reported to stimulate keratinocyte differentiation, thereby reinforcing the skin barrier (Gao et al., 2025). As components of the structure of the skin as well as important actors in the skin's immune response, keratinocytes are not merely structural components of the skin but also significant players in the skin's immune response. These cells possess various pattern recognition receptors that enable them to identify pathogens and coordinate immune responses, thus acting as the first line of defense in cutaneous immunity. Upon stimulation, keratinocytes can secrete pro-inflammatory cytokines and chemokines that recruit immune cells into the site of infection or injury, thus playing a significant role during skin repair and inflammation. Moreover, their interaction with immune cells highlights the dynamic function of keratinocytes beyond structural purposes. As research continues to reveal the multifunctional nature of keratinocytes, it is increasingly evident that maintaining them in a healthy and functional state is imperative not just for the integrity of the skin but also for overall physiological health (Al-Dhubaibi et al., 2025) (Figure 1.12).

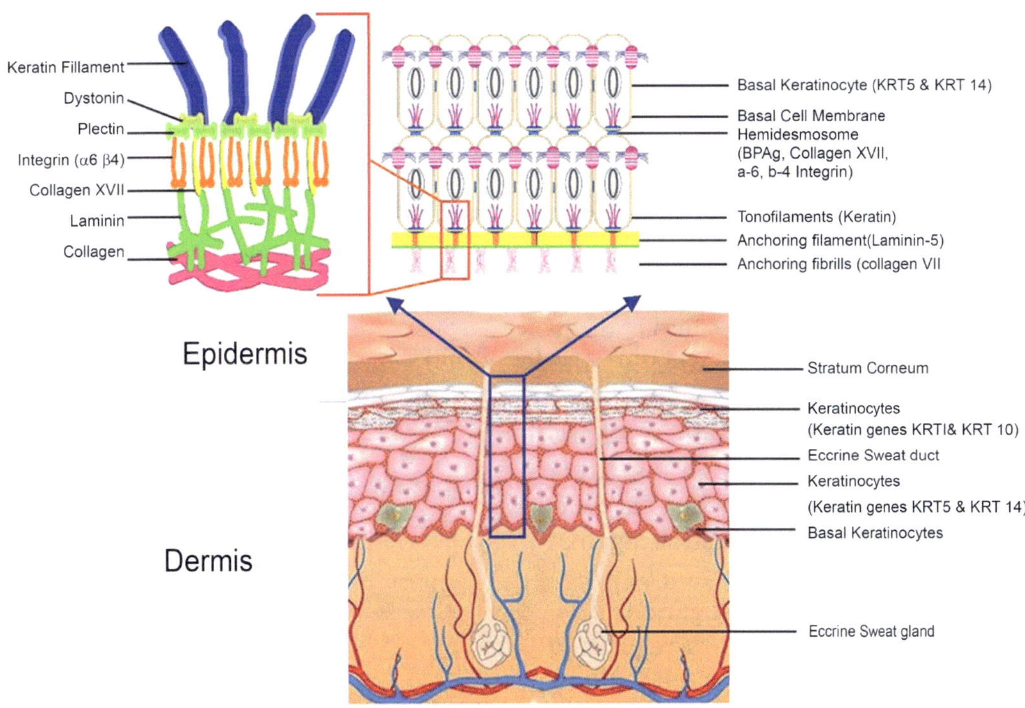

Figure 1.12. Differentiated keratinocytes in the structure of human skin.

Source: https://www.researchgate.net/publication/353313095/figure/fig1/AS:1046549832421378@1626528332333/Differentiated-Keratinocytes-in-Structure-of-Human-Skin.ppm.

1.4.2. Melanocytes: Pigment Production

Melanocytes, the cells responsible for melanin production, play the most crucial role in skin anatomy and physiology. Present predominantly in the basal layer of the epidermis, they originate from embryonic neural crest cells and are intrinsically linked with skin pigmentation. Their primary function is to produce melanin through the melanogenesis pathway, in which the enzyme tyrosinase catalyzes the reaction between the amino acid tyrosine into melanin precursors. Variations in the activity and quantity of melanocytes contribute significantly to variations in skin color in various individuals. In addition, exposure to UV radiation stimulates melanocyte activity, leading to increased production of melanin as a protective response against UV-induced DNA damage. The biochemical process of melanin synthesis is important in pigmentation as well as in the protection of the skin. Melanin is a natural sunblock that absorbs UV radiation and protects the skin against damage and the eventual development of skin cancers. Melanocyte dysfunction can result in hypopigmentation or hyperpigmentation disorders that reflect conditions like vitiligo and melasma, respectively. These pigment production changes indicate that knowledge of melanocyte biology is crucial both cosmetically and clinically. Emerging developments in therapeutic intervention have targeted melanin synthetic pathways either for stimulating or inhibiting pigment formation, according to the purpose, i.e., whitening the skin or protection against UV and exposed a complex interaction between therapy and biology. Recent investigations have underscored heterogeneous factors regulating melanocyte function and melanogenesis, e.g., oxidative stress and antioxidant activity. Antioxidants like resveratrol have been shown to be capable of inhibiting the activity of tyrosinase and blocking melanin synthesis in melanocytes. Resveratrol's ability to influence multiple inflammation and oxidation-related signaling pathways positions it not only as a potential agent for skin lightening but also as a possible ingredient for anti-aging cosmetics. Studies have indicated that derivatives of the compound resveratrol were found to improve skin texture and color, hinting at their promise for application in the treatment of pigmentation disorders and overall skin health. With ongoing studies uncovering new ways to regulate melanocyte activity, increased understanding of these mechanisms will be essential in developing effective therapeutic interventions against various skin diseases and in optimizing the overall dietetic and topical regimes for the management of the skin (Boo, 2019; Kolimi et al., 2022) (Figure 1.13).

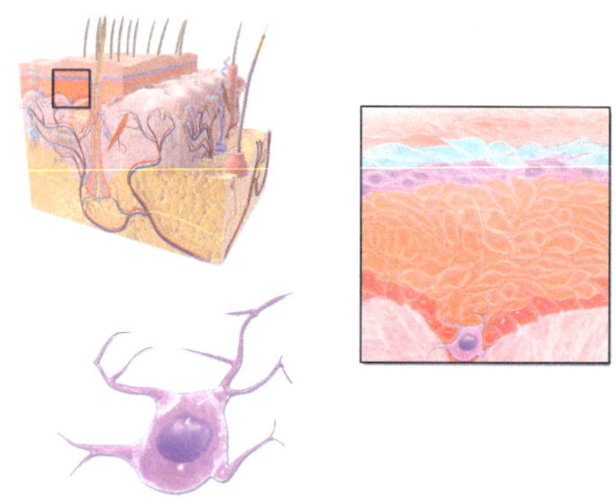

Figure 1.13. Illustration of a melanocyte.

Source: https://upload.wikimedia.org/wikipedia/commons/thumb/3/36/Blausen_0632_Melanocyte.png/800px-Blausen_0632_Melanocyte.png.

1.4.3. Langerhans Cells: Immune Response

LCs are essential epidermal antigen-presenting cells, playing a central role in skin immune response. As a unique lineage of dendritic cells, LCs are sentinels that can detect pathogens and trigger immune responses. By being at the outermost layer of the skin, LCs can immediately respond to environmental insults like infections and allergens. Upon such encounters with danger, LCs mature, moving from the epidermis to local lymph nodes where they process and present antigens to T cells. This enables the induction of an effective adaptive immune response since it enables selective activation of the pathogen while the tissue remains immunotolerant to self-antigens, which ensures tissue homeostasis and prevents unnecessary inflammation in the skin. Cross-communication between LCs and other extracellular cues, particularly endocannabinoids, exerts considerable influence on immune regulation. By research, endocannabinoids such as anandamide have been found to regulate the function and cytokine release of LCs, suggesting a subtle regulatory mechanism of immune functions in the skin. For instance, studies show that exposure to anandamide results in reduced production of pro-inflammatory cytokines such as IL-6 and IL-12 from LCs after stimulation by toll-like receptor (TLR) ligands. This is significant as it can suppress excessive inflammation, usually seen in skin conditions. Moreover, LCs that are differentiated in the presence of anandamide show retained ability to activate naïve T cells, important for the orchestration of a strong immune response and possibly preventing the hyperactive inflammatory processes that can worsen diseases such as psoriasis and atopic dermatitis (Pénzes et al., 2024). Also, LCs have an important role to play in the case of melanoma, the most aggressive form of skin cancer. Being key components in the immune system's ability to recognize and respond to cancer, LCs have a pivotal role within the tumor microenvironment, most prominently in sentinel lymph nodes (SLNs). The study highlights that dysfunction of LCs within SLNs can compromise effective anti-tumor immunity and facilitate immune tolerance to melanoma antigens. This tumor immune evasion enables tumors to proliferate, highlighting the significance of LCs in providing immune surveillance against cancer cells. Efforts to restore the activity of LCs in this environment provide promising avenues for immunotherapeutic approaches. By stimulating these cells, it is conceivable to restore the immune response against melanoma, reinforcing the critical intersection of LCs and immunological processes in skin morphology and physiology in general (Gerlini et al., 2024) (Figure 1.14).

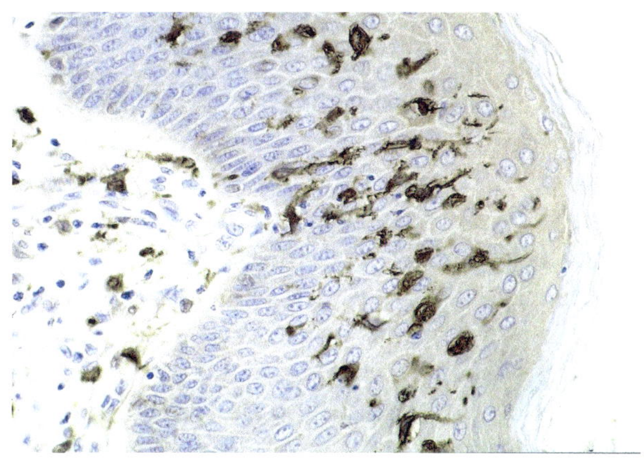

Figure 1.14. Section of skin showing large numbers of dendritic (Langerhans) cells in the epidermis.

Source: https://upload.wikimedia.org/wikipedia/commons/thumb/2/2e/Dendritic_cells.jpg/1024px-Dendritic_cells.jpg.

Test Your Knowledge

1. What are the main types of cells found in the epidermis?
2. What is the primary role of keratinocytes in the skin?
3. How do melanocytes and keratinocytes work together to protect the skin from UV damage?

1.5. Skin Appendages

Learning Outcome

1. Understand hair follicles and hair growth
2. Discuss sweat glands and thermoregulation
3. Describe sebaceous glands and oil production

Skin appendages like hair follicles, sebaceous glands, sweat glands, and nails are crucial in the overall physiology and function of the skin. All these appendages are derived from the epidermis but extend into the underlying dermal tissues, reflecting the complex interdependence of different skin structures. Hair follicles not only provide insulation and protection from the outside world but also contain a variety of sensory receptors that help the skin in its capacity to respond to stimuli. Sebaceous glands contribute to skin well-being by secreting sebum, a natural oil that maintains moisture integrity while having the function of protecting from invading pathogens. Understanding the intricate interplay between these appendages is essential in formulating treatment for skin diseases and optimizing skin health according to Lotfollahi (2024). In addition, the physiological function of sweat glands takes center stage in the skin's capacity to regulate body temperature and eliminate waste substances. The glands are classified into eccrine and apocrine glands and have different functions in thermoregulation and body odor. Eccrine glands, which are found primarily on the palms of the hands and soles of the feet, enable the body to cool down through the secretion of sweat. Apocrine glands, which are found in large numbers along the armpits, secrete a thicker secretion that smells after having been broken down by bacteria. Both types of glands are regulated by hormonal changes and environmental stimuli because of their function in homeostasis and the general health of the skin. With scientists exploring the importance of these appendages, a deep understanding becomes increasingly critical to extend skin treatment processes further, as touched on in current research into skin anatomy and physiology. Skin appendages also play a vital role in the aging process, illustrating the continuously evolving nature of skin physiology. With age, the structure and function of these appendages can become poor, leading to changes such as thinning of hair, decreased activity of sebaceous glands, and slowed nail growth. The epidermis becomes thinner, with decreased resilience and a higher susceptibility to injury and infection. Further, the diminished regenerative capacity of hair follicles is the basis for typical forms of hair loss in older individuals. Aging of skin appendages is a vibrant field of investigation, which illuminates the processes underlying such change and provides opportunities for targeted intervention capable of restoring or enhancing skin function. This emphasizes the need for ongoing research into skin appendages as intrinsic components of skin regeneration and health to guide future clinical applications to reverse the aging process, as emphasized in recent reviews of skin biology (and advancements in bioprinting technologies (Lotfollahi, 2024).

1.5.1. Hair Follicles and Hair Growth

Hair follicles are the essential element in the complex mechanism of hair growth, a process significant to the skin's anatomy and physiology. Each follicle is an intricate structure consisting of several cell types and tissues working together to produce hair. The follicle itself is rooted in the dermis and extrudes through the epidermis, establishing a microenvironment for hair growth. These follicles proceed through periodic phases of development known as the hair growth cycle, which consists of the anagen (growth), catagen (recession), and telogen (resting) phases. Understanding these cycles, as well as the biological signals and molecular pathways that regulate them, is of significant value to hair health and dermatological disorders. This recurrent nature, along with the influence of hormones and external conditions, points towards the advanced physiology of hair follicles that is responsible for the overall health of the skin (Axel et al., 2023). Moreover, the dialogue between hair follicles and the surrounding skin cells is also vital to the regulation of hair growth. Specifically, stem cells residing in the hair follicle are critical in the maintenance of hair regeneration, repair ability, and response to various injuries. In addition to contributing to the development of the different cellular elements of the hair shaft, these stem cells contribute also to the cycling capability of the follicle through the growth phases. In addition, melanocytes within follicles color hair, while fibroblasts and other dermal papilla mesenchymal cells are involved in signaling pathways that regulate hair cycle dynamics. Such multi-cell synergy creates a unitary network that sustains the health of hair and supports the structural integrity of the skin, exemplifying the sophistication of hair follicle physiology in the context of skin anatomy (Chenthamara et al., 2019). Several disorders can disrupt the functioning of hair follicles and lead to baldness or thinning of the hair, and this is a common issue in dermatology. Androgenetic alopecia, alopecia areata, and telogen effluvium are some of the disease conditions that significantly alter the physiology of hair follicles and result in a variety of patterns of hair thinning or baldness. Such diseases typically have their origins in genetic, autoimmune, or environmental factors acting on the health and regeneration of follicles. Secondly, improvements in the biology of hair follicles have paved the way for new therapeutic interventions aimed at hair restoration or the prevention of hair loss. New therapeutic modalities, such as targeted therapies that address the central cellular and molecular abnormalities, are an expression of the ongoing development of the field of dermatology in its efforts to continue learning about hair follicles and their essential role in skin physiology (Axel et al., 2023) (Figure 1.15).

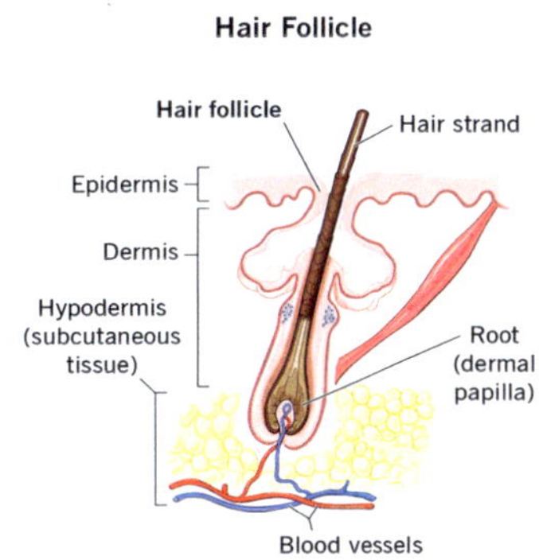

Figure 1.15. Hair follicle.

Source: https://my.clevelandclinic.org/-/scassets/images/org/health/articles/23435-hair-follicle.

1.5.2. Sweat Glands and Thermoregulation

Sweat glands also play a critical role in the skin's thermoregulatory functions for the establishment of homeostasis in the human body. The skin is the largest body organ and consists of various structures like eccrine and apocrine sweat glands, which regulate temperature. Eccrine glands, found mainly in the palms of hands, the soles of the feet, and the forehead, are stimulated by heat and emotional stimuli and create a very effective cooling system through evaporation of the sweat. This mechanism not only cools the surface of the skin but also has effects on core body temperature, demonstrating the interaction between the integumentary system and thermoregulation (Yamashita et al., 2023). By facilitating the release of excess heat through sweating, the body can effectively counteract this change in environmental temperature and metabolic requirements. Suboptimal physiological function is avoided in this way. The intricate biological process of sweat secretion is controlled through a highly developed system of signaling pathways and cellular processes. Important factors, such as the pituitary adenylate cyclase-activating polypeptide (PACAP), that induce sweat secretion through multiple receptors, such as PAC1R, have been identified in research more recently. Experiments have proved that PACAP causes the translocation of aquaporin 5 (AQP5) to the cellular membrane, which enhances the transport of water and eccrine gland secretions of sweat (Vestita et al., 2022). PACAP also regulates genetic expressions for sweating, such as those encoding ion channels and transporters, accounting for the molecular mechanism whereby the body regulates sweat production.

Understanding these intricate signaling pathways not only contributes to our knowledge of thermoregulation but also presents the potential for the development of rational therapies for disorders of sweat. Moreover, alterations in the secretion of sweat can lead to significant disturbances in health, such as hyperhidrosis or anhidrosis, that disrupt normal thermoregulatory processes. Hyperhidrosis, or excess sweating, may give rise to skin irritations and social embarrassment, whereas anhidrosis, decreased ability to sweat, presents risks of heat exposure and heat disorders (Yamashita et al., 2023).

This identification underscores the importance of discovering sweat gland physiology in the context of the broader topic of skin anatomy. By investigating mechanisms of sweat production and regulation, researchers aim to enhance therapy for these disorders. This not only contributes to improved quality of life for the concerned subjects but also asserts the significant role played by sweat glands in the overall physiology of the integumentary system, demonstrating the interconnected nature between integumental well-being and overall well-being (Vestita et al., 2022) (Figure 1.16).

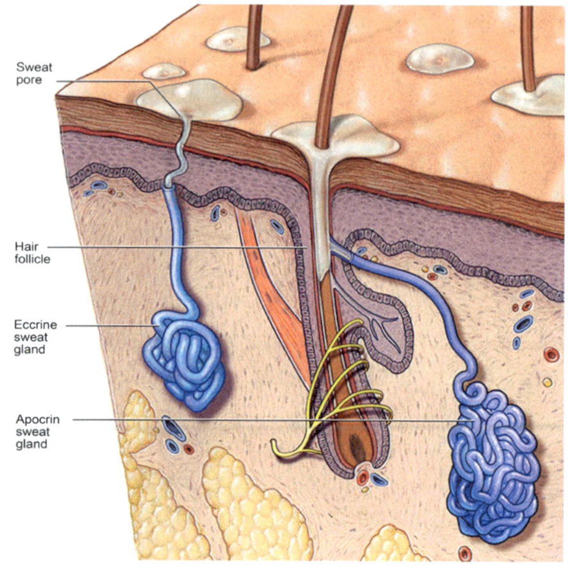

Figure 1.16. Sweat glands.

Source: https://www.mayoclinic.org/-/media/kcms/gbs/patient-consumer/images/2013/08/26/10/41/_bhtestimage.jpg.

1.5.3. Sebaceous Glands and Oil Production

Sebaceous glands play a role as well in maintaining healthy skin through the secretion of sebum, an oily secretion that is core to skin biology. Sebaceous glands are located primarily within the dermis, associated with hair follicles, and extend to most of the body's surface, except for the palms and soles. Sebum, composed of lipids such as triglycerides, wax esters, and squalene, plays a number of roles, including hydrating the skin, providing a barrier against external stressors, and possessing antimicrobial activity capable of inhibiting the growth of pathogenic microorganisms. The volume and makeup of sebum may also be determined by factors such as age, hormonal function, and disease. It is important to understand this variation since sebum secretion changes are associated with skin diseases like acne and seborrheic dermatitis, demonstrating the relevance of sebum gland function research within the broader frame of skin anatomy and physiology.

The biochemical composition of sebum has also been of interest due to its implications for skin barrier function and dermal health in general. Recent studies have established that the lipid profile is altered in individuals with sensitive oily skin as opposed to normal skin. For example, elevated levels of sphingolipids and aberrant ratios of glycerophospholipids have been detected in individuals who have sensitive dry skin, suggesting a correlation between sebum composition and compromised ability of the skin to act as a barrier. These compositional changes affect the physical structure of the stratum corneum and hydration levels, leading to increased TEWL. Therefore, the role of sebaceous glands is more than the secretion of oil; they have an important role to play in maintaining skin barrier integrity, hydration, and protection against damage from the outside environment, highlighting the subtle interaction between sebaceous gland activity and general skin health (Xie et al., 2025). In addition to their protective and lubricating role, sebaceous glands react to various hormonal stimuli, regulating the secretion of oil. The interaction between androgens such as testosterone and dehydroepiandrosterone and sebaceous gland activity is of particular interest. Proliferation of sebocytes and sebum secretion are both stimulated by a rise in androgen levels, whereas hormonal changes can lead to conditions like acne vulgaris. It has been found that manipulation of these endocrine mechanisms can benefit the treatment of acne. Apart from this, the new idea of dermal white adipose tissue (dWAT) suggests that it is able to engage with sebaceous glands and regulate oil production during skin repair processes. The dedifferentiation potential of dWAT and secretion of inflammatory mediators make it difficult to regulate sebaceous glands and open new venues for therapy for encouraging healing of the skin and resuscitation of sebum homeostasis (Li et al., 2024) (Figure 1.17).

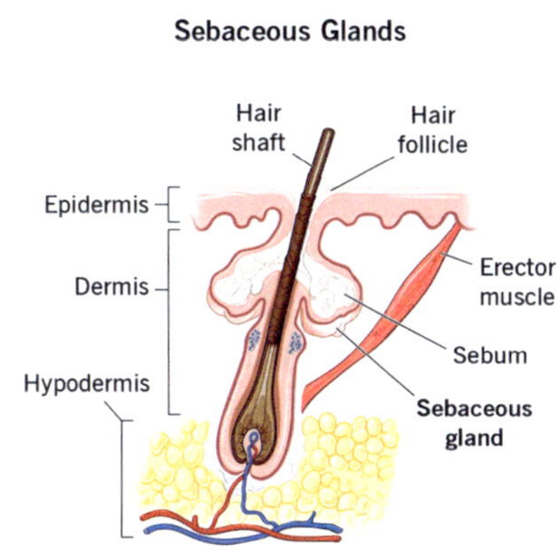

Figure 1.17. Sebaceous glands.

Source: https://my.clevelandclinic.org/-/scassets/images/org/health/articles/24538-sebaceous-glands.

Test Your Knowledge

1. What are three major skin appendages?
2. What is the function of sebaceous glands?

1.6. Skin Health and Disorders

Learning Outcome

1. Understand common skin conditions
2. Explain the effects of aging on skin
3. Discuss the importance of skincare and protection

The skin's health is significantly influenced by a number of physiological parameters, most significantly the structure and function of the skin barrier. The stratum corneum, the outermost layer of the skin, is the main defense against the environment and the pathogens. When the barrier is compromised, it is liable to enhance TEWL, which, based on evidence, may be exacerbated by disorder states such as sleep fragmentation (SF). SF has been proven by research to markedly enhance TEWL, demonstrating a damaged barrier and suggesting potential mechanisms whereby defective sleep can result in dermatoses and early aging. Hence, optimal skin barrier function is essential for the overall health of skin, and the intricate interaction between general health determinants and dermatological outcomes is emphasized (Lee et al., 2025). In addition, skin aging is associated with a wide range of structural and functional changes that may predispose to several skin diseases. With increasing age, there is a remarkable diminution in collagen density and epidermal thickness that are essential in maintaining skin resilience as well as elasticity. Aquaporin expression alterations, the essential proteins that are engaged in water transport as well as other essential mechanisms in skin physiology, have been associated with these mechanisms of aging. Research has indicated that aquaporin dysfunctions may lead to impaired hydration and integrity of the barrier function and hence, exacerbate the manifestation of skin diseases such as psoriasis and eczema. Clarification of such molecular events not only clarifies the mechanism of skin aging but also identifies potential therapeutic targets that may inhibit the detrimental effects of age-related skin diseases (Karimi et al., 2024). Examination of several pathophysiological processes at the molecular level is necessary in achieving a complete concept of skin health as well as skin disease development. For instance, research on the role of fatty acid metabolism has unveiled significant findings of how chronic stressors affect skin physiology. In experiments of SF, dramatic gene expression changes related to fatty acid pathways were found to impair skin barrier function negatively. These results highlight the imperative to combat lifestyle factors likely to trigger the onset of skin diseases. Further, identification of crucial pathways regulated by both internal body conditions and external environmental conditions provides a foundation for the design of new interventions that will ensure skin health maintenance and avoid the appearance of dermatological issues (Lee et al., 2025).

1.6.1. Common Skin Conditions (e.g., Acne, Eczema)

Acne is the most prevalent of all the skin conditions, affecting a high percentage of the adolescent population and commonly persisting into adulthood. Accommodating comedones, inflammatory lesions, and sometimes cysts, acne results from a complex mixture of forces like fluctuating hormone levels, increased sebum production, and Cutibacterium acnes bacterial growth on the skin. These contribute to hair follicle obstruction, leading to the characteristic acne lesions. Pathophysiology of acne highlights the importance of understanding skin anatomy, particularly the sebaceous glands and hair follicle structures, which constitute the foundation of its formation. Moreover, the condition can have its emotional effects, leading to lower self-esteem and social anxiety (referring to the need for comprehensive management plans that cover both the physical and emotional health involved with acne). Another very common skin disorder is eczema, or atopic dermatitis, and is characterized by dry, red, and itchy skin. The condition is typically seen in individuals who are genetically predisposed and is connected to dysfunctions in the skin barrier, which cannot retain water inside or protect against allergens and irritants. The immune systems of individuals with eczema tend to overreact to environmental stimuli, leading to inflammation and aggravation of symptoms. This chronic condition can vary widely in severity and is most commonly precipitated by the stress of illness, climate change, and allergens. A solid understanding of the physiology behind the skin, especially relating to the stratum corneum and how it preserves moisture, is vital in order to devise successful therapeutic interventions. Interventions typically involve topical corticosteroids and moisturizers, and therefore, there is a need for more study into more sustainable and whole-systems approaches to management. In the management of widespread dermatological ailments such as acne and eczema, cosmetic technology plays a critical role. Chemicals such as alpha-hydroxy acids (AHAs) have been placed in the spotlight for their skin rejuvenating and healing abilities. AHAs such as glycolic acid dissolve the topmost layer of the skin and enhance cell turnover, of huge advantage to conditions such as acne and photoaging. Their ability to improve skin texture and glow sees them being demanded by both dermatology clinics as well as cosmetic skincare. Additionally, the use of plant oils, being antioxidants, is a feasible option in maintaining skin health. Not only do the oils provide hydration, but they also have anti-inflammatory and antimicrobial activities that can be used to treat symptoms of skin disease (Rahim et al., 2023; Almeman, 2024). With advances in skin studies, the focus on the use of effective plant-based components can open the door to innovative therapies that enhance the skin and overall well-being (Figure 1.18).

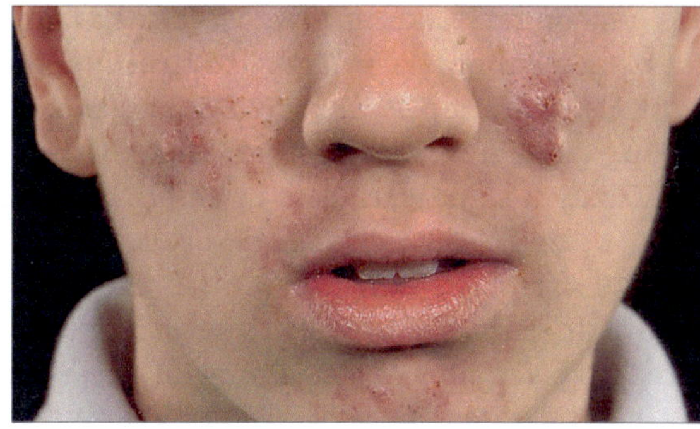

Figure 1.18. Adolescent acne vulgaris.

Source: https://ars.els-cdn.com/content/image/1-s2.0-S2352464222003145-gr1.jpg.

1.6.2. Effects of Aging on Skin

With time, skin undergoes numerous physiological changes that significantly influence its function and organization. Arguably, the most significant impact of getting older is a decrease in collagen and elastin production, the two proteins most responsible for giving skin firmness and elasticity. As they are diminished, the skin can no longer maintain its tautness and therefore starts sagging and wrinkling. Moreover, the hydration of skin decreases as a result of decreased sebaceous gland function, rendering it vulnerable to dryness and irritation. All these elements portray a visible contrast between young and older skin, in turn making it essential to comprehend the physiological process of this aging process within the overall scenario of skin anatomy and physiology. Aging can also be seen at the cellular level through the slow turnover rate of skin cells. In youth, the skin is renewed approximately every 28 days; however, this activity also gets longer with age and makes the skin dull and lackluster. The decline in the rate of cell regeneration not only in the appearance of the skin but also makes the skin inept at healing wounds and external injuries. Furthermore, age affects the fat redistribution in the skin to create a thinner dermis and lower cushioning, which accentuates the visibility of underlying structures such as bones and veins. An understanding of these cellular and structural changes is vital in controlling the overall contribution to skin health and beauty with aging. Further, lifestyle and external factors play a significant role in amplifying the impact of aging on the skin. Exposure to UV radiation from the sun accelerates the aging of the skin through a process referred to as photoaging, leading to darkening of the skin, rough texture, and loss of elasticity. Smoking and diet also contribute to the aging of the skin because they result in collagen breakdown and overall decline of the skin. The coming together of intrinsic factors such as genetics and extrinsic forces like lifestyle habits results in the variation of skin aging among various individuals, necessitating personalized skincare and preventive therapy. This point reflects the plight of the aging skin and aligns with the ongoing research towards improved treatments and interventions (Rosander, 1985; Pedersen et al., 2021) (Figure 1.19).

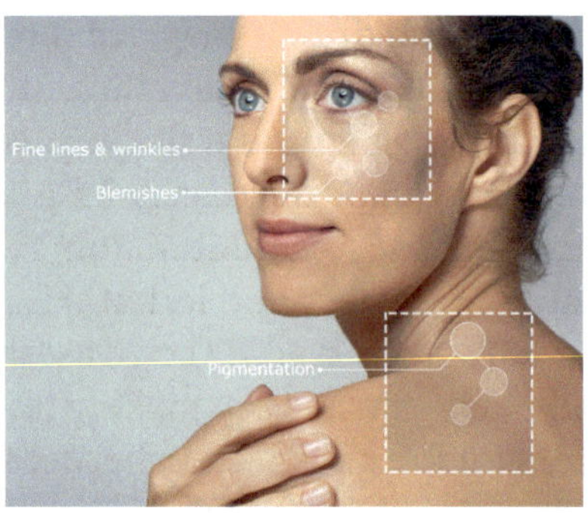

Figure 1.19. Aging skin.

Source: https://www.cutislaserclinics.com/wp-content/uploads/2018/05/Prevent-Aging-Skin.jpg.

1.6.3. Importance of Skincare and Protection

The significance of protective care cannot be exaggerated when it comes to studying skin anatomy and physiology. The skin is the body's first line of defense against external irritants like UV light, toxins, and microbes. Maintenance of a healthy barrier skin is the most crucial step in preventing conditions like dermatitis and premature aging. An optimally formulated skincare system that integrates protective with repair components can enhance skin strength. For instance, the application of alpha-hydroxy acids (AHAs), discussed in current dermatological literature reviews, is said to stimulate skin renewal and texture. The products not only stimulate the synthesis of collagen but also possess a defensive action on environmental aggressors, which shows the double role of skincare being preventive and corrective in effect (Almeman, 2024). Hence, awareness of the products is essential in order to gain the utmost benefit and ideal skin health. Skincare is not only a cosmetic issue; it is a significant component of the general health and well-being. Comprehensive skincare regimens lead to improved self-esteem and self-confidence, particularly for individuals afflicted with some skin diseases like acne or hyperpigmentation. The psychological importance of having healthy skin is profound in the sense that it forms the basis of social interaction and personal identity. Furthermore, there is a growing awareness of the link between body health and skin health. Poor skincare leads to aggravation of conditions, for instance, in diabetic patients who may develop complications such as diabetic foot syndrome due to a lack of proper care and education (Krawiec et al., 2023). This emphasizes the importance of holistic education about skincare that includes lifestyle determinants and disease management. Secondly, the confluence of skincare and health places significance on it as part of overall individual care. Finally, an appreciation of the role of expert guidance and learning in promoting effective skincare is necessary. Dermatologists and skin care specialists are increasingly being tasked not just with curing skin diseases but with teaching individuals how to perform proper skin protection and rejuvenation. Natural ingredient use in cosmetics, as highlighted in a publication, brings to the forefront the significance of thorough research in product safety and efficacy (Krawiec et al., 2023). Consumers are best served with well-managed products that optimize their skin's health without compromising on safety. This renders informed choices in skincare of utmost importance, leading to responsible citizens who can proactively maintain their skin health. Finally, the complex nature of skincare has to be comprehended for the flourishing of not just physical appearances but mental wellness and overall quality of life.

Test Your Knowledge

1. What is the most common skin disorder?
2. How does eczema affect the skin?
3. What is the importance of skincare and protection?

SUMMARY

In summarizing skin anatomy and physiology, it is evident that understanding the intricate structure and functions of the skin is essential in driving medical and therapeutic research forward. Being the largest body organ, the skin serves as a defensive layer with varying physiological processes like thermoregulation and sensation being housed. Its interactive nature of its different layers, including the epidermis, dermis, and the subcutaneous tissue, is indicative of the intricacy of the role that it plays in overall homeostasis. As medical technology continues to advance, searching further into the physiological nature of the skin can possibly reveal new avenues of treatment, particularly in dermatological disorders. Such growing understanding is a key step towards devising more targeted and more effective treatments. Furthermore, the promotion of newer techniques, such as ultrasound, emphasizes the importance of precision in procedures on the skin. For instance, in cases of neuraxial anesthesia during cesarean section, proper identification of the depth of the epidural space is essential to minimize complications. Studies have reported using ultrasound to improve the accuracy of needle positions, a point of great relevance in pregnant women due to changing anatomical values resulting from physiological changes. Knowing how technologies offer real-time data regarding skin anatomy has extremely significant implications for optimizing clinical outcomes and patient safety, representative of the reality that continuous innovation remains at the forefront of medical practice and research (Moktan et al., 2024). With improvements in medical procedures comes the incorporation of new approach methodologies (NAMs) in skin irritation tests as evidence of further evolution of knowledge concerning the physiology of the skin. With older testing techniques occasionally falling short of expectation, particularly concerning consistency of yield and transferability to human anatomy, alternative models reflecting human-relevant systems are promising. Not only do such models enhance the accuracy of skin response prediction, but they also aid in ethical reasoning by minimizing animal testing. From a thorough analysis of such new methodologies, there is evidence of synchrony with the physiological reactions that are seen in human subjects. Lastly, the adoption of such advancements both in research and clinical settings is essential for promoting an educated, efficacious rationale towards skin well-being and disease control (Raabe et al., 2024). The skin serves various functions, including protection against infection, thermoregulation, and sensory perception. Comprised of three major layers—the epidermis, the dermis, and the subcutaneous tissue—the skin has a varied representation of cells, including keratinocytes, melanocytes, and fibroblasts, each contributing to its total function and integrity. In addition, the vascular supply of the skin plays a vital role in thermoregulation and healing, indicating its function in homeostasis. It is necessary to know these fundamental facts of skin structure in learning how physiological responses are provoked and how skin diseases may be caused by structural or functional disorders, which is helpful for the overall thesis regarding the role of the skin in health.

KEY TERMS FROM THIS CHAPTER

Aging skin	Antioxidants	Biochemical processes
Broad-spectrum sunscreen	Collagen synthesis	Dermatological disorders
Elastin production	Langerhans cells	Microenvironment
Skin cancers	Skin diseases	Skin elasticity
Skin harmony	Skin physiology	Skin texture
Skincare	Social relationships	Structural integrity

CRITICAL THINKING QUESTIONS

1. **Which layer of the skin is primarily responsible for producing new skin cells?**
   a. Epidermis
   b. Dermis
   c. Hypodermis
   d. Subcutaneous layer
2. **Which of the following is NOT a function of the skin?**
   a. Protection from environmental damage
   b. Regulation of body temperature
   c. Production of vitamin C
   d. Sensory reception
3. **Which of the following cells is responsible for the production of melanin in the skin?**
   a. Keratinocytes
   b. Melanocytes
   c. Langerhans cells
   d. Merkel cells
4. **The dermis is primarily composed of which type of tissue?**
   a. Stratified squamous epithelium
   b. Adipose tissue
   c. Smooth muscle tissue
   d. Dense connective tissue
5. **Which of the following is the primary function of sebaceous glands in the skin?**
   a. Produce sweat for cooling
   b. Produce sebum for lubricating the skin and hair
   c. Detect pain and temperature changes
   d. Regulate body temperature through perspiration

Short Answer Questions

1. What are the three primary layers of the skin, and what are the key functions of each layer?
2. What is the role of keratinocytes in the epidermis, and how do they contribute to skin protection?
3. Explain the difference between eccrine and apocrine sweat glands, including their location and function.
4. How does the skin regulate body temperature, and what role do blood vessels play in this process?
5. Describe the structure and function of the dermis, and how it supports the epidermis?
6. What are melanocytes, and how do they contribute to skin color?
7. What is the role of the subcutaneous layer (hypodermis) in the skin, and how does it contribute to overall skin function?
8. How does the skin act as a barrier against pathogens and environmental damage, and what role do lipids and tight junctions play in this function?

Answer to Critical Thinking Questions

1. (a); 2. (c); 3. (b); 4. (d); 5. (b)

REFERENCES

1. Abaci, H. E., Guo, Z., Doucet, Y., Jackow, J., & Christiano, A. M. (2017). Next generation human skin constructs as advanced tools for drug development. *Experimental Biology and Medicine, 242*, 1657–1668. https://doi.org/10.1177/1535370217712690 (accessed on 11th June 2025).
2. Aggarwal, N., Kitano, S., Puah, G. R. Y., Kittelmann, S., Hwang, I. Y., & Chang, M. W. (2022). Microbiome and human health: Current understanding, engineering, and enabling technologies. *Chemical Reviews, 123*, 31–72. https://doi.org/10.1021/acs.chemrev.2c00431 (accessed on 11th June 2025).
3. Al-Dhubaibi, M., Mohammed, G. F., Bahaj, S., AbdElneam, A. I., Al-Dhubaibi, A. M., & Atef, L. M. (2025). The role of keratinocytes in skin health and disease. *Dermatological Reviews.* https://www.semanticscholar.org/paper/9b700272bb2ceaa05a4d8bc77e54c38a99e5917b (accessed on 11th June 2025).
4. Almeman, A. (2024). Evaluating the efficacy and safety of alpha-hydroxy acids in dermatological practice: A comprehensive clinical and legal review. *Clinical Cosmetic and Investigational Dermatology, 17*, 1661–1685. https://doi.org/10.2147/ccid.s453243 (accessed on 11th June 2025).
5. Almet, A. A., Yuan, H., Annusver, K., Ramos, R., Liu, Y., Wiedemann, J., Sorkin, D. H., et al. (2023). A roadmap for a consensus human skin cell atlas and single-cell data standardization. *Journal of Investigative Dermatology, 143*, 1667–1677. https://doi.org/10.1016/j.jid.2023.03.1679 (accessed on 11th June 2025).
6. Bandodkar, A. J., Jeerapan, I., & Wang, J. (2016). Wearable chemical sensors: Present challenges and future prospects. *ACS Sensors, 1*, 464–482. https://doi.org/10.1021/acssensors.6b00250 (accessed on 11th June 2025).
7. Boo, Y. C. (2019). Human skin lightening efficacy of resveratrol and its analogs: From *in vitro* studies to cosmetic applications. *Antioxidants, 8*, 332–332. https://doi.org/10.3390/antiox8090332 (accessed on 11th June 2025).
8. Chenthamara, D., Sadhasivam, S., Ramakrishnan, S. G., Krishnaswamy, S., Essa, M. M., Lin, F. H., & Qoronfleh, M. W. (2019). Therapeutic efficacy of nanoparticles and routes of administration. *Biomaterials Research, 23.* https://doi.org/10.1186/s40824-019-0166-x (accessed on 11th June 2025).
9. Cozart, D., Hesse, D., Nichols, R., & Szymik, et al. (2017). *UGA Anatomy and Physiology 1 Lab Manual* (3rd ed.). https://core.ac.uk/download/217306564.pdf (accessed on 11th June 2025).
10. Delafield-Butt, J., & Trevarthen, C. (2013). Theories of the development of human communication. https://core.ac.uk/download/9040032.pdf (accessed on 11th June 2025).
11. Fan, Y., Wei, C., Su, N., Ma, Y., Liu, W., Sun, P., & Shan, S. (2025). Correlation study of facial lipid profile differences and skin physiological characteristics in Chinese women aged 19–33 years. *International Journal of Cosmetic Science.* https://www.semanticscholar.org/paper/cdadfd03e3c10624a8b6b6fb872ff8d45c9decaa (accessed on 11th June 2025).
12. Fulgione, D., Maselli, V., Rivieccio, E., Aceto, S., Salvemini, M., & Buglione, M. (2023). Evolutionary plasticity in insular lizard, adapting over reproduction, metabolism, and color variation. *Biology, 12.* https://www.semanticscholar.org/paper/1c238ab82076307819098e20d07d98d49e86981d (accessed on 11th June 2025).

13. Gao, J. F., Li, T. X., & Zhang, G. Q. (2025). Myricetin enhances keratinocytes differentiation via TRPV4 channel activation in mouse primary keratinocytes. *International Journal of Immunopathology and Pharmacology, 39.* https://www.semanticscholar.org/paper/6876ac1c01489c7d2a2010f3c6f091c19ae81fb6 (accessed on 11th June 2025).

14. Gerlini, G., Susini, P., Sestini, S., Brandani, P., Giannotti, V., & Borgognoni, L. (2024). Langerhans cells in sentinel lymph nodes from melanoma patients. *Cancers, 16.* https://www.semanticscholar.org/paper/40f0639ee52e75d93dd72f33eabca1b5df092e9f (accessed on 11th June 2025).

15. Goadsby, P. J., Holland, P. R., Martins-Oliveira, M., Hoffmann, J., Schankin, C. J., & Akerman, S. (2017). Pathophysiology of migraine: A disorder of sensory processing. *Physiological Reviews, 97*, 553–622. https://doi.org/10.1152/physrev.00034.2015 (accessed on 11th June 2025).

16. Habib, G., Lancellotti, P., Antunes, M. J., Bongiorni, M. G., Casalta, J. P., Del Zotti, F., Dulgheru, R., et al. (2015). 2015 ESC guidelines for the management of infective endocarditis. *European Heart Journal, 36*, 3075–3128. https://doi.org/10.1093/eurheartj/ehv319 (accessed on 11th June 2025).

17. Heng, W., Solomon, S. A., & Gao, W. (2021). Flexible electronics and devices as human-machine interfaces for medical robotics. *Advanced Materials, 34.* https://doi.org/10.1002/adma.202107902 (accessed on 11th June 2025).

18. Hofmann, E., Schwarz, A., Fink, J., Kamolz, L. P., & Kotzbeck, P. (2023). Modelling the complexity of human skin *in vitro*. *Biomedicines, 11*, 794–794. https://doi.org/10.3390/biomedicines11030794 (accessed on 11th June 2025).

19. Igarashi, T., Nayar, S. K., & Nishino, K. (2005). *The Appearance of Human Skin.* https://core.ac.uk/download/161437173.pdf (accessed on 11th June 2025).

20. Karimi, N., & Ahmadi, V. (2024). Aquaporin channels in skin physiology and aging pathophysiology: Investigating their role in skin function and the hallmarks of aging. *Biology, 13.* https://www.semanticscholar.org/paper/177adb6db8adf7daa36fd408b3f0eb8f8ab592b7 (accessed on 11th June 2025).

21. Kastl, A., Terry, N. A., Wu, G. D., & Albenberg, L. (2019). The structure and function of the human small intestinal microbiota: Current understanding and future directions. *Cellular and Molecular Gastroenterology and Hepatology, 9*, 33–45. https://doi.org/10.1016/j.jcmgh.2019.07.006 (accessed on 11th June 2025).

22. Kolimi, P., Narala, S., Nyavanandi, D., Youssef, A. A. A., & Dudhipala, N. (2022). Innovative treatment strategies to accelerate wound healing: Trajectory and recent advancements. *Cells, 11*, 2439–2439. https://doi.org/10.3390/cells11152439 (accessed on 11th June 2025).

23. Krawiec, A., Czerwińska-Ledwig, O., Kita, B., & Piotrowska, A. (2023). Active ingredients and natural raw materials used in foot care in diabetic patients—A literature review. *Cosmetics, 10*, 96–96. https://doi.org/10.3390/cosmetics10040096 (accessed on 11th June 2025).

24. Lee, D. B., Yoo, S. L., Heo, J. S., Lim, J. Y., Pyo, S. S., Moon, J. S., Lee, M. R., et al. (2025). Skin transcriptomic analysis reveals altered fatty acid metabolism pathways in mice subjected to sleep fragmentation. *Skin Pharmacology and Physiology.* https://www.semanticscholar.org/paper/16017f36e3b387402d8659599bdd2c85a4b131d5 (accessed on 11th June 2025).

25. Levine, J. M., Delmore, B., & Cox, J. (2022). Skin failure: Concept review and proposed model. *Advances in Skin & Wound Care, 35*, 139–148. https://doi.org/10.1097/01.asw.0000818572.31307.7b (accessed on 11th June 2025).

26. Li, Y., Long, J., Zhang, Z., & Yin, W. (2024). Insights into the unique roles of dermal white adipose tissue (dWAT) in wound healing. *Frontiers in Physiology, 15.* https://www.semanticscholar.org/paper/306e809e3e3df3d6a0c587bfd88dd4740f28874b (accessed on 11th June 2025).

27. Lotfollahi, Z. (2024). The anatomy, physiology and function of all skin layers and the impact of ageing on the skin. *Wound Practice and Research.* https://www.semanticscholar.org/paper/b3db7cfbe4873d19551c35bc557886a941aaf91c (accessed on 11th June 2025).

28. Lu, G., & Fei, B. (2014). Medical hyperspectral imaging: A review. *Journal of Biomedical Optics, 19*, 010901–010901. https://doi.org/10.1117/1.jbo.19.1.010901 (accessed on 11th June 2025).

29. Madsen, R. R., Vanhaesebroeck, B., & Semple, R. K. (2018). Cancer-associated PIK3CA mutations in overgrowth disorders. *Trends in Molecular Medicine, 24*, 856–870. https://doi.org/10.1016/j.molmed.2018.08.003 (accessed on 11th June 2025).

30. Männer, J. (2024). The functional significance of cardiac looping: Comparative embryology, anatomy, and physiology of the looped design of vertebrate hearts. *Journal of Cardiovascular Development and Disease, 11.* https://www.semanticscholar.org/paper/f81b4e760a36767c905093690cc89889a2f58c47 (accessed on 11th June 2025).

31. Marcinkowska, E. (2020). The vitamin D system in humans and mice: Similar but not the same. *Reports–Medical Cases Images and Videos, 3*, 1–1. https://doi.org/10.3390/reports3010001 (accessed on 11th June 2025).

32. Moktan, S., Thapa, M. K., Shrestha, U., & Subedi, P. (2024). Ultrasonographic measurement of skin to lumbar epidural space depth in pregnant women undergoing elective cesarean section: An observational study. *JNMA: Journal of the Nepal Medical Association, 63*, 42–46. https://www.semanticscholar.org/paper/0553b317ebe61bc17c046fef78f807cfc0ff2206 (accessed on 11th June 2025).

33. Murphy, C. M. (2015). *Principles of Toxicology.* https://www.semanticscholar.org/paper/d87929cd0acbb3b1bae363754849812d2aac7f23 (accessed on 11th June 2025).

34. Pedersen, C., Rechnitzer, C., Andersen, E., Kenborg, L., Norsker, F. N., Bautz, A., Baad-Hansen, T., et al. (2021). Somatic disease in survivors of childhood malignant bone tumors in the Nordic countries. *Cancers, 13.* https://www.semanticscholar.org/paper/01712c584fa0b7adb24d1851adf218732a470b9b (accessed on 11th June 2025).

35. Pénzes, Z., Horváth, D., Molnár, P., Fekete, T., Pázmándi, K., Bácsi, A., & Szöllősi, A. (2024). Anandamide modulation of monocyte-derived Langerhans cells: Implications for immune homeostasis and skin inflammation. *Frontiers in Immunology, 15.* https://www.semanticscholar.org/paper/69e43044bc02040e320cf971c8d1d63d819240b4 (accessed on 11th June 2025).

36. Raabe, H., Costin, G. E., Allen, D. G., Lowit, A., Corvaro, M., O'Dell, L., Breeden-Alemi, J., et al. (2024). Human relevance of *in vivo* and *in vitro* skin irritation tests for hazard classification of pesticides. *Cutaneous and Ocular Toxicology.* https://www.semanticscholar.org/paper/24ecddb55a4f7fba930a5cb286463c56e3ab1cbd (accessed on 11th June 2025).

37. Rahim, M. A., Ayub, H., Sehrish, A., Ambreen, S., Khan, F. A., Itrat, N., Nazir, A., et al. (2023). Essential components from plant source oils: A review on extraction, detection, identification,

and quantification. *Molecules, 28*, 6881–6881. https://doi.org/10.3390/molecules28196881 (accessed on 11th June 2025).

38. Reis, C. P. da S. e S. (2011). *P2 purinoceptors Signaling in Fibroblasts of Rat Subcutaneous Tissue.* https://core.ac.uk/download/15568458.pdf (accessed on 11th June 2025).

39. Rosander, A. (1985). Applications of quality control in the service industries. https://www.semanticscholar.org/paper/801dda77a223a41f618d1195abecabd3b9a5d3e2 (accessed on 11th June 2025).

40. Said, K. B., Al-Otaibi, A., Aljaloud, L., Al-Anazi, B., Alsolami, A., Alreshidi, F., & On Behalf of the Ha'il Com Research Unit Group. (2022). The frequency and patterns of post-COVID-19 vaccination syndrome reveal initially mild and potentially immunotropic signs in primarily young Saudi women. *Vaccines, 10.* https://www.semanticscholar.org/paper/c63905250d1767ca4ec9752f5f5f6527aebc32dd (accessed on 11th June 2025).

41. Serra, O., Mähönen, A. P., Hetherington, A. J., & Ragni, L. (2022). The making of plant armor: The periderm. *Annual Review of Plant Biology, 73*, 405–432. https://doi.org/10.1146/annurev-arplant-102720-031405 (accessed on 11th June 2025).

42. Singhal, K., Azizi, S., Tu, T., Mahdavi, S. S., Lee, J., Chung, H. W., Scales, N., et al. (2023). Large language models encode clinical knowledge. *Nature, 620*, 172–180. https://doi.org/10.1038/s41586-023-06291-2 (accessed on 11th June 2025).

43. Smolarz, B., Szyłło, K., & Romanowicz, H. (2021). Endometriosis: Epidemiology, classification, pathogenesis, treatment and genetics (Review of literature). *International Journal of Molecular Sciences, 22*, 10554–10554. https://doi.org/10.3390/ijms221910554 (accessed on 11th June 2025).

44. Tharakan, M. and Lonczak, L. (2024) Supporting Skin Structure and Its Barrier Functions with Evidence-Based Skin Care Ingredients. *Journal of Cosmetics, Dermatological Sciences and Applications*, **14**, 200-210. doi: 10.4236/jcdsa.2024.142013.(accessed on 11th June 2025).

45. Torres, T., Filipe, P., Menezes Brandão, F., Figueiredo, A., Pinto Soares, A., Sousa Basto, A., Rebelo, C., et al. (2023). Epidemiology of psoriasis in Portugal: A population-based study. *Acta Medica Portuguesa.* https://www.semanticscholar.org/paper/2212b929e6450009dba9de42612fb8b74f852eb1 (accessed on 11th June 2025).

46. Vandenberg, L. N., Zoeller, R., Prins, G., & Trasande, L. (2023). Evaluating adverse effects of environmental agents in food: A brief critique of the US FDA's criteria. *Environmental Health, 22.* https://www.semanticscholar.org/paper/e0e1e33e209f1984a95674605e86897df2f3a34a (accessed on 11th June 2025).

47. Vestita, M., Tedeschi, P., & Bonamonte, D. (2022). Anatomy and physiology of the skin. In *Textbook of Plastic and Reconstructive Surgery.* https://www.semanticscholar.org/paper/638aba2a9c843d3cd15d0435fea385db4bb0f9bb (accessed on 11th June 2025).

48. Woods, A. J., Antal, A., Bikson, M., Boggio, P. S., Brunoni, A. R., Celnik, P., Cohen, L. G., et al. (2015). A technical guide to tDCS, and related non-invasive brain stimulation tools. *Clinical Neurophysiology, 127*, 1031–1048. https://doi.org/10.1016/j.clinph.2015.11.012 (accessed on 11th June 2025).

49. Xie, A., Zhang, X., Huang, Q., & Wu, J. (2025). Utilizing untargeted lipidomic technology to elucidate differences in lipid compositions among sensitive dry, sensitive oily and healthy

skin types. *Metabolites.* https://www.semanticscholar.org/paper/88100f14301ac320d68b3c8adfa06284bd959641 (accessed on 11th June 2025).

50. Yamashita, M., Shibato, J., Rakwal, R., Nonaka, N., Hirabayashi, T., Harvey, B., Shioda, S., et al. (2023). Molecular and physiological functions of PACAP in sweat secretion. *International Journal of Molecular Sciences, 24.* https://www.semanticscholar.org/paper/ea95b8bb6c752fafc10ae2b5105f7977eced774f (accessed on 11th June 2025).

51. Yokum, E. E., Goldstein, D. L., & Krane, C. M. (2025). Winter is coming: Integrative analysis of cold acclimation in a freeze tolerant frog. *Integrative Organismal Biology, 7.* https://www.semanticscholar.org/paper/6afc3d81234cbab678290d8cc1eb146fad77e034 (accessed on 11th June 2025).

SKIN AGING AND PHOTOAGING

2

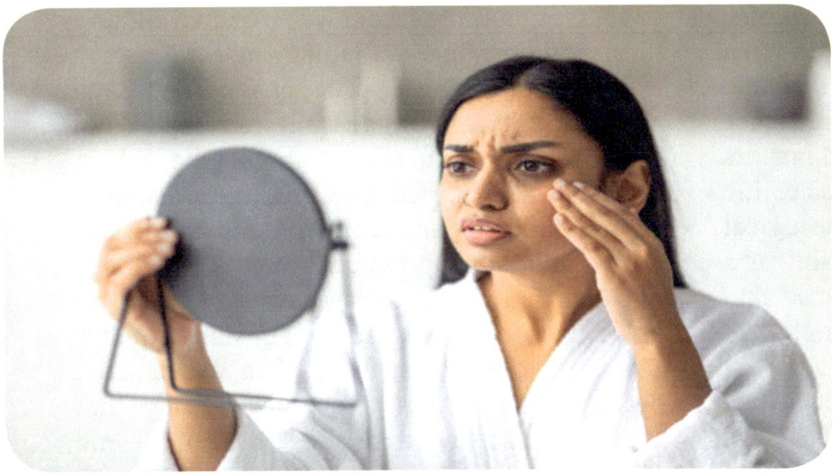

LEARNING OBJECTIVES

After studying this chapter, you will be able to:

1. Describe the biological mechanisms of skin aging
2. Explain environmental factors contributing to skin aging
3. Discuss the role of genetics in skin aging
4. Understand signs and symptoms of skin aging
5. Describe prevention strategies for skin aging
6. Focus on treatment options for skin aging and photoaging

Introduction

Admiration of the intricate process of aging skin demands careful examination of the intrinsic and extrinsic causes of aging skin. Aging skin is a natural consequence of biological aging, which is governed by genetic predisposition, hormonal changes, and metabolism. However, extrinsic factors such as ultraviolet (UV) radiation, environmental pollution, and lifestyle are indeed responsible for imparting a boosted pace to the aging process, a theory known as photoaging. The interplay of these variables renders the chronological age a poor predictor for the skin status, pointing towards the necessity of a more complex approach. A closer look at mechanisms of skin aging reveals that it comprises alterations in the structure and function of the skin, which ultimately affect appearance and overall skin health. Thus, the research on various interventions is important because they can reduce the impacts of aging and increase skin resilience (Fernández-Varela-Gómez et al., 2024). Overexposure to UV radiation is a major cause of photoaging and can lead to a range of skin issues, from wrinkles and fine lines to pigment disorders. The additive effects of sunlight not only accelerate the aging process but also compromise the skin barrier function, causing a drop in hydration and elasticity. Traditional preventive measures have been largely accomplished with the aid of synthetic sunscreens; however, concerns about potential adverse effects have created interest in more natural alternatives. This growing amount of evidence investigates compounds of natural origin, such as Bombyx mori, that have been hypothesized to possess certain photoprotective impacts. Through the integration of such new interventions with conventional skincare practices, there is a high likelihood of promoting skin well-being and resilience towards the photoaging process's harmful impacts (Damayanti et al., 2023). Integrating scientific understanding and advanced dermatological practices allows for the implementation of a holistic approach to the struggle against skin aging and photoaging. The understanding of the dual effect of intrinsic aging and photoaging allows individuals to make intelligent decisions regarding their skincare and lifestyle. This introduction lays the groundwork for further investigation of successful interventions like retinoids and natural photoprotective agents, in turn providing a foundation for grasping the intricacies of skin aging. Generally, focusing on both basic research and pragmatic solutions equips individuals with the ability to implement active measures, possibly resulting in healthier skin and a better quality of life later in life. The heightened consciousness of skin aging points to the importance of an integrative approach that facilitates both protection and rejuvenation (Fernández-Varela-Gómez et al., 2024).

Definition of Skin Aging

Skin aging is a complex process with a gradual loss in the structural stability and functional effectiveness of the skin over time. With age, the skin undergoes a chain of physiological changes that appear as evident signs of aging, including fine lines, wrinkles, and loss of elasticity. This process is determined by factors inherent to it, such as genetics, hormonal imbalance, and cellular ageing, which undermine the skin's capacity to repair and regenerate. Secondly, the continuous degeneration of essential components such as collagen and elastin plays an important role in contributing to giving the skin its aged appearance. While the aging process in itself is irreversible, it can indeed occur very differently from one person to another, depending on a myriad of interactive processes, among them environmental and lifestyle determinants that may be accelerators or brakes of the aging process. Environmental determinants are significant for explaining skin aging, particularly in photoaging, which is specifically caused by chronic exposure to UV radiation. Experiments have shown that UV radiation not only produces direct DNA damage but also induces oxidative stress, leading to inflammation and degradation of skin proteins. The oxidative stress results in accelerated degradation of elastin and collagen fibers that are essential to avoid loss of skin elasticity and turgor. Besides, environmental pollutants such as particulate matter (PM), along with harmful habits such as smoking and excessive alcohol consumption, hasten the process of skin aging by contributing to oxidative damage. All these highlight the complex interconnectivity between external exposures and intrinsic mechanisms of aging, highlighting the role of protective measures, including the use of sunscreen and antioxidant diets, in the preservation of skin integrity and reversibility of premature aging effects (Dorosz et al., 2025). In recent years, there has been growing interest in harnessing the potential of marine-derived cosmetic active ingredients to assist in fighting skin aging. Marine organisms, in particular some algae, carry significant bioactive compounds with antioxidant and anti-inflammatory activities. Marine ingredients can potentially offset the negative effects of environmental determinants of skin aging. Despite the enormous variety of such products available in the cosmetic industry, the therapeutic potential of marine compounds is still not fully explored (Amaral et al., 2023). Further research into these natural substances is required to define their mechanisms of action, safety, and effectiveness. Through collaborative work between academia and the cosmetics sector, there exists enormous potential for creating innovative solutions that embrace sustainable practice in addition to addressing the intricate issues of skin aging and photoaging (Figure 2.1).

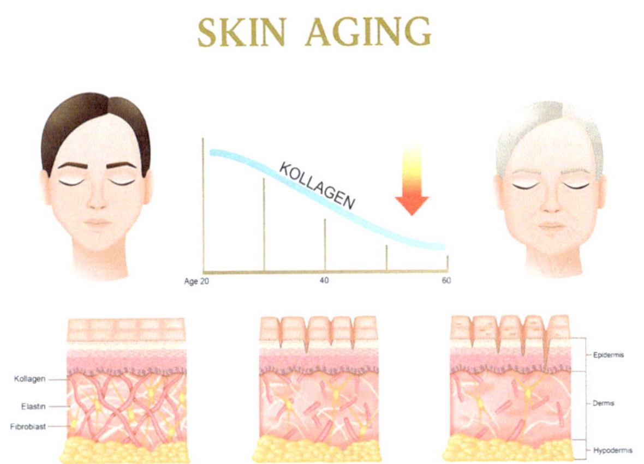

Figure 2.1. Skin aging.

Source: https://cdn.shopify.com/s/files/1/0053/8866/4950/files/2__0000s_0003_causes_of_skin_aging_1024x1024.jpg?v=1676389140.

Importance of Studying Skin Aging

The significance of studying skin aging extends well beyond cosmetic concerns with appearance, such as having significant broader implications for health and well-being, particularly with aging populations. Understanding what causes the biological mechanisms of skin aging is vital to being able to develop effective interventions to reverse the detrimental effects of intrinsic and extrinsic aging. Given that the skin is the body's first line of defense against extrinsic stressors, defects in its integrity can have the effect of increasing vulnerabilities to infections, UV damage, and skin cancers. Not only do the above considerations underscore the benefits of prioritizing dermatological research, but aging skin's impacts on self-esteem and social interaction are also of profound psychological significance. By examining these parameters, scientists can lay the foundation for novel treatments and prevention strategies, which subsequently enhance the quality of life among individuals with the issues of skin aging and associated conditions. The investigation of skin aging also provides us with insight into how the intrinsic factors, such as genes, mix with extrinsic factors, primarily UV radiation. Intrinsic aging, that is, the chronological change, is largely manifested as thinner skin, loss of elasticity, and compromised wound healing. On the other hand, extrinsic aging or so-called photoaging is an accumulated environmental stress, in which UV radiation is cumulated, and dermal matrix changes, including collagen and elastin, are induced. The cross-talk between these two processes of aging has been quite insightful as far as molecular pathways to skin breakdown are concerned. A comprehension of this is key to developing goal-specific therapies that not just cure the apparent indicators of aging but also reverse the underlying skin health issues. Knowing how the extrinsic and intrinsic mechanisms cause aging of the skin can more specifically delineate treatment modalities and improve patient outcomes overall. Investigating the mechanisms of skin aging has also emerged as the impetus for the development of therapeutic techniques, including advancements in techniques such as photodynamic therapy (PDT). Studies have demonstrated that the effectiveness of such treatments is influenced by type and skin age, with findings suggesting greater penetration of light through older skin, particularly lighter skin types, and therefore potentially more effective treatments. The results of these studies reveal the potential for daylight to be a viable light source for PDT, which may offer more cost-effective alternatives for treatment. With the population aging and dermatological conditions on the increase, research into skin aging remains top of the agenda to enable the medical fraternity to devise methods ensuring healthier skin across life. Ultimately, the building of an understanding and response to the multifaceted nature of skin aging is central to furthering dermatological treatment, in addition to overall quality of life.

Overview of Photoaging

Photoaging refers to skin changes and injury brought about by exposure over many years to UV radiation, accelerating the typical process of aging. Contrary to intrinsic aging, which is hereditary, photoaging has environmental causes and manifests in the form of wrinkles, uneven pigmentation, and loss of skin elasticity. This premature aging is a cumulative damage on the cellular level, whereby UV light induces the creation of reactive oxygen species (ROS) and inflammatory mediators that compromise the integrity of the skin. Geographic location, lifestyle, and protective practices all contribute to the degree of photoaging that an individual experiences. It is most significant, though, that the adverse impact of UV radiation on the skin highlights the necessity of protective action, such as the use of broad-spectrum sunscreen and protective clothing, in preventing long-term damage and promoting healthier skin down the line.

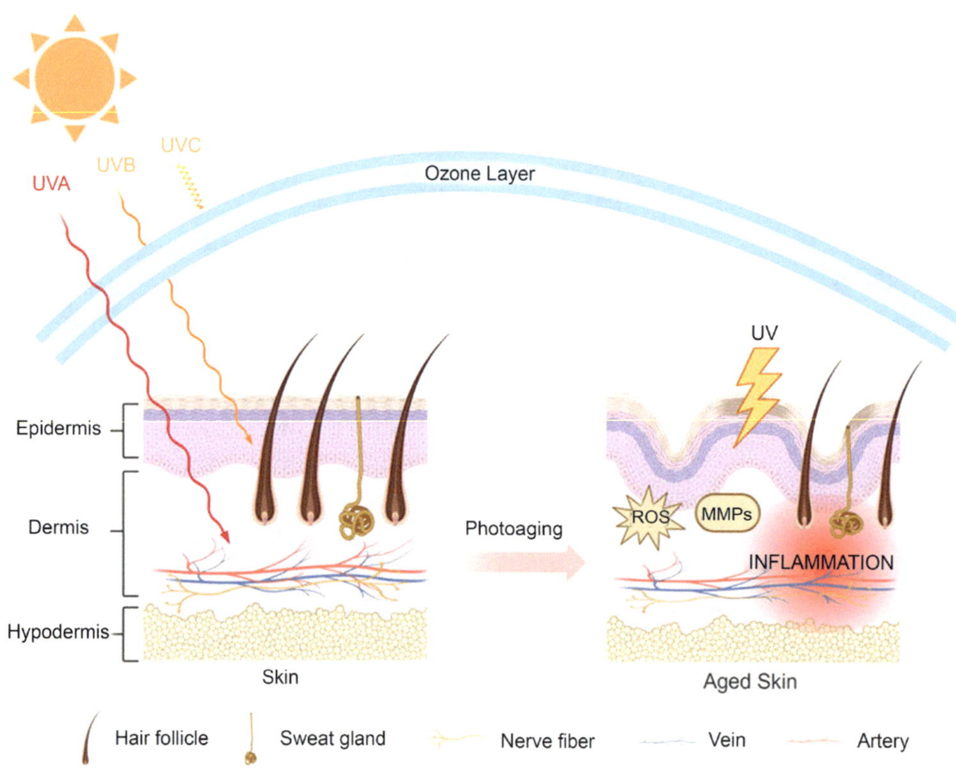

Figure 2.2. Mechanisms of skin photoaging caused by UV radiation.

Source: https://www.researchgate.net/publication/378479009/figure/fig1/AS:11431281230846748@1711123700691/Mechanisms-of-skin-photoaging-caused-by-UV-radiation-The-skin-can-be-divided-into-three.jpg.

The interaction between hormonal change and photoaging is another critical area of study in terms of considering skin health. Experimental research has revealed that estrogen deficiency may enhance the effects of UV-induced skin damage through heightened oxidative stress and decreased collagen production. Most crucially, topical 17β-estradiol (E2) treatments have been investigated for their capacity to curtail numerous features of skin aging. Unfortunately, these efficacies are often constrained by challenges related to bioavailability as well as side effects. The development of new delivery systems, such as Au/E2@mPDA-HCG nanoparticle composite hydrogels, demonstrates novel methods of enhancing the therapeutic action of estrogen against UV-induced deformities. Such developments constitute a revolution in targeted therapy aimed at reducing the severity of photoaging, in addition to intervention in the underlying biological processes that lead to skin degradation (Li et al., 2025). Apart from that, research on natural products in cosmetics is increasingly significant to prevent photoaging. Recent studies focused on the use of upcycled food waste-derived products, specifically low-molecular-weight anionic peptides (LMAPs) derived from Citrus Junos TANAKA seeds. The peptides were found to have protective effects against UV, enhancing the resistance of the skin against damage through the depletion of ROS and the suppression of inflammation. By stimulating collagen production and blocking melanin formation in response to UV exposure, LMAPs are a suitable alternative to conventional anti-aging treatments. The potential of such bioactive molecules speaks to the importance of sustainable operations in the cosmetics sector while defining skin health concerns. With the constant advancement in technology and research, these innovative measures may prove to be a valuable tool in improving the overall efficacy of anti-photoaging treatments (Ko et al., 2024) (Figure 2.2).

2.1. Biological Mechanisms of Skin Aging

Learning Outcome

1. Explain the term cellular senescence
2. Discuss decreased collagen production
3. Understand the changes in skin elasticity

It is crucial to know the biological mechanisms of skin aging so that effective interventions can be designed to optimize skin health. Skin aging exhibits a highly heterogeneous breakdown characterized by loss of collagen and elastin, critical proteins that provide structural integrity and elasticity to the skin. This loss is also augmented by extrinsic factors, namely UV radiation, that encourage the degradation of these proteins by activating matrix metalloproteinases (MMPs) that break down the extracellular matrix. The synergistic effects of intrinsic aging and these extrinsic factors enhance the observable effects of aging, such as wrinkles and sagging skin. Interestingly enough, chronological age is now being regarded more as an insufficient indicator for assessing skin condition because genetic influence and lifestyle also have a colossal impact on aging. Therefore, a better appreciation of these determinants of a biological nature is important to be able to counteract skin aging effectively (Fernández-Varela-Gómez et al., 2024). Oxidative stress is a force that cannot be overstressed in the aging of skin because it is one of the key contributors to cellular senescence and tissue damage. Reactive oxygen species (ROS), which are both endogenous metabolic products and extrinsic harmful stimuli like UV radiation, cause oxidative damage to the structures in cells, including lipids, proteins, and DNA. This injury initiates the activation of pro-inflammatory cascades that add to chronic inflammation, a characteristic of senescent skin. Scientific study has demonstrated that the buildup of oxidative stress enhances marks of photoaging, appearing as increased pigmentation, fine wrinkles, and lost skin elasticity. The use of antioxidant treatments, which can reverse the action of oxidative stress, has been demonstrated to be an effective strategy to reverse skin aging and improve skin health. These therapies focus on the importance of understanding the intricate interaction between skin aging and oxidative stress (Damayanti et al., 2023). Furthermore, recent advances in the understanding of biological processes have opened up potential windows for novel therapies targeting skin aging. For instance, the use of biological peptides, for instance, Bombyx mori, has become a potential way to enhance skin rejuvenation processes. These peptides possess intrinsic antioxidant and anti-inflammatory activity, which can reverse the deleterious actions of UV radiation and thus prevent photoaging. Research suggests that these compounds not only protect skin cells from oxidative stress but also stimulate collagen formation and improve overall skin texture. As the demand for improved, nature-based solutions to conventional anti-aging therapies rises, such findings place emphasis on leveraging the biological activity of some natural products in cosmetic treatments. Although research is ongoing, an understanding of the underlying mechanisms behind these activities will be critical to improving such treatments (Damayanti et al., 2023; Fernández-Varela-Gómez et al., 2024).

2.1.1. Cellular Senescence

Cell senescence is an essential biological process characterized by the permanent activation of cell growth and shutdown, and it has a significant influence on skin aging under photoaging. When skin cells such as fibroblasts are treated with stressors such as ultraviolet (UV) light, they are apt to become senescent, which consequently causes weakens extracellular matrix. This matrix is responsible for maintaining the integrity, elasticity, and appearance of the skin. Senescent cells trigger a cascade of molecular processes through pro-inflammatory cytokines and MMPs secretion, implicated in the degradation of collagen and elastin. Senescence-associated secretory phenotype (SASP) not only encourages local tissue damage but also generates a chronic inflammatory microenvironment, a feature of aged skin. Consequently, cellular senescence is an integral participant in both intrinsic aging and photoaging, necessitating targeted therapeutic interventions to oppose its activity. Cellular senescence's participation in the aging process thus signifies the multifaceted relationship between genetic susceptibility and environmental insult. Based on investigation, it has been shown that oxidative stress, primarily caused by UV radiation, significantly contributes to determining the establishment of senescence among skin cells. Elevated levels of ROS as a result of exposure to UV light are responsible for the oxidative damage that accelerates cellular aging. The oxidative environment is often altered by other factors, including way of life and inherent genetic factors, that, when combined, determine the extent of photoaging that an individual experiences. While chronological age is somehow related to aging, the accumulation of senescent cells reflects the real biological age of the skin. Therefore, it is important to understand the molecular outcomes of cellular senescence for the development of an efficient anti-aging strategy that can enhance resistance to photoaging (Fernández-Varela-Gómez et al., 2024). Addressing cellular senescence is at once a challenge and a prospect in dermatology and anti-aging medicine. Treatment approaches to rejuvenating senescent skin cells hold out the possibility to counteract some of the effects of photoaging by alleviating the SASPs. Targeting and eliminating methods for senescent cells, including senolytic therapies, have been considered for their potential to rejuvenate senescent tissue and facilitate function. Moreover, topical agents that modulate the senescence pathways can potentially mitigate inflammation and promote the regeneration of extracellular matrix. In addition, such therapies combined with lifestyle interventions such as rigorous sun avoidance practices and antioxidant-containing skincare may cumulatively enhance skin health and resilience to environmental stressors. Lastly, embracing a multi-faceted understanding of cellular senescence in the pathogenesis of skin aging and photoaging is key to developing new therapeutic approaches to generate healthier, more youthful skin (Pilán et al., 2023) (Figure 2.3).

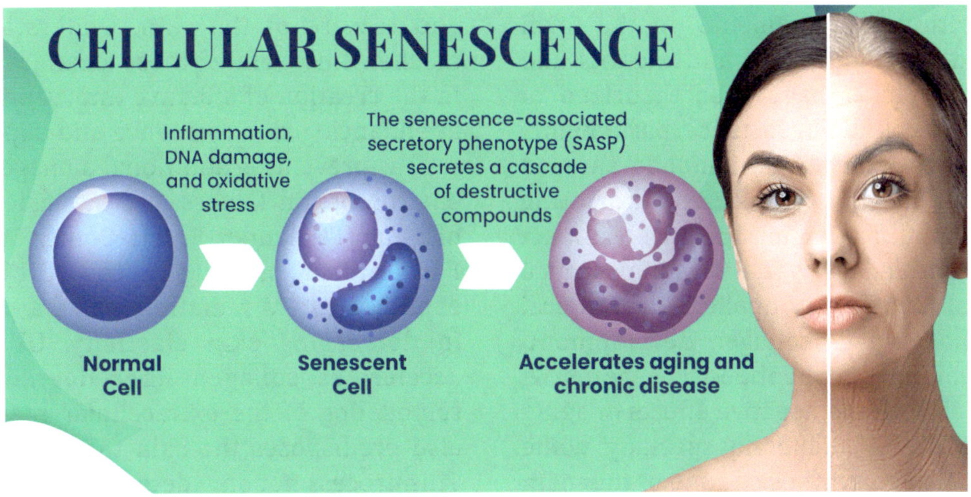

Figure 2.3. Cellular senescence.

Source: https://thenutritioninsider.com/wp-content/uploads/2022/08/Cellular-Senescence-Graphic-1536x1040.png.

2.1.2. Decreased Collagen Production

With age, there is a significant decrease in collagen synthesis, which is reflected in many changes that can be seen. Collagen, as a significant structural protein within the dermal matrix, maintains the significance of ensuring skin's elasticity, moisture, and overall strength. As the aging process takes place, particularly among postmenopausal women, the production of collagen decreases due to intrinsic causes such as hormonal changes and extrinsic causes such as stress caused by the environment. This decrease results in the development of wrinkles, skin sagging, and lower structural integrity. Furthermore, research has shown that collagen breakdown speeds up simultaneously, which furthers the effects of aging and makes a circle where it continues to degrade skin health and appearance. With the knowledge of these intrinsic processes, it is clear that reduced collagen production is a key component of aging skin, which becomes more brittle and less resilient to damage as people mature in age. External influences, particularly sun exposure and environmental contaminants, significantly enhance the decline of collagen, a process termed as photoaging. Sunlight induces UV radiation that leads to inflammation and oxidative stress that may negatively affect dermal collagen and lead to its degradation at an enhanced rate. The structural integrity of the skin is, therefore, disrupted, and wrinkles become more frequent, in addition to a loss of firmness. The dynamic interaction between intrinsic aging and photoaging adds to the fact that both enhance collagen depletion in the skin. Further, the population that is aging has higher risks of such expressions with lifestyle factors such as diet and exposure to toxic chemicals. A general understanding of photoaging makes inevitable skin protection against UV damage even more crucial, and with this need comes the promotion of interdisciplinarity in the approach to skin care for prevention as well as treatment of collagen loss. Research has indicated that lifestyle measures can reverse the loss of collagen content and offer hope to those concerned with photoaging and skin aging. Nutritional supplements, in the form of increased consumption of antioxidants and essential fatty acids, have been theorized to keep the skin healthy. For instance, participants in research who consumed almonds showed improvement in wrinkle severity, indicating that dietary modification may positively impact collagen retention and overall skin appearance (Burney et al., 2019). Also, application of topical products that trigger collagen development, such as retinoids and peptides, has potential for turning around the negative effects of aging (Hwang et al., 2011). Generally speaking, while decreased collagen synthesis is one of the main issues of skin aging, active measures can be used to enhance resilience, retain beauty, and ultimately, support healthier skin aging (Figure 2.4).

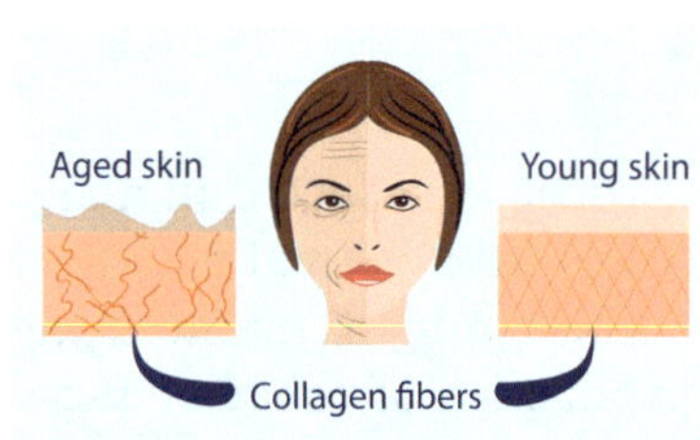

Figure 2.4. Collagen fibers.

Source: https://yonboon.ae/storage/upload/1153201786.jpg.

2.1.3. Changes in Skin Elasticity

When the skin ages, the most noticeable alteration may be a decrease in elasticity, or the capacity of the skin to return to normal after stretching and shrinking. The major cause of such a loss of elasticity is a decline in the production of collagen and elastin, the two prominent proteins that provide a structural framework to the skin. The process of aging, which has been hastened by sun exposure, pollution, and lifestyle, leads to structural changes within the dermis. These changes can lead to sagging, wrinkles, and fine lines, which play a significant role in determining the overall appearance and texture of the skin. Understanding the mechanisms behind these changes is critical in the creation of effective interventions aimed at enhancing skin resilience and appearance as well as preventing additional damage caused by environmental factors and intrinsic processes of aging (Fernández-Varela-Gómez et al., 2024). Furthermore, photoaging, caused by extended exposure to UV radiation, plays a pivotal role in decreasing skin elasticity. UV radiation accelerates collagen fiber degradation and remodeling of the extracellular matrix, which also predisposes the skin to structural injury. This process not only deteriorates the elasticity of the skin but also decreases its hydration level and increases roughness to create a textured effect that is typically observed in aged skin. In addition, photoaging may lead to the formation of deep wrinkles and abnormalities of pigmentation, again emphasizing the need for full sun protection practices. Effective interventions need to include both preventive and restorative interventions to mitigate the pathological effects of UV exposure to preserve the elasticity and overall integrity of the skin (Ziobro et al., 2024). Treatment and prevention strategies for skin elasticity alterations are based on a multi-modal approach that includes topical, oral, and procedural interventions. Topical therapies like retinoids are known to effectively stimulate the synthesis of collagen and enhance skin texture. Antioxidants also suppress free radicals, preventing oxidative stress that will further result in loss of elasticity. Supplementation of nutraceuticals orally or systemic retinoids has also been in the limelight for promoting skin wellness from the inside out. Along with that, procedural therapies such as laser, microneedling, and chemical peels are known to significantly improve skin elasticity by promoting collagen production and cellular turnover. Lastly, an extended treatment regimen that includes preventive measures such as adequate sun protection along with individually tailored treatment regimens can yield better outcomes in the maintenance of skin elasticity as well as in the prevention of intrinsic as well as extrinsic aging (Fernández-Varela-Gómez et al., 2024; Ziobro et al., 2024) (Figure 2.5).

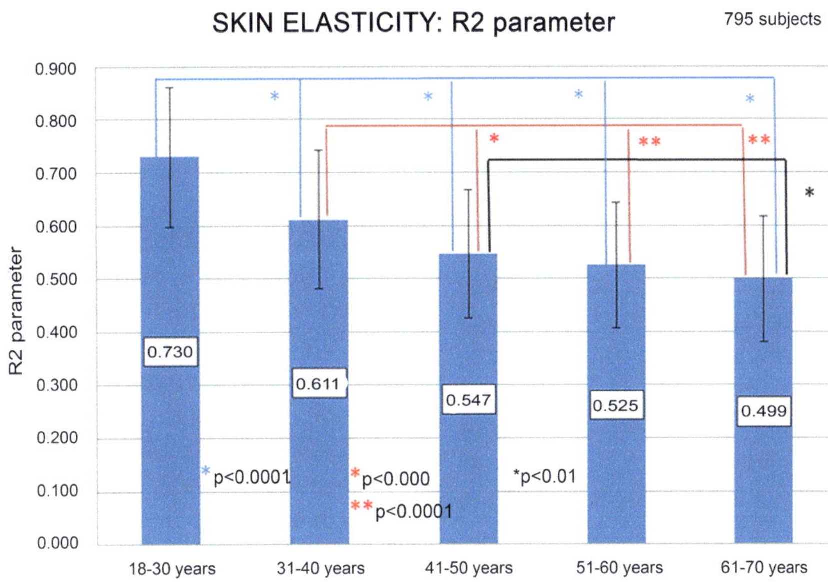

Figure 2.5. Skin elasticity basal values (R2 parameter) as a function of the age group. Statistical comparison among the age groups: * p < 0.0001 (18–30 vs. 31–40 years; 18–30 vs. 41–50 years; 18–30 vs. 51–60 years; 18–30 vs. 61–70 years); * p < 0.001 (31–40 vs. 41–50 years); ** p < 0.0001 (31–40 vs. 51–60 years; 31–40 vs. 61–70 years); * p < 0.01 (41–50 vs. 61–70 years).

Source: https://www.researchgate.net/publication/276034459/figure/fig2/AS:340610646069255@1458219314265/Skin-elasticity-basal-values-R2-parameter-as-a-function-of-the-age-group-Statistical.png.

Test Your Knowledge

1. How does cellular senescence contribute to the structural and functional decline of aging skin?
2. What are the primary cellular and molecular mechanisms responsible for decreased collagen production in aging skin?

2.2. Environmental Factors Contributing to Skin Aging

Learning Outcome

1. Explain the effects of UV radiation exposure on skin aging
2. Understand the relationship between pollution and skin aging
3. Discuss how lifestyle choices influence skin aging and photoaging

Among the range of environmental reasons for skin aging, UV radiation is the major cause and contributes significantly to deep damage to skin cells and acceleration of the aging process. Exposure to sunlight, primarily from the sun, breaks down collagen and elastin fibers and leads to wrinkles, loss of elasticity, and irregular pigmentation. This extrinsic form of aging, photoaging, results in noticeable alterations that differ significantly from genetically controlled intrinsic aging. The link between exposure to UV radiation and cutaneous harm also emphasizes the greatest importance of sun protection practices. These practices, including the use of broad-spectrum sunscreens and protective clothing, can significantly diminish the negative effects of UV radiation. Thus, knowing how UV light works in aging the skin becomes crucial in taking preventive action to ensure healthy skin throughout life, as emphasized by evidence for proper skin care routines and interactions with the environment (Fernández-Varela-Gómez et al., 2024). Pollution is another major environmental factor influencing skin aging, especially in urban environments where air quality has reached alarming levels. Toxic substances such as PM, heavy metals, and volatile organic compounds can migrate across the skin barrier and induce oxidative stress. Oxidative damage leads to premature aging by triggering inflammation and degradation of cellular components, thereby producing prematurely aged skin. The clinical significancc of this ccological poison is supported by scientific evidence illustrating a direct correlation between pollution exposure and various skin disorders, including eczema and premature aging. Due to the expense of pollutants in modern societies, the addition of anti-pollution skincare products and the implementation of cleaner air initiatives become imperative components of an integrated model of dermatological health. Treating these environmental aggressors is crucial to mitigating their harmful effects on skin health and integrity, as proven in previous research (Tri,2018). Finally, lifestyle habits that are compounded by environmental components are major contributors to the aging of skin. Cigarette smoking, for instance, not only has serious physical health consequences but also negatively impacts the skin through constricted blood vessels and limited oxygen and nutrient supply. This leads to pale skin, premature wrinkles, and overall premature skin aging. Lifestyle diet also has a significant role to play; high intake of sugar and processed foods can lead to glycation, which breaks down collagen and leads to skin aging. The synergy between these lifestyle habits with environmental exposures also highlights the need to adopt a balanced diet, regular exercise, and abstinence from smoking as main components of skin conservation measures. With increasing proof of complex determinants of skin aging, it is increasingly clear that a holistic grasp of environmental determinants and lifestyle choices is needed in order to have effective skincare practices (Fernández-Varela-Gómez et al., 2024).

2.2.1. UV Radiation Exposure

The effects of UV radiation exposure on skin aging are profound and widespread, and they play a crucial role in photoaging. Upon exposure to ultraviolet light, skin triggers a series of biological effects that lead to changes on the structural and functional levels. Repeated exposure may lead to overt manifestations such as wrinkles, abnormal pigmentation, and loss of skin elasticity. This damage is primarily due to UV radiation's ability to induce DNA mutations and interrupt repair mechanisms, leading to premature aging. Experimental evidence indicates that constituents in exosomes are capable of modulating cellular responses against UV stress, giving hints on potential therapeutic strategies for reducing the signs of photoaging (Li et al., 2025). Understanding the mechanisms involved in UV-induced skin damage is key to developing successful prevention and treatment strategies that preserve skin integrity over time. Furthermore, UV division into UVA and UVB wavelengths illustrates the way in which these rays affect the skin. UVB rays, which produce sunburn, affect DNA directly as well as play a role in skin cancers. Compared to UVB, UVA penetrates deeper into the skin, causing oxidative stress and contributing significantly to the aging process through the breakdown of collagen and elastin fibers. Cumulative damage from these rays is compounded by additional environmental factors like geography and season, which can potentially affect levels of exposure. Sunscreens have an important role in avoiding exposures deleterious effects but are quite variable in effectiveness based on SPF ratings and types (Mishra, 2024). Establishing the holistic awareness of UV radiation components is thus essential in creating the appropriate protective measures to combat photoaging effectively. The body's response to UV radiation is dependent on complex regulation processes by numerous molecules, of which some are long non-coding RNAs (lncRNAs). They have been shown in recent research to modulate stress response to UV exposure and, consequently, influence cellular survival and apoptosis. The findings of research studies on UV-exposed rats showed widespread changes in the expression profiles of lncRNA and mRNA, which suggest their significant contributions to the cellular protection mechanism against UV-induced injury (Li et al., 2025). Further, transcriptomic studies reveal that lncRNAs not only modulate inflammation and apoptosis but also oxidative stress responses. This discovery foregrounds the possibility of targeting such regulatory molecules for therapeutic interventions in the direction of countering the harmful effects of photoaging. As continued research matures, how lncRNAs interact with other cellular constituents could find new ways to enhance skin resistance to UV light and, thus, increase the health and longevity of the skin (Figure 2.6).

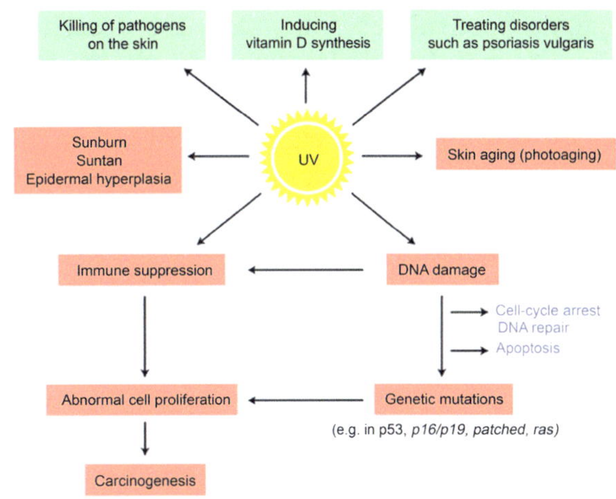

Figure 2.6. Effects of UV radiation on human skin.

Source: https://www.researchgate.net/profile/Ninon-Etsassala/publication/332632357/figure/fig2/AS:751493049241600@1556181313047/Effects-of-UV-radiation-on-human-skin.ppm.

2.2.2. Pollution and Environmental Toxins

The link between skin aging and pollution is clearer with modern research, showing how environmental toxins intensify this natural process. Environmental factors such as UV radiation and air pollution play a significant role in affecting the structural stability and general well-being of the skin. Both are responsible for the accelerated breakdown of elastin and collagen, proteins essential in maintaining the firmness and elasticity of the skin. According to

Dorosz et al (2025), environmental stresses such as UV and air pollution induce oxidative stress, the central driving force for skin aging. Oxidative damage not only creates apparent signs of aging, such as wrinkles and fine lines, but also disrupts vital cellular processes. As a result, it is important to understand how pollution aggravates these alterations to effectively combat its effects on aging skin and promote general dermatologic health. Pollutants in the air, including a mix of toxic particulates and gases, are a serious threat to skin health. Studies have shown that toxins such as particulate matter (PM), nitrogen oxides, and ozone are capable of entering the skin, causing inflammation and oxidative stress. Particularly, PM2.5, which are the smallest particles, have been linked to more extensive cellular damage and faster aging processes. Notably, Sieradocha et al. (2024) recognize that the pollutants destabilize the extracellular matrix, which maintains skin elasticity and hydration. Moreover, air pollution disrupts the skin's microbiome, leading to dysbiosis that can exacerbate a variety of skin conditions, including eczema and acne. Hence, the importance of knowing the role played by air pollution in the health of the skin is based on a complex skincare routine that encompasses protection from such environmental toxins and the demand for public measures against exposure. To reverse the impact of pollution and its role in skin aging, a balanced skincare routine must be adopted. Preventive steps consist of the application of antioxidants, such as vitamins C and E, to suppress free radicals caused by oxidative stress. Aside from this, moisturizers also offer a strengthening function against the skin barrier to minimize the side effects of environmental factors. Along with the application of topical products, lifestyle changes, such as consuming an antioxidant-dense diet and sun protection, are important in keeping general skin health intact. The review conducted by Dorosz et al. (2025) highlights the importance of a healthy lifestyle to counteract the negative effects of environmental factors on aging. Further, current research into the efficacy of night care products that restore damaged skin while sleeping holds hope against the effects of pollution. In conclusion, it will become essential to create an integrated strategy comprising skincare along with sensitization towards environmental factors in order to maintain youthful skin (Figure 2.7).

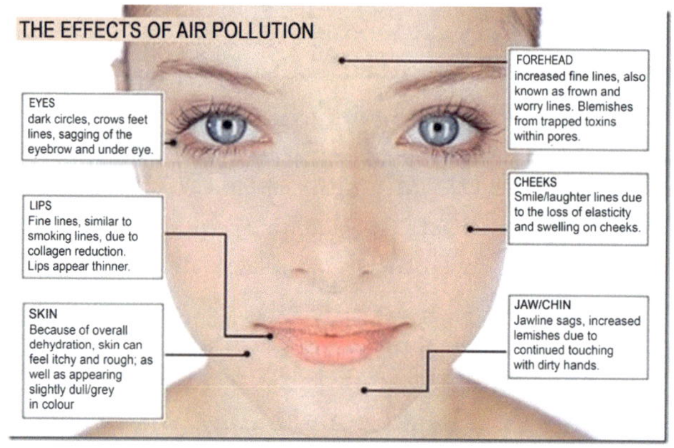

Figure 2.7. The effect of air pollution.

Source: https://parsikhabar.net/wp-content/uploads/clip_image002_thumb-76.jpg.

2.2.3. Lifestyle Choices (Smoking, Diet)

Lifestyle plays a significant role in skin aging and photoaging, with diet and smoking being significant contributors. Smoking is not healthy for the skin and is largely to be blamed due to tobacco's chemicals that cause oxidative stress and decrease blood circulation. The poor circulation affects the supply of oxygen and nutrients to skin cells, leading to a pale appearance and premature wrinkle development. Moreover, the process of smoking mechanically, such as pursing lips and squinting eyes to keep out the smoke, creates dynamic wrinkles around the mouth and eyes. Thus, smoking cessation not only halts skin aging but also can create some regions of improvement in complexion, emphasizing the significant impact of this life choice on dermatologic well-being as detailed in the literature concerning the environmental aspect of skin aging (Dorosz et al., 2025). Diet is another important determinant of skin health and a main provider of the nutrients needed for repair and regeneration. A diet rich in antioxidants, including vitamins C and E, has been shown to reverse damage due to oxidative stress caused by environmental triggers, including UV light and pollution. Foods that are high in omega-3 fatty acids, such as fish and flaxseeds, keep the lipid layer of the skin enriched, keeping the skin hydrated and elastic. A poor diet with high sugar and processed foods, however, hastens skin aging by inducing glycation, causing damage to collagen and elastin fibers. The connection between nutrition and skin shows the importance of including balanced and nutrient-dense food to fight the evident outward signs of aging and encourage overall skin care (Dorosz et al., 2025). Topical dermatocosmetic products, on the other hand, may aid or work against a healthy lifestyle in the fight against skin aging. While the cosmetic industry has produced a huge variety of skin care creams, both chemical and herbal, designed for various types of skin, their effects are extremely vulnerable to the health of the skin and lifestyle. Organic cosmetics have organic ingredients that may be beneficial to the skin without any ill effects compared to synthetic products. However, this apparent transformation is achievable only with the simultaneous application of such creams and proper lifestyle patterns. Last but not least, healthy lifestyle habits, like smoking cessation and a healthy diet, can be synergized with topical skincare to retard the aging process and improve skin quality in the long run.

Test Your Knowledge

1. How does chronic exposure to UV radiation contribute to photoaging at the cellular and molecular levels?
2. What is the role of air pollution, particularly particulate matter and ozone, in accelerating skin aging?

2.3. The Role of Genetics in Skin Aging

Learning Outcome

1. Describe hereditary factors influencing skin aging
2. Discuss about genetic predisposition to photoaging
3. Understand family history and skin health

The genetic predisposition to skin aging is a key area to understand how biological processes influence the process of aging. Genetic determinants are held accountable for the individual differences in skin aging among individuals and shape traits such as elasticity, pigmentation, and resistance to environmental variables in general. While chronological age can be used as a general framework for assessing skin aging, it cannot reflect the individual differences shaped by genetic determinants. Researchers are identifying specific genetic markers for various signs of aging that could lead to targeted interventions that seek to inhibit unwanted aging effects. The identification of such markers allows individualized skincare regimens to be developed, more potent, considering the particular genetic makeup of a person and addressing the intricate interplay between genes and epidermal well-being (Fernández-Varela-Gómez et al., 2024). The advancement in Genome-Wide Association Studies (GWAS) has come a long way in enhancing our understanding of the genetic factors of skin aging. The studies have identified several single-nucleotide polymorphisms (SNPs) that are associated with pigmentation as well as other aspects of aging across different populations. For instance, IRF4, MC1R, and ASIP genes have been implicated in differences in pigmentation that affect skin aging. Though GWAS has proven to be helpful, more research is still a priority. The current pool of knowledge is pointed towards the prevalence of certain ethnic groups, with the issue of under-represented populations being covered in genetic research. Thus, an expanded strategy for GWAS is warranted in order to permit a comprehensive perspective into genetic diversity and its influence on skin aging processes among various populations (Shabihah & Paramita,2023). An insight into the intrinsic genetic mechanisms of skin aging has the promise of enhancing not only scholarly inquiry but even applied dermatological and cosmetic use. Through interpreting the genetic signals being taken in by the skin during aging, scientists can better understand the way these factors function in conjunction with environmental stresses, such as UV exposure and lifestyle. This integrated picture perspective extends the conversation beyond the visual to include the physiological changes in skin function and structure with aging. Ultimately, it is a goal to work toward integral measures that incorporate genetic information following preventative regimes to enable healthier skin throughout life. Emphasizing a multi-sighted approach will not only enhance comprehension of skin aging, but it will also provide the foundation from which innovative treatments tailored to individual genetic profiles will be created (Fernández-Varela-Gómez et al., 2024).

2.3.1. Hereditary Factors Influencing Skin Aging

The intricate interaction among the genetic and skin aging variables highlights the multifaceted processes that underlie not only the appearance of the skin but also its internal function and resistance. Genetic predispositions are responsible for how one ages the skin, including inherited tendencies to shape the texture, elasticity, and color of the skin. These characteristics are often the result of polymorphisms in genes that regulate the synthesis of collagen, cell repair, and apoptosis regulation, all vital processes for maintaining skin's youth. Consequently, people who possess genetic variations that enhance these processes may experience postponed signs of aging, indicating the contribution of genetic variation to the aging process. In addition, knowledge of these hereditary factors offers a basis for creating specific interventions, as it indicates that individualized skincare programs might be programmed based on genetic susceptibility, which may be used to counteract the signs of aging (Fernández-Varela-Gómez et al., 2024). GWAS are now shedding light on the contribution of genetics to skin aging, specifically with regard to pigmentation traits. By identifying SNPs in IRF4, MC1R, and ASIP genes, researchers are able to determine how certain genetic profiles impact the aging process in different populations. Such studies indicate that varying gene expression among these genes can cause variations in the appearance of the skin, such as age spots and mottled pigmentation, with age. However, while there has been incredible advancement, the current research exemplifies the deplorable lack of sample diversity in populations studied, tending to study primarily European and East Asian populations. This gap necessitates more representative research approaches that incorporate a greater variety of genetic backgrounds in order to offer a more extensive understanding of hereditary skin aging drivers (Shabihah & Paramita,2023). The implications of genetic influence extend into clinical practice and product development for skincare products, underscoring the need for personalized dermatological care. With the growing recognition that genetics play a role in aging, cosmetic and pharmaceutical companies are beginning to provide genetic testing as part of their services so that anti-aging treatment can be specially prepared according to the unique genetic characteristics of the person. Such technology may lead to more efficient skincare products that address the unique needs of multicultural populations and perhaps change the mode of anti-aging treatment. Through the integration of genetic insights in dermatology, doctors are better placed to advise patients about the importance of early prevention and treatment based on their genetic predisposition. Overall, a complex understanding of how genetic factors interact with environmental influences is needed to extend the science of skin aging and photoaging to new and personalized skincare practices (Fernández-Varela-Gómez et al., 2024) (Figure 2.8).

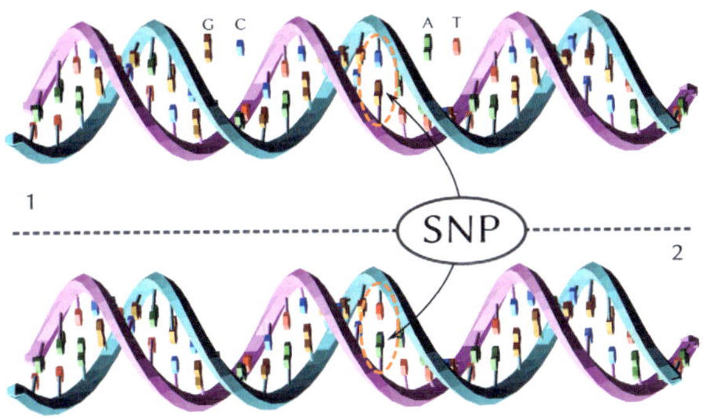

Figure 2.8. A single nucleotide polymorphism (SNP).

Source: By SNP model by David Eccles (gringer), CC BY 4.0, https://commons.wikimedia.org/w/index.php?curid=2355125

2.3.2. Genetic Predisposition to Photoaging

The photoaging process, as manifested through wrinkles, pigmentation, and texture changes, is not only dependent on environmental exposures but also largely on genetic susceptibility. Genetic variation can play a critical role in predetermining how the skin responds to UV radiation. Specific genes are known to control the processes of skin repair and antioxidant protection and thus influence the susceptibility to the injurious effects of sun exposure. Understanding these genetic factors is central to the development of specific therapies that may reverse photoaging effects. Certain alleles, for instance, may enhance the ability of the skin to repair DNA damage provoked by UV radiation, which identifies a genetic pathway that can be harnessed in dermatological treatment. As science progresses, a more nuanced knowledge of the intricately complex genetic mechanisms of photoaging will assist in creating customized skincare regimens for maximizing skin health throughout an individual's lifetime. In addition to DNA repair mechanisms, genetically regulated individual variation in collagen production and epidermal barrier function will further enhance the influence of photoaging. Collagen, a vital component that lends strength to the skin's structure, decreases with age and further with photoaging. Genetic factors could play a role in the quality and quantity of collagen synthesis, hence impacting sun-induced aging of the skin. Gene action can also influence sebum secretion and hydration, both of which impart elasticity and overall skin appearance. Studying these phenotypes has shown that certain genetically defined individuals tend to develop accelerated photoaging symptoms more so than others, reflecting the necessity for an individualized approach to dermatologic treatment that takes into account these genetic factors. These findings also emphasize the need for early intervention, such as sun protection practices tailored to genetically determined skin types, to counteract the effects of photoaging. New research continues to illuminate the functions of the genetic determinants of photoaging, revealing potential pathways for new treatments. As an example, the role of antioxidants in counteracting oxidative stress, a significant causative agent of photoaging, has been studied as a function of genetic susceptibility. The harmful effects of UV light can be especially common among individuals whose genetic predispositions tend towards low antioxidant levels. This association has led to an increasing tendency to use natural ingredients, including those rich in antioxidants, in the form of topical formulations. Studies have found that plant-derived antioxidants, with the use of innovative formulations with gold nanoparticles, can enhance the penetrability of such agents, thus providing better anti-aging outcomes. These findings show the possible utility in integrating genetic information into designing individualized skincare treatments for photoprotection and overall skin well-being, highlighting the way the complicated interdependence of genetics and lifestyle drives the skin's aging process (Permatasari et al., 2023; Fernández-Varela-Gómez et al., 2024).

2.3.3. Family History and Skin Health

The influence of genetic factors on the skin state is significant, particularly regarding skin aging and photoaging effects. Genetic susceptibility decides how individuals age, including wrinkle development and skin elasticity. There are indications that certain genetic markers influence the skin's characteristics, stressing the necessity for individuals to pay attention to their lineage when assessing their skin state. For instance, studies have identified specific genetic variants linked with skin aging traits, e.g., microtopography of the skin, which demonstrate the genetic determinants of the skin status of an individual. By investigating the family history and genetic traits, dermatologists can better predict the course of their patients' skin health, which requires prevention measures tailored to genetic makeup (Burney et al., 2019). Family history not only determines individual genetics but also affects lifestyle patterns, which could influence a great deal towards skin health. Lifestyle and surroundings and family habits usually move together in accord with hereditary influences, creating a complex interaction of heredity and behavior. For example, if one has a sun-sensitive family history, he or she will automatically be adopting protective measures against sun exposure at an early stage, which would forestall the effect of photoaging. The common family histories of skin conditions, such as rosacea or eczema, can also inform preventive care in the next generations. Thus, the knowledge of one's family skin health history enables an individual to make sensible decisions on sun exposure, skin care habits, and diet that could potentially render the skin healthier in the long term (Burney et al., 2019). In addition, more recent research is increasingly looking at the interface between skin health and familial genetics using twin pairs and large cohorts of data analysis. Investigation has determined significant correlations between specific genetic loci and visible signs of aging skin, including pigmentation and texture. For instance, genetic variations such as those linked with the MC1R gene determine individual reactions to sun exposure and the process of skin aging, demonstrating the influence of genetic factors on the status of skin. Such observations not only confirm family history involvement in the process of skin aging but also enable individuals to take active roles in their skincare routines based on their genetics. This new model places a lot of emphasis on incorporating genetic counseling and dermatologic care as key aspects in achieving increased skin health outcomes (Barbour et al., 2017) (Figure 2.9).

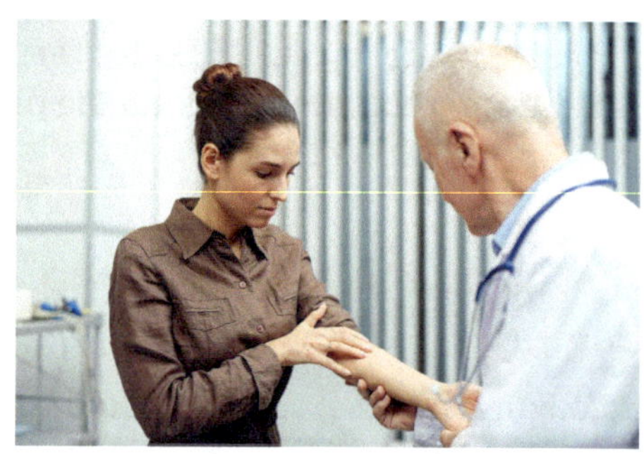

Figure 2.9. A dermatologist examining a patient's forearm, illustrating the importance of professional skin evaluations in diagnosing and managing dermatological conditions.

Source: https://www.health.com/thmb/j05U--EQnUu5uIGjpWJKqYT311Q=/2121x0/filters:no_upscale():max_bytes(150000):strip_icc()/Health-GettyImages-886098366-5a2b34568cc04e26ac9e1e72ce19c589.jpg.

Test Your Knowledge

1. How do specific genetic variations influence the rate and visible signs of skin aging?
2. Which specific genes have been identified as key regulators in the skin aging process?

2.4. Signs and Symptoms of Skin Aging

Learning Outcome

1. Explain wrinkles and fine lines
2. Discuss about age spots and pigmentation changes
3. Understand dryness and texture changes

The symptoms and signs of aged skin can be divided into a number of groups that account for both extrinsic and intrinsic causes. Intrinsic aging, or chronological aging, is when the skin slowly loses elasticity, loses its collagen production, and overall gets thinner in the dermis. Normal aging causes wrinkling, fine lines, and sagging skin. In contrast, extrinsic aging, which is precipitated by environmental factors such as UV radiation, hastens these expressions, leading to photoaging. Photoaged skin is usually characterized by irregular pigmentation, coarse texture, and deep wrinkles, particularly in sun-exposed areas. In understanding these diverse manifestations, one is more able to offset the impact through targeted interventions that address genetic susceptibility and environmental influences, which explains why having a holistic strategy to skin health over the lifespan is as much a part of skin aging science and intervention work as has been argued (Fernández-Varela-Gómez et al., 2024). In addition to physical shifts, there should not be disregard for the psychological and emotional consequences of skin aging. When individuals begin noticing skin imperfections, they may feel a loss of confidence and a greater awareness of their appearance. Research indicates that beauty norms are not innate but rather societal, and the resultant emotional response of aging skin leads to a feeling of insufficiency or worry. This need-based response compels individuals to seek solutions through cosmetic procedures or topical creams, which would favor the industry promoting anti-aging solutions. Furthermore, mass distribution of marketing claims on skin products has the tendency to create unrealistic expectations, which consequently results in dissatisfaction. Lastly, the identification of the intricate link between skin aging and subjective perception is crucial in the communication of mental well-being alongside physical treatments in the hope of creating a comprehensive insight into the aging process (Mohiuddin, 2020). Prevention and therapy of signs and symptoms of skin aging require individualized strategies that involve both lifestyle changes and preventive interventions. Every day use of broad-spectrum sunscreen, for example, is essential in preventing the skin from harmful UV radiation, a leading cause of extrinsic aging. The skin care industry has responded to this need with new products that, in addition to providing photoprotection, contain active ingredients that promise to rejuvenate the skin. As consumer understanding of skin wellness continues to grow, effective anti-aging products that contain new actives are emerging, allowing men and women to combat visible signs of aging through preventative measures. Research highlighted the necessity of integrating sun protection with other skin care rituals, such as moisturizing and antioxidant use, to promote overall skin health and resilience to the aging process. Thus, an interdisciplinary approach, harmonizing personal care and dermatological treatments, would be most beneficial in guaranteeing youthful skin (Fernández-Varela-Gómez et al., 2024).

2.4.1. Wrinkles and Fine Lines

Wrinkle and fine-line development is one of the more visible indicators of skin aging, particularly in the case of the photoaging phenomenon. Not merely surface changes, they reflect more in-depth changes in the integrity of the skin. Wrinkles are likely to develop through an interaction of intrinsic aging, or normal skin aging, and extrinsic factors like sunlight exposure. Since the collagen and elastin fibers deteriorate with age, the skin loses its tautness and elasticity and is more prone to the formation of fine lines and deeper creases. Also, the loss of subcutaneous fat results in a concave face, and therefore, the prominence of these signs of aging increases. Interestingly, fine lines and wrinkles are capable of affecting individuals' self-concept and social relationships, demonstrating the significant psychological consequences of aging. The influence of environmental stressors, particularly UV radiation, plays a central role in causing the acceleration of skin aging and wrinkle and fine line development. Chronic exposure to UV light evokes a multi-step cascade of molecular events that damage the skin's connective tissues, leading to cellular changes that take the form of photoaging. Photoaging is clinically evident in the form of fine and coarse wrinkles, among other phenotypic features such as roughness and irregular pigmentation. Surprisingly, sun-exposed areas such as the face, neck, and hands exhibit these signs of aging more rapidly. This accentuates the significance of sun protection as a prophylactic intervention to minimize the long-term effects of photoaging, maintaining the integrity of the skin and delaying the onset of wrinkles and fine lines. Awareness of the biological underpinnings of wrinkle formation calls for a comprehensive discussion of intrinsic and extrinsic mechanisms of aging. Intrinsic aging is characterized by a gradual slowing down of skin and cellular metabolism, with consequent thinning of the epidermis and reduced dermal thickness, ultimately leading to fine wrinkles. Extrinsic aging, or photoaging, accelerates this timetable, and hence, there is a pressing need for such interventions. Interventions that include the application of topical retinoids, antioxidants, and adequate sun protection can fortify the skin against such aging. Embracing an integrated approach with preventive and corrective solutions is necessary to provide long-term skin well-being. In that context, the understanding of skin aging complexities and creation of efficient strategies can significantly enhance the appearance and quality of life of the skin, emphasizing the necessity for ongoing research and educational activity in the area of dermatological sciences (Figure 2.10).

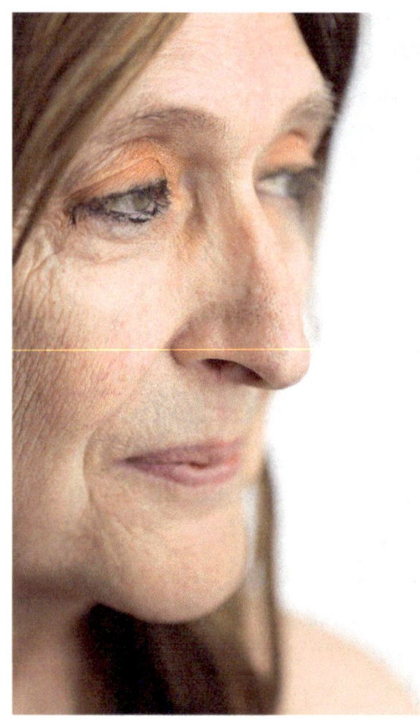

Figure 2.10. A woman of European origin with facial wrinkles.

Source: https://upload.wikimedia.org/wikipedia/commons/thumb/e/e0/Nose_%E2%80%93_Caisa.jpg/800px-Nose_%E2%80%93_Caisa.jpg.

2.4.2. Age Spots and Pigmentation Changes

During the lifetime, the skin experiences a variety of changes, most significant among them being pigmentation alterations and age spots. These alterations, often considered signs of aging skin, are largely due to the cumulative photo damage from sunlight and the intrinsic biological alterations. Age spots, also referred to as lentigines, are flat, darkened macules on sun-exposed areas of the skin, reflecting the reaction of the skin to UV radiation damage. This color change is due to augmented melanin production, a protective natural function intended to cloak lower layers from harmful UV light. However, despite the protective nature of the process, excessive exposure to UV light leads to abnormal pigmentation distribution, resulting in visible age spots, which can affect not only the external appearance of the skin but also overall self-esteem. Moreover, the influence of environmental factors and genetic susceptibility also plays a significant role in determining the dynamics of pigmentation alterations with aging. As highlighted in recent research, the identification of specific genetic markers linked to aging skin has shed light on the question of how internal factors control the function of the skin. Studies have revealed candidate genes that have been linked to pigmentation, such as IRF4 and MC1R, which act with environmental stressors to exacerbate or mitigate pigmentation changes over time (Shabihah & Paramita,2023). This explains why genetic susceptibility and lifestyle elements, such as sun protection and skincare routines, are crucial to controlling skin appearance. Hence, it is significant to be aware of these multi-factorial factors in planning means to prevent or minimize the formation of age spots. The treatment and prevention of age spots and color alterations consist of a multi-factorial strategy involving both prevention and treatment modalities. Preventive measures such as aggressive sun protection through the use of sunscreen can reduce the formation of age spots by limiting UV exposure. In addition, progress in dermatologic treatments like topical creams like retinoids and peels has been promising at stimulating skin rejuvenation and evening out pigmentation (Fernández-Varela-Gómez et al., 2024). These treatments handle the cell turnover activities of the skin and make the present blemishes fade away and give way to new and healthy skin growth. By combining protective strategies with proactive interventions, it is possible to effectively manage the external manifestations of aging, resulting in healthier and more youthful-looking skin throughout the aging process (Figure 2.11).

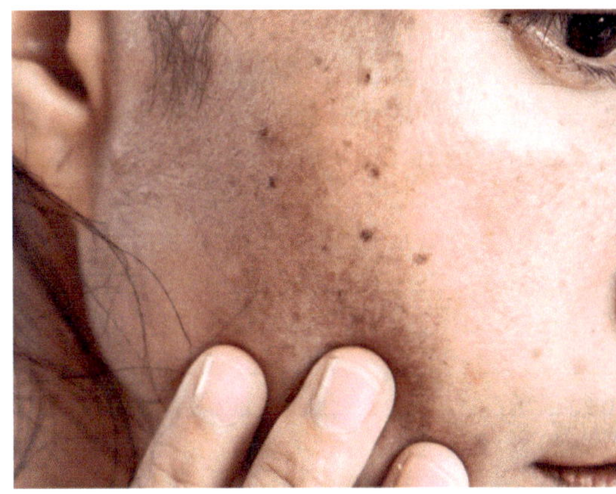

Figure 2.11. Age spots.

Source: https://cdn-gghej.nitrocdn.com/NTlqTaLbBUEcKxxKRwpFvizWChNtFXfq/assets/images/optimized/rev-f6724c6/drtheva.com.au/wp-content/uploads/2024/01/Age-Spots.png.

2.4.3. Dryness and Texture Changes

The effect of aging on the skin is manifested visibly by dryness and textural disturbances that visibly impact its overall health and appearance. As a person ages, the natural moisture content of the skin declines due to various factors such as impaired sebaceous gland activity and reduced ceramide levels. These lead to compromised skin barriers, which are required to retain moisture and provide protection against environmental stressors. The skin is then more susceptible to various irritants, which make it rough to the touch and worse for fine lines and wrinkles. This deterioration serves to appreciate how intrinsic and extrinsic characteristics can contribute to such changes, as improper skincare routines can aggravate dryness and render effective control schemes impossible (Fernández-Varela-Gómez et al., 2024). Besides dryness loss, textural alterations become apparent as age progresses. The structural makeup of the dermis, which is basically collagen and elastin, changes due to lower synthesis and higher breakdown. This results in loss of firmness and elasticity, causing a drier, more brittle texture. The roughness and irregular texture of old skin may be due to a lowering of the turnover rate of the skin cells, leading to a buildup of dead skin. This exacerbation not only enhances the sense of dryness but also strips away the skin's radiance and youthful glow. Highlighting such features brings about the critical need for targeted treatments that aim to revive both texture and moisture, thus improving skin quality when proceeding through the natural process of aging (Barnawi & Barnawi, 2021). Dryness and textural changes need to be addressed properly by utilizing a combination of methods involving both preventive and active intervention. Holistic skincare regimens with hydration-focused ingredients such as glycerin and hyaluronic acid have been effective in enhancing moisture retention within the skin. Topical retinoid application has also been found to be effective in triggering the production of collagen and cell turnover, which can reverse aging's impact on dryness and texture of the skin. However, it is important to approach these treatments with realistic expectations since their potency may vary from one individual to another depending on their personal skin types and the circumstances of their lives. With regard to the importance of personalized skincare regimens, the ability to effectively deal with the aging process is enhanced while simultaneously addressing the specific concerns of dryness and texture change (Fernández-Varela-Gómez et al., 2024) (Figure 2.12).

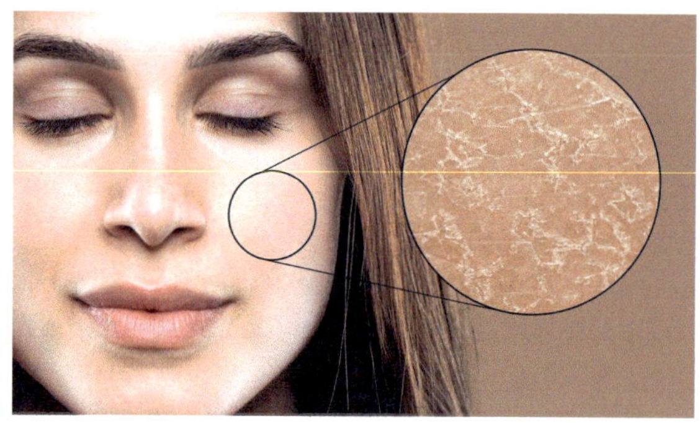

Figure 2.12. Dry skin.

Source: https://cdn.shopify.com/s/files/1/0648/1955/files/large-main_magnified_dry_skin.jpg?v=1636095114.

Test Your Knowledge

1. What are the most common visible signs of natural skin aging?
2. How does the structure and function of the skin change over time, and what symptoms indicate these underlying changes?

2.5. Prevention Strategies for Skin Aging

Learning Outcome

1. Discuss sun protection measures
2. Understand skincare routines and products
3. Explain how healthy lifestyle choices play a critical role in mitigating the effects of skin aging

Adequate prevention of skin aging is a multi-faceted process that entails lifestyle change coupled with new dermatological therapies. The most crucial aspect of preventing skin aging is the regular use of broad-spectrum sunscreens. UV light, particularly UVA radiation, plays a significant role in photoaging and thus reduces skin elasticity and wrinkle formation. Research highlights the importance of taking into account UVA exposure, as it takes part in collagen degradation and inflammatory responses. Preventive measures such as the use of sunscreen with a high SPF daily and remaining under shade during peak hours reduce these injurious effects and preserve skin integrity for a duration of time. These preventive habits, aside from reducing the risk of immediate sunburn, promote long-term skin health, thereby slowing down visible signs of aging. Aside from sun protection, antioxidative use in skincare regimens is vital to neutralize oxidative stress, which accelerates the aging process. Antioxidants such as vitamins E and C play a significant role in neutralizing free radicals resulting from UV radiation and environmental pollutants. The application of antioxidants can contribute significantly to fortifying the natural defenses of the skin and improving the overall appearance of the skin through stimulation of collagen synthesis and increased hydration in the skin. New advancements in skincare products have begun to include new ingredients that have been synthesized from nature, such as plant-derived exosome-like nanoparticles (PDNPs). Such molecules, including aloe-derived exosome-like nanoparticles (ADNPs), have been shown to decrease oxidative stress and reverse signs of aging by initiating significant molecular pathways. The data here underscore the need for implementing evidence-based ingredients in daily skincare as a strategy for preventing and alleviating skin aging. Furthermore, recent research into molecular processes involved in skin aging, in particular related to collagen maintenance and repair, offers new possibilities for emerging prevention strategies. For instance, recombinant type XVII collagen has been found to be promising in undoing UVA-induced skin aging by altering collagen dynamics and regulating vital signaling pathways. This research illustrates how molecular treatments targeted towards specific molecules can undo damage incurred due to environmental insults. By enhancing collagen production and regulating MMP expression, these treatments could possibly delay the onset of the manifestation of aging by several orders of magnitude. With our knowledge of these molecular mechanisms further understood, it opens doors to the creation of new anti-photoaging products with a solid theoretical foundation for efficacious interventions that fight skin aging and support long-term skin health (He et al., 2025; Sun et al., 2025).

2.5.1. Sun Protection Measures

Effective sun protection habits are crucial in preventing skin aging and photoaging due to the fact that they directly reverse the damaging actions of UV light. Prolonged and regular application of broad-spectrum sunscreens with a high SPF is one of the best habits recommended. Besides shielding the skin from UVA and UVB light, such products also prevent the degradation of elastin and collagen which leads to skin aging. In addition, the wearing of protective clothing, including long sleeves and hats, creates an external barrier to further reduce exposure to sunlight. Studies have found that individuals who consistently practice these barriers to protection exhibit much healthier skin and less evidence of aging compared to individuals who do not practice sun protection. Therefore, incorporating these basic yet powerful techniques into everyday practices can have far-reaching long-term consequences for skin integrity. Besides sunscreen and protective gear, behavioral interventions are very important in terms of facilitating sun protection in populations at risk, e.g., outdoor workers. Well-planned educational interventions on the risks of UV exposure and the cumulative impact of sun protection failures can trigger substantial changes in attitude and behavior. A trial of male outdoor workers, for instance, revealed that participants given UV photography as a complement to education videos had improved sun protection cognitions, which translated to healthier behaviors such as increased sunscreen use and the wearing of protective clothing. This emphasizes a heavy reliance on actively involving individuals in the learning process of their risk of sun exposure and informing them to become proactive about it. Through heightened awareness and self-efficacy regarding sun protection, such interventions can prevent photoaging and ultimately lead to healthier skin. Furthermore, public health campaigns that focus on widespread awareness surrounding the importance of sun protection are able to exert significant influence on community behaviors and ultimately skin health outcomes. Preventive campaigns that promote awareness of the risks of exposure to UV, the importance of routine skin checks, and the benefits of sun protection can make a culture of prevention possible. Skin health awareness community activities, combined with free and available screenings as well as educational workshops, have the ability to create an environment where sun safety is a community issue. Also, because skin aging is propelled by myriad determinants, including lifestyle and genetic factors, an integrated action that can include sun protection activities can help individuals better manage their own skin health. By addressing the multi-factorial nature of skin aging, such programs can encourage a preventive approach to sun protection among various groups, thereby tackling both public and individual health (Figure 2.13).

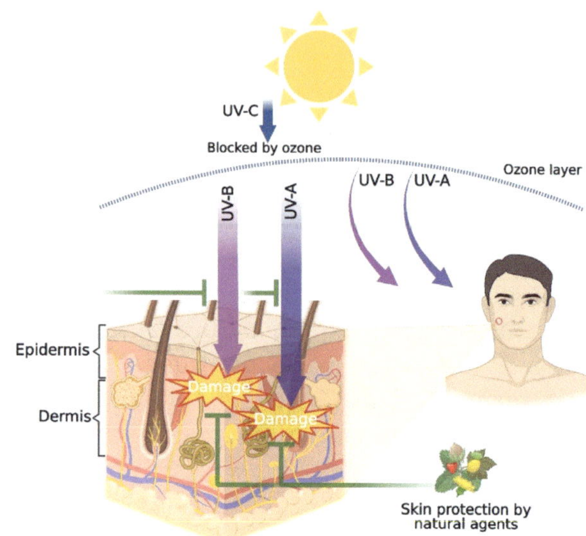

Figure 2.13. Penetration of the skin by ultraviolet radiation of different wavelengths.

Source: https://media.springernature.com/full/springer-static/image/art%3A10.1007%2Fs10311-023-01649-4/MediaObjects/10311_2023_1649_Fig1_HTML.png?as=webp.

2.5.2. Skincare Routines and Products

A serious skincare routine is necessary in the management of aging skin and photoaging and consists of a variety of products targeted at various types of skin and conditions. With more cosmeceuticals available to consumers, a consumer is bound to be overwhelmed by the number of products provided. The products range from regular daily moisturizers to focused serums that exploit active ingredients such as retinoids and antioxidants. These types of compounds are being hailed for their anti-aging properties, as they work to activate collagen production and reverse oxidative damage caused by outside influences, most notably UV radiation. With all that, though, a sophisticated appreciation of how these products cross over and impact various skin types must exist, especially in younger age groups who will be tempted to try these higher-strength products. Dermatologists emphasize prudent choice based on the respective skin conditions in order to reduce the risk of side effects and realize maximum efficacy, especially in children and adolescents who will be more prone to some of the ingredients (Goff et al., 2025). In addition, the effect of skincare products extends beyond mere surface-level cosmetic effects; they also reflect broader consumerism patterns and the pursuit of effective anti-aging outcomes. Existing studies emphasize that the performance of whitening products, which are traditionally over-advertised based on their anti-aging features, can vary significantly based on ingredient combinations and individual skin reactions. Skin color, type, and concerns are factors in product performance. Therefore, understanding these variations is crucial to developing a personalized skincare routine that not only pleases one's preference but also delivers optimum outcomes (Chu et al., 2024). It is advised that customers seek guidance from professional skincare professionals who can help individualize regimens that address specific aging concerns, taking into account the unique needs of each user. Engaging a holistic approach to skincare also involves recognizing the role lifestyle plays in aging. Beyond treatments applied at the surface level, aspects such as diet, hydration, and sun protection are significant in maintaining healthy skin and decelerating aging signs. Application of broad-spectrum sun lotion every day, for example, is among the most effective ways of fighting photoaging, supporting the importance of education for proper, consistent use. Additionally, more recent preventive research addresses internal well-being and skin appearance as mutually beneficial, with an antioxidant-balanced diet also playing a part in the skin's capacity to resist the aging process. Ultimately, a consistent skincare routine that is preventative and restorative, combined with intelligent product use and lifestyle adjustment decisions, is instrumental in the fight against skin aging and photoaging.

2.5.3. Healthy Lifestyle Choices

Healthy lifestyle choices are embraced to serve a significant role in minimizing the effects of photoaging and aging of the skin. The skin is the body's largest organ and reflects the overall health, being equally susceptible to outside factors from exposure to the sun, pollutants, etc. Guarding against UV radiation must be practiced on a regular basis. For instance, application of broad-spectrum sunscreen every day decreases the extent of photoaging by inhibiting photo-induced damage, one of the leading causes of wrinkles and color shifts. Finally, it should not be stressed more that antioxidants in foods neutralize oxidative stress induced by environmental factors, thereby ensuring skin integrity. The synthesis of major proteins like collagen and elastin, which ensure the firmness and elasticity of the skin, is enhanced through a lifestyle that emphasizes good nutrition and moisturization, further developing the skin's resistance to the effects of aging (Fernández-Varela-Gómez et al., 2024). Regular exercise is always cited as the foundation for a healthy lifestyle, with the direct effect on skin condition and aging. Exercise enhances blood circulation, which maximizes oxygen and nutrient delivery to skin cells essential for cell repair and regeneration. Exercise also helps control stress levels that have been known to cause aging through increased inflammation and oxidative stress. The body's efficient detox processes when exercising also lead to clearer skin and fewer blemishes. In addition, research shows that those who exercise regularly appear younger, due in part to the physiological effects of exercise, such as enhanced collagen production and lower fat volume of subcutaneous structures, which resist sagging skin (Dorosz et al., 2025). Adding a well-balanced diet fortified with vitamins, minerals, and healthy fats will be the key to maintaining young and smooth skin and combating the degenerative mechanisms of aging. Vitamins C and E are vital in collagen stimulation and providing antioxidant protection from environmental toxins, hence enhancing the resilience of the skin. Omega-3 fatty acids, found in fish and certain plant oils, help to keep the skin hydrated and pliable, reducing the visibility of fine wrinkles and lines by a considerable amount. Also, good hydration helps balance the water in the skin, creating a rich and healthy look. Overall, these vitamins and fatty acids work in synergy to promote healthy skin and resistance to age-related decline. The addition of a wholesome dietary lifestyle is not only a temporary solution but a sustained dedication to overall skin health, reminding us once again of the value of sustainable lifestyle habits for graceful aging (Fernández-Varela-Gómez et al., 2024) (Figure 2.14).

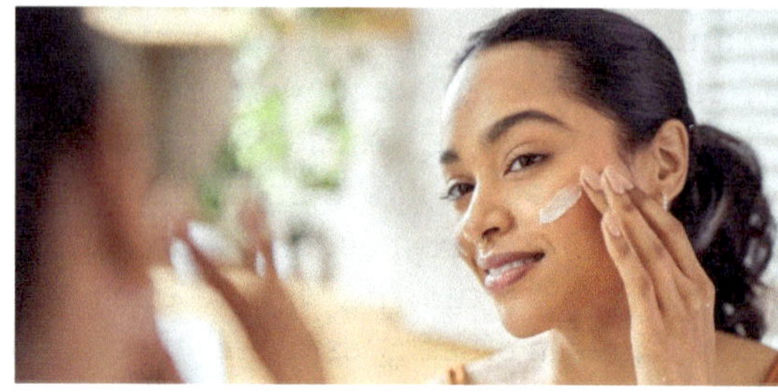

Figure 2.14. A woman applying skincare cream to her face, representing a common daily routine aimed at maintaining skin hydration, barrier function, and overall dermatological health.

Source: https://images.news18.com/ibnlive/uploads/2024/04/img-2-2024-04-02t182107.833-2024-04-827c90c9d5480427ec645eb7fd90e3f8-3x2.jpg.

Test Your Knowledge

1. What role does daily sun protection play in preventing premature skin aging, and how effective are different types of sunscreen?
2. What lifestyle habits have been scientifically shown to delay skin aging, and how do they interact with genetic risk factors?

2.6. Treatment Options for Skin Aging and Photoaging

Learning Outcome

1. Discuss topical treatments for skin aging and photoaging
2. Understand cosmetic procedures
3. Explain emerging technologies in skin rejuvenation

The treatments of photoaging and skin aging cover both topical and systemic therapies aimed at reversing the environmental and chronological signs of aging. Some of the most well-known treatments are retinoids, vitamin A derivatives that have been discovered to stimulate collagen production, enhance cell turnover, and reduce fine line visibility. These drugs have been effective in treating photoaging by improving skin texture and tone. Moreover, studies show that the efficacy of these agents may be enhanced by using them in combination with broad sun protection measures. By combining topical retinoids with widely researched photoprotective agents, clinicians can provide a more efficient answer to the risky effects of UV radiation, aligned with the contemporary definition of skin aging as an interaction between genetic and environmental factors, as highlighted in González et al. (2023). Aside from retinoids, plant extracts are also gaining popularity as effective treatment agents for skin aging. Fernblock®, one of the extracts derived from the fern *Polypodium leucotomos*, has been shown to be a potential adjunct treatment to conventional photoaging therapy. This extract has also been found to be not only potentially preventative of UV damage but also protective against infrared and visible light, increasingly implicated in skin decline, as reviewed by González et al. (2023). Its use of natural substances like Fernblock® can enhance patient outcomes through complementing topical treatments and procedural interventions, e.g., photodynamic treatment. This overall philosophy can address various areas of skin aging, thereby having a healthier appearance and improving overall skin resilience. Moreover, the use of novel technologies such as lasers and chemical peels provides an adjuvant modality to address skin aging effectively. Treatments are designed for action on multiple layers of the skin, leading to rejuvenation and the management of fine lines, hyperpigmentation, and textural irregularities. Laser therapy, for instance, can induce controlled damage to the dermal layer to initiate a wound healing process that leads to collagen synthesis. Chemical peels, on the other hand, remove the surface layer of dead skin cells to reveal smoother underlying skin. Combined with consistent use of sun protection and topical antioxidants, these technological treatments can significantly enhance the appearance and survival of the skin. An awareness of the multifactorial aspect of skin aging highlights the relevance of including diverse treatments and education for patients to achieve the best outcomes as proposed by Fernández-Varela-Gómez et al. (2024).

2.6.1. Topical Treatments (Retinoids, Antioxidants)

Skin aging and photoaging pathogenesis is a multifaceted process that is influenced by intrinsic and extrinsic factors, necessitating effective intervention strategies. From the numerous topical treatments, retinoids have garnered significant attention due to their potential to stimulate the regeneration of the skin and promote cellular turnover. Such vitamin A derivatives do this by inducing the exfoliation of old skin cells and stimulating collagen, which ultimately increases the quality of the skin and reduces the appearance of fine lines and wrinkles. Retinoids also reverse UV radiation-induced photoaging, a leading causative factor of photoaging, by promoting the healing of sun-damaged tissue. Studies have attested that long-term use of retinoids brings drastic alterations to the look of skin and therefore they are a cornerstone in premature skin aging treatment (Ziobro et al., 2024). The above-mentioned facts justify the application of retinoids as part of complete skincare. Antioxidants are contained in products that give foundational protection against skin aging, particularly in the mitigation of oxidative stress caused by environmental stressors such as pollution and UV radiation. These types of compounds, which include vitamins C and E, green tea constituents, and other polyphenols, work synergistically to neutralize free radicals and inhibit cell damage. The application of topical antioxidants not only can suppress the formation of signs of aging but also to activate mechanisms of repair of the skin. Clinical trials have established that routine application of antioxidant preparations leads to higher skin elasticity and moisture content, additionally combating the formation of signs of aging (Fernández-Varela-Gómez et al., 2024). In general, the incorporation of topical antioxidants into a skincare routine every day increases the resilience of the skin and offers a preventive measure against photoaging. The use of both retinoids and antioxidants in skincare routines represents a comprehensive method for managing skin aging and photoaging. Each category of treatment provides its own advantages with its own adjunctive benefits to the overall skin health. Where retinoids take the lead in cell turnover and collagen stimulation, antioxidants serve to protect the skin from further insult by the environment. This double-barreled assault not only corrects current signs of aging, but also fortifies the skin's defenses against future insult. To this end, complemented by the increasing evidence from new research highlighting the merit of tailored skincare regimens, the combination of such surface treatments may also be tailored to suit individual skin types and conditions (Ziobro et al., 2024). Collectively, a full identification and integration of such treatments are the building blocks of effective care regimens against skin aging and photoaging (Figure 2.15).

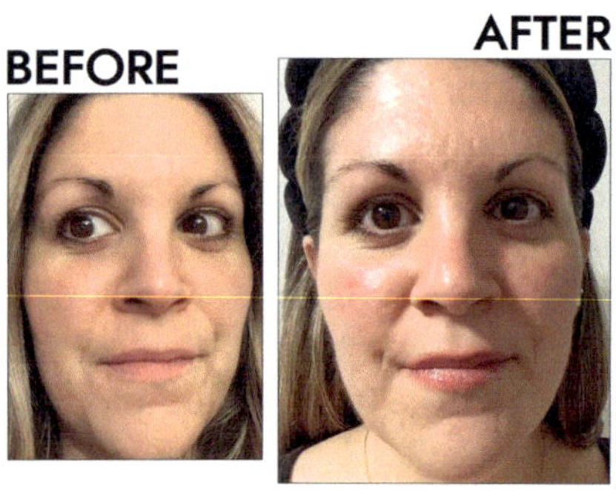

Figure 2.15. Before and after topical treatments.

Source: https://www.byrdie.com/thmb/AgKUiSNUJHbRBJtoKfbeUq_R_PU=/750x0/filters:no_upscale():max_bytes(150000):strip_icc():format(webp)/byr-anti-aging-serums-test-dennis-gross-advanced-retinol-ferric-texture-renewal-before-after-karah-rosa-53073aef97c04a8aa45d4acd5a17dc9e.jpeg.

2.6.2. Cosmetic Procedures (Laser Therapy, Fillers)

Cosmetic treatments have evolved to the point where laser treatment and dermal fillers are the most common interventions used in reversing skin aging and photoaging. Low-level laser therapy (LLLT) has been studied extensively on its ability to rejuvenate the skin. The method uses specific wavelengths, such as 660 nm, to penetrate the skin layers, activating the function of cells and boosting the production of collagen. A clinical trial in Syrian females revealed a staggering gain in skin elasticity and wrinkle reduction after a series of LLLT treatments, supporting its utility as a safe and effective treatment option (Shurrab et al., 2024). By provoking deeper skin regeneration, laser therapy corrects common signs of photoaging, such as dyspigmentation and structural deterioration, offering patients the opportunity for dramatic cosmetic improvement. Used in combination with laser therapy, dermal fillers have become popular for their capacity to restore volume and soften skin texture. These non-surgical injections are capable of correctly addressing volume loss in the face due to aging as well as improving facial contours, making one look generally youthful. Of note are the hyaluronic acid fillers, which are acclaimed for their safety and biocompatibility, with results seen instantaneously and minimal downtime. Filler treatments have demonstrated good physical appearance and mental health improvement in patients, leading to higher satisfaction levels and quality of life (Ku et al., 2024). Moreover, the treatments can be customized according to the individual facial structure and aging concerns of the patient, thereby being highly versatile in treating the differentiated signs of aging skin. The synergy of these treatments not only addresses the visible consequences of photoaging and skin aging but also fosters an interdisciplinary treatment approach to integrative skin health. By combining the restorative effects of LLLT with the volumizing properties of dermal fillers, providers can create synergistic treatment protocols that lead to the best outcomes. This multi-modal treatment strategy maximizes patient satisfaction and the efficacy of aesthetic treatments. Also, ongoing study and technology advancements promise to further improve these techniques, leading to improved outcomes and safety profiles. With growing familiarity and acceptance of these procedures, individuals seeking to reverse signs of aging will increasingly seek out these state-of-the-art treatments, eventually remapping the landscape of cosmetic dermatology in the coming decades (Figure 2.16).

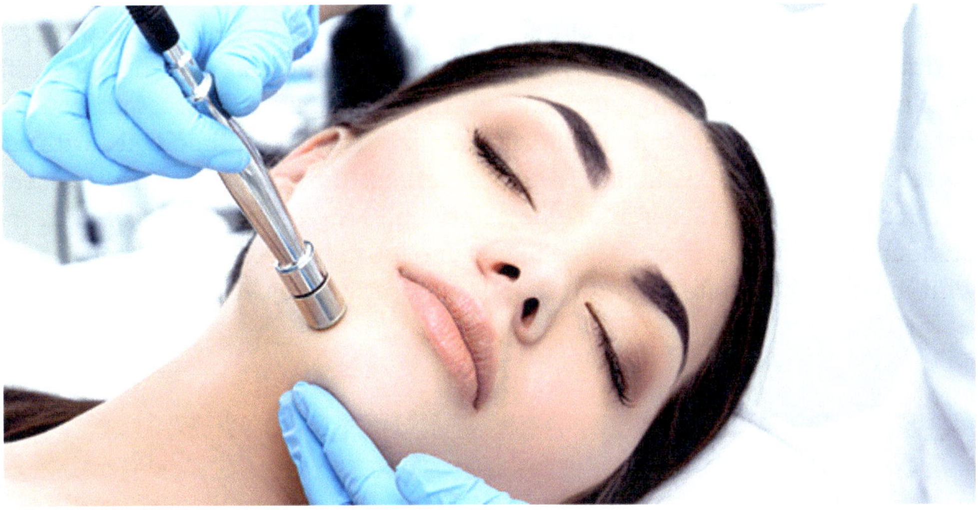

Figure 2.16. A patient undergoing a microdermabrasion procedure, a non-invasive cosmetic treatment aimed at exfoliating the skin to improve texture, tone, and overall appearance.

Source: https://www.thenewyou.in/wp-content/uploads/2017/03/Microdermabrasiona.jpg.

2.6.3. Emerging Technologies in Skin Rejuvenation

The quest for the best skin rejuvenation has led to several new technologies aimed at combating skin aging and photoaging. Procedural therapies such as laser treatments, microneedling, and chemical peels are possibly the most important breakthroughs. All these treatments treat signs of aging through stimulation of cellular turnover, enhanced production of collagen, and improved skin texture. For instance, laser treatments utilize intense beams of light to stimulate the underlying dermal layers, thereby promoting regeneration as well as creating an impressive aesthetic enhancement. Additionally, expanding understanding of the skin's biological processes emphasizes the importance of such advanced modalities, which, as recent studies indicate, can provide exceptional results when combined with surface treatments like retinoids and antioxidants. Therefore, there is a need to study the implementation of such technologies in comprehensive management techniques for effective skin rejuvenation (Ziobro et al., 2024). In recent times, the role of extracellular vesicles (EVs), in particular, exosomes, has been a breakthrough area in skin rejuvenation technology. These small membrane-bound vesicles form the focal point of intercellular communication and have been greatly promising in regenerative medicine.

It has been seen in studies that EVs can deliver bioactive molecules that trigger skin regeneration and therefore, are a candidate for treating age-related skin diseases such as wrinkles and loss of skin elasticity. Use of EVs in clinics indicates they can not only be used for skin aging, but also for other skin diseases such as acne scars and alopecia. Though current studies demonstrate the efficacy of EVs for therapies in the skin, there are some issues left, like making them standardized and requiring large randomized trials to confirm their benefits (Ziobro et al., 2024). Integrating new technologies with old-school therapeutic regimes may pave the way for additional individualized and effective skin rejuvenation methods. The integration of age-old topical treatments with advanced approaches like EV treatments has the potential to optimize the overall effectiveness of rejuvenation therapy. Individualized medicine, considering genetic, environmental, and lifestyle influences, is especially applicable while designing personalized interventions to address targeted skin aging problems. By facilitating the understanding of the combination of new technologies with conventional treatments, researchers are in a position to further customize the therapy protocols based on patient requirements. Besides, further research on the safety and long-term efficacy of such treatment is critical to standardize in clinical practice. Thus, a model that incorporates new and traditional modalities will most likely dictate the future landscape of skin rejuvenation (Ziobro et al., 2024).

Test Your Knowledge

1. What are the most effective medical and cosmetic treatments currently available for reversing signs of photoaging, and how do they work?
2. How do non-invasive treatments (e.g., topical agents) compare to invasive procedures (e.g., fillers, laser resurfacing) in terms of results, risks, and recovery time?

SUMMARY

Conclusion of the discussion regarding skin aging and photoaging caps the salient points learned throughout this examination. Skin aging can primarily be categorized as intrinsic and extrinsic determinants, of which the latter is widely driven by environmental factors such as UV radiation. Understanding the mechanisms of skin aging is required because with such knowledge, interventions may be designed with particular challenges to reverse its effects. For instance, dietary change interventions, including dietary supplements such as almonds, have been discovered to be effective in enhancing the look of the skin. As per the study, every day almond eating might reduce wrinkle severity among postmenopausal women, which points towards the potential significance of nutritional treatment in skin aging management and the attainment of healthier skin outcomes (Burney et al., 2019). Furthermore, new dermatological therapies bring with them new avenues to address photoaging, emphasizing the need for coupling scientific advances with applied realities. The simultaneous application of amniotic membrane stem cell metabolite products (AMSC-MP) and vitamin E, with microneedling, is a potent method for achieving maximum skin rejuvenation. This multi-modal therapy treats all the elements of photoaging, demonstrating statistically significant improvement in skin texture, pore size, and wrinkle depth (Ardhaninggar et al., 2020). This kind of multi-disciplinary research highlights the necessity of future research in dermatology, and the way the different components work synergistically to bring youth to the skin and reverse photoaging. In conclusion, the mutual interaction of intrinsic and extrinsic factors of skin aging underlines the specificity of the process and the simultaneous need for comprehensive approaches. Additional research on diet, novel treatments, and protective measures against UV irradiation is required in order to enhance the knowledge on skin aging. While research demonstrates the effectiveness of new treatments and diet interventions to reduce the signs of aging, this is a dermatological revolution. The revelations gained from these studies not only aid in the formulation of particular cures but also help individuals make decisions about their skin care routine, fostering skin health and wellbeing among diverse groups (Burney et al., 2019; Rahmadewi et al., 2020).

The skin aging process is inherently related to several biological processes that are time-dependent. Both extrinsic and intrinsic causes lead to derangement in skin function and structure. Senility occurs intrinsically due to gene predisposition and metabolism, and this lessens the production of collagen and elastin. This leads to signs characteristic of aging, such as wrinkles and skin sagging. Extrinsic causes, specifically photoaging, result from exposures to the environment, specifically UV radiation of the sun, that significantly accelerate such aging events. Environmental trauma results in altered architecture in the skin, with loss of elasticity and increased pigmentation. Collating information from different studies, it is evident that both environmental and genetic influences play a crucial role in unravelling the mechanisms of skin aging and photoaging, forming a basis for future investigation into possible treatments and interventions. Photoaging forms a significant component of skin aging, which is primarily promoted by chronic exposure to UV radiation. This is a process that disrupts normal skin function, primarily by breaking down collagen and by creating abnormal elastin fibers, leading to wrinkle and fine line formation. Furthermore, exposure to UV also causes inflammatory responses that may result in photo-damage, including hyperpigmentation and precancerous lesions. The severity of photoaging also varies between individuals, based on individual lifestyles and sun exposure levels. As identified in recent literature, photoaging necessitates a multi-faceted treatment, integrating preventative measures such as sunscreen usage and skin protection with therapeutic advances aimed at the repair of damaged skin. Effective treatments for reversing photoaging have widespread implications for the enhancement of skin well-being and health, further supporting the importance of sun protection in daily routines. The intersection of medical research and dermato-clinical practice places emphasis on the need for effective countermeasures to counteract photoaging and skin aging. Advances in treatments, such as LED-RL therapies, offer new avenues to avert fibrotic responses and increase skin resilience. As well put in recent research, the application of targeted light therapies has been shown to produce beneficial results in promoting skin healing and reducing scarring following dermatological procedures (Heilman et al., 2019). Moreover, evidence-based skin cancer prevention programs also emphasize the central role played by education and behavior interventions in the development of protective behaviors among high-risk populations, such as athletes and lifeguards (Yancey, 2014). These programs entail increasing awareness of the necessity of sun safety practice and promoting positive behavior change towards UV exposure. Collectively, this publication demonstrates that a combined approach, with preventive education complemented by therapeutic development, is essential in addressing the complexities of skin aging and photoaging successfully.

KEY TERMS FROM THIS CHAPTER

- Oxidative stress
- Aging skin
- Bioactive compounds
- Biological mechanisms
- Chronological change
- Compromised skin
- Cosmeceuticals
- Dermatological health
- Microdermabrasion
- Particulate matter (PM)
- Aesthetic treatments
- Antioxidants
- Biocompatibility
- Cellular ageing
- Collagen formation
- Conventional treatments
- Cosmetic dermatology
- Environmental influences
- Moisturization
- Photoaging

CRITICAL THINKING QUESTIONS

1. **Which of the following is a primary factor responsible for skin aging?**
   a. Genetics
   b. Hormonal changes
   c. Ultraviolet (UV) radiation
   d. Lack of sleep
2. **What is the main effect of UV radiation on the skin that leads to photoaging?**
   a. Increased production of melanin
   b. Breakdown of collagen and elastin
   c. Enhanced skin cell turnover
   d. Increased sebum production
3. **Which of the following is a common visible sign of skin aging?**
   a. Decreased oil production
   b. Increased skin elasticity
   c. Reduced pore size
   d. Wrinkles and fine lines
4. **Which layer of the skin is most affected by photoaging?**
   a. Epidermis
   b. Dermis
   c. Hypodermis
   d. Subcutaneous fat layer
5. **What is the term used to describe the skin aging process caused by exposure to UV radiation?**
   a. Intrinsic aging
   b. Environmental aging
   c. Photoaging
   d. Hormonal aging

Short Answer Questions

1. What is the difference between intrinsic aging and photoaging, and how do they contribute to the overall aging of the skin?
2. How does UV radiation cause structural damage to the skin at the cellular level, and what are its long-term effects on collagen and elastin?
3. What role does oxidative stress play in both intrinsic aging and photoaging of the skin, and how can antioxidants help mitigate this damage?
4. How does the skin's ability to repair itself decline with age, and how does this affect the severity of photoaging?
5. What are the clinical signs of photoaging, and how do they differ from the typical signs of intrinsic skin aging?
6. How effective are modern sunscreen formulations in preventing both intrinsic aging and photoaging, and what factors should individuals consider when choosing a sunscreen?
7. What are some of the most common treatments for photoaging, and how do they work to restore youthful skin appearance?

Answer to Critical Thinking Questions

1. (c); 2. (b); 3. (d); 4. (b); 5. (c)

REFERENCES

1. Hwang, K. A., Yi, B. R., & Choi, K. C. (2011). Molecular mechanisms and in vivo mouse models of skin aging associated with dermal matrix alterations. *Laboratory animal research*, *27*(1), 1–8. https://doi.org/10.5625/lar.2011.27.1.1 https://core.ac.uk/download/pdf/8600426.pdf (accessed on 11th June 2025).
2. Amaral, M. N., Fonseca, S. L., et al. (2023). Marine natural products as innovative cosmetic ingredients. https://core.ac.uk/download/560853254.pdf (accessed on 11th June 2025).
3. Rahmadewi, R., Retha, R., Pitasari, D. A., Kusumastanto, V. A., Ardhaninggar, A. A. A., Citrashanty, I., Sari, M., Umborowati, M. A., & Prakoeswa, C. R. S. (2020). The Efficacy of Amniotic Membrane Stem Cell (AMSC) Metabolite Product and Vitamin E for Wrinkles, Spots, and Pores in Photoaging. *Dermatology research and practice*, *2020*, 1584541. https://doi.org/10.1155/2020/1584541(accessed on 11th June 2025).
4. Barbour, J. M., Bataille, V., Duffy, D. L., Glass, D., et al. (2017). Genome-wide association reveals pigmentation genes play a role in skin aging. https://core.ac.uk/download/586952770.pdf (accessed on 11th June 2025).
5. Barnawi, A. M., & Barnawi, G. M. (2021). Truths and myths about marketed anti-aging skin products: A systematic review. https://core.ac.uk/download/539910780.pdf (accessed on 11th June 2025).
6. Brown, C. T. A., Campbell, C. L., Christison, C., Moseley, H., et al. (2015). 3D Monte Carlo radiation transfer modelling of photodynamic therapy. https://core.ac.uk/download/30319719.pdf (accessed on 11th June 2025).
7. Burney, W. A., Chodur, G. M., Foolad, N., Newman, J. W., et al. (2019). Prospective randomized controlled pilot study on the effects of almond consumption on skin lipids and wrinkles. https://core.ac.uk/download/323062627.pdf (accessed on 11th June 2025).
8. Ziobro, A., Camlet, K., Kocur, K., & Lis, P. (2024). Comprehensive Management of Premature Skin Aging: Current Strategies, Treatments, and Emerging Therapies. *Journal of Education, Health and Sport*, *68*, 55295. https://doi.org/10.12775/JEHS.2024.68.55295(accessed on 11th June 2025).
9. Chu, P. (2024). Comprehensive evaluation of the regulation of skin pigment deposition by active ingredients based on whitening products. https://core.ac.uk/download/616936880.pdf (accessed on 11th June 2025).
10. Damayanti, P. A. A., & Djunaidy, A. (2023). *Bombyx mori* as a potential sunscreen to prevent photoaging. https://core.ac.uk/download/599384318.pdf (accessed on 11th June 2025).
11. Domaszewska-Szostek, A., Krzyżanowska, M., Polak, A., & Puzianowska-Kuźnicka, M. (2025). Effectiveness of extracellular vesicle application in skin aging treatment and regeneration: Do we have enough evidence from clinical trials? https://core.ac.uk/download/650323067.pdf (accessed on 11th June 2025).
12. Dorosz, A., Skoczeń, A., Kulesza, M., Wawrzynów, W., Jakubowska, M. M., Kruk, A., ... Kaczmarek, B. (2025). The Impact of Environmental Factors on Skin and Tissue Ageing: Mechanisms, Effects, and Preventive Strategies. *Journal of Education, Health and Sport*, *79*, 58282. https://doi.org/10.12775/JEHS.2025.79.58282(accessed on 11th June 2025).
13. Fernández-Varela-Gómez, F., Sandoval-García, A., & Valeria Cabrera-Rios, K. (2024). Signs of

skin aging: a review. *International Journal of Research in Medical Sciences, 12*(7), 2674–2679. https://doi.org/10.18203/2320-6012.ijrms20241935(accessed on 11th June 2025).

14. Girgis, A., Geller, A. C., Rowe, A. K., Levy, A. S., Armstrong, B. K., Ramirez, C. C., Holman, C. D. J., et al. (2009). Sun protection intervention for highway workers: Long-term efficacy of UV photography and skin cancer information on men's protective cognitions and behavior. https://core.ac.uk/download/pdf/8376824.pdf (accessed on 11th June 2025).
15. Goff, K., & Stein, S. L. (2025). Cosmeceuticals in the pediatric population Part I: A review of risks and available evidence. https://core.ac.uk/download/640805204.pdf (accessed on 11th June 2025).
16. González, S., Juarranz de la Fuente, Á., Rodríguez-Luna, A., Zamarrón, A., et al. (2023). Clinical applications of *Polypodium leucotomos* (Fernblock®): An update. https://core.ac.uk/download/619331991.pdf (accessed on 11th June 2025).
17. He, Y., Yin, S., Xu, R., Zhao, Y., Du, Y., Duan, Z., & Fan, D. (2025). Recombinant type XVII collagen inhibits EGFR/MAPK/AP-1 and activates TGF-β/Smad signaling to enhance collagen secretion and reduce photoaging. *Cosmetics.* https://www.semanticscholar.org/paper/45246c71a7704aaa0e90071ad45b7fb8bb3de659 (accessed on 11th June 2025).
18. Heilman, E., Isseroff, R. R., Jagdeo, J. R., Jakus, J., et al. (2019). A dose-ranging, parallel group, split-face, single-blind phase II study of light emitting diode-red light (LED-RL) for skin scarring prevention: Study protocol for a randomized controlled trial. https://core.ac.uk/download/323070347.pdf (accessed on 11th June 2025).
19. Jusuf, N. K., & Zulfa, R. A. (2024). Skin care in dermatology: Between organic versus synthetic products. https://core.ac.uk/download/617167601.pdf (accessed on 11th June 2025).
20. Ko, H. J., Sim, S. A., Park, M., Ryu, H. S., Choi, W. Y., Park, S. M., Lee, J. N., et al. (2024). Anti-photoaging effects of upcycled *Citrus junos* seed anionic peptides on ultraviolet-radiation-induced skin aging in a reconstructed skin model. *International Journal of Molecular Sciences, 25.* https://www.semanticscholar.org/paper/d54ab7e6da4a2ed2121789b87068dc75c197e940 (accessed on 11th June 2025).
21. Kuźma, K., Jakubowska, E., Hoppe-Mitera, E., Sionek, I., Pakuła, A., Ślemp, J., Bierć, K., et al. (2024). Enhancing athletic recovery: Scar treatment using microneedling, dermal fillers, and lasers. *Quality in Sport.* https://www.semanticscholar.org/paper/2cbf5761be2557b29fb18b72a26a0e5e207f0d80 (accessed on 11th June 2025).
22. Li, D., Wang, Y., Zhao, W., Li, L., & Zhang, P. (2025). Gold@mesoporous polydopamine nanocomposite hydrogel loaded with estrogen for the treatment of skin photoaging. *International Journal of Nanomedicine, 20*, 4571–4587. https://www.semanticscholar.org/paper/e74adef2331351cf4d322495f58bf06212a18f8e (accessed on 11th June 2025).
23. Li, K., Lin, S. F., Zhou, P., Guo, Y. N., Lin, S., & Ji, C. (2025). The role of exosome lncRNAs in mediating apoptosis and inflammation in UV-induced skin photoaging. *Frontiers in Cell and Developmental Biology, 13.* https://www.semanticscholar.org/paper/941204562cc13a293aeb8cdd3dbb3c1887d609c3 (accessed on 11th June 2025).
24. Mishra, A. (2024). Know your sunscreen. *International Journal for Multidisciplinary Research.* https://www.semanticscholar.org/paper/31ea2b7e8b103726f1b7ff9a33fc1bcfdf2d4b71 (accessed on 11th June 2025).

25. Mohiuddin, A. K. (2020). An extensive review on sunscreen and suntan preparations. https://core.ac.uk/download/482242155.pdf (accessed on 11th June 2025).
26. Farah Shabihah & Rafika Indah Paramita(2023). Genome-wide association study in pigmentation as one of skin aging characteristics. VOLUME 24NO 02 2023, pp 237-248ISSN : Print 1411-3724 —Online 2549-7464DOI : https://doi.org/10.24036/eksakta/vol24-iss02/412. https://core.ac.uk/download/567890570.pdf (accessed on 11th June 2025).
27. Permatasari, A. D., Syukri, Y., & Werdyani, S. (2023). Gold nanoparticles with natural ingredients as anti-aging: A systematic review. https://core.ac.uk/download/578287503.pdf (accessed on 11th June 2025).
28. Pilán Vázquez, R. (2023). *In vitro* and *ex vivo* characterization of skin photoaging and its effects on skin aging biomarkers. https://core.ac.uk/download/586345568.pdf (accessed on 11th June 2025).
29. Shurrab, K., & Alzghayar, J. N. (2024). Low-level laser therapy for skin rejuvenation: A safe and effective solution baked by data and visual evidence. *Journal of Cosmetic Dermatology.* https://www.semanticscholar.org/paper/7c8a77a50e89b5b6520f0f0664e87cde34edac12 (accessed on 11th June 2025).
30. Sieradocha, K. (2024). Air pollution and skin aging. https://core.ac.uk/download/636385461.pdf (accessed on 11th June 2025).
31. Sjerobabski-Masnec, I., & Šitum, M. (2010). *Starenje kože lica.* https://core.ac.uk/download/14451789.pdf (accessed on 11th June 2025).
32. Sun, Z., Zheng, Y., Wang, T., Zhang, J., Li, J., Wu, Z., Zhang, F., et al. (2025). Aloe vera gel and rind-derived nanoparticles mitigate skin photoaging via activation of Nrf2/ARE pathway. *International Journal of Nanomedicine, 20*, 4051–4067. https://www.semanticscholar.org/paper/c6c887f39c157e89534152c992b1e73d762f9637 (accessed on 11th June 2025).
33. Tri, P. P. (2018). *Hubungan Kadar Nitrit Oksida Serum Dengan Derajat Keparahan Photoaging Berdasarkan Klasifikasi Glogau Pada Petani Perempuan di Alahan Panjang.* https://core.ac.uk/download/231035702.pdf (accessed on 11th June 2025).
34. Yancey, J. P. (2014). *Doctor of Philosophy.* https://core.ac.uk/download/276264126.pdf (accessed on 11th June 2025).

COSMECEUTICALS AND TOPICAL AGENTS

3

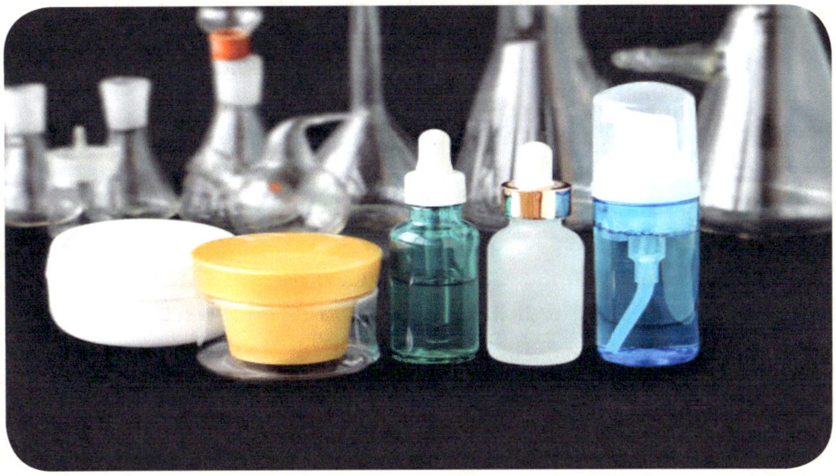

Introduction

The emerging and new category of cosmeceuticals, a blend of pharmaceuticals and cosmetics, is the innovative range of skincare and beauty. These products are designed not only for appearance but also for therapy, offering themselves as effective solutions to skin problems. With the cosmetics market still seeing tremendous growth, projected to hit over US$800 billion by 2023, determining the role of active ingredients in such products gains further significance. A heightened awareness among consumers over product performance and safety has generated a substantial demand for product ingredients that come from natural sources. This increasing interest in natural products is reflective of a shift in consumer patterns whereby individuals are more inclined towards formulations that benefit skin well-being with the least probable side effects attributed to synthetic components. Hence, the study of bioactive compounds included in cosmeceuticals is warranted in order to support this trend and advance the product further within the market

LEARNING OBJECTIVES

After studying this chapter, you will be able to:

1. Discuss about historical background of cosmeceuticals
2. Understand mechanisms of action within cosmeceuticals and topical agents
3. Describe common ingredients in cosmeceuticals
4. Explain the efficacy of cosmeceuticals and topical agents
5. Deal with the safety and side effects of cosmeceuticals and topical agents
6. Focus on market trends and consumer awareness

(Ji-Liu, 2022). The inclusion of ingredients with reported biological activity is at the center of cosmeceutical evolution. Compounds like seaweed extract, which have been long revered as sacred for their many health benefits, now find themselves under the microscope. Recent research has brought to light the possibility of seaweed as a vehicle for obtaining extremely bioactive compounds rich in vitamins, minerals, and antioxidants. These ingredients have multi-faceted therapeutic applications ranging from anti-inflammatory to anti-aging properties that target any skin care maladies. The research into seaweed not only reveals its medicinal and nutritional applications but also divulges its broader role in cosmetics. Its bi-function facilitates cosmeceuticals to access the beneficial attributes of natural ingredients while ensuring users have a holistic approach to skincare. With the industry set to expand further, accessing the potential of natural agents like seaweed is top of the agenda for future product design (Hossam et al., 2022). The marriage of cutting-edge scientific investigation with traditional cosmetic procedures is enhancing the efficacy and safety of topical preparations. While the increasingly informed and discerning consumer population continues to demand transparency regarding the source of ingredients and their performance, in fact, it is increasing all the time. The awareness has not only driven the growth of the industry called cosmeceuticals but also encouraged companies to adopt sustainable practices in choosing ingredients. By focusing on the sustainability of natural ingredients and emphasizing the efficacy of the bioactive compounds, the industry can meet consumer needs and be a responsible environmental steward. Additionally, an understanding of what the natural products do will lead the way to the development of even more sophisticated formulations. Lastly, the debate on cosmeceuticals and dermal agents underscores the call for creativity in addressing the complexity of skin health and personal care (Ji-Liu, 2022; Hossam et al., 2022).

Definition of Cosmeceuticals

Cosmeceuticals are a unique intersection of pharmaceuticals and cosmetics that possess the power to provide aesthetic pleasure along with therapeutic value to the skin. With active components shown in treating skin diseases or improving the well-being of the skin, cosmeceuticals transcend mere surface beautification. Employing bioactive molecules, such as antioxidants, vitamins, and peptides, cosmeceuticals treat skin issues like acne, hyperpigmentation, and aging. This utilitarian strategy is backed by growing scientific proof testifying to the efficacy of a number of ingredients used in cosmeceuticals, positioning cosmeceuticals at the intersection of consumer demand for effective skin care products and regulatory requirements, otherwise the preserve of pharmaceutical products. Growing awareness of skin health and the need for self-care habits on the part of consumers correlates with the intensified popularity of cosmeceuticals. Because people are seeking products that not only enhance their appearance but also address skin issues on a deeper scale, there has been a growing demand for products containing natural and sustainable ingredients. For instance, there has been a clear trend towards the utilization of plant-based materials and by-products within the product. Under the antioxidant and anti-inflammatory action of bioactive compounds derived from citrus and other sources, companies are developing more sustainable and cleaner products that serve consumers' beauty and wellness interests, hence meeting effectiveness as well as sustainability and education requirements (Cristina et al., 2024). Such convergence of effectiveness, sustainability, and consumer education continues to drive cosmeceuticals in the skincare industry. The role of the skin microbiome in cosmeceutical formulation indicates the sophisticated nature of skin health management. As more indications are being made of the relationship between microbial equilibrium and healthy skin, researchers are looking at microbiome-targeted approaches that enhance the efficacy of cosmeceuticals. Prebiotics and probiotics, for instance, are being looked at as the principal ingredient in optimizing functional microbial processes on the skin, which leads to healthier-looking skin appearances and conditions. Understanding the delicate equilibrium among these microorganisms and skin health can yield more effective treatments appropriate for specific dermatological diseases (Al-Smadi et al., 2023). With ongoing development in the cosmeceutical science, integration with such scientific information will further shape future innovation to produce products that both possess therapeutic benefits and improved skincare outcomes (Figure 3.1).

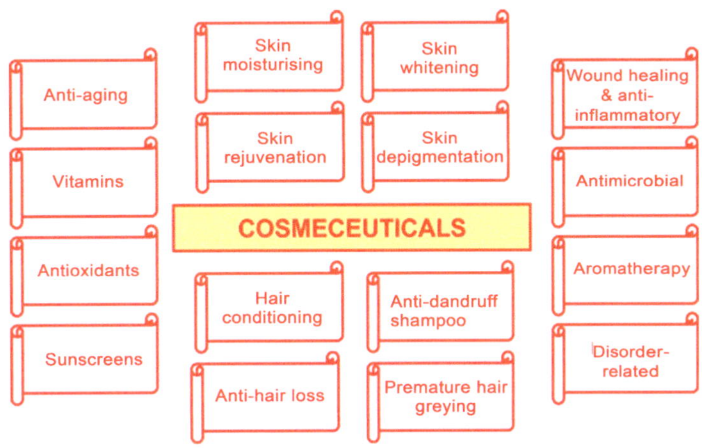

Figure 3.1. Cosmeceuticals.

Source: https://ars.els-cdn.com/content/image/3-s2.0-B9780323996846000070-f04-01-9780323996846.jpg.

Importance of Topical Agents in Skincare

Topical agents are the basis of skin care, primarily due to the fact that they are applied directly to the skin, thus enabling specific treatment of various dermatological conditions. Topical agents like creams, gels, and ointments are applied for their therapeutic value in the treatment of conditions such as dryness, inflammation, acne, and aging. The creation of cosmeceuticals, which combine cosmetic and pharmaceutical characteristics, highlights the importance of these agents to improve skin health and appearance. The cosmetic industry has evolved over recent years with the response to demand for natural and synthetic products from consumers, producing products that are customized to address the specific needs of unique skin types. This progress has been facilitated by the fact that good topical agents will significantly cure the skin condition without significant side effects, which is a critical factor for users and dermatology practitioners alike (Jusuf et al., 2024). Topical agents are more than cosmetic value because they play a crucial role in managing chronic skin conditions like rosacea. This inflammatory facial condition, with its redness and sensitivity, is a challenge to both physicians and patients. Topical preparations designed specifically for rosacea try to reduce inflammation while addressing symptoms of erythema and irritation. Cosmeceuticals formulated specifically for sensitive skin not only address the aesthetic appearance but also rebalance the skin and improve texture overall. Through delivering symptom relief from the root inflammatory cause while maintaining skin integrity of the barrier, such topical treatments hold the potential to lead to significant quality-of-life improvement for rosacea patients and those with related conditions (Gonçalves et al., 2017). Moreover, choosing organic over synthetic topical products is also important in determining their effectiveness and safety for consumers. Though both have been effective in multiple applications, the origin and components can produce varying effects on different skin types. Organic products, being derived from natural sources, are more liked by customers who seek gentler options, especially those with sensitive skin that can easily get irritated. Synthetic products may bring intense effects through well-formulated ingredients that directly cater to problems. However, both types carry with them the potential side effects, which necessitate informed consumer choice as well as professional advice. Knowledge of the pros and cons of the formulas makes tailored skincare routines necessary and reiterates the need for ongoing research in the domain of dermocosmetics (Jusuf et al., 2024).

3.1. Historical Background of Cosmeceuticals

Learning Outcome

1. Understand the evolution of skincare products
2. Describe key milestones in cosmeceutical development
3. Discuss regulatory changes affecting cosmeceuticals

The name cosmeceuticals was coined in the 1980s by combining the fields of cosmetics and pharmaceuticals. The new name was coined to describe products that profess to possess medicinal virtues, with the main objective being cosmetic. The initial products were characterized by being made of basic ingredients to improve the skin; however, with the growth of science, the biological effects of various ingredients began to be discovered. The emerging understanding of skin physiology and the proliferation of new technologies in drug delivery propelled the integration of active ingredients into dermatological products forward. This shift dramatically grew the cosmeceutical market, satisfying consumers' demands for functional skincare products with active functionalities that were greater than superficial enhancements. The stage was thus set for a fast-growing industry that couples cosmetic beauty with therapeutic efficacy, transforming the landscape of personal care products forever. Throughout history, natural products have been the core of cosmeceutical formulation, with societies applying their unique characteristics to heal and enhance the skin. Botanicals, minerals, and animal-derived products have been incorporated into ancient civilizations, which indicates an initial finding of the therapeutic attributes of these materials. Egyptian creams, for instance, had oils and resins that provided aesthetic and protective properties. With the elapse of time, these traditions led to modern formulations and greater emphasis on the pharmacological activities of active constituents. Recent emphasis on naturally occurring constituents, such as those from seaweed, has renewed these traditional practices. The complex bioactive constituents present in these ingredients have antioxidant, anti-inflammatory, and antimicrobial activities, indicating their high therapeutic potential as explained in current literature. This lasting correlation between old practices and new applications amplifies the role of nature in cosmeceutical development. Moreover, the interplay between the human microbiome and dermal well-being broadened the discussion of cosmeceuticals, paving the way for emerging treatment modalities. The skin microbiome, as a collective of varied microorganisms, plays a key role in maintaining dermal balance and arresting skin diseases. The realization of this association has led to the application of prebiotics and probiotics in cosmeceuticals for correcting skin resilience and addressing issues associated with microbiome disturbance.

This new trend not only induces healthy skin but is also part of an expanding drive towards microbiome-guided remedies in dermatology. Research has shown that tapping into the power of these helpful microbes can develop successful remedies for a range of skin ailments, broadening the perception of cosmeceuticals to go beyond aesthetics and achieve overall skin health, thereby being an example of the growth and future direction of this complex industry as depicted in current studies (Al-Smadi et al., 2023).

3.1.1. Evolution of Skincare Products

The development of skincare products mirrors the shifting attitudes towards beauty, health, and environmentalism in modern society. Early skincare was the use of natural ingredients like plant extracts and oils for maintaining skin integrity across varied climates. When scientific knowledge about dermatology grew, so did the formulation of skincare products. The arrival of cosmeceuticals was a turning point; these cosmetics occupy the liminal space between pharmaceuticals and cosmetics, featuring active ingredients that are proven to exert therapeutic benefits. Consumers therefore began to pay attention not only to the enhancement of appearance but also to skin well-being, creating an expanding market for creative topical products aimed at treating specific skin problems. This shift is a testament to growing recognition of the biological link between skin health and general well-being, setting the stage for products designed with emerging scientific techniques. Over the past several years, the explosion of microbiome-focused solutions has further remade the landscape of skin care, putting the constantly evolving relationship between human skin and its microbial communities in the spotlight. Research has illuminated the critical roles of skin-resident microbes, particularly in regulating the skin's inflammatory responses and maintaining its barrier function. Of specific interest is that Malassezia yeasts, as reported in recent reviews, possess the possibility of synthesizing lipid mediators with highly potent anti-inflammatory activities, which are capable of against common skin issues inherent in inflammation. Skin care products that take advantage of such microbial interactions signal a paradigm shift toward a more integrated understanding of skin care, one that is tantamount to growing consumer demand for natural and biologically compatible ingredients.

Such a shift is a call for the application of microbiome science in formulating products, suggesting the potential for more effective and helpful skin care options attractive to today's health-conscious consumers (Pagac et al., 2024). Further, the pursuit of sustainability has significantly influenced the way skincare products evolve, and one observes the trend towards clean and sustainable products. The changing demands from customers have propelled the industry into more sustainable paths, such as employing natural, biodegradable actives with a lowered waste regime. Among the outstanding examples is the valorization of citrus by-products, which not only offers a chance to reduce environmental burdens but also to collect bioactive compounds. Hesperidin, which is a flavonoid that is found abundantly in orange peels, illustrates the promise of these by-products since it has numerous therapeutic qualities that are beneficial to skin health, such as antioxidant and anti-inflammatory activities. Taking into consideration both skin health and environmental sustainability, today's skincare industry reflects a holistic ethos that has current societal realities in mind. These advances not only indicate the ongoing evolution of skin care formulation but also emphasize the incorporation of sustainability into the essence of cosmetic and therapeutic formulation (Cristina et al., 2024) (Figure 3.2).

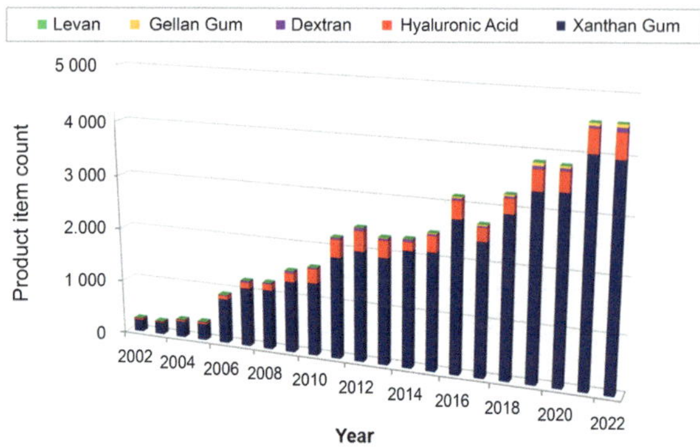

Figure 3.2. Evolution of new skincare products containing bacterial EPS over 20 years on three markets: France, the USA and China.

Source: https://www.researchgate.net/publication/375476944/figure/fig2/AS:11431281420804204@1746262905451/Evolution-of-new-skincare-products-containing-bacterial-EPS-over-20-years-on-three.tif.

3.1.2. Key Milestones in Cosmeceutical Development

Cosmeceutical development is a milestone in dermatological science, marking the synthesis between cosmetics and drugs. In the second half of the 20th century, the increasing interest in the health of the skin stimulated considerable work on bioactive molecules that produce therapeutic effects. The second half of the 20th century witnessed the introduction of topical actives such as retinoids and alpha hydroxy acids (AHAs), and their chief function was to enhance the smoothness of the skin and combat the signs of aging. These initial blends established a precedent for cosmeceuticals as being able to achieve both health- and beauty-based goals. Additionally, the incorporation of antioxidants like vitamin C served to further emphasize the cosmeceutical's capacity to fight against oxidative stress, a core component of aging and skin damage. These innovations established the precedent for a new product line that bridges beauty and health, ultimately changing the way that consumers perceive skincare products. With the development of science, the beginning of molecular biology and biotechnology began to revolutionize cosmeceutical formulation. The discovery of peptides, growth factors, and plant extracts with defined skin-enhancing properties was unveiled at the start of the 21st century, and with it came formulation addressing more specific skin concerns such as inflammation and photodamage. In particular, green tea catechins (GTCs) were identified with strong antioxidant and anti-inflammatory properties, which offered great benefits to skin health beyond conventional approaches. GTCs' efficacy in suppressing UV-induced skin aging and regulating inflammation offers a powerful direction for future research in cosmeceuticals. Not only did these bioactive ingredients enhance the therapeutic potency of topical products, but they also prompted the cosmetic industry to re-evaluate and label products based on their scientific merit, indicating a transition from promotional to evidence-based marketing. Ongoing research into vitamin D's health impact further illustrates a seismic shift in the cosmeceutical sector. Once considered only essential for bone formation, vitamin D is now involved with skin health and the prevention of skin conditions, including psoriasis and acne (Neonilli et al., 2025). This has resulted in the development of topical products that contain high concentrations of vitamin D, intended to alleviate these conditions as well as overall skin health. These trends point to the convergence of emergent scientific discovery and consumer demand for multi-action skincare products. Ingredient safety and performance have been the attention that drove rigorous testing and quality assurance across the industry, promoting greater consumer trust and facilitating cutting-edge formulation in the cosmeceutical sector. Eventually, these tipping points represent a broader paradigm shift towards merging scientific investigation with pragmatically effective dermatology solutions in order to decide the future of cosmetic and therapeutic dermatology (Figure 3.3).

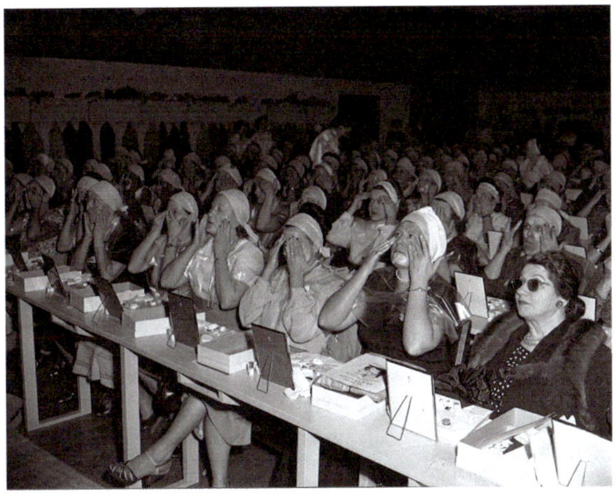

Figure 3.3. Audience applying makeup at a lecture by a beautician in Los Angeles in 1950.

Source: https://upload.wikimedia.org/wikipedia/commons/thumb/c/c5/Cosmetic_Class%2C1950.jpg/800px-Cosmetic_Class%2C1950.jpg.

3.1.3. Regulatory Changes Affecting Cosmeceuticals

The evolving regulatory environment of standards impacting cosmeceuticals is a key factor in both product formulation and consumer protection. As the official definition of cosmeceutical does not exist under the present Food, Drug, and Cosmetic Act, this uncertainty leaves manufacturers with the autonomy to term products cosmetic or drug-like just for marketing. This lack of strict definitions can be both useful and dangerous, as today more than ever, consumers require products that promise to have a therapeutic impact. Companies will generally exploit this grey area to market their products without clear support for their effectiveness, and thus many products that fail to meet established standards of safety will end up on the shelves. As demand for cosmeceuticals grows, driven by a population eager for better skincare solutions, the demand for more open, tighter regulatory oversight becomes critical to safeguard consumers and track efficacy in the marketplace (Anuradha et al., 2015). Acting on mounting consumer and regulatory pressure, recent policy shifts have already begun to address the disconcerting prevalence of unsubstantiated claims concerning cosmeceuticals. Regulatory bodies are starting to realize the imperative necessity of creating guidelines that draw demarcating lines between cosmetic and pharmaceutical characteristics clearly. This regulatory shift not only seeks to protect consumers but also to build credibility for the new cosmeceutical sector. Furthermore, through analysis of the active ingredients common in these products, regulatory agencies can establish standards for substantiation and safety testing, thus enhancing scientific rigor in product formulation. Such reforms eventually result in a more responsible industry environment where consumers and manufacturers can engage with higher confidence in the safety and effectiveness of cosmeceuticals (Sachs et al., 2013).

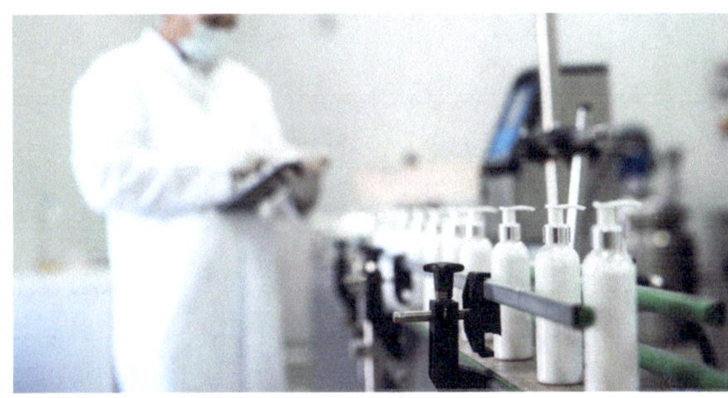

Figure 3.4. A technician monitoring the production line in a cosmetics manufacturing facility, ensuring compliance with good manufacturing practices (GMP) for product safety and quality control.

Source: https://cisema.com/wp-content/uploads/2022/08/Cosmetics-GMP.jpg.

Furthermore, the emerging regulatory change in the cosmeceutical industry is significant in determining public health and increasing market transparency. As the industry expands, particularly in ethnically diverse ethnic and demographic communities, establishing claims according to scientific evidence is becoming more critical. Regulatory measures are being formulated to ensure the cosmeceutical marketing does not mislead consumers about potential benefits. Greater regulatory oversight is able to assist in debunking inflated claims and guard against unforeseen outcomes that are likely to arise from misuse or over-reliance on such products. As a buffer between product performance and consumer education, regulatory agencies are able to aid in preventing the spread of unverifiable cosmeceutical solutions and enhance the overall integrity of the skincare industry (Anuradha et al., 2015) (Figure 3.4).

Test Your Knowledge

1. What were some of the earliest examples of cosmeceutical products?
2. How have regulatory challenges and the lack of standardized definitions for cosmeceuticals shaped the growth and marketing of these products over time?

3.2. Mechanisms of Action

Learning Outcome

1. Explain how active ingredients work on the skin
2. Define the role of penetration enhancers
3. Discuss the interaction of cosmeceuticals and topical agents with skin cells and receptors

Understanding mechanisms of action in cosmeceuticals and dermatologic products is essential to appreciating both their therapeutic potential and efficacy. These mechanisms are often complex biochemical pathways that influence skin physiology and address a multitude of dermatologic problems. Botanics, for instance, have been more highly valued for their multifunctional properties, such as anti-inflammatory activity. In the setting of central centrifugal cicatricial alopecia (CCCA), a current series of cases demonstrated the efficacy of a new botanical formulation, which pointed to certain phytoactive ingredients aimed at attacking inflammation and fibrosis. Notably, the development inhibited proinflammatory cytokines with enhancement of pathways associated with cellular energy and lipid metabolism, such as AMP-activated protein kinase and peroxisome proliferator-associated receptor-gamma activity, emphasizing the significance of these pathways for the control of CCCA (Umar et al., 2022). The benefits of marine-derived cosmeceuticals also reflect the striking heterogeneity in mechanisms of action of topical agents. The marine-derived chemical compounds offer new biological activities that are capable of improving skin health. The extraction of such compounds from seas is an emerging field in the development of cosmeceuticals. A majority of marine compounds have functionalities not found in land-based ingredients to enable them to be involved in various biological reactions in the skin. For example, some marine molecules can modulate skin barrier function, enhance hydration, and display antioxidative activity. This adds to the therapeutic value of cosmeceuticals derived from the ocean, making them effective substitutes in skincare products (Habeeba, 2022). Furthermore, a comprehensive analysis of the mechanism of action of topical agents is critical to inform clinical and consumer decisions in skincare. Understanding how these agents act at the molecular level on the skin educates practitioners and consumers alike in making prudent decisions regarding treatments. Effective cosmeceuticals rely not only on their active moiety but also on their ability to produce a desirable biological response. Mechanism insights can lead to optimization of existing formulations and the design of new agents with increased efficacy and stability. Moreover, as research continues to advance in this field, there is substantial potential for the discovery of new therapeutic targets and optimization of therapies that could have significant effects upon the treatment of many dermatological conditions.

3.2.1. How Active Ingredients Work on the Skin

Active cosmeceutical ingredients act through several mechanisms that have deep impacts on skin appearance and health. Active ingredients pass through the epidermis and engage in intricate biochemical interactions. For instance, retinoids are good cell turnover products that enhance skin texture and decrease aging signs. Concurrently, antioxidants like vitamin C and E fight free radicals and protect the skin from oxidative stress, the chief causative agent in early aging. This multi-step skin care regimen underlines the importance of selecting products that do not just promise but use scientifically proven active ingredients that act synergistically with skin cell functions towards bestowing a healthier and more vibrant-looking complexion. Besides, applications of nanotechnology in formulations have also become more prominent in cosmeceutical formulations, offering higher delivery of the active ingredients. Nanoparticles enhance the penetration of the compounds through the skin, thus greater bioavailability and activity. For instance, entrapment of the active ingredients in nanoparticles facilitates higher dermal penetration and targeted release, achieving maximum therapeutic effect of the compounds. Research has indicated that nanomaterials possess the capability to increase moisturizing properties and UV protection in products, hence becoming the most important movers in skincare technology. With nanotechnology, product formulators can formulate products not just to provide but to excel beyond customers' performance and aesthetic expectations. Further exploration of the developments has the prospect of redesigning the future of topical agents in the health and beauty industries (Salvioni et al., 2021). Active ingredient interaction with target skin receptors and biological mechanisms is essential to the achievement of desired therapeutic effects. For instance, compounds isolated from seaweed exhibit diverse bioactive activities, such as anti-inflammatory and antioxidant properties, which are affected through their typical phytochemical compositions. This underlines the importance of knowing how such interactions take place, particularly in skin permeability and even the potential behavioral responses of skin cells to such active ingredients. A better knowledge of the pharmacological action of such ingredients can offer possible pathways to more efficient treatment of diseases such as hyperpigmentation and acne. As the demand for improved cosmeceuticals grows, ongoing research into the active mechanisms of action of these ingredients will prove essential to their use in effective skincare products designed to improve overall skin health (Hossam et al., 2022) (Figure 3.5).

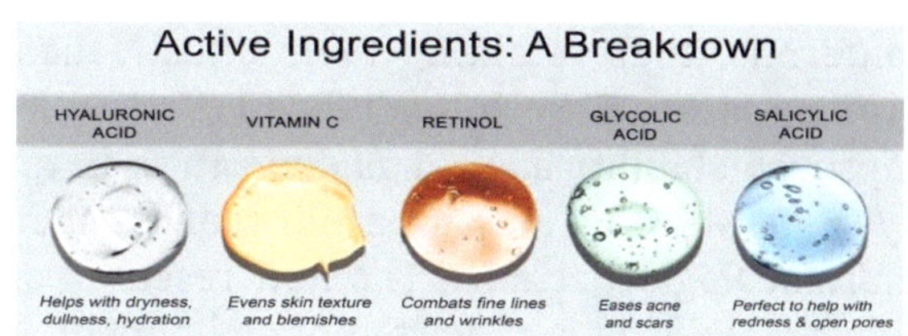

Figure 3.5. Active ingredients.

Source: https://www.zicail.com/wp-content/uploads/2024/09/Skincare-infographic-active-ingredients-and-benefits-500x281.webp.

3.2.2. Role of Penetration Enhancers

Delivery of cosmeceuticals and drugs has been significantly enhanced through the use of penetration enhancers, which facilitate efficient molecule transport across the skin barrier. The stratum corneum of the skin is an excellent barrier since it is lipophilic in nature and therefore presents a barrier to the delivery of hydrophilic molecules like peptides. Emerging advances in penetration enhancement technologies like cell-penetrating peptides and microneedles demonstrate remarkable enhancements in the permeability of such molecules. For instance, methods like Dermaportation utilize pulsed electromagnetic fields to increase the permeability of small molecules and demonstrate considerable therapeutic potential by circumventing the skin's barrier function. These approaches not only improve delivery but also have the potential for an enhanced safety profile of varied topically applied therapies, becoming the cornerstone of their decisive contribution to the future of cosmeceuticals and topical agents (Mohammed et al., 2012). Moreover, the use of lipoamino acid (LAA) conjugation techniques has found applications in enhancing dermal delivery significance. These LAA conjugates, tailored to increase the physiological properties of therapeutic peptides, offer increased penetration efficiency as well as biological activity. Experiments revealed that lipophilic LAA conjugation to peptides enhances their permeation across the epidermis, thus retaining their effectiveness upon application. Such modifications allow for improved stability as well as deposition in the layers of skin for increased duration of their pharmacological actions. The new research on the stereoselectivity of diastereomer lipopeptide demonstrates the difference in permeation, indicating that optimal molecular design can provide significantly enhanced skin permeation patterns, demonstrating an important step forward in the development of cosmeceutically applied topical formulations (Namjoshi et al., 2009). Finally, investigation into new penetration enhancement strategies has shown great promise for enhanced drug delivery systems in dermatology and cosmetic use. Methods such as electroosmosis and sonophoresis also show the extensive range of methods used in improving transdermal delivery of active substances. Such new delivery methods are particularly beneficial in instances where normal topical delivery is not as effective as desired therapeutic outcomes, especially for bulky or water-soluble molecules. Notably, cyclization of peptides has been found to not just improve stability but also enhance skin penetration mechanisms. With this continuous progress, these technologies are expected to play a crucial role in the formulation of future-generation cosmeceuticals that depict a harmonious blend of efficacy, safety, and patient compliance that profoundly redefine the face of topically delivered treatments (Namjoshi et al., 2009) (Figure 3.6).

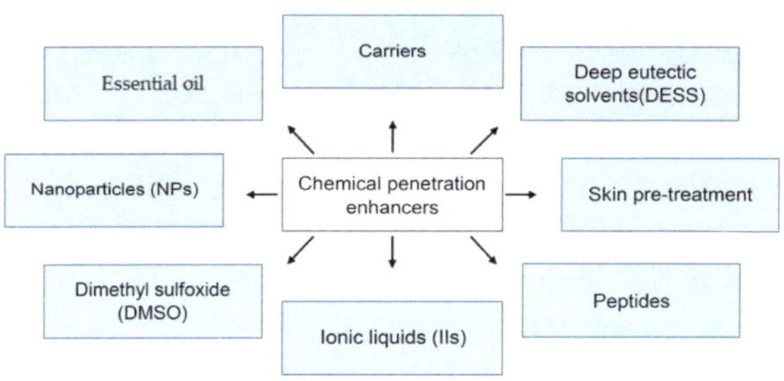

Figure 3.6. Different types of chemical penetration enhancers.

Source: Sugumar V, Hayyan M, Madhavan P, Wong WF, Looi CY. Current Development of Chemical Penetration Enhancers for Transdermal Insulin Delivery. Biomedicines. 2023; 11(3):664. https://doi.org/10.3390/biomedicines11030664

3.2.3. Interaction with Skin Cells and Receptors

The degree of interaction between cosmeceuticals and topical products and skin cells and receptors is instrumental in determining their efficacy. Certain of the constituents of the preparations, such as hyaluronic acid (HA), play multifunctional roles in the appearance and condition of the skin. HA, a matrix molecule of central importance, demonstrates its importance by influencing not only moisture but also cell migration and cell proliferation. Its ability to bind water molecules aids in the maintenance of the hydration level of the skin, and its interaction with some cell surface receptors could regulate intracellular signaling pathways responsible for tissue repair and inflammation. These mechanisms highlight the therapeutic potential of HA and the requirement for targeted formulations that are able to interact effectively with skin receptors for optimal skin function and regeneration, as well as react appropriately to aging signs and environmental stress conditions, thereby enhancing the overall impact of cosmeceuticals (Ashrafi et al., 2024). Apart from HA, the role of many extrinsic factors in skin aging cannot be overlooked, and more so in terms of how topical products interact with skin cells. The UV radiation and environmental pollutants trigger the production of reactive oxygen species (ROS), leading to collagen degradation and reduced skin elasticity. This degradation is contributed largely through matrix metalloproteinases (MMPs), which are induced due to injury or damage. Cosmeceuticals that aim to reverse these effects of toxicity have to communicate with skin receptors, inhibit MMP activity, and activate intrinsic collagen synthesis in fibroblasts. Understanding overlapping pathways through which intrinsic and extrinsic forces cause skin aging provides vital information for clinicians and researchers in the development of successful treatments. Focus on interference with these mechanisms allows for restoration of skin integrity and health, leading eventually to healthier skin (Kim et al., 2016). The development of cosmeceuticals that interact strategically with receptors in the skin indicates the growing sophistication of skin care science. Products designed to enhance receptor activity can have synergistic effects that optimize the function and look of the skin. For instance, the use of antioxidants and peptides in topical products may maintain the body's own system of defenses in the skin. Targeted interaction of such agents with cellular receptors not only protects against UV radiation or pollutant-induced oxidative stress but also triggers skin renewal processes. The science unfolding, the potential for creating next-generation cosmeceuticals that are more personalized and effective grows. With the assistance of our growing knowledge of skin biology and its receptors, the formulator can create products that are not only preventive but also therapeutic, setting a new standard for skincare efficacy and consumer satisfaction, which is essential to address the multiform challenge of aging skin (Ashrafi et al., 2024) (Figure 3.7).

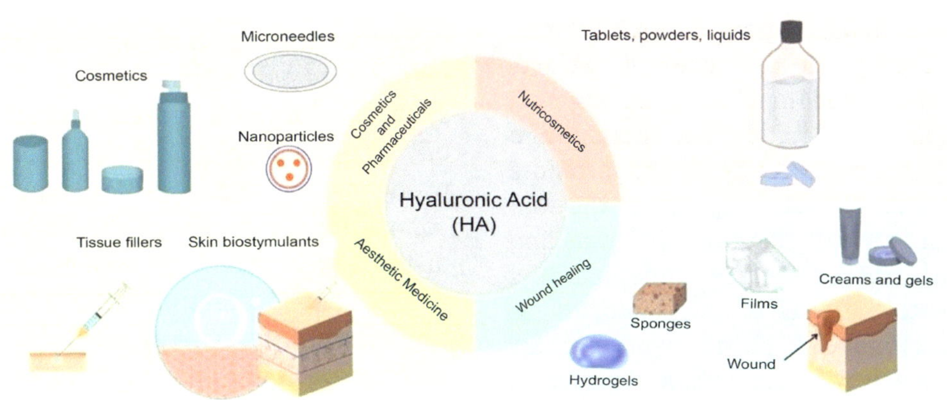

Figure 3.7. Hyaluronic acid (HA).

Source: Chylińska N, Maciejczyk M. Hyaluronic Acid and Skin: Its Role in Aging and Wound-Healing Processes. Gels. 2025; 11(4):281. https://doi.org/10.3390/gels11040281

Test Your Knowledge

1. How do active ingredients work on the skin?
2. What are the receptors in the skin cells?

3.3. Common Ingredients in Cosmeceuticals

Learning Outcome

1. Describe antioxidants and their benefits
2. Explain peptides and their role in skin repair
3. Define retinoids and their effects on aging

The composition of cosmeceuticals sometimes entails a collection of biologically active substances, among them being extracts of marine organisms, particularly seaweeds. Such natural substances have been found to contain high levels of bioactive substances like vitamins, minerals, and polysaccharides that make them effective in topical applications. Based on current reviews, the anti-inflammatory, antioxidant, and antimicrobial properties of seaweed extracts make them highly beneficial in managing skin issues like aging and irritation. The vitamins and minerals inherent in seaweeds not only promote health in the skin but also help supply the skin with essential nutrients that can rejuvenate and nourish. With further studies, understanding the mechanistic impacts of these substances in cosmeceuticals can unveil even greater potential, hence demanding further exploration in their therapeutic application and green source methods within the cosmetics industry (Hossam et al., 2022). Yet another leading cosmeceutical ingredient is the incorporation of nanoparticles (NPs) that have garnered immense interest since they provide great enhancements in the delivery and activity of active ingredients. The nanomaterials are the leading players in formulations developed to improve skin penetration, control the release of active ingredients, and thus contribute to the overall bioavailability of the product. This technology is most useful in the field of skincare, where whether or not an agent is able to penetrate can be the determining factor in how well it works to combat specific skin ailments. Research has revealed that NPs can increase moisture binding, provide superior UV protection, and stabilize products, demonstrating their multifunctional role in modern cosmeceutical formulation. However, ongoing debate about the safety and long-term effects of nanotechnology on cosmetics mandates large-scale studies to ensure consumer safety and effectiveness (Salvioni et al., 2021).

Furthermore, the use of plant-based extracts continues to remain a focal point in cosmeceuticals, addressing consumer demand for organic and natural products. Ingredients such as aloe vera, green tea, and essential oils give a variety of benefits, from anti-aging to hydrating and soothing. Their chemical composition maximizes the barrier function of the skin, accelerates healing, and provides antioxidant protection from environmental aggressors. The synergy between these plant extracts not only maximizes the physiological benefits of the skin but also resonates with consumers who wish for integrated solutions for skincare. As regulatory regimes evolve, ingredient provenance and bioactive properties is the name of the game when it comes to building trust and loyalty among consumers by brands. The synergy that exists among these common ingredients is proof of the sophistication that has grown in cosmeceuticals as they bridge the gap between pharmaceuticals and cosmetics to serve an informed and discerning public.

3.3.1. Antioxidants and Their Benefits

The addition of antioxidants to cosmeceutical formulations represents a groundbreaking advance in the fields of skin care and topical therapy. Antioxidants such as vitamins C and E, coenzyme Q10, and other plant extracts are very effective in protecting against oxidative stress, the pivotal mechanism of skin aging and damage. Oxidative stress in the context of skin well-being is caused by an imbalance between antioxidant defenses and ROS within the body, thereby causing cellular destruction and inflammation. Antioxidants slow down these processes by neutralizing free radicals, and thus they are imperative in preserving skin integrity and looks. Furthermore, the application of antioxidants in topical products has been shown to enhance skin hydration and texture, thereby demonstrating their varied properties in cosmeceutical applications. Amongst the abundant natural antioxidant sources are berries, found to have notable beneficial effects on the skin, aligning with cosmeceutical aims. These phenolic fruits, which consist of anthocyanins and polyphenols, have anti-inflammatory and antioxidant properties that relate directly to skin health. Systematic reviews observe that berry extracts reduce oxidative stress markers and inflammation in skin tissues, leading to increased production of collagen and elastin, which are crucial to skin firmness and elasticity.

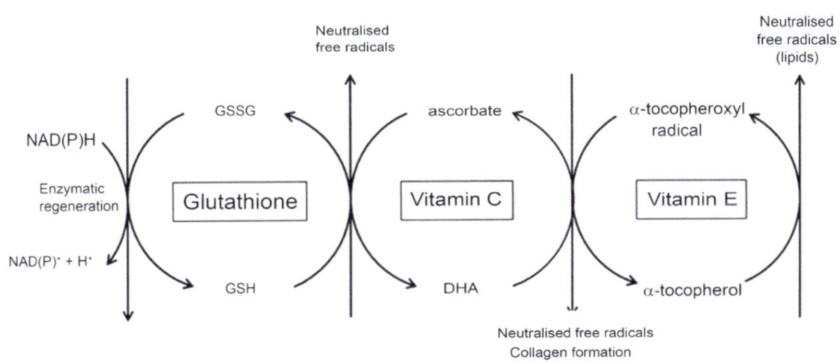

Figure 3.8. The central role of vitamin C and other antioxidants pertinent to the skin. The interdependence of vitamins E and C, and glutathione, in the scavenging of free radicals and regeneration of the reduced antioxidants, is shown. Vitamin E is in the lipid fraction of the cell, whereas vitamin C and glutathione are water-soluble and present in the cytosol.

Source: Pullar JM, Carr AC, Vissers MCM. The Roles of Vitamin C in Skin Health. Nutrients. 2017; 9(8):866. https://doi.org/10.3390/nu9080866

The benefits derived from berry-derived antioxidants not only promote better wound healing but also enhance the extracellular matrix composition, thereby benefiting individuals seeking effective topically applied remedies for skin restoration and revitalization. Thus, the presence of such bioactive molecules in cosmeceuticals lends strength to their role in skin care treatments. In times of transformation with cosmeceuticals, transference of antioxidant benefits into effective topical products is also backed by formulation technology advancements. Progresses, above all in nanotechnology, enhance the stability, penetration, and bioavailability of antioxidant molecules, ensuring their optimal therapeutic effects on the skin. Through microencapsulation methods, among others, formulators can cause antioxidants to remain effective and active while using them, thus enhancing their ability to fight oxidative damage. In addition, the popularity of such types of formulations is rising, which reflects a heightened consumer interest in products that not only offer aesthetic enhancement but also physiological benefit. With the regulatory framework shifting to address safety and efficacy concerns, the future of cosmeceuticals with antioxidants is good, offering preventive as well as therapeutic interventions for skin issues (Azevedo et al., 2025; Khavate & Chougule, 2025) (Figure 3.8).

3.3.2. Peptides and Their Role in Skin Repair

Peptides, which are brief chains of amino acids, play a vital role in skin repair as they facilitate a sequence of biological activities responsible for maintaining healthy skin. Bioactive peptides are able to pass through the outer layers of the skin and exert immediate effects on cellular activities such as collagen synthesis, wound healing, and modulating inflammation. Through the activation of skin cells to enhance their regenerative capacity, peptides are increasingly being recognized as functional cosmeceutical agents and topical products.

Through the mimicking of naturally occurring cellular behavior signals, peptides can effectively address a vast range of skin concerns, including aging, dryness, and damage caused by external aggressors. More application of peptides in cosmeceuticals is in accordance with the industry's shift towards products that deliver drug-like results alongside traditional cosmetic benefits, and this is a mirror of the evolving trends in skin repair and care (Anuradha et al., 2015). Different studies have repeatedly validated the effectiveness of some peptides in boosting skin repair. For instance, peptides like palmitoyl pentapeptide induce collagen production, tightening up the skin and reducing the visibility of wrinkles and fine lines. Certain peptides also have anti-inflammatory properties that can soothe inflammatory skin and accelerate the healing process following injury or dermatological procedures. This multi-pronged approach not only enhances the appearance of the skin but also enhances its structural integrity, making it more resilient to environmental stress. The complementarity of these biological processes gives rise to a general healthier skin barrier, which is critical to preventing the loss of moisture and protecting against pathogen invasion.

Therefore, the therapeutic potential of peptides has placed them on the center stage in the development of advanced cosmeceutical products to rejuvenate and restore aged and compromised skin (Lee et al., 2012). Moreover, the use of peptides in topical products is an exemplary step in the intersection of cosmetics and therapeutic modalities. With cosmeceuticals gaining more popularity, the science behind peptide action gains importance for formulators and consumers alike.

The regulatory setting, as described in cosmeceutical reviews, is that, while the products constitute cosmetics, the pharmacological nature complicates safety and efficacy testing. Regulation of peptides, then, is thus difficult under current frameworks, which could potentially fail to adequately reflect the complex benefits, resulting in calls for improved classification under current legislation. Through successful manipulation of both clinical and cosmetic outcomes, peptides are a testament to the potential of cosmeceuticals to speed up healing in the skin, underlining the need for intense scientific examination and regulatory oversight in this new field (Anuradha et al., 2015) (Figure 3.9).

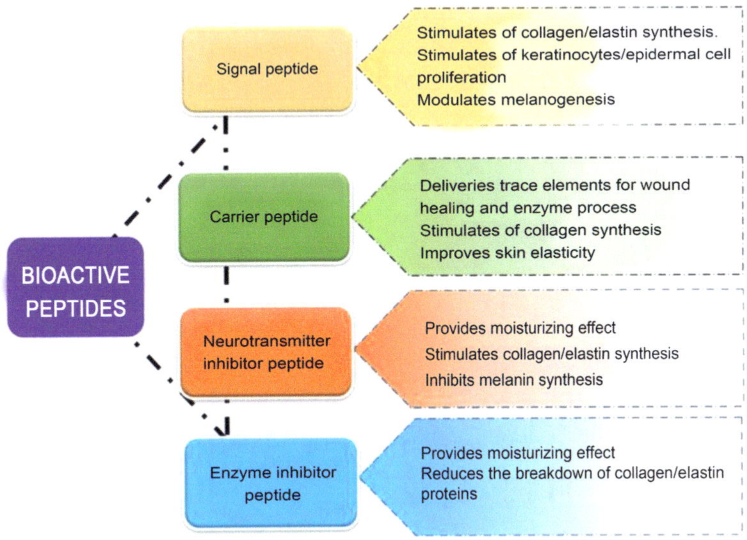

Figure 3.9. Classification of bioactive peptides based on cosmetic properties.

Source: Ngoc LTN, Moon J-Y, Lee Y-C. Insights into Bioactive Peptides in Cosmetics. Cosmetics. 2023; 10(4):111. https://doi.org/10.3390/cosmetics10040111

3.3.3. Retinoids and Their Effects on Aging

The skin aging process is multifactorial and has both intrinsic and extrinsic factors that contribute to its deterioration. Unlike one of the factors, retinoids, derivatives of vitamin A, are one of the best methods of resisting these processes. One of the most noteworthy functions of retinoids is their ability to enhance cellular turnover, leading to the elimination of dead cells and the stimulation of new, healthier layers. Such regenerative action not only improves the tone and texture of the skin but also plays a significant role in decelerating the aging signs, such as fine lines and wrinkles. Retinoids also stimulate retinoid receptors, which play a significant role in preserving cutaneous elasticity, thereby bringing about a youthful appearance in the long run (Draelos et al., 2024). In the context of photoaging, resulting from cumulative ultraviolet exposure, retinoids' activities are even more important. The medications have been found to stimulate collagen synthesis and restore elastin fibers, thereby making the skin firmer and more elastic. Topical retinoids have been found to correct the activity of melanocytes and keratinocytes in such a manner as to correct pigmentation abnormalities that are common with aging. For instance, studies indicate that retinoids prescribed, such as tazarotene and tretinoin, were the most effective agents to employ to correct the changes defining photoaging, with excellent results in skin texture and tone in reported clinical trials (Neil et al., 2023). This indicates the relevance of retinoids not only as cosmetics but also as essential drugs in aging skin treatment. Nevertheless, while retinoids possess vast benefits, their utilization is not without potential disadvantages. Side effects like erythema, peeling, and dryness are common and are more often seen with more concentrated preparations. Irritative reactions to these responses can cause avoidance of daily use, which is necessary to achieve optimal benefits. Therefore, ongoing research attempts to maximize retinoid formulations and develop ways to maximize their safety and tolerability. More recent formulations, such as lower-potency tazarotene creams, have been formulated, and these are promising to reduce marks of photoaging with fewer side effects (Neil et al., 2023). With more interest in anti-aging products that work, information on finding a balance between tolerability and efficacy will be key to consumers as well as medical professionals when selecting the correct retinoid-based drug (Figure 3.10).

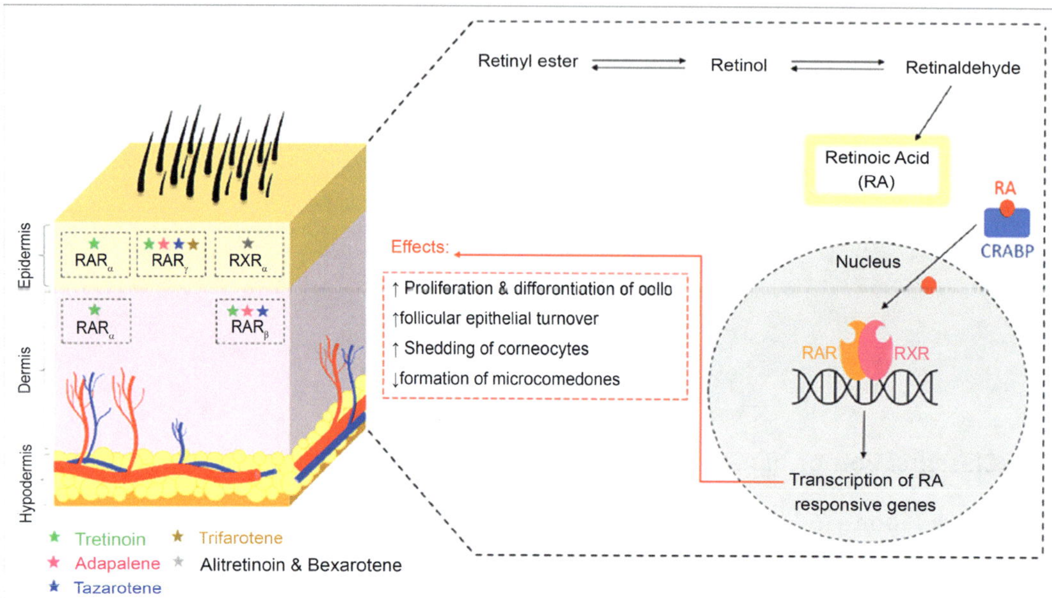

Figure 3.10. Biological pathway of natural retinoids and target sites of synthetic retinoids.

Source: https://www.researchgate.net/publication/353398594/figure/fig1/AS:1048598405976065@1627016750586/Biological-pathway-of-natural-retinoids-and-target-sites-of-synthetic-retinoids.png.

Test Your Knowledge

1. What role do antioxidants play in cosmeceuticals, and how do they benefit the skin?
2. What are peptides, and how do they function in cosmeceuticals to stimulate collagen production and improve skin firmness?

3.4. Efficacy and Clinical Evidence

Learning Outcome

1. Focus on studies supporting the use of cosmeceuticals
2. Understand the comparison with traditional pharmaceuticals
3. Explain the limitations of current research surrounding cosmeceuticals and topical agents

Efficacies of cosmeceuticals and topical treatments are often supported by levels of clinical evidence obtained through valid studies. Essential to this conversation is the understanding that not all agents are equal; therapeutic effects often can be greatly influenced by the biochemical nature of active ingredients and their preparations. For example, recent evidence points to differences in performance between particular agents, like S-1 plus cisplatin (SP) versus capecitabine plus cisplatin (XP), in the case of gastric cancer, according to histological types. This suggests that treatment stratification by tumor type can be made to improve clinical results, implying the value of personalization in the broader application of topical agents in dermatology. Such a refined recognition is a critical foundation for further exploration into the clinical efficacy of various cosmeceutical products. Moreover, the issue of drug resistance in clinical practice inevitably renders it highly challenging to quantify topical agents. Topical antibacterials are regularly employed to cure skin infections, for example, but greater usage has to be matched with the rise in multidrug-resistant strains, in particular *Staphylococcus aureus*. This resistance not only challenges the long-term effectiveness of these antibiotics but also points to the urgent need for judicious use in therapy. As seen in studies comparing community-acquired strains, indiscriminate use of topical agents actually selects for multidrug resistance, thus narrowing therapy options in the long run. Thus, the clinician is faced with the urgent requirement of addressing efficacy and safety to an equal extent, necessitating strict evidence-based guidelines for the use of these products. Finally, an efficient critique of the clinical evidence about cosmeceuticals should include both systemic absorption and local effects since the latter decides the final therapeutic success of these products. Most cosmeceuticals include active ingredients whose activity is greatly boosted by their formulation, stability, and penetration characteristics. The rate of absorption of some agents, for example, can vary substantially, which can influence their clinical performance and practical effectiveness. The consequences of this difference serve to emphasize the necessity of carefully designed studies that are not only used to test individual compounds, but also to examine the overall synergy in the entire formula. As research in this field continues to progress, the development of a better understanding of such intricacies will be crucial to the development of valid benchmarks for effectiveness and clinical proof in cosmeceuticals and topicals.

3.4.1. Studies Supporting the Use of Cosmeceuticals

The new trend of cosmeceuticals has generated wide interest due to the increasing number of studies affirming their efficacy in enhancing dermatological health as well as appearance. Research has determined that bioactive molecules such as vitamins, minerals, and fatty acids are the primary molecules accountable for skin rejuvenation and dermatological health. Specifically, these molecules are accountable for the major skin properties such as elasticity, firmness, and hydration, as well as the treatment of skin conditions due to aging. For instance, the literature attests to the instant action of such bioactive compounds on indicators like wrinkles and senile dryness. Aggregating such findings, it is certain that the use of cosmeceuticals can bring about quantifiable improvements to skin well-being, hence inclining towards their incorporation in daily and nighttime regimens to support a healthier and more youthful complexion (Michalak et al., 2021). When evaluating the therapeutic potential of specific ingredients used in cosmeceuticals, polyunsaturated fatty acids (PUFAs) are central. Omega-3 and omega-6 fatty acids have been researched for their beneficial effects on chronic inflammatory skin diseases like atopic dermatitis and acne. Studies indicate that these fatty acids can alter cellular metabolism and signal transduction and thereby modulate inflammation. The combination of gamma-linolenic acid (GLA) and omega-3 long-chain PUFAs appears particularly potent in de-escalating inflammation, something strongly relevant to the treatment of numerous dermatological ailments. This suggests a critical field of ongoing research where dietetic and supplementing protocols utilizing these factors could optimize individual skin health outcomes, underlining the need for balanced dermatology styles incorporating cosmeceutical innovation in everyday regimens (Bali et al., 2020). Given the variety of evidence in support of cosmeceutical use, it is important to adopt individualized approaches in integrating these agents into dermatological care. The variations in skin type and genetic background that define each subject necessitate individualized approaches that are capable of proportionally modulating inflammatory response while boosting strength. Current studies elucidate that while certain cosmeceutical procedures can create universally beneficial effects, there most often will exist individual-specific outcomes that must be carefully thought out concerning skin biology. Investigating this further permits that optimal nutrition and supplementation with bioactive materials specifically targeted, particularly in individuals at risk for skin issues, can create the greatest outcomes. As research continues to uncover the complexity of skin aging and health, cosmeceuticals will likely evolve to include more sophisticated and customized modalities of therapy, solidifying their position in contemporary dermatological science (Bali et al., 2020; Michalak et al., 2021).

3.4.2. Comparison with Traditional Pharmaceuticals

The introduction of cosmeceuticals has developed great interest, with particular reference to traditional pharmaceuticals with a long tradition in dermatologic therapy. Traditional pharmaceuticals have the tendency to address symptomatic relief by systemic treatment, with satisfactory solutions for various skin diseases. Side effects, however, may limit patient compliance and satisfaction. Cosmeceuticals, however, bridge the gap between drugs and cosmetics as they offer benefits to the skin without the potentially damaging side effects typical of conventional drugs. This allows consumers to enhance their skincare routine and, at the same time, address specific concerns or needs, such as hydration, anti-aging, or pigmentation. Thus, as consumers become more health-conscious and educated, the demand for a product that is effective and safe takes precedence, and hence, cosmeceuticals are a desirable alternative to traditional treatments. Talking about effectiveness, comparing cosmeceuticals with traditional drugs brings out some of the special positives and negatives. For instance, traditional drugs tend to be rigorously tested under laboratory conditions, and as a result, an exact understanding of the therapeutic impact and risks is known. On the other hand, cosmeceuticals do not normally include lengthy clinical trials due to regulatory problems, perhaps diminishing their perceived function as therapeutic medications. Despite this, research has been able to indicate favorable results for certain active ingredients of cosmeceuticals that are comparable to their pharmaceutical counterparts. Particularly, the use of antioxidants and peptides in cosmeceuticals has been seen to be highly effective in improving skin texture and luster without eliciting the adverse side effects normally associated with pharmaceutical treatments. This dramatic safety profile inevitably makes cosmeceuticals a popular choice among consumers who seek effective yet non-irritating treatments (Li et al., 2019). However, the growing popularity of cosmeceuticals does pose the challenges of standardization and regulation of cosmeceuticals. Traditional drugs are tested thoroughly and receive regulatory approval, which provides a guarantee of safety and efficacy. Yet the cosmeceutical industry remains relatively unregulated, and that leaves doubt regarding consistency in product formulation and claims made by manufacturers. This variance can cause a gap in consumer confidence as the similar nomenclature of cosmetics and pharmaceuticals muddies treatment modalities. It is essential that healthcare providers and consumers are able to grasp these nuances because they can direct treatment plan decisions for skin disease. Lastly, even though cosmeceuticals provide an enticing option, one must weigh their application thoroughly, specifically in relation to the way their efficacy and safety compare to traditional pharmaceutical interventions (Delgado et al., 2023) (Figure 3.11).

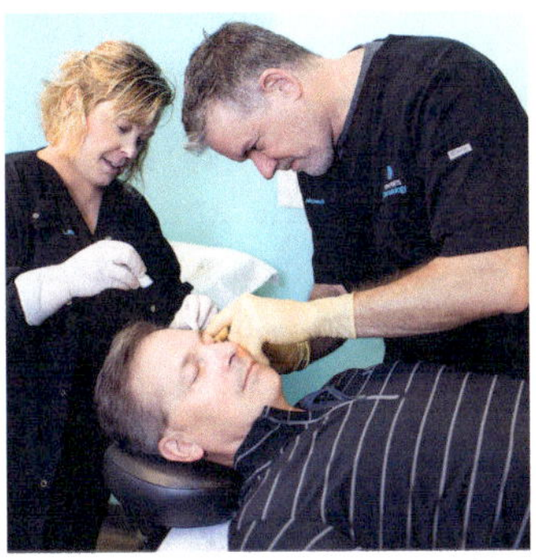

Figure 3.11. A dermatologist performing a cosmetic procedure on a patient, highlighting the clinical precision and expertise involved in dermatological treatments compared to med spa services.

Source: https://www.twinportsderm.com/wp-content/uploads/2024/09/Med-Spa-vs-Dermatologist_-Which-is-Best_contentimage-e1725904760433.png.

3.4.3. Limitations of Current Research

The scientific environment covering cosmeceuticals and topical preparations reflects a variety of dominant limitations that hinder the development of this industry. One of the major challenges is the often-inadequate understanding of the processes through which the active ingredients actually function. Much of the research focuses on clinical outcomes without sufficient examination of the processes producing them, resulting in oversimplification. In addition, the chemical sophistication of such formulations may make analysis tricky to separate out the effects of each component. In particular, the use of newly emerging delivery systems like microneedles is two-edged; on the one hand, they offer promising pathways towards enhanced penetration and action, whereas on the other hand, they are also plagued by drawbacks like poor drug loading capabilities and plugged pores that serve as barriers to their widespread applicability in practice (Sartawi et al., 2022). Furthermore, regulatory policies for cosmeceuticals remain uncertain, which presents yet another obstacle for researchers. The lack of standardized testing procedures, therefore causes variation in product safety and efficacy profiles, and thus consumer skepticism and hesitation. The characterization of new materials, e.g., nanoparticles, also adds another layer of complexity; while they have a vast potential for several advantages in cosmetics, the limited availability of effective safety data raises the anxiety of the public regarding their toxicity (Salvioni et al., 2021). This fragile balance between potential benefits and intrinsic risks continues to limit investment in research. It is for this reason that the requirement for an expansive regulatory framework becomes increasingly obvious, as it would provide a standard basis for measuring the safety and effectiveness of such emerging technologies. Finally, the salience of marketing claims tends to obscure scientific rationales, thereby leading both consumers and practitioners into a knowledge gap. Today's studies tend to focus on the good things about new ingredients and technologies with minimal concern for long-term effects or overall safety assessments. This trend creates a marketplace where products might be marketed on the grounds of perceived innovation, not scientifically proven outcomes. As the technology improves, it will be essential that robust studies that establish both the advantages and disadvantages of cosmeceuticals and topical therapies take priority, therefore opening the door for more informed consumers and encouraging practitioners to make evidence-based recommendations. Indeed, the future of the industry will rest in bridging the gap between marketing and science, so that innovations become practical and effective treatments with an assurance of safety (Figure 3.12).

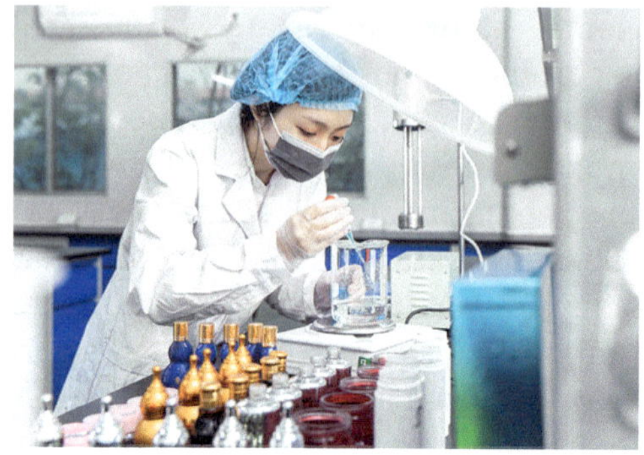

Figure 3.12. A researcher formulating cosmetic products in a laboratory setting, emphasizing the role of research and development (R&D) in ensuring product efficacy, safety, and innovation in the skincare industry.

Source: https://www.djmskin.com/wp-content/themes/mml-theme/dist/img/p05-2-r&d/p052-s02-img02.jpg.

Test Your Knowledge

1. What are the uses of cosmeceuticals?
2. What are the challenges in conducting clinical studies to assess the long-term effectiveness and safety of topical cosmeceuticals?

3.5. Safety and Side Effects

Learning Outcome

1. Describe common adverse reactions to topical agents
2. Explain the importance of patch testing
3. Focus on regulatory standards for safety

Side effects and safety of cosmeceuticals and topical drugs are the most important considerations of their efficacy and popularity with consumers. As the products occupy the boundary area between pharmaceuticals and cosmetics, the awareness of the potential adverse effects is of utmost significance to healthcare professionals and consumers alike. The majority of topical agents are designed for a specific dermatologic condition, e.g., acne or hyperpigmentation, and can induce responses ranging from mild irritation to anaphylactic reaction. Exploratory research into oral mucositis, a non-curable side effect of oncologic treatments, searched for several topical agents, such as natural and antimicrobial ones, to be assessed for efficacy and safety profile (Coppini et al., 2024). This would imply that while some agents could prove to be beneficial in the management of some conditions, safety needs to be established by extensive clinical trials so that patients can use them safely with no harmful consequences to health. For topically applied antifungal drugs like terbinafine hydrochloride, safety issues are even more pertinent. In a trial of topical use of this drug, patients experienced very little systemic exposure, with plasma levels well below what is observed with oral administration (Tavakkol et al., 2024). This stark contrast highlights the inherent advantage of topical drugs, where the application is not at risk of causing systemic side effects. Surprisingly, very few side effects were reported, suggesting an acceptable safety profile for topical treatments when proper use recommendations are taken into account. Nevertheless, even mild side effects such as headaches or local irritation must be closely monitored, emphasizing the significance of proper safety testing before cosmeceutical use. Besides, ongoing monitoring of side effects and safety in cosmeceuticals informs consumers about potential dangers in the use of such products. Companies are increasingly being called upon to conduct thorough safety assessments to comply with regulations, including the identification of any harmful effects to be experienced from prolonged use. These preventive measures not only create user confidence but also render cosmeceuticals overall more efficacious in the management of skin conditions. With newer products being developed, ongoing studies of the safety profiles will be instrumental, again calling for the preservation of efficacy while reducing risks with topical agents. In this way, consumer needs are more effectively met by the cosmetics and drug industries while an atmosphere of safety and trust in product choice is encouraged.

3.5.1. Common Adverse Reactions to Topical Agents

The use of topical drugs, especially those designated as cosmeceuticals, has become widely popular because of their claimed advantages regarding the health and beauty of the skin. It is important to consider, though, that these products can cause any number of negative reactions, posing difficulties to users as well as medical practitioners. Common side effects include irritation, allergic reactions, and photosensitivity in the form of redness, swelling, burning, or rashes over the area of application. These reactions will compromise the desired effects of topically applied treatments and lead to poor adherence and patient dissatisfaction. It is important to understand the mechanisms of these adverse effects to face the concerns of consumers and to assist clinicians in choosing and recommending suitable products for patients. Studies show that the absence of extensive studies comparing the safety profiles of such agents usually places practitioners dealing with these frequent problems under-equipped to make decisions based on evidence-based guidelines (Prakoeswa et al., 2024). Furthermore, there may be some side effects that can be linked to active ingredients contained in cosmeceuticals. For instance, excessive dryness, peeling, and irritation of the skin, particularly in sensitive skin types, can be caused by excessive concentrations of AHAs and retinoids, which are typically promoted as possessing anti-aging benefits. The occurrence of such side effects underlines the utmost need for individualization of skin care regimens. It is desirable for a person to do patch testing when introducing new topical preparations in an effort to minimize the risk of severe reactions. It is also helpful to know one's own skin type and condition so that agents likely to have less effect in causing unpleasant effects can be selected. Aside from that, consumer education campaigns about ingredient listings, instructions for use, and possible side effects can significantly encourage secure usage and trust in cosmeceuticals (Prakoeswa et al., 2024). In certain situations, side effects might propagate beyond local dermal irritation to produce psychological distress, particularly when there are occurrences of hyperpigmentation. This effect not only affects the look of the skin but also causes increased anxiety and low self-esteem in individuals, further complicating the psychological effects of the use of topical treatments. Studies have noted that complications such as hyperpigmentation often require careful management to avoid aggravation through the use of improper topical treatments. New medications like miglitol have been shown to be promising in minimizing hyperpigmentation with fewer side effects; further studies are necessary, however, to identify complete profiles of such medications. The pursuit of efficient and safe topical medications necessitates ongoing studies of the mechanism of their efficacy and concomitant risk so that patients are treated with cosmetic enhancement along with preservation of cutaneous health in a balanced manner (Figure 3.13).

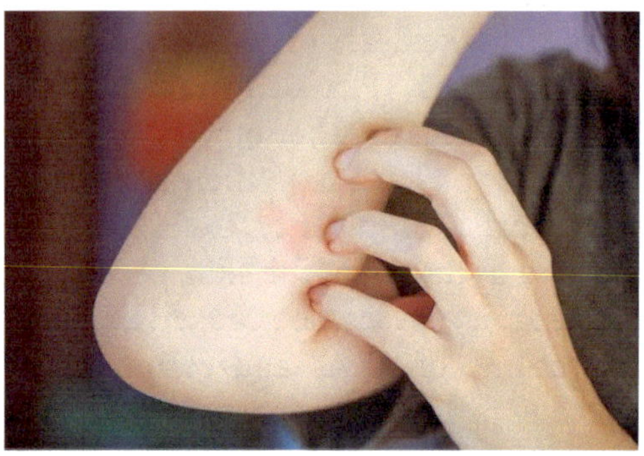

Figure 3.13. Rashes by using topical agents.

Source: https://www.beckerentandallergy.com/wp-content/uploads/2024/03/woman-is-scratching-red-blistere-beckerent-nj.webp.

3.5.2. Importance of Patch Testing

Patch testing is a critical component of cosmeceuticals and topical product analysis and their safe application. Patch testing involves the application of tiny amounts of potential allergens on the skin to find out if one is sensitive or allergic before applying a product in full. With an increasing market for personal care products, which is now valued at US$500 billion in 2017 and is poised to reach more than US$800 billion by 2023, the value of skin compatibility testing cannot be overstated (Ji-Liu, 2022). When individuals use ineffective or irritating products, not only can it lead to skin illnesses such as dermatitis, but, more importantly, it may make them hesitate to use beneficial treatments. With patch testing, businesses are able to ensure consumer safety, enhance product formulae, and foster trust in the competitive beauty market. Natural and organic skincare products have gone on to further highlight the necessity of patch testing. As consumer awareness of ingredients in their cosmetics increases, with increasing demands for natural remedies, potential allergic reactions to plant extracts and ingredients must be extensively tested (Ji-Liu, 2022). Patch testing allows the identification of individual sensitivities to these ingredients and promotes a policy of skincare that is individualized. With the diversity of skin types and idiosyncratic reactions individuals will have, patch testing is not merely a precaution; it is a necessary part of responsible cosmetic practice. Further, since most products are a mixture of several active ingredients, it is critical to analyze their interaction by performing patch tests to reduce the chances of adverse reactions that might occur due to such multiplicity. With new delivery systems such as dissolvable microneedles rapidly becoming popular in the beauty segment, the significance of patch testing becomes more prominent. Given their ability to administer therapeutic agents transdermally successfully, such systems must undergo rigorous testing for safety, especially considering developments in formulations. The microneedle applications must not invoke any untoward reactions through thorough patch testing, thus safeguarding the consumer's health. Moreover, with cosmetic products now possessing innovative ingredients or using novel delivery mechanisms, patch testing will still remain the indispensable tool in alleviating uncertainties in relation to their safety. By doing this, it not only preserves consumer protection integrity but also protects the continued development of successful and safe cosmetic innovations, ultimately adding value to user and manufacturer experience in the ever-evolving cosmeceutical landscape (Figure 3.14).

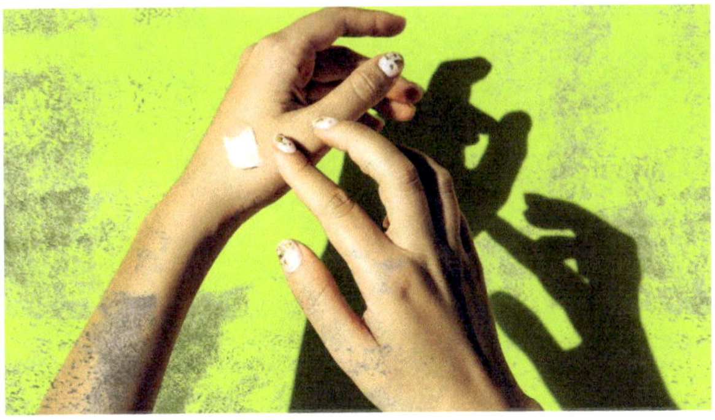

Figure 3.14. A patch test for skincare products.

Source: https://i0.wp.com/post.medicalnewstoday.com/wp-content/uploads/sites/3/2022/01/patch_testing_GettyImages1337523320_Header-1024x575.jpg?w=1155&h=1528.

3.5.3. Regulatory Standards for Safety

The growing use of cosmeceuticals and topical products has created the need for strict regulatory standards to guarantee consumer safety. Regulatory agencies, including the Food and Drug Administration (FDA) in the United States, are responsible for assessing the safety and efficacy of such products before they are made available on the market. With the market size of cosmetics and topical drugs growing notably, estimated to reach over $800 billion by 2023 (Ji-Liu, 2022), the requirement for rigorous safety assessment becomes increasingly important. This includes ingredient evaluation, product formulation screening, and clinical testing to protect public health from potential adverse effects, especially considering the growing consumer interest in natural ingredients. Moreover, the social media explosion has heightened consciousness regarding the health issues of certain cosmetic chemicals, highlighting the need for transparent regulatory processes that give precedence to effectiveness and safety. Besides regulatory oversight, the incorporation of new delivery systems enhances cosmeceutical and topical agents' safety profile. For instance, dissolving microneedles are emerging as an effective transdermal drug delivery system with distinct advantages of drug loading and patient compliance (Sartawi et al., 2022). In facilitating controlled delivery of active components, the technology minimizes the risk of skin irritation and systemic absorption of harmful substances. Such innovations offer a significant shift towards combining safety with efficacy in product development. Moreover, biocompatibility in such systems is also a priority for ensuring active ingredients work as expected without compromising the health of the users. As technology improves, it remains crucial for regulatory policies to keep up with integrating these new-age approaches while always keeping the welfare of consumers in mind. Cosmeceutical regulation never stands still; it always evolves based on evolving scientific research and consumer needs. More scrutiny of product ingredients and ingredient sourcing is common, primarily because consumers are still becoming more conscious of the potential consequences of synthetic ingredients versus natural alternatives (Ji-Liu, 2022). This has led to an increase in a trend towards the regulation of herbal and botanical ingredients so that they are safe and effective for use in topical form. Secondly, these organizations are establishing wide standards for testing new delivery systems, such as microneedles, for safety and side effects (Sartawi et al., 2022). Last but not least, the dynamic nature of regulation ensures that the safety of the consumers is of the highest priority, with an environment developed where successful and innovative cosmeceuticals can bloom simultaneously while avoiding health dangers.

Test Your Knowledge

1. What are the side effects of cosmetic products?
2. What is the function of a patch test?

3.6. Market Trends and Consumer Awareness

Learning Outcome

1. Understand the growth of the cosmeceutical market
2. Explain the influence of social media on consumer choices
3. Discuss the importance of education and transparency

The increasing popularity of cosmeceuticals is fueling profound changes in market trends as consumers increasingly seek products that offer cosmetic and therapeutic benefits in balance. With more knowledgeable consumers becoming aware of the ingredients in their skincare products, there is a sense of change toward transparency and effectiveness. This development points to the growing role of bioactive ingredients of natural origin, including seaweeds and fermentation derivatives. The presence of compounds with documented biological activities, such as antioxidants and anti-inflammatory compounds, encourages such products in the minds of discerning consumers. As highlighted in recent studies, consumer demand for products containing active ingredients such as those from seaweed grows on the basis of their well-documented health benefits, thus prompting companies to invest in R&D in order to tap into such consumer-led demand (Hossam et al., 2022). At the same time, increasing consumer interest in sustainability and ethical sourcing is shaping the cosmeceuticals market. Today's consumers no longer simply care about the quality of a product but also about the social and environmental footprint that their purchasing decision will generate. This changing attitude has brought about sustainable practices, including the utilization of by-products such as spent brewers yeast, which not only supports environmental stewardship but also yields powerful bioactive peptides that contribute to skin health (Oliveira et al., 2022). The circular economy concept is gaining popularity in the industry, making it push brands towards innovation while minimizing waste and maximizing resource use. Effective communication of such green practices is crucial for businesses to build trust and loyalty, considering that consumers increasingly desire products that are aligned with their values. Moreover, merging digital marketing approaches has increased consumer education, enabling more effective targeting of approaches to engage health-focused populations. Social media and influencer partnerships have emerged as significant platforms for information dissemination about cosmeceutical efficacy and safety. Brands that successfully access these platforms not only expand their reach but also create a consumer base of engaged buyers who will share their experience and point of view. With the heightening of consumer awareness comes the demand for science-driven claims of product efficacy, and only the best survive in this competitive market. The constant interaction between research on new ingredients, consumer attitudes, and innovation in marketing steers the direction of the cosmeceuticals market, evidencing the key role played by informed consumers in furthering industry standards.

3.6.1. Growth of the Cosmeceutical Market

The cosmeceutical market has experienced vast growth over recent years owing to increased consumer interest in products that have cosmetic and therapeutic properties. This demand stems from an overall awareness of skin health and desire for products that address a multitude of skin complaints, such as aging, acne, and inflammation. As there is greater awareness by consumers of the interconnect between health and skincare in general, their demands are better suited to be on products that have active ingredients with efficacy. This resulting mass will compel producers to innovate their formula to incorporate improved compounds, such as antimicrobial peptides, that have been said to have potential usage and hence there will be a trend of being part of a series of cosmeceuticals (Mazurkiewicz-Pisarek et al., 2023). Thus, consumers are more willing to spend on items that not only look good for cosmetic purposes, but also for their therapeutic benefits. According to market research, the cosmeceutical market is also heavily influenced by the accelerating rate of self-care and wellness trends. As individuals concentrate on individual well-being, there is a concomitant interest in products that contribute to healthier skin and radiance. This is a reflection of changing consumer behavior, whereby consumers are more likely to discover and invest in high-quality products that resonate with their health objectives. The commonality of diseases such as skin irritation, premature aging, and environmental damage attributable to causes such as pollution has fueled the quest for solutions. Thus, the application of natural ingredients like polyphenols and probiotics possessing immune-modulating activity is becoming more prevalent in products found in the market. Such trends identify a holistic approach preferred by consumers, enhancing the charm and development potential of the cosmeceutical industry (Andreia et al., 2023). Further, the online environment has heightened the growth of the cosmeceutical industry, providing customers with greater access to information along with greater choices in products. Online retailers and social media are the key touch points for brand interaction and customer education, raising the level of awareness of cosmeceuticals. Products claiming cosmetic value as well as treatment are typically recommended by celebrities and dermatologists, heavily influencing consumer choice. The recognition of issues such as inflammation and oxidative stress in skin well-being has driven increased interest in products that offer protection and recovery benefits. As the market moves in this direction, businesses are more under pressure to build credibility and transparency around the efficacy and safety of their ingredients. It presents opportunities and challenges to grow, requesting constant innovation and research in the cosmeceutical field (Andreia et al., 2023; Mazurkiewicz-Pisarek et al., 2023) (Figure 3.15).

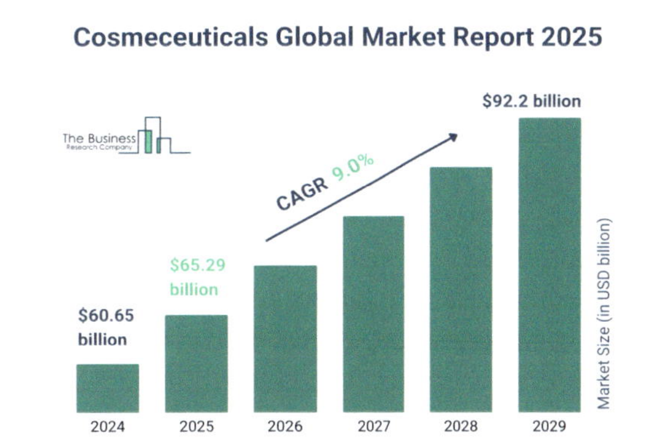

Figure 3.15. Cosmeceuticals global market report 2025.

Source: https://www.thebusinessresearchcompany.com/graphimages/Cosmeceuticals_Global_Market_Report_2024_Market_2025_Graph.webp.

3.6.2. Influence of Social Media on Consumer Choices

The intersection of consumer choice and social media within the cosmeceutical sector has profound implications for brands and consumers alike. Social media sites are online battlegrounds where consumers post opinions, reviews, and tips on skincare treatments and products. Consumers can make informed decisions based on opinions from peers rather than relying on traditional forms of advertising in this culture of immediacy. Through influencers, dermatologists, and enthusiasts promoting what they have tried, the products are given more exposure, reinforcing one another through a ripple effect of market demand. For instance, the rising movement towards natural and marine-inspired cosmeceuticals is typically traced to social media trends that began on these sites, demonstrating how these sites drive consumers' choices and drive industry innovation, which, in turn, impacts product offerings by manufacturers (Nimisha et al., 2024). Also, social media is the best facilitator of consumer engagement and customer loyalty within the cosmeceutical sector. Instagram and TikTok allow businesses to not only demonstrate how good their products are but also the story behind them. User-generated content is utilized by various brands to build credibility and a sense of community among customers. Engagement tactics—such as promotions, how-to guides, and participatory polls—increase brand presence while developing loyal customer communities. This fundamental transformation towards a consumer-focused model is also reflected in the manner in which corporations are becoming increasingly product-specific in response to insights derived from social media engagement. As businesses adapt to serve the expressed wants of their customers, the feedback mechanism is a constant power for product innovation and marketing enhancement, underscoring the important contribution of social media as a driver of consumer choice (Kyriakoudi et al., 2024). Enduring, as well, is the psychological aspect of the influence of social media on consumers. Visual imagery and pleasing aesthetics are paramount in the way cosmeceuticals are perceived. The images that usually accompany social media updates make products more attractive, appealing to dreams of health and beauty from customers. The clean beauty and sustainability trends have compelled customers to shift towards brands that, besides providing efficacy, appeal to their values as well. As peer pressure and social approval are injected into consumer choice-making, the cosmeceutical sponsor, through social media, increasingly shapes what products are popular in a competitive market. This aspect is an indicator of how social media has extended beyond traditional modes of advertising, transforming the terrain of consumer preference for both brands and products within the cosmeceutical industry (Nimisha et al., 2024).

3.6.3. Importance of Education and Transparency

In the new field of cosmeceuticals and topicals, education and honesty are of the highest importance. As there is more consumer demand for products having not just cosmetic but therapeutic potential, there needs to be extensive awareness regarding these products. Education involves equipping consumers with the knowledge to enable them to sort out effective product formulations from those that are full of deceitful information. Ingredient sourcing transparency, production methods, and scientific efficacy promote consumer confidence and facilitate intelligent choice. The recent emphasis on vitamin D's role in healthy skin provides an example of the necessity for clear communication about active ingredients and benefits. Literature discusses the bio-functionality of vitamin D in curing various cutaneous diseases, highlighting labeling transparency about its effectiveness and applications in topical preparations and cosmeceuticals (Neonilli et al., 2025). This allows consumers to make educated decisions that beautify but also feed the skin in general. Cosmeceutical education campaigns should also extend to healthcare professionals and manufacturers. During a climate of fast-paced development and competing demands, practitioners would benefit significantly benefited by being current with the latest developments in ingredients, formulations, and treatment regimens. Education provides a consensus environment wherein healthcare professionals can serve their patients to the best advantage through safe and effective products. One such example is the heightened need for aromatherapy as an optimal vehicle for practitioners to expand their treatment armamentarium. By discovering how phytoconstituents in essential oils may supplement conventional therapy, practitioners can administer integrated care that honors science while also honoring patients' desires (Lalitkumar et al., 2024). Finally, organized education among industry leaders is necessary for promoting a culture of transparency that serves the consumer and the wider healthcare family as a whole. Secondly, the commingling of regulatory frameworks with consumer awareness is critical to the protection of the integrity of the cosmeceutical industry. Regulators should uphold stringent standards for marketing and distribution and penalize firms for misrepresentative data and unsubstantiated claims. Transparent regulation establishes a culture whereby educational campaigns can thrive because consumers grow to trust products under rigid oversight. Equilibrating innovation with responsibility is critical to preserving credibility in the industry. As the importance of vitamins, like vitamin D, and natural remedies, including essential oils, increasingly increases, being proactively involved in informing consumers about possible benefits, risks, and usage will make these products more effective. Developing a foundation in education and transparency is imperative to encouraging a responsible, consumer-oriented model for cosmeceuticals and topical agents and, in turn, public health and safety.

Test Your Knowledge

1. What factors are driving the rapid expansion of the global cosmeceuticals market?
2. How has social media, particularly platforms, influenced consumer awareness and demand for cosmeceuticals?

SUMMARY

The probe is initiated on cosmeceuticals and topical agents, but it reveals an astonishing overlap between skincare and therapeutic interventions. Different studies have revealed the effectiveness of the agents in treating numerous skin conditions and bringing significant improvement in the patient's overall skin condition. For instance, recent meta-analyses reveal that some topical preparations can influence significant clinical outcomes such as probing pocket depth and clinical attachment levels of periodontal therapy. This is imperative given the increasing demand for non-surgical treatments in dermatology. Nevertheless, even as proof supports the efficacy of some agents, it also points to a requirement for more studies to standardize interventions and solidify their place in clinical practice. Perception of complex roles of cosmeceuticals means its significance not only in aesthetic practice but on general therapeutic strategies. In dermatology, cosmeceuticals have much more significant roles than cosmetics alone. Cosmeceuticals containing active ingredients such as sucralfate have already been found to be useful in the prevention and management of complications of cancer treatment, e.g., oral mucositis. They bestow the required cytoprotection and nurturing to patients who undergo aggressive treatments. Moreover, systematic reviews have shown natural and antimicrobial agents to have great benefits, supporting the necessity to include scientifically proven preservatives in clinical practice. Such findings reiterate the importance of evaluating the totality of topical agents and biological activities. With healthcare evolving, awareness about the efficacy of cosmeceuticals will be the foundation in maximizing patient outcomes, making them very useful in prevention as well as treatment. In the end, the convergence of clinical practice and scientific evidence is what underpins cosmeceuticals and topical drugs. As highlighted by recent review articles, demands for optimal control of conditions continue to remain the driving force to advance research efforts. Numerous clinical trials have established convincing benefits from their use in combination with standard treatments, further supporting their inclusion into routine practice. The striking achievements of interventions, as illustrated in treatment studies for diseases like oral mucositis and periodontal disease, reflect their therapeutic potential. With advancing scientific research, the establishment of guidelines pertaining to both safety and efficacy increases in importance. Therefore, generating a harmonized notion of cosmeceuticals can aid towards more holistic, patient-centric treatment approaches, ultimately optimizing quality of care in dermatology and beyond.

In the area of cosmeceutics and topical agents, advances reflect the central role played by antioxidants in avoiding oxidative stress and maintaining healthy skin. The skin, being the body's defense, is repeatedly exposed to assault from environmental aggressors that are part of the production of ROS. This oxidative stress leads to disease of the skin, making it necessary to have effective antioxidant therapy. To enhance the delivery of such important compounds, new methodologies have emerged, primarily the incorporation of nanotechnology. Nanocarrier systems such as nanoemulsions and liposomes have significant potential to facilitate penetration across the skin by antioxidants, thus maximizing their therapeutic effect. This marriage of biotechnology in cosmetics is a shocking shift towards more effective topical therapy, as discussed below under the headings of clinical implications and the dermatological future of antioxidant therapy (Zazuli et al., 2025). In addition to antioxidants, utilization of natural compounds, particularly from macrofungi, has also become increasingly popular in the development of anti-aging cosmetic products. Mushroom traditional usage in cosmeceuticals focuses on their potential application in the future against the effects of aging, which are exaggerated by environmental and lifestyle factors. A review seems to cite numerous active components present in the fruiting bodies of a variety of mushrooms, such as polysaccharides, phenolic compounds, and triterpenes. These substances possess a range of beneficial properties such as antioxidant activity, photoprotection, and collagen stabilizing, making them very valuable to the production of modern cosmeceuticals. With the continued search for natural anti-aging agents, the evidence around mushroom extracts is a highly promising avenue towards enhancing skin resistance to aging (Paterska et al., 2024). The use of these findings in cosmeceuticals is only one step of a larger trend towards multidisciplinary approaches to skincare. By integrating knowledge from dermatology, biochemistry, and natural product science, the development of topical agents can be optimized. The growing recognition of the importance of antioxidants when blended with other natural agents such as mushroom extracts is an evolutionary pattern in dermatology doctrine wherein not only short-term cosmetic benefit is at stake but long-term skin health. With each new technique being continually unveiled by means of continued research for the improvement in delivery and efficacy of these agents, ever-increasing hope for improved outcomes in dermatology enters the limelight. This determination to harness traditional as well as non-traditional approaches will most likely define the future cosmeceutical and topical agents market, with customers being offered science-backed, natural solutions to their skin concerns (Paterska et al., 2024; Zazuli et al., 2025).

KEY TERMS FROM THIS CHAPTER

- Anti-inflammatory compounds
- Bioactive compounds
- Biocompatibility
- Collagen synthesis
- Cosmeceuticals
- Dermatological health
- Environmental aggressors
- Extracellular matrix
- Gamma-linolenic acid (GLA)
- Antioxidant
- Bioactive ingredients
- Biological mechanisms
- Compromised skin
- Dermatological diseases
- Dissatisfaction
- Environmental stress
- Food and Drug Administration
- Green tea catechins (GTCs)

CRITICAL THINKING QUESTIONS

1. **Which of the following is the primary purpose of cosmeceuticals?**
   a. To treat medical conditions
   b. To enhance the aesthetic appearance of the skin
   c. To provide deep hydration for hair
   d. To protect the skin from UV radiation
2. **Which of the following ingredients is commonly used in topical agents for anti-aging benefits?**
   a. Retinoids
   b. Benzoyl peroxide
   c. Salicylic acid
   d. Hydrocortisone
3. **Which of these is a common function of sunscreens, a type of topical agent?**
   a. To reduce acne formation
   b. To promote collagen synthesis
   c. To protect the skin from UV damage
   d. To hydrate the skin
4. **What is the role of peptides in cosmeceuticals?**
   a. They act as antioxidants to reduce inflammation.
   b. They stimulate collagen production, improving skin elasticity.
   c. They provide exfoliation for the skin.
   d. They prevent fungal infections of the skin.
5. **Which of the following is a key difference between cosmeceuticals and traditional cosmetics?**
   a. Cosmeceuticals are solely used for aesthetic purposes.
   b. Traditional cosmetics always contain SPF.
   c. Cosmeceuticals are only available through a prescription.
   d. Cosmeceuticals contain active ingredients that may have therapeutic effects on the skin.

Short Answer Questions

1. What is the difference between cosmeceuticals and traditional cosmetics?
2. How do topical agents such as retinoids function in the treatment of acne and aging?
3. Explain the role of antioxidants in cosmeceuticals. How do they benefit the skin?
4. How do peptides in cosmeceuticals contribute to skin rejuvenation and repair?
5. What is the significance of the skin's barrier function in the efficacy of topical agents?

Answer to Critical Thinking Questions

1. (b); 2. (a); 3. (c); 4. (b); 5. (d)

REFERENCES

1. Al-Smadi, K., Leite-Silva, V. R., Andréo-Filho, N., Lopes, P. S., & Mohammed, Y. (2023). Innovative approaches for maintaining and enhancing skin health and managing skin diseases through microbiome-targeted strategies. *Antibiotics, 12*, 1698–1698. https://doi.org/10.3390/antibiotics12121698 (accessed on 11th June 2025).
2. Ashrafi, H., Baseer, A. Q., Hassand, M. H., Hejran, M., et al. (2024). *The Importance of Hyaluronic Acid in Biological Systems.* https://core.ac.uk/download/603903802.pdf (accessed on 11th June 2025).
3. Azevedo, F. S., Pires, A. R., Lila, M., Valacchi, G., Hoskin, R., Sarandy, M. M., Novaes, R., et al. (2025). Berry fruit extracts as topical cosmeceuticals for skin health applications: A systematic review. *Cosmetics.* https://www.semanticscholar.org/paper/ed48aac6fef95b12e1586a4c59ea7d68fe18f7b0 (accessed on 11th June 2025).
4. Balić, A., Vlašić, D., Žužul, K., Marinović, B., & Bukvić Mokoš, Z. (2020). Omega-3 versus omega-6 polyunsaturated fatty acids in the prevention and treatment of inflammatory skin diseases. *International Journal of Molecular Sciences, 21*, 741–741. https://doi.org/10.3390/ijms21030741 (accessed on 11th June 2025).
5. Carter, G., Schultz, M. B., Baines, S. L., Gonçalves da Silva, A., Heffernan, H., Tiong, A., Pham, P. H., et al. (2017). Topical antibiotic use corselets for the carriage of mobile genetic elements conferring resistance to unrelated antimicrobials in *Staphylococcus aureus. Antimicrobial Agents and Chemotherapy, 62.* https://www.semanticscholar.org/paper/e7b586dda3b7adef54616c72ae7188f36adb3b06 (accessed on 11th June 2025).
6. Sachs, D. L., Rittié, L., Chubb, H. A., Orringer, J., Fisher, G., & Voorhees, J. J. (2013). Hypo-collagenesis in photoaged skin predicts response to anti-aging cosmeceuticals. *Journal of cosmetic dermatology, 12*(2), 108–115. https://doi.org/10.1111/jocd.12037(accessed on 11th June 2025).
7. Coppini, M., Caponio, V., Mauceri, R., Bizzoca, M. E., Laino, L., Lorenzo-Pouso, A., Russo, D., et al. (2024). Efficacy of topical agents in oral mucositis prevention: Systematic review and network meta-analysis. *Oral Diseases.* https://www.semanticscholar.org/paper/134daf6375be30e5d723f46d2cc253c1b13e3287 (accessed on 11th June 2025).
8. Cotas, J., Lomartire, S., Gonçalves, A. M. M., & Pereira, L. (2024). From ocean to medicine: Harnessing seaweed's potential for drug development. *International Journal of Molecular Sciences, 25*, 797–797. https://doi.org/10.3390/ijms25020797 (accessed on 11th June 2025).
9. Delgado, A., Cornett, B., Choi, Y. J., Colosimo, C., Stahel, V. P., Dziadkowiec, O., & Stahel, P. (2023). Investigational medications in 9,638 hospitalized patients with severe COVID-19: Lessons from the "fail-and-learn" strategy during the first two waves of the pandemic in 2020. *Patient Safety in Surgery, 17.* https://www.semanticscholar.org/paper/cf2f5a9805c8b14a1ae1ad2c89bda79b6eee4734 (accessed on 11th June 2025).
10. Draelos, Z. D., Bogdanowicz, P., & Saurat, J. H. (2024). Top weapons in skin aging and actives to target the consequences of skin cell senescence. *Journal of the European Academy of Dermatology and Venereology, 38*, 15–22. https://doi.org/10.1111/jdv.19648 (accessed on 11th June 2025).

11. El-Beltagi, H. S., Mohamed, A. A., Mohamed, H. I., Ramadan, K. M. A., Barqawi, A. A., & Mansour, A. T. (2022). Phytochemical and potential properties of seaweeds and their recent applications: A review. *Marine Drugs, 20*, 342–342. https://doi.org/10.3390/md20060342 (accessed on 11th June 2025).

12. Fernandes, A. S., Rodrigues, P., Pintado, M., & Tavaria, F. K. (2023). A systematic review of natural products for skin applications: Targeting inflammation, wound healing, and photo-aging. *Phytomedicine, 115*, 154824–154824. https://doi.org/10.1016/j.phymed.2023.154824 (accessed on 11th June 2025).

13. Gonçalves, M. M. B. M., & Pina, M. E. S. R. T. de. (2017). *Dermo Cosmetic Care for Rosacea.* https://core.ac.uk/download/268265254.pdf (accessed on 11th June 2025).

14. Jusuf, N. K., & Zulfa, R. A. (2024). Skin care in dermatology: Between organic versus synthetic products. https://core.ac.uk/download/617167601.pdf (accessed on 11th June 2025).

15. Kawakami, H., Nishikawa, K., Shimokawa, T., Fujitani, K., Tamura, S., Endo, S., Kobayashi, M., et al. (2022). Histology classification highlights differences in efficacy of S-1 versus capecitabine, in combination with cisplatin, for HER2-negative unresectable advanced or recurrent gastric cancer with measurable disease. *Cancers, 14.* https://www.semanticscholar.org/paper/26a84641b3d4e79f6e8a85461429a7d2ea745db8 (accessed on 11th June 2025).

16. Khavate, S. B., & Chougule, S. S. (2025). Exploring cosmeceuticals: A comprehensive review of skin-boosting science. *International Journal of Pharmaceutical Research and Applications* Volume 10, Issue 2 Mar–Apr 2025, pp: 1270-1275. https://www.semanticscholar.org/paper/0802ef24a8fcb2eb7b8d0514da1f54cf9315a069 (accessed on 11th June 2025).

17. Kim, H. M., & Hyun, C. (2022). Miglitol, an oral antidiabetic drug, downregulates melanogenesis in B16F10 melanoma cells through the PKA, MAPK, and GSK3β/β-catenin signaling pathways. *Molecules, 28.* https://www.semanticscholar.org/paper/22f788e821683a07f093d2b8141827a6a1531acb (accessed on 11th June 2025).

18. Kim, M., & Park, H. J. (2016). *Molecular Mechanisms of Skin Aging and Rejuvenation.* https://core.ac.uk/download/322426446.pdf (accessed on 11th June 2025).

19. Kyriakoudi, A., Redovniković, I. R., Vidović, S., Radošević, K., Andreou, T., Mourtzinos, I., & Cvjetko Bubalo, M. (2024). Coupling deep eutectic solvents with innovative extraction techniques towards plant derived bioactive compositions. *RSC Sustainability, 2*, 1675–1691. https://doi.org/10.1039/d4su00111g (accessed on 11th June 2025).

20. Lee, M. (2012). *The Expanding "Cosmeceutical" Conundrum: The Growing Need for Heightened FDA Regulations in The Face of Modern-Day Cosmeceuticals.* https://core.ac.uk/download/28938428.pdf (accessed on 11th June 2025).

21. Li, Y., Stewart, D. A., Ye, X., Yin, L., Pathmasiri, W., McRitchie, S., Fennell, T., et al. (2019). A metabolomics approach to investigate Kukoamine B—A potent natural product with anti-diabetic properties. *Frontiers in Pharmacology, 9.* https://www.semanticscholar.org/paper/e9c4ef2ea6fc857c6905c0659062a7277ac9e12d (accessed on 11th June 2025).

22. Liu, J. K. (2022). Natural products in cosmetics. *Natural Products and Bioprospecting, 12.* https://doi.org/10.1007/s13659-022-00363-y (accessed on 11th June 2025).

23. Mazurkiewicz-Pisarek, A., Baran, J., & Ciach, T. (2023). Antimicrobial peptides: Challenging journey to the pharmaceutical, biomedical, and cosmeceutical use. *International Journal of*

Molecular Sciences, 24, 9031–9031. https://doi.org/10.3390/ijms24109031 (accessed on 11th June 2025).

24. Michalak, M., Pierzak, M., Kręcisz, B., & Suliga, E. (2021). Bioactive compounds for skin health: A review. *Nutrients, 13*, 203–203. https://doi.org/10.3390/nu13010203 (accessed on 11th June 2025).

25. Mohammed, Y. H. (2012). *Targeted Topical Delivery of Peptides and Small Molecules to The Skin.* https://core.ac.uk/download/195692716.pdf (accessed on 11th June 2025).

26. Namjoshi, S. M. (2009). *Development of Novel Carriers for Transdermal Delivery of Peptides.* https://core.ac.uk/download/195632962.pdf (accessed on 11th June 2025).

27. Nimisha, & Singh, A. (2024). Exploring marine-derived bioactive for innovative cosmeceutical applications: A review. *Journal of Applied and Natural Science, 16*, 478–494. https://doi.org/10.31018/jans.v16i2.5433 (accessed on 11th June 2025).

28. Oliveira, A. S., Ferreira, C., Pereira, J. O., Pintado, M., & Carvalho, A. P. (2022). Spent brewer's yeast (*Saccharomyces cerevisiae*) as a potential source of bioactive peptides: An overview. *International Journal of Biological Macromolecules, 208*, 1116–1126. https://doi.org/10.1016/j.ijbiomac.2022.03.094 (accessed on 11th June 2025).

29. Pagac, M., Gempeler, M., & Campiche, R. (2024). A new generation of postbiotics for skin and scalp: *In situ* production of lipid metabolites by *Malassezia*. *Microorganisms, 12*, 1711–1711. https://doi.org/10.3390/microorganisms12081711 (accessed on 11th June 2025).

30. Papadopoulou, S. N. A., Anastasiou, E. A., Adamantidi, T., Ofrydopoulou, A., Letsiou, S., & Τσούπρας, A. (2025). A comprehensive review on the beneficial roles of vitamin D in skin health as a bio-functional ingredient in nutricosmetic, cosmeceutical, and cosmetic applications. *Applied Sciences, 15*, 796–796. https://doi.org/10.3390/app15020796 (accessed on 11th June 2025).

31. Pardo, A., Fiorini, V., Zangani, A., Faccioni, P., Signoriello, A., Albanese, M., & Lombardo, G. (2024). Topical agents in biofilm disaggregation: A systematic review and meta-analysis. *Journal of Clinical Medicine, 13.* https://www.semanticscholar.org/paper/c206f8a204363c2f208f838773fe5e1a2fa8da56 (accessed on 11th June 2025).

32. Paterska, M., Czerny, B., & Cielecka-Piontek, J. (2024). Macrofungal extracts as a source of bioactive compounds for cosmetical anti-aging therapy: A comprehensive review. *Nutrients, 16*, 2810–2810. https://doi.org/10.3390/nu16162810 (accessed on 11th June 2025).

33. Prakoeswa, F. R. S., Maharani, F., Satria, Y. A. A., Awanis, G. S., & Febrianty, A. F. (2024). Topical anti-aging agents: State-of-the-art review. *Journal of the Medical Sciences (Berkala Ilmu Kedokteran).* https://www.semanticscholar.org/paper/cbc16555a73843d916493c7c9ae5e5dfe4cdd859 (accessed on 11th June 2025).

34. Rodrigues, C. V., & Pintado, M. (2024). Hesperidin from orange peel as a promising skincare bioactive: An overview. *International Journal of Molecular Sciences, 25*, 1890–1890. https://doi.org/10.3390/ijms25031890 (accessed on 11th June 2025).

35. Sadick, N. S., Pannu, S., Abidi, Z., & Arruda, S. (2023). Topical treatments for photoaged skin. *PubMed, 22*, 867–873. https://doi.org/10.36849/jdd.7753 (accessed on 11th June 2025).

36. Salvioni, L., Morelli, L., Ochoa, E., Labra, M., Fiandra, L., Palugan, L., Prosperi, D., et al. (2021). The emerging role of nanotechnology in skincare. *Advances in Colloid and Interface Science, 293*,

102437–102437. https://doi.org/10.1016/j.cis.2021.102437 (accessed on 11th June 2025).

37. Sartawi, Z., Blackshields, C., & Faisal, W. (2022). Dissolving microneedles: Applications and growing therapeutic potential. *Journal of Controlled Release, 348*, 186–205. https://doi.org/10.1016/j.jconrel.2022.05.045 (accessed on 11th June 2025).

38. Shaikh, H. S. (2022). Cosmeceutical from marine origin and their collection, isolation and extraction: A review. *Research Journal of Topical and Cosmetic Sciences.* https://www.semanticscholar.org/paper/d477aa72fae03d2ff0a334bb919805e9a98a39a9 (accessed on 11th June 2025).

39. Tavakkol, A., DuBois, J. C., & Gupta, A. K. (2024). Systemic absorption and safety of topical terbinafine hydrochloride 10% solution (MOB015B): A phase 1 maximal usage trial in patients with moderate-to-severe onychomycosis. *Antimicrobial Agents and Chemotherapy, 68.* https://www.semanticscholar.org/paper/75efaa2c245f48c5e8cfde0bb482bb37964ffc47 (accessed on 11th June 2025).

40. Umar, S., Kan, P., Carter, M., & Shitabata, P. (2022). Treatment-refractory central centrifugal cicatricial alopecia responsive to a novel botanical treatment. *Clinical, Cosmetic and Investigational Dermatology, 15*, 609–619. https://www.semanticscholar.org/paper/fb0e3dae69888392c377053e6b0d6ffd672e0e8a (accessed on 11th June 2025).

41. Vora, L. K., Gholap, A. D., Hatvate, N. T., Naren, P., Khan, S. S., Chavda, V. P., Balar, P. C., et al. (2024). Essential oils for clinical aromatherapy: A comprehensive review. *Journal of Ethnopharmacology, 330*, 118180–118180. https://doi.org/10.1016/j.jep.2024.118180 (accessed on 11th June 2025).

42. Zazuli, Z., Hartati, R., Rowa, C. R., Asyarie, S., & Satrialdi, S. (2025). The potential application of nanocarriers in delivering topical antioxidants. *Pharmaceuticals, 18*, 56–56. https://doi.org/10.3390/ph18010056 (accessed on 11th June 2025).

43. Zheng, X. Q., Zhang, X. H., Gao, H., Huang, L., Ye, J., Ye, J. H., Lu, J. L., et al. (2024). Green tea catechins and skin health. *Antioxidants, 13*, 1506–1506. https://doi.org/10.3390/antiox13121506 (accessed on 11th June 2025).

PHOTOPROTECTION AND SUNSCREENS

4

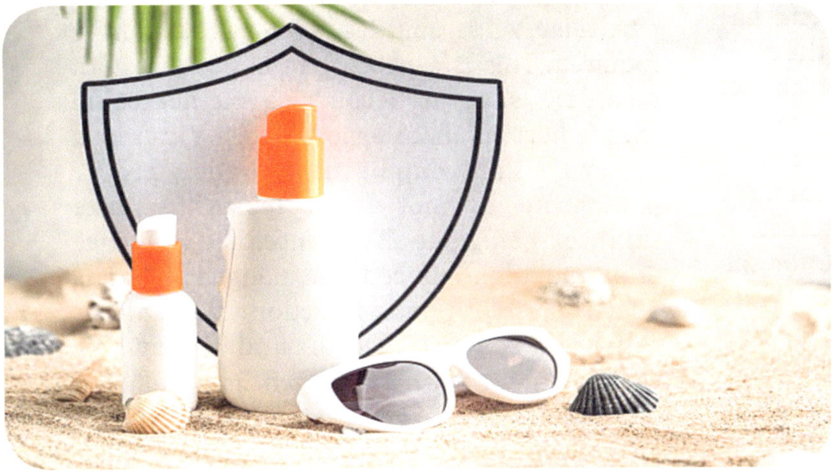

LEARNING OBJECTIVES

After studying this chapter, you will be able to:

1. Understand the science of UV radiation
2. Discuss the mechanisms of photoprotection
3. Explain the types of sunscreens
4. Describe sunscreen protection factor (SPF) and its significance
5. Focus on application and usage guidelines
6. Deal with controversies and misconceptions

Introduction

In the science of dermatology, the importance of photoprotection and the application of sunscreens cannot be overstated. The human skin is exposed to all kinds of environmental stressors around the clock, and among them the ultraviolet (UV) radiation that the sun emits is extremely harmful. This kind of exposure can lead to a whole array of damaging effects, ranging from photoaging, immune suppression, to even skin malignancies. Sunscreens function as a crucial line of defense by either absorbing or reflecting UV light, hence minimizing its penetration into the skin. Because of the escalating incidence rates of skin cancer and other related diseases, an educated awareness of photoprotection practices is invaluable. The task of developing effective sunscreens is a formidable one; they must be broad-spectrum protectors and yet cosmetically pleasing, and this puts extreme demands upon research and development in this field. Recent developments in sunscreen formulation have taken advantage of a range of bioactive chemicals that not only enhance photoprotection but also confer other benefits to the skin. The application of ferulic acid, for instance, is becoming more actively sought after due to its generalized benefits to the skin. It also acts as a potent antioxidant that combats free radicals formed under UV light, which otherwise enhance skin damage and aging. Ferulic acid further preserves the structural integrity of the skin by protecting against keratinocytes and fibroblasts, thereby avoiding loss of collagen and elastin. As a photoprotectant, ferulic acid has uses beyond its use as a protectant for the skin. It also facilitates wound healing and inhibits melanogenesis, suggesting that modern-day sunscreens are shifting towards having a more holistic philosophy of skincare that addresses both protection and anti-aging. This interaction of active ingredients is full of promise for the battle against skin aging and damage. While major advances have been achieved in the understanding of photoprotection and the efficacy of sunscreens, the exposome itself offers a compelling new horizon in skin health research. The exposome is not only UV radiation but also encompasses other environmental and lifestyle exposures that together impact skin aging and health. Elucidation of the exposome will be necessary to design more effective sunscreens and preventive strategies against skin damage. The newest studies target the identification of these diverse factors and their complex interactions to finally tackle the individual needs of the skin in a sophisticated manner. As the environmental exposures and aging of the skin a better comprehension, technology in photoprotection programs will be forced to continue to evolve to develop solid coverages for skin integrity in an increasingly demanding environment (Krutmann et al., 2016). Increasing our understanding of the skin's exposome will be the future guide in defining the direction of sun care products and practices.

Definition of Photoprotection

Photoprotection is the biological and therapeutic process employed in shielding the skin against harmful UV radiation, which has been proven to speed up skin damage and cancer risk. Photoprotection may have natural or man-made explanations, such as employing sunscreens. The natural barrier property of the skin, in addition to pigments like melanin, provides some protection against UV. However, in circumstances of heightened sun exposure or in patients with particular vulnerabilities, added protection is required. This is especially so in patients with disorders such as xeroderma pigmentosum (XP), where minimal exposure to UV can lead to severe skin complications. Hence, proper photoprotection not only helps to maximize skin well-being but also reduces the incidence of UV radiation-induced skin malignancies. The effectiveness of photoprotection interventions relies on environmental and behavioral determinants. Recent research has examined individually targeted interventions, specifically concerning patient experience among high-risk groups. A case in point is research among patients with XP, where they evaluated the XPAND program for increasing adherence to various photoprotection behaviors, such as frequent sunscreen application and protective clothing. Participants showed increased self-confidence as well as higher participation in protective behaviors, proving the contribution of psychosocial factors to the use of proper measures (Walburn et al., 2023). Tailored interventions such as these illustrate the importance of individualized measures to enhance photoprotection, which can result in better outcomes for persons with varying exposure to risk. In addition, the shift in the composition of cosmetic products is due to a heightened sensitivity to the environment and health consequences associated with photoprotection products. Traditional sunscreens made up of organic UV filters have come under criticism based on ecotoxicity concerns, which has necessitated the innovation of inorganic filters as safer substitutes. Despite being environmentally friendly, there are application and conformity problems with consumers. The performance of such contemporary sunscreens is often reliant on the physical aspects of the product, with careful particle morphology choice and evaluation for efficacy and stability (Tortini et al., 2022). An understanding of these forces is crucial when creating sustainable photoprotection solutions that safeguard not only individual skin wellness but also broader environmental issues with respect to cosmetic products (Figure 4.1).

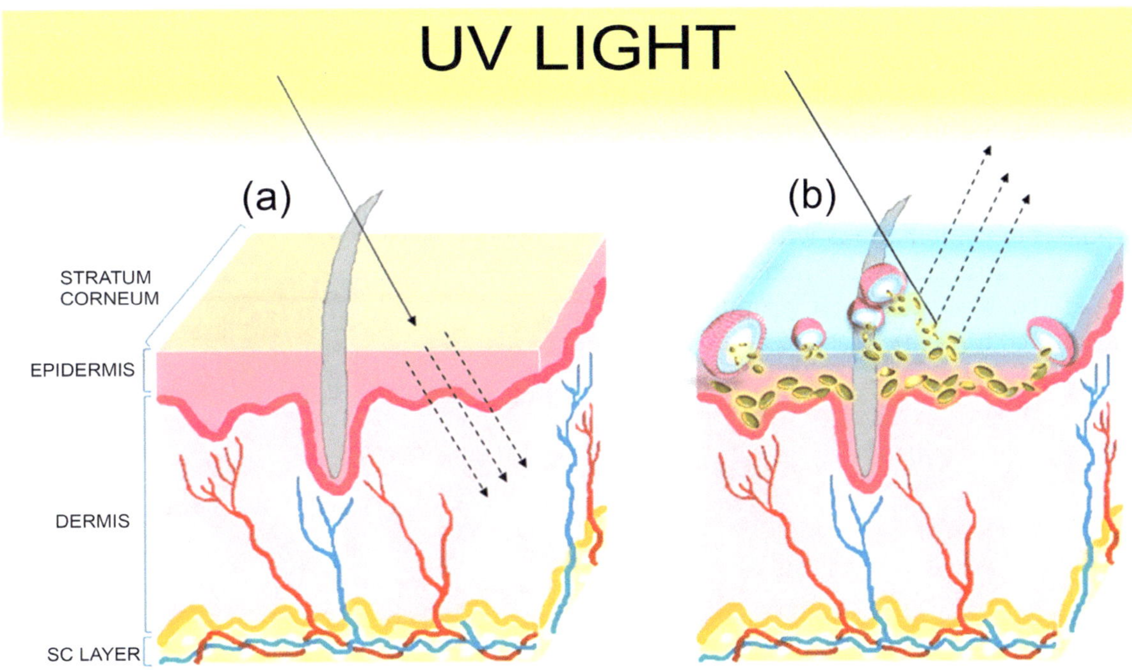

Figure 4.1. Mechanism of photoprotection. (a) Unprotected skin exposed to UV light absorbs the harmful radiation; and (b) In skin protected with phytoactive nanoformulations.

Source: https://www.researchgate.net/publication/343483634/figure/fig3/AS:941839058223123@1601563338843/Mechanism-of-photoprotection-a-Unprotected-skin-exposed-to-UV-light-absorbs-the-harmful.png.

Importance of Sunscreens in Skin Health

Sunscreens are important in the maintenance of skin health through the protection from the harmful effects of UV light. The risk for developing various types of skin cancers, including melanoma and non-melanoma cancers, is significantly increased by exposure to UV light, which is significantly linked to sunburns as well as chronic UV exposure. This toxic insult not only initiates the processes of carcinogenesis but also increases the process of photoaging, involving wrinkles, loss of turgor, and color changes. Through competent absorption or reflection of UV light, sunscreens are a first line of defense against cutaneous damage. The importance of the correct application of sunscreen is underscored by the concurrence that chronic exposure to UV light is the most widespread etiology for skin cancer worldwide, contributing to the necessity of enacting this protective measure as a routine skin care regimen (Maier & Korting, 2005). Sunscreens' effectiveness, however, varies with the application and formulation efficiency. Some users do not apply sunscreens in correct quantities or do not apply them at intervals as required, and this more or less nullifies their protective benefits. There are issues with the range of sunscreens as they are available, because some of them do not protect the full spectrum of UV light. Inorganic sunscreens such as zinc oxide and titanium dioxide are broad-spectrum protective but potentially less cosmetically elegant than organic analogues that have the potential to elicit allergic reactions. Recent developments in sunscreen technology, such as micronization of minerals and the development of combinations with DNA repair enzymes and antioxidants, are indicative of the ongoing efforts to render these products more efficient and convenient (Masnec et al., 2010).

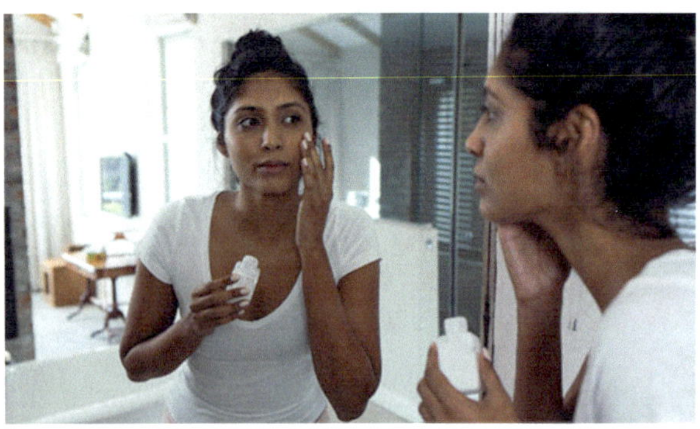

Figure 4.2. A woman applying skincare product while looking into a mirror, emphasizing the importance of daily skincare routines such as sunscreen application for maintaining healthy and protected skin.

Source: https://www.hopkinsmedicine.org/-/media/images/health/3_-wellness/skin-and-hair-care/sunscreen-teaser.jpg.

Moreover, it should be noted that sunscreens need to be part of a comprehensive photoprotection policy. While sunscreens are highly effective against the penetration of hazardous UV wavelengths, they also have their disadvantages, such as the susceptibility to photoinactivation, where UV exposure deactivates the product's protective effect. Combining other types of protection, such as sun avoidance, use of protective clothing, and antioxidants, will aid in facilitating healthy skin. The additive action of these protective practices not only reduces the incidence of skin cancers but also reverses some signs of prior photodamage. In turn, ensuring adequate photoprotection through the use of sunscreen application and other adjunctive practices is vital to preserving the integrity of the skin and stopping the long-term consequences of excessive exposure to sunlight (Maier & Korting, 2005) (Figure 4.2).

4.1. The Science of UV Radiation

Learning Outcome

1. Explain the types of UV radiation
2. Discuss the effects of UV radiation on skin cells
3. Understand the role of UV radiation in skin aging and cancer

The relationship between UV radiation and skin well-being constitutes a crucial area of study under photoprotection, therefore indicating the need to minimize its detrimental effects by using effective mechanisms. UV radiation, primarily categorized into UVA and UVB, poses a number of risks to human skin. UVA radiation penetrates deeply and causes oxidative stress and long-term effects such as photoaging and skin cancer. On the other hand, UVB radiation affects predominantly the outer skin layers and induces erythema or sunburn. The mechanisms that cause such damages, like the destruction of collagen and DNA modification, highlight the necessity for protection against UV-induced damage. Experiments have established the effectiveness of some antioxidants and plant extracts against the deleterious phototoxicity of

UV radiation, and these have formed a foundation for advanced photoprotection technology based on these natural agents in favor of dermal well-being (Sharma, 2024). Sunscreen formulation and performance are also central to effective photoprotection against UV radiation. Sunscreens contain active ingredients that function as UV filters, reflecting or absorbing harmful radiation before skin penetration. It plays a vital role in preventing immediate damage, such as sunburn, and long-term skin disease caused by UV exposure. Recent scientific findings have promoted interest in the synthesis of nature-based, microbial UV filters, which hold promise to be less toxic to both human health and the environment. This paradigm shift addresses not only safety concerns with traditional chemical sunscreens but also underscores the potential of innovative solutions in photoprotection. Consequently, current research aims to enhance sunscreen products for more efficient and safer consumption by consumers for effective protection against UV radiation (Schalka et al., 2014). The addition of antioxidants to sunscreens represents an emerging trend toward improved photoprotection. Beyond their classic role as UV filters, antioxidants possess the ability to neutralize free radicals generated by UV exposure, thereby providing a second line of defense against photodamage. This complementary approach underscores the utility of a multi-pronged approach to the protection of skin health, as antioxidants would also be expected to be anti-inflammatory and to enhance mechanisms of skin repair. Furthermore, studies on novel photoprotective compounds, such as mycosporine-like amino acid-type UV filters, shed light on advanced mechanisms of protection beyond traditional methods. With ongoing advancements of scientific research into the complexities of the impact of UV radiation on the skin, the future promise of photoprotection will aim towards an integrated approach that combines conventional sunscreens with nature-derived and biomimetic materials to enhance optimal skin health and resistance to UV-induced damage (Schalka et al., 2014; Sharma, 2024).

4.1.1. Types of UV Radiation: UVA and UVB

The understanding of UV radiation and its subdivisions holds central relevance in the context of photoprotection and sunscreens. The sun's UV radiation consists predominantly of UVA and UVB radiation, both of which have different roles in the induction of skin damage. UVA with a longer wavelength penetrates deeper into the skin and is predominantly responsible for inducing oxidative stress, leading to photo-aging of the skin and photocarcinogenesis. This type of radiation can cause indirect DNA damage through the production of reactive oxygen species (ROS), which poses a risk to skin disease, including melanoma and non-melanoma cancers. Although extensively engaged in skin pathology, UVA rays have previously not been given as much attention as UVB rays under sun protection, producing a gap in public awareness and preventive interventions (Denisa et al., 2020). On the other hand, UVB radiation with its smaller wavelength in essence attacks the outermost skin layers and leads to sunburns and erythema. They are the ones that directly induce DNA damage in the form of pyrimidine dimers that ultimately lead to genetic mutations and skin cancer. UVB rays are also critical in the body's synthesis of vitamin D; that said, an enormous amount of UVB exposure is harmful since it induces a strong immune reaction that causes inflammation of the skin as well as an increased risk of skin malignancies. The dual character of UVB justifies that complete sun protection should embrace UVA as well as UVB protection for effectively countering the damage to the skin and promoting the health of the skin (Denisa et al., 2020). An efficient photoprotective effect is required when one considers the synergistic effects of antivirus and antioxidant molecules in sunscreen products. The incorporation of phytochemicals, such as ferulic acid, has also been remarked upon as an effective approach to enhancing photoprotection. Ferulic acid includes a number of protective functions on the skin, including antioxidant effects, that can counteract the detrimental activity of both UVA and UVB light. The ability of ferulic acid to suppress melanogenesis and induce angiogenesis further supports the value of adding such compounds to sunscreens. This sun-break-through formulation not only broaches traditional UV protection but also offers potential benefits to skin rejuvenation and anti-aging, making phytochemicals a key research area in the field of photoprotection (Figure 4.3).

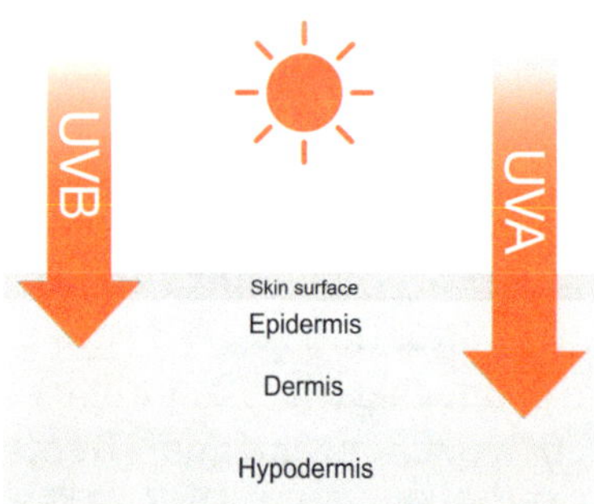

Figure 4.3. Types of UV radiation.

Source: https://www.iqskintelligence.com/home/wp-content/uploads/2018/04/IQ_UVAUVB_3.jpg.

4.1.2. Effects of UV Radiation on Skin Cells

The action of UV light on skin cells is profound in that it is one of the primary causes of both acute and chronic damage to the skin. Chronic exposure to UV light, for instance, leads to various forms of skin cancer, from malignant melanoma to non-melanoma skin cancers such as squamous cell carcinoma and basal cell carcinoma. The damage caused by UV radiation initiates a chain of cellular changes, especially in the DNA of skin cells, resulting in mutations that can initiate tumorigenesis. Also, exposure to UV radiation brings about photoaging as wrinkles, decreased elasticity of the skin, and mottling of the skin color, making an understanding of the cellular dynamics all the more critical. The perennial threat from UV radiation necessitates effective photoprotection strategies, hence highlighting the urgent need for sunscreens in neutralizing such detrimental impacts on skin cells, as evidenced by rising demand for new defense products (Maier & Korting, 2005). New research explains the mechanisms through which UV radiation damages the skin, particularly among those with heightened sensitivity, e.g., victims of lupus disorder. Patients with cutaneous and systemic lupus erythematosus experience more severe skin lesions following exposure to UV light, which predicts a close association between the underlying pathophysiology and UV radiation. Photosensitivity reactions in such patients demonstrate that UV light can trigger immune mechanisms leading to inflammation of the skin and cell apoptosis. Standardized assays have been defined to classify patients with photosensitive disease, and they offer a clinical rationale for treatment. Understanding these mechanisms not only explains the risk UV light presents to vulnerable individuals but also emphasizes the importance of effective photoprotection measures, including the development of certain sunscreens that will defend delicate skin and minimize UV-induced damage (Cazenave et al., 1997). Sunscreen technology has evolved, allowing for full-spectrum protection against both UVA and UVB radiation that causes skin injury. In recent years, inorganic sunscreens such as zinc oxide and titanium dioxide have gained more popularity since they are broad-spectrum and less likely to cause allergic reactions compared to their organic counterparts. Though they are better, sunscreens lose their effectiveness through poor application and evolving ideas regarding how UV light damages the skin at the cellular level. The introduction of innovations in sunscreen technology, such as encapsulation and micronization, seeks to enhance photoprotection as well as address consumer expectations for cosmetic acceptability. Nevertheless, continued revelation of systemic toxicity concerns related to organic sunscreens still occurs, and thus the demand for ongoing studies that ensure protective products' safety and efficacy with new scientific data regarding UV radiation's detrimental effects on skin cells (Maier & Korting, 2005) (Figure 4.4).

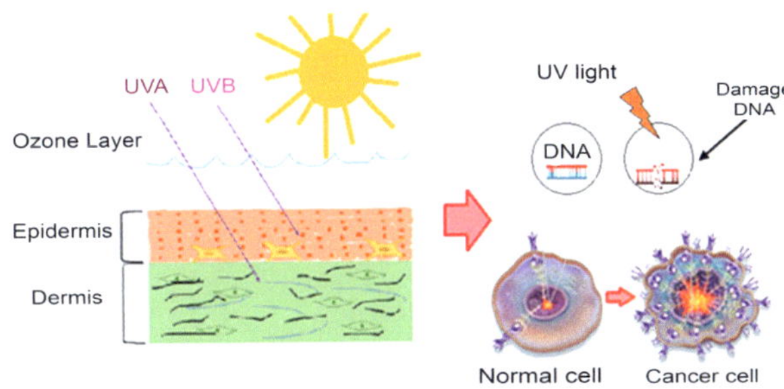

Figure 4.4. Effect of UV radiation on human skin. UV: ultraviolet; UVA: ultraviolet A; UVB: ultraviolet B.

Source: https://www.researchgate.net/publication/373205849/figure/fig2/AS:11431281212401830@1702597265950/Effect-of-UV-radiation-on-human-skin-UV-ultraviolet-UVA-ultraviolet-A-UVB.tif.

4.1.3. Role of UV Radiation in Skin Aging and Cancer

The role of UV radiation in skin aging and the development of skin cancer is a key area of research in photoprotection. UV radiation, primarily classified as UVA and UVB rays, is harmful to the health of the skin. UVA rays penetrate deeply into the skin and promote photoaging by inducing collagen degradation and the development of free radicals. Meanwhile, the UVB radiation is mainly responsible for sunburn and plays a direct role in initiating damage to the DNA at the cellular level. This damage has the potential to cause mutations leading to derangement of normal cellular function and, consequently, skin cancer formation. The understanding of these mechanisms stresses the importance of effective photoprotection mechanisms, as it is apparent that acute and chronic exposure to UV has cumulative effects compromising the integrity of the skin and elevating oncogenic risk. As such, taking adequate protective measures against UV radiation becomes an imperative in preventing its harmful effects. Current studies have provided insight into the multifaceted impact of UV radiation on skin health, highlighting the interaction between UV radiation and natural aging processes. The evidence suggests that, while sunburn is a definitive risk factor for the development of skin cancer, chronic exposure to moderate UV radiation in the long term may not be directly linked to an increased risk of skin aging. This train of thought opposes conventional thought regarding sunlight exposure and proposes that moderate, long-term sun exposure may possess some protective mechanisms against skin cancer through inducing a sort of adaptive response in skin cells. However, this relative understanding necessitates a cautious practice of sun exposure, as it should be realized that moderate exposure may not be detrimental, but prolonged and acute exposure remains a grave risk that necessitates aversive sunscreens and measures to maintain skin well-being in varied circumstances (Chiou, 2024). The addition of antioxidants and plant preparations to sunscreen formulations is gaining greater recognition as a novel approach to enhancing skin protection against damage induced by UV. Research has proved that phytochemical molecules, such as polyphenols found in green and black tea, play significant photoprotective functions. Not only do these antioxidants neutralize free radicals induced by UV, but they also fortify the skin's own protective mechanisms against oxidative stress (Sharma, 2024). Botanical-based sunscreens are, therefore, emerging as a go-green option for those seeking to adopt healthy skincare without sacrificing the protection offered by UV radiation. Furthermore, the development of products blending traditional sunscreen chemistry with herbal infusions signals a shift in paradigm towards more natural, effective photoprotection strategies. This union of science and herbal remedy shows the call for continued investigation on new means of preserving skin integrity and preventing the degenerative effects of UV radiation (Figure 4.5).

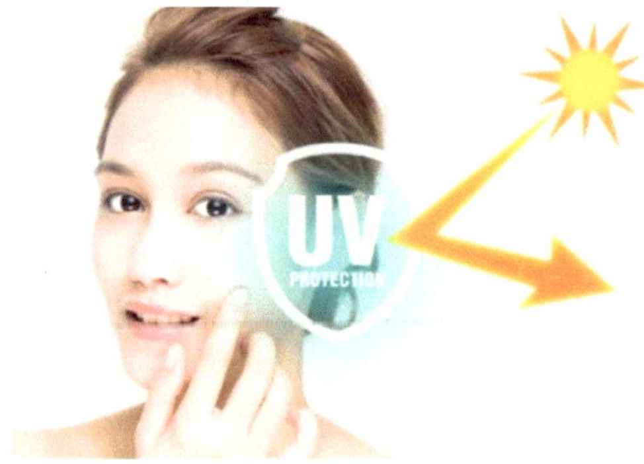

Figure 4.5. Conceptual image illustrating ultraviolet (UV) protection.

Source: https://www.shutterstock.com/image-photo/beautiful-woman-sunscreen-uv-protection-260nw-558756334.jpg.

Test Your Knowledge

1. What are the different types of UV radiation (UVA, UVB, UVC), and how do they each affect the skin?
2. How does melanin protect the skin from UV-induced damage, and what are its limitations?

4.2. Mechanisms of Photoprotection

Learning Outcome

1. Describe biological photoprotection mechanisms
2. Understand chemical photoprotection through antioxidants
3. Define physical barriers in photoprotection

Photoprotection processes are multifaceted and also play the critical function of safeguarding the skin against harmful ultraviolet (UV) light. The primary function of photoprotection is its ability to absorb or deflect UV radiation so that it cannot penetrate the skin. Traditional sunscreens typically contain chemical compounds that absorb UV light and transform it into less harmful wavelengths of energy. Through continued study, there is, nevertheless, increased interest in the plant- and microalga-derived natural photoprotectants that possess UV-absorbing properties. These compounds not only protect a physical shield against systemic damage to the skin but also strengthen the skin's own repair mechanisms, thus evading the hazard of premature skin aging and skin cancers due to UV exposure. The ongoing research on these natural compounds and their mechanisms of action underscores the importance of enhancing the efficacy of the conventional sunscreen products in the management of most skin conditions caused by UV radiation (Gupta et al., 2023). Apart from the chemical barriers, the second major aspect of photoprotection involves the presence of endogenous mechanisms within the skin to regulate the action of UV radiation. When exposed to UV radiation, cells in the skin initiate repair mechanisms by way of signaling pathways, one of them being to activate enzymes for DNA repair. These enzymes work diligently to repair the damage induced by UV light, hence preserving cell integrity and preventing malignancies. Photoprotective intervention research highlights the importance of supplementing these natural repair mechanisms, particularly for individuals at high risk of UV-induced damage, such as those with rare genetic disorders, including xeroderma pigmentosum (XP). In XP patients, photoprotection is crucial because their ability to repair DNA damage induced by UV light is severely compromised. Thus, activation and comprehension of such endogenous mechanisms represent a new frontier to facilitate photoprotection practices among healthy people as well as individuals with inherited susceptibility (Sainsbury et al., 2017). Moreover, the role of behavioral interventions in facilitating effective photoprotection cannot be overemphasized. Adherence to photoprotection advice, including routine use of sunscreen and protective clothes, is crucial for the attainment of optimal results. Behavioral psychology offers data on the determinants of individuals' sun protection behavior and makes recommendations for specific interventions to modify perception of UV risk and the importance of photoprotection. As is observed in investigations in populations with augmented susceptibility to UV damage, such as XP patients, individually tailored education programs can effectively raise awareness and enhance compliance with protective practices. By combining psychological understanding with the science of photoprotection, we can develop integrated approaches that not just address the physical aspects of protection of the skin but also the behavioral drivers that facilitate long-term engagement in safe sun practices. This two-pronged strategy can potentially make a significant impact on health outcomes by reducing the incidence of skin conditions resulting from UV radiation exposure (Sainsbury et al., 2017).

4.2.1. Biological Photoprotection Mechanisms

The skin's biological photoprotection mechanisms are invaluable in maintaining defense against the harmful effect of UV radiation. One of the primary protectors is melanin, as it absorbs UV radiation and prevents DNA damage by reducing oxidative stress. The amount and structure of melanin vary considerably between individuals based on susceptibility to disease and damage of the skin. Fair skin types, which contain lesser amounts of melanin, inherently possess a SPF of about 3.3 and are thus more prone to photoaging and UV radiation-induced skin cancers. On the other hand, those who possess darker skin types, which contain greater amounts of eumelanin, may possess increased photoprotection but remain at risk for the development of diseases like post-inflammatory hyperpigmentation (PIH). It is necessary to recognize these differences to develop individualized strategies for photoprotection that correspond to the unique needs of various skin types (Brar et al., 2025). In addition to melanin, structural components of the skin also play a role in the intrinsic photoprotection of the skin. The epidermis is a physical barrier that reflects and absorbs UV radiation, and other cellular processes, such as DNA repair functions, also fight UV-induced damage. Keratinocytes, the predominant cell type of the epidermis, play a pivotal role in these repair processes since they employ DNA photolyases and other repair enzymes to fix damage caused by UV. Moreover, antioxidants in the skin, such as ascorbic acid and tocopherols, detoxify the ROS generated by UV irradiation and consequently decrease oxidative stress and hinder cellular damage. These biological defense mechanisms serve to emphasize the role of inherent properties of the skin in the management of UV risks and suggest the requirement for the incorporation of antioxidants within skin care regimes to enhance the resistance of the skin to photodamage (Gabbanini et al., 2024). Parallel to this, photoprotection by biological means extends to the application of topical photoprotective agents, e.g., sunscreens, to further enhance the natural defenses of the skin. These agents function by absorbing, reflecting, or scattering UV radiation, and thus diminishing its penetration into the skin. Broad-spectrum preparations that protect against both UVA and UVB rays are especially useful because each has its own mechanisms of injury; UVA plays a role in chronic aging of the skin and collagen degradation, whereas UVB causes sunburn and carcinogenesis. The effectiveness of sunscreens can be enhanced even further by incorporating compounds that enhance the biological photoprotection pathways of the skin, such as vitamins and phytochemicals with antioxidant activity. Synergizing the biochemical effects of biological photoprotection using topical products offers individuals total measures of skin protection that deal with all the detrimental effects of UV radiation (Gabbanini et al., 2024; Brar et al., 2025) (Figure 4.6).

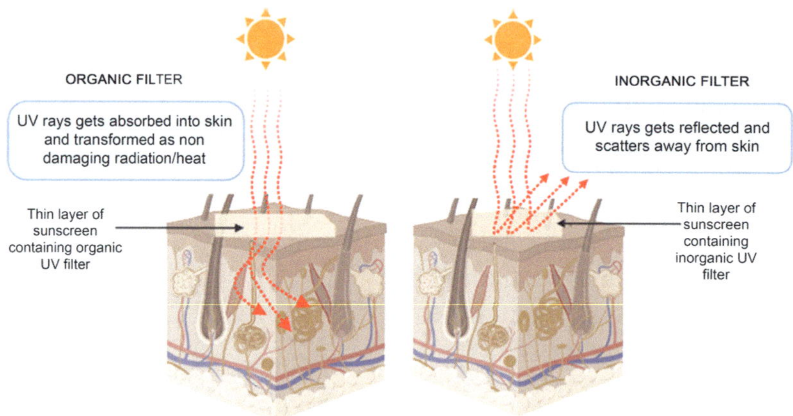

Figure 4.6. Mechanism involved in photoprotection.

Source: https://www.researchgate.net/publication/380939544/figure/fig3/AS:11431281252589297@1718777861060/Mechanism-involved-in-photoprotection-provided-by-inorganic-and-organic-sunscreens.png

4.2.2. Chemical Photoprotection Through Antioxidants

The interaction of visible light with skin cells has posed the risk of oxidative stress and consequent cellular damage, primarily by photosensitization of melanin. Current studies have highlighted the protective role of antioxidants against this risk by demonstrating photoprotective activity. Antioxidants such as apigenin, chrysin, and beta-carotene have demonstrated great potential in scavenging radical chain reactions and singlet oxygen produced during visible light irradiation. This protective role is relevant as oxidative stress has been implicated in diseases like the aging of the skin and even skin cancer. It has been revealed by studies that these antioxidants not only function via scavenging ROS but are also capable of enhancing the viability of the skin cells against melanin damage, thereby playing a crucial role in their application in topical preparations. Accordingly, the inclusion of these compounds in sunscreens may offer more protection beyond the conventional UV filters (Freitas et al., 2018). Additionally, ferulic acid is an imperative antioxidant with multi-potential benefits in skin health and photoprotection. Being of low toxicity, ferulic acid has different physiological activities, such as anti-inflammatory and antimicrobial activities. Its role as a free radical scavenger renders it a key component in anti-stress skin care preparations, counteracting the actions of environmental stressors such as UV. Through the inhibition of enzymes catalyzing the formation of free radicals, ferulic acid not only inhibits oxidative stress but also enhances the body's natural antioxidant defense systems. Apart from that, its shield also protects the skin's crucial structures, such as keratinocytes and collagen, thus exhibiting an anti-photoaging effect. Addition of ferulic acid to a sunscreen is an amazing breakthrough in photoprotection since it offers another layer of protection against skin damage caused by exposure to both UV-induced and visible light-induced damage (Zdu et al., 2018). The challenge facing the development of photoprotective is balancing antioxidant performance and stability. While beneficial, some antioxidants like ferulic acid are also prone to rapid oxidation, which could undermine their protective functions in the long term. To address this shortcoming, researchers are exploring advanced delivery mechanisms that facilitate stabilization and bioavailability of the antioxidants in skin care products. These technologies could bring to market sunscreens that not only absorb lethal UV radiation but also combat oxidative stress through extended antioxidant activity. Furthermore, the synergistic effect of blends of various antioxidants can reasonably improve protective actions while taking advantage of their modes of action against the multiple types of skin damage. In short, collaboration among chemical photoprotection by antioxidants and cutting-edge formulation strategies will be the future of sun care, towards more holistic solutions to skin health protection against environmental aggressors.

4.2.3. Physical Barriers in Photoprotection

Physical barriers used in photoprotection form a crucial component of effective sun protection, primarily through the use of mineral-based agents, such as titanium dioxide and zinc oxide. These agents work by forming a reflective coating that deflects and scatters UV light away from the skin and hence prevents cellular damage. Unlike chemical sunscreens, which are absorbed and released as heat, physical barriers create an immediate, protective barrier when applied. This feature is especially good for individuals who have sensitive skin or allergic tendencies because these mineral products are better tolerated and less likely to irritate. The widespread use of titanium dioxide, as detailed in the literature, has advanced due to its unique optical properties and performance in absorbing UV light, making it a norm in the majority of sunscreens today (Murase et al., 2017). In addition to the capacity to safeguard, physical sunscreens have been successful in lowering the likelihood of skin disease associated with UV radiation. Studies have proved that the major cause of sunburns and nonmelanoma carcinomas is the exposure of the skin to UV irradiance. Therefore, by employing physical sunscreens, one would not only be benefiting himself/her/hemself with short-term photoprotection but also would aid in maintaining long-term skin integrity and health. Their frequent use in everyday life is the established treatment for preventing photodamage currently, but issues remain regarding their proper use and application among consumers (Martinez, 2023). Educating consumers regarding the use and benefits of physical barriers to attain maximum effectiveness and thereby their photoprotective action is imperative. Also, the formulations developed with nanoparticles of titanium dioxide are important because they yield added cosmetic beauty as well as protective efficacy. The nanoparticles allow for a more transparent use without the usual white cast from traditional mineral sunscreens. Formulation development has helped to improve consumer acceptability and compliance, and they provide an easy way for people to incorporate photoprotection into their lifestyle. However, controversy over the safety and efficacy of nanoparticles continues, as more studies need to be conducted to ensure that these kinds of formulations do not pose systemic risks. Understanding the physics of physical sunscreens will provide a basis for better appreciating the need for considerable research and development in sun protection technologies, both safety and effectiveness in sun avoidance of UV-induced skin injury, and satisfying diverse consumer needs (Murase et al., 2017).

Test Your Knowledge

1. How do antioxidants contribute to photoprotection at the cellular level?
2. How do photostabilizers enhance the efficacy and durability of sunscreen formulations?

4.3. Types of Sunscreens

Learning Outcome

1. Understand chemical sunscreens and their active ingredients
2. Describe physical (mineral) sunscreens and their properties
3. Differentiate between broad-spectrum and non-broad-spectrum sunscreens

The broad range of sunscreens can be generally classified into two broad groups: chemical and physical (or mineral) sunscreens. Chemical sunscreens are based on the principle of absorption of UV radiation through active ingredients such as avobenzone, octisalate, or octocrylene. These chemicals emit a chemical reaction that transforms harmful rays into harmless heat, which is then removed from the skin. By comparison, physical sunscreens consist primarily of mineral ingredients like zinc oxide or titanium dioxide that sit on top of the skin and reflect the UV rays off the skin. This is important in that it controls how effective the product is, how suitable it is for various skin types, and how much it can irritate. With these features, physically sun-protected persons can also use physical sunscreens since they have a gentle composition reducing the frequency of unwanted effects typical in chemical equivalents, pointing to the significance of individualized sun protection routines. Apart from this, amongst these varieties, sunscreens further differ according to the spectrum of protection, whether broad-spectrum or single-spectrum. Broad-spectrum sunscreens defend the skin against both UVA and UVB radiation and thus provide broad protection against sunlight damage. UVA rays penetrate deep into the skin and induce photoaging and risk of skin cancer, while UVB rays induce sunburn and are a leading cause of skin cancer occurrence. Insofar as evidence shows, integration of broad-spectrum sunscreen habit in regular practice significantly decreases the risk of harmful skin diseases brought about by UV radiation, such as photodamage and cancers, emphasizing the importance of evidence-based sunscreen application choices in ensuring better skin health (Kotowicz et al., 2024). It is through an understanding of the variations between these properties that consumers can make better choices regarding their sun protective habits. Other than the active ingredients and protection spectrum, formulation and application of sunscreen influence its overall effectiveness. Sunscreen also comes in various forms, including sprays, lotions, gels, and sticks, with differences in ease of application and coverage. For instance, lotion forms can provide more comprehensive coverage, especially on large areas, while sprays can facilitate quick application. But proper application frequency and quantity are significant factors too often overlooked, most individuals apply too little sunscreen to achieve the labeled SPF protection. Research has shown that individuals underapply sunscreen, leading to suboptimal protection and increased risk of skin harm (Martinez, 2023).

Therefore, educating consumers on these points is critical to maintaining quality sun protection. Emphasizing comprehensive strategies, including adequate sunscreen application together with protective equipment, can substantially limit the harmful effects of UV rays on skin health.

4.3.1. Chemical Sunscreens and Their Active Ingredients

Chemical sunscreens are efficient due to their active ingredients, which are designed to absorb ultraviolet (UV) radiation and thus prevent harmful effects from taking place on the skin. Common ultraviolet filters such as octinoxate, avobenzone, and octisalate function by a chemical reaction that converts UV light to heat, which is removed from the skin. This photochemical transformation is subtle; it entails ultrafast molecular motion that could occur on femtosecond timescales, underscoring the rapidity of energy interconversion within these compounds upon exposure. Although noteworthy advancements have been made regarding how these ingredients work, knowledge gaps still linger regarding the nature of individual interactions and molecular mechanisms underpinning their activity. Studies continue to analyze the inherent characteristics of these chemicals to render them more protective in nature and less likely to cause skin irritation, and enhance skin compatibility, both crucial in providing consumer safety and efficacy (Rodrigues et al., 2018). The sun care industry has expanded exponentially in the last decade and has been fueled by growing consumer awareness of the dangers arising from UV exposure. This awareness has led to the demand for sun protection that is broad-spectrum and protective against both UVA and UVB radiation. As a result, professionals are continuously developing better formulations with newer active ingredients and delivery systems meant to offer optimum photoprotection. While various active ingredients can be employed, regulatory systems greatly influence the selection process in the creation of good sunscreens. For example, regulatory bodies in the European Union and Australia have approved a far broader group of effective agents than their counterparts in America, where the FDA, in turn, oversees sunscreens as drugs and under strict controls (Mohiuddin, 2020). As skin cancer rates rise, the addition of new actives in sunscreens grows more vital in the fight to maximize sun protection for the skin.

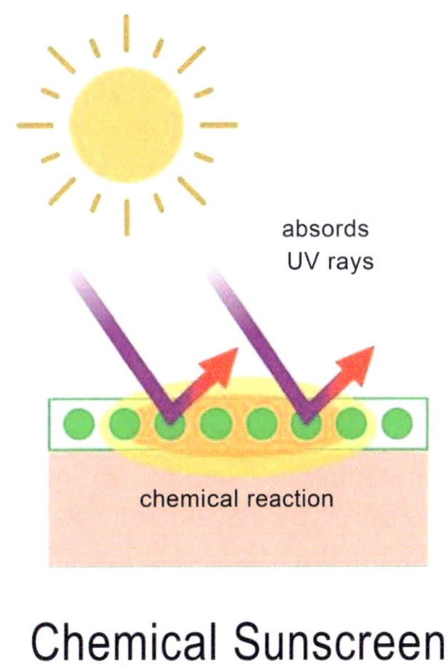

Figure 4.7. Chemical sunscreen.

Source: https://setsukobeauty.com/wp-content/uploads/2022/03/Chemical-vs-Physical-sunscreen.webp.

The relationship between innovation and regulation within the sun care sector is also made more complex by patent constraints as well as safety trials that local regulatory authorities put chemical active ingredients through. For instance, while the US FDA will allow fewer UV filters, others have embraced a broader and more diverse selection of ingredients. The difference highlights the ongoing challenge presented to formulators who want to deliver broad sun protection while complying with legally mandated standards. Moreover, the scientific community continues to call for further research on the long-term effects of the active ingredients of dominant sunscreens on human health as well as the environment. Owing to the growing demand for sunscreen products worldwide, resolving such regulatory and scientific concerns is important in order to provide consumers with safe, efficient, and science-based protection against the damaging effects of UV radiation (Mohiuddin, 2020). This union of innovation with efficacy and safety will ultimately shape the destiny of chemical sunscreens and their active ingredients, further upholding enhanced photoprotection practices worldwide (Rodrigues et al., 2018) (Figure 4.7).

4.3.2. Physical (Mineral) Sunscreens and Their Properties

Physical (or mineral) sunscreens are constituted mainly of naturally occurring minerals like zinc oxide and titanium dioxide. Mineral agents neither absorb UV radiation as chemical sunscreens do, but they work by creating a physical barrier on the skin that scatters and reflects cancerous UV rays. This unique mechanism not only provides broad-spectrum protection against UVA and UVB radiation but also diminishes skin irritation, a unique advantage for individuals with sensitive skin or rosacea-like conditions. Physical sunscreens' performance relies on a number of variables, including particle size and formulation viscosity.

Smaller particles, for instance, are likely to result in a more transparent application with preservation of protective functions. In addition, these physical sunblocks are also photostable, that is, they are not required to be reapplied as frequently as some chemical sunblocks, ultimately making them a viable option for long-term sun protection regimens. Studies have established that the incorporation of natural components into physical sunblocks can enhance their properties and overall effectiveness. Studies illustrate the ability of plant oils, such as açaí oil, to increase stability and cosmetic appeal in sunscreen products. For example, there has been a study of the preparation of O/W/O multiple emulsions that contained açaí oil and formed stable systems with desirable rheological properties. Astonishingly, the new formulations did not show a significant difference in their *in vivo* SPF from traditional formulations. This suggests that the inclusion of natural oils does not have to be at the cost of efficacy, thus providing a twin benefit of photoprotection plus skin nutrition. Improved formulation methods with natural ingredients represent a growing trend toward more all-encompassing sunscreens that balance efficacious protection with skin health. Additional technologies in sunscreens have led to the exploration of innovative delivery systems that maximize product effectiveness. New strategies include encapsulating sunscreen chemicals in nanocarriers or hydrogels, which may dramatically increase stability and penetration into the skin of active ingredients. These technologies are not only aiming towards improved UVA and UVB protection but also against the new issues regarding longer wavelengths, such as blue light. When scientists are learning about new types of radiation's biological effects, they are looking for effective physical filters that can have the potential to give protective capabilities from these newly recognized risks. The search for natural substances as photoprotectors, e.g., mycosporines and other flavonoids of plant origin, is an encouraging avenue towards safer and more effective sunscreen actives, emphasizing the synergy between science-driven innovation and nature-driven breakthroughs in photoprotection and sunscreens (Ferrari et al., 2011; Aguilera et al., 2023) (Figure 4.8).

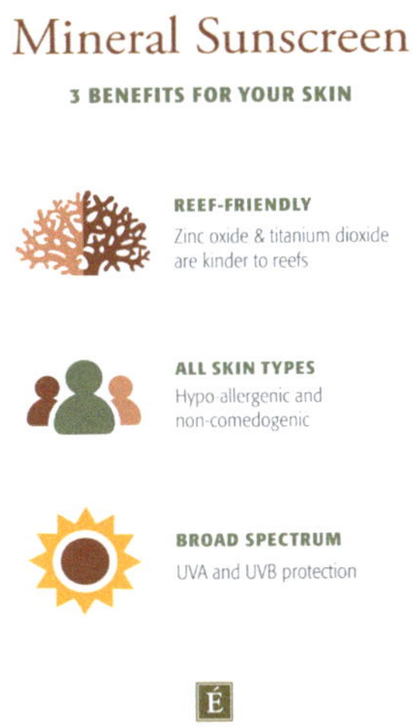

Figure 4.8. Benefits of mineral sunscreen.

Source: https://eminenceorganics.com/sites/default/files/content/blog/2025/3_benefits_of_mineral_sunscreen-1500x2250.jpg.

4.3.3. Broad-Spectrum vs. Non-Broad-Spectrum Sunscreens

The distinction between broad-spectrum and non-broad-spectrum sunscreens carries significant implications for protecting the skin from UV radiation. Broad-spectrum sunscreens are formulated to guard against both UVA and UVB radiation, which have been found to produce skin damage, photoaging, and the development of skin cancer. Non-broad-spectrum sunscreens, however, primarily shield the skin from UVB radiation, which is largely responsible for sunburn. While UVB protection is essential, the absence of UVA protection in non-broad-spectrum products might expose consumers to other ill effects, such as photoimmunosuppression and premature skin aging. The need for comprehensive photoprotection serves to emphasize the need to use broad-spectrum products to guard against a spectrum of damaging UV rays, exposing the limitation of using SPF levels alone as a gauge of sunscreen efficacy. The effectiveness of sunscreens is usually determined by their SPF, which is mainly for protection against UVB. Increasing acceptance of UVA contribution to causing skin damage, however, has seen a rethinking of the determination of sunscreen effectiveness. Current debate highlights that numerous non-filtering substances are capable of increasing sunscreen protection against numerous skin diseases other than erythema, including skin carcinogenesis and disorders of pigmentation. While standard SPF testing won't fully encompass the protection potential of such agents, adding others like UVA-PF would provide a more comprehensive feel for photoprotection offered by broad-spectrum and non-broad-spectrum products.

Thus, sunscreens' analysis has to be altered to consider the whole UV and visible light spectrum effect on the skin to ensure access to product performance information for both users and dermatologists (Gonz et al., 2022). Recent studies highlight the importance of formulating broad-spectrum sunscreens not only to shield against UV radiation but also against extrinsic reasons for skin aging, including pollution-generated oxidative stress and visible light-induced skin harm. Broad-spectrum sunscreens with antioxidant and anti-aging ingredients have proven to be effective in countering the actions of said stressors, providing consumers with a two-in-one advantage. There is evidence to suggest that the inclusion of pigments, such as iron oxide, in broad-spectrum sunscreens can provide further skin protection against diseases like melasma, broadening the protective spectrum above and beyond that provided by standard UV filters. This all-encompassing photoprotection approach becomes increasingly significant with our growing understanding of the synergy among environmental exposures and skin health. With the discussion of everyday photoprotection evolving, it is apparent that broad-spectrum products tailored with other active ingredients are required to minimize the look of aging and enhance overall skin wellness, as indicated by recent photoprotection study results (Krutmann et al., 2021) (Figure 4.9).

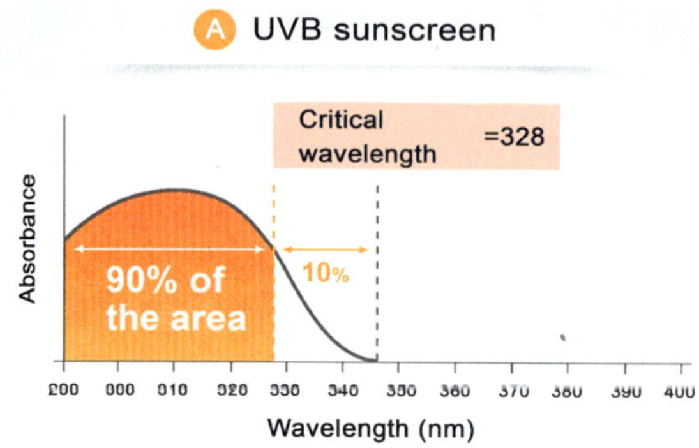

Figure 4.9. Broad spectrum sunscreens.

Source: https://www.researchgate.net/publication/357854018/figure/fig6/AS:1156035834327040@1652631829518/Critical-wavelength-is-a-quality-characteristic-and-allows-for-a-statement-about-the.jpg.

Test Your Knowledge

1. What are the main differences between physical (mineral) and chemical sunscreens in terms of ingredients and how they protect the skin?
2. List common active ingredients in chemical sunscreens and describe how they absorb UV radiation.

4.4. SPF and Its Significance

Learning Outcome

1. Understand sun protection factor (SPF)
2. Explain the limitations of SPF ratings
3. Deal with recommendations for SPF usage

The definition of SPF extends much further than marketing mumbo-jumbo; it is an important standard of measure of a sunscreen's ability to shield skin from destructive UV radiation. SPF indicates how long one may remain under the sun without harming skin relative to being without sunscreen. For example, SPF 30 in theory implies one can stay out in the sun 30 times longer than without protection. This figure is important, especially because UV exposure has increased in the last several decades due to climatic alterations. Higher SPF sunscreens are more protected from sun-induced harm to the skin, i.e., photoaging and skin cancers, and are hence an essential element in a regular skin care regimen, particularly for zones with high UV index values or people with lighter skin types who are more susceptible to damage from UV radiation. Current advances in photoprotection measurement have shed light on the significance of SPF in protection measurements against DNA damage. Research employed new methods such as DNA dosimetry to define the SPF for DNA. This measurement only determines how effective sunscreens are in preventing CPD and oxidized DNA base formation, indicators of genetic damage from UV radiation, from control samples with no sunscreen used versus test samples with sunscreen applied. Such studies project that several commercial SPF 30 products offer sufficient protection from simulated sunlight genotoxicity. This particular evaluation is important, not just in its advice to consumers about the effectiveness of their sun protection, but also in providing incentives for manufacturers to optimize their product formulations for better photoprotection against genetic damage, further highlighting the central role of SPF in contemporary dermatological practice (Tewari et al., 2012). In addition to protection against DNA damage, the applicability of SPF stands out dramatically for vulnerable individuals, such as autoimmune disease patients suffering from lupus erythematosus. These patients are often found to be more sensitive to ultraviolet rays in the skin, resulting in painful lesions that can significantly affect their quality of life. As highlighted in the clinical literature, there have been standardized testing methods developed to establish photosensitivity among such patients. These findings point to the need for high SPF ratings to offset the risks that are part of UV exposure. For individuals who have compromised skin protection mechanisms, correct sunscreen use is vital not only to prevent harm but also to reduce the potential danger of skin cancer in the long run. Therefore, SPF serves as a barometer of safety that has serious and far-reaching public health meanings among risk groups (Cazenave et al., 1997).

4.4.1. Understanding Sun Protection Factor (SPF)

The SPF idea is an extremely significant gauge of the effectiveness of sunscreens at preventing destructive UV radiation. SPF refers to the amount of time a person can stay in the sun before sunburn compared to being bare-skinned. An example would be an SPF of 30, which equates to a person being able to stay in sunlight 30 times longer than bare skin. However, the interaction is made more complex in practice because efficacy is influenced by conditions like skin type, application thickness, and weather (Maier & Korting, 2005). In a study, it was illustrated that improper application and reapplication left one with less than full protection, and therefore, public health education on proper sunscreen use and application is a necessity. Further, although SPF is the most widely recognized measure, it protects against only one aspect of UV radiation, so broader evaluations are required for whole-spectrum photoprotection. Despite its limitations, however, SPF is consumers' best information to date for proper sun protection. Without context, the correspondence between SPF values and protective capacity can be confusing. For instance, products with higher SPF do not necessarily lead to proportionally greater protection. A 50 SPF provides an extremely minor boost in protection over a 30 SPF, but customers tend to expect that the more numbers, the better they are going to be protected. The customer must realize this fact, considering the increased number of cases of skin cancer related to exposure to sunlight (Schalka et al., 2014). The linkage between chronic UV exposure and skin cancer places a focus on understanding SPF about other preventive measures. This is why constant research plays a vital role not only to enhance the methods of testing SPF but also to enhance consumer awareness of photoprotection procedures, ultimately yielding better outcomes for health. The increasing occurrence of skin cancers makes proper photoprotection measures a priority, particularly in highly sun-exposed regions, such as Brazil. Epidemiological data indicate a rise in nonmelanoma and melanoma skin cancers on the basis largely of a mix of strong solar radiation and cultural attitudes toward sun exposure. The Brazilian Society of Dermatology has responded to this challenge to public health through the creation of the Brazilian Consensus on Photoprotection, specifically tailored to meet the needs of the particular population and climate of Brazil (Schalka et al., 2014). The consensus addresses the application of SPF as a matter of cultural practice and environmental considerations rather than simply adopting other countries' guidelines. These interventions are needed to raise awareness and compliance with sun protection measures among populations that have a high burden of UV exposure, thereby aiming to reduce the risks posed by UV radiation and improve public health status (Figure 4.10).

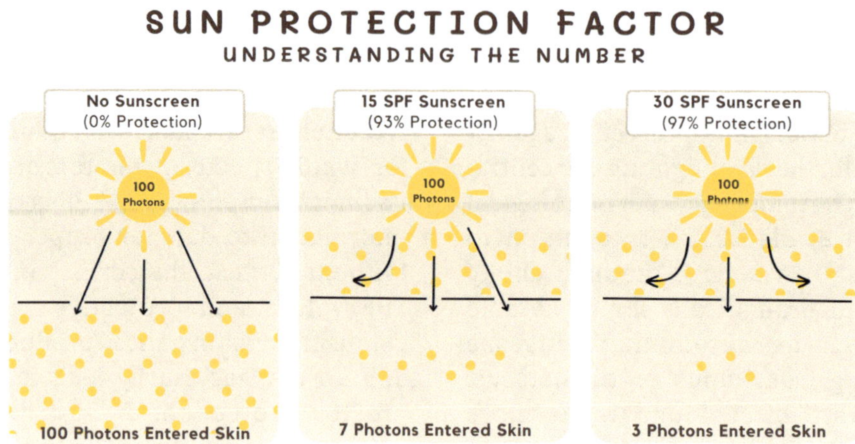

Figure 4.10. Sun protection factor (SPF).

Source: https://s.guavahealth.com/article-img/decoding-spf/spf-explained.png.

4.4.2. Limitations of SPF Ratings

The limitations of SPF values are a serious concern to consumers seeking efficient photoprotection. Although SPF values were intended to protect against UVB radiation, they should be biased towards overlooking other crucial determinants, such as the broad-spectrum protection needed against UVA radiation. The majority of consumers incorrectly believe that higher SPF equates to proportionally greater protection without regard to the intricate reality that SPF bears no connection to duration of protection or extent of UVA protection. This can lead to inefficient sun protection practice with consumers overestimating protection from high SPF products and not using them as often as necessary, thereby inadvertently being exposed to more cumulative skin damage. Apart from that, unregulated SPF labeling can cause miscommunication, and as such, it becomes very important for the regulatory agencies to provide clear guidance on sunscreens and their protection against a range of UV radiation (Tuchayi et al., 2023). Variability in application technique and adherence by the users is another important limitation with profound influence on the effectiveness of SPF scores. Several individuals apply sunscreen poorly, specifically fail to reapply it after two hours, or use less than the recommended amount, usually one ounce to cover the full body. This invalidates the protective effectiveness of the SPF value. Other aspects, including skin type, sweating, water exposure, and duration of sunlight, influence the effectiveness of sunscreen. Even water-resistant products are not completely protective because they typically must be applied again after some interval of being exposed to water. Thus, the functional effectiveness of SPF values can be less than values determined in the laboratory, even showing an expectation for repeated application and better education about the necessity for complete sun protection measures, including clothing and shade (Fonseca et al., 2023). Further, the health and environmental issues associated with certain sunscreen chemicals may negate their perceived benefits even when they possess high SPF levels. With rising awareness of the ill effects of chemicals, such as their potential toxicological effects on the environment and human health, consumers are becoming increasingly fussy about the chemicals in sunscreens. This analysis challenges the general efficacy of sunscreens since several commonly used UV filters have been implicated in endocrine disruption and negative ecological effects.

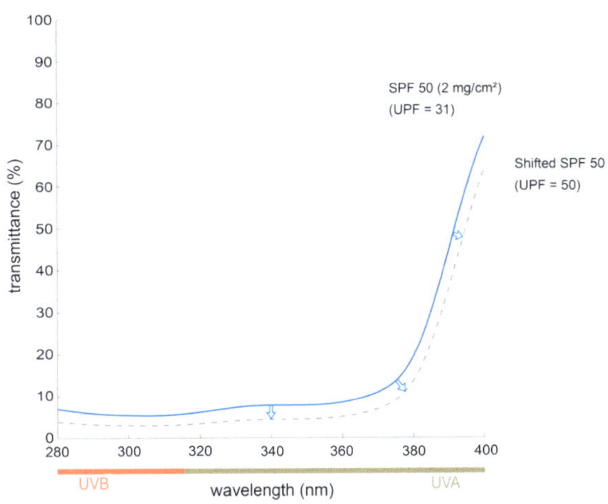

Figure 4.11. Illustration of the limitations of current measures of sun protection. The solid curve shows the measured transmittance of Sunscreen B applied at 2 mg/cm^2, which has an SPF rating of 50 but had a measured UPF of only 31. The dashed curve was generated using a shifting function to simulate a transmittance curve with an average UPF of 50. For both the measured and simulated curves, the rapid increase in transmittance in the UVA region represents reduced protection from UVA radiation.

Source: https://www.researchgate.net/publication/358048960/figure/fig6/AS:11431281210550173@1702052769686/Illustration-of-the-limitations-of-current-measures-of-sun-protection-The-solid-curve.tif.

For instance, while the preparations might display high SPF, the formulations could contain additives that offer inadequate photoprotection for prolonged or cumulative exposure. Hence, there is a need to develop safer and more effective sunscreen products with high SPF values standardized to safe formulations, ensuring improved public health outcomes while addressing sustainability concerns in the photoprotection arena (Fonseca et al., 2023) (Figure 4.11).

4.4.3. Recommendations for SPF Usage

The increase in skin cancer, particularly in sun-exposed regions, underscores the necessity of applying sunscreen correctly. In Brazil, for instance, environmental and cultural determinants tend to maximize UV exposure, and prevention efforts for skin cancer become difficult in the public health context. The Brazilian Society of Dermatology has reported extensively on these disorders, resulting in the creation of the Brazilian Consensus on Photoprotection. This form of agreement establishes clear guidelines for SPF use, where application is advised using broad-spectrum sunscreens with a minimum SPF of 30. Brazil's geographical position and its long exposure to the sun make the guidelines an adaptable approach towards photoprotection rather than accrediting others' methods as being directly applicable to Brazil but emphasizing the need for local guidelines based on the country's unique demographic and climatic conditions (Schalka et al., 2014). In selecting sunscreen, consumers are best served by opting for products that deliver broad-spectrum protection against both UVA and UVB radiation because double-duty is needed in reducing skin injury. The growing worldwide demand for sunscreen has fueled innovation in the marketplace, which has produced improved products featuring advanced sun-blocking ingredients. Research has brought about an increased diversity of active ingredients that synergize to improve photoprotection, as highlighted in recent reports from the industry. These developments also signify a growing consumer understanding of the importance of overall protection from the sun, rather than just sunburn prevention—a factor that cannot be underrated given the rising incidence of skin cancers related to UV exposure. Besides, regulatory bodies like the FDA have established standards to give the product safety and efficacy, which can more efficiently allow consumers to make their own choices in the market. Keeping up with such developments is necessary to maximize sun protection practices (Mohiuddin, 2020). Aside from selecting a proper sunscreen, application is just as crucial in the effectiveness of the sunscreen. Dermatologists recommend applying sunscreen generously, using an ounce (the amount that fills a shot glass) to cover all the exposed skin adequately. The sunscreen must be applied a minimum of 15 minutes before sun exposure to allow adequate absorption and functioning. Additionally, sunscreen also has to be applied every two hours, or more frequently after swimming or sweating, to maintain protective cover. The reapplication must be accorded top priority, particularly in areas of high UV indices. Awareness of one's environment and the strength of the sun throughout the day is pertinent, as the sun at midday is most hazardous. Such mundane advice is elementary in the avoidance of both acute and long-term damage to the skin as well as combating the rising figures of skin cancer (Schalka et al., 2014; Mohiuddin, 2020) (Figure 4.12).

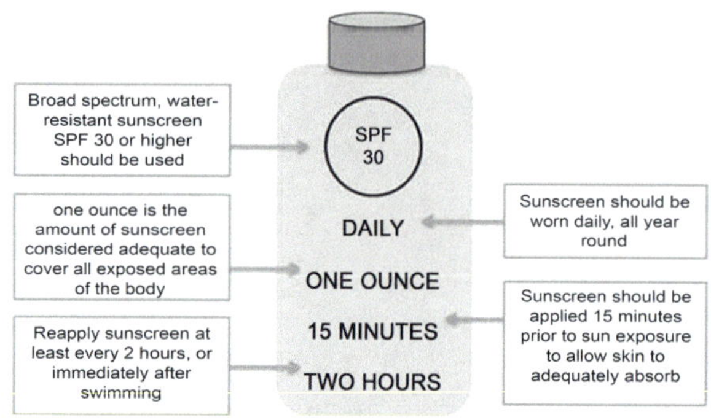

Figure 4.12. Dermatology guidelines for proper sunscreen application.

Source: https://jcadonline.com/wp-content/uploads/VasicekFigure2Jan2018.jpg.

Test Your Knowledge

1. What does SPF measure, and how is it calculated in terms of UVB protection?
2. Why does SPF not provide a complete measure of protection against UVA radiation?

4.5. Application and Usage Guidelines

Learning Outcome

1. Discuss about proper application techniques for effective protection
2. Deal with frequency of reapplication
3. Focus on considerations for different skin types and conditions

The use and application of sunscreens are the most important factors of effective photoprotection. To be at maximum effectiveness, sunscreens should be applied liberally and evenly to all exposed areas of skin. A general rule is to use roughly an ounce, or the shot glass equivalent, to adequately cover the body. Furthermore, timing also plays a crucial role; sunscreens have to be applied between 15 and 30 minutes before exposure so that the working ingredients get time to lock in. Other than how much and when, the interval at which reapplication occurs is also vital: experts recommend applying every two hours, or after a swim or excessive sweating. This broad-spectrum method of application guarantees the protective properties of sunscreen are preserved, a valuable decrease in the risk of UV-precipitated skin impairment and concomitant disorders of health, such as skin cancer and photoaging, highlighted in recent reviews (Kotowicz et al., 2024). Apart from correct application, an appreciation for the value of broad-spectrum protection maximizes sunscreen utilization. Broad-spectrum sunscreens protect against UVA and UVB rays, which result in several types of skin damage. UVA rays are primarily associated with aging of the skin and result in long-term skin damage, whereas UVB rays result in sunburn and are the biggest cause of skin cancer. Consumers must scrutinize product labels very carefully for this broad-spectrum description in order to give complete protection to the skin. Also, the selection of the appropriate SPF levels matters; current guidelines are to use products with an SPF value of 30 and higher for sufficient protection. Despite the availability of high SPF products, there are restrictions on labeling in how high the SPF can be above 30+, a sign of the FDA's efforts at standardization of sunscreen efficacy (Mohiuddin, 2020). This underlines the importance of educating the user about factors influencing good product choice and use. Secondly, integrating the use of sunscreen into a broader photoprotection strategy is essential to overall skin health. Approaches in this respect could include wearing protective clothing, seeking shade, and avoiding sunlight when solar radiation is most intense. The benefits of sun-protective clothing, such as garments containing a high ultraviolet protection factor (UPF), have been empirically validated, significantly reducing exposure and potential skin damage (Kotowicz et al., 2024). Public campaigns will increase the level of awareness concerning these combined measures, ultimately increasing regular sunscreen use alongside other protection measures. Moreover, the evolving landscape of sunblock research, along with stringent regulatory requirements, ensures that the consumer is offered advanced products designed for peak performance against carcinogenic UV rays. It is important that one stays well informed about such advancements in sun protection technology to maximize skin health and prevent skin cancer.

4.5.1. Proper Application Techniques for Effective Protection

For successful photoprotection, the right method of application of sunscreen is important. Evidence shows that most people use too little sunscreen, which seriously detracts from its protective effect. To get the best out of it, the recommendation is to use a broad-spectrum sunscreen with SPF 30 or higher and apply one ounce, which is the amount required to fill a shot glass, divided equally over all exposed body parts. This application needs to be done about 15 to 30 minutes before sun exposure to provide sufficient time for proper absorption, which promotes the sunscreen's protective effects from damage by destructive UV radiation. In addition, the sunscreen needs to be reapplied after every two hours or soon after swimming or perspiring, as water and sweat can dilute the effectiveness of the sunscreen, increasing the risk for UV-induced damage and development of skin cancer (Maier & Korting, 2005). One of the most overlooked aspects of proper application is making sure to pay attention to certain areas of the body. Often, forgotten places are the ears, the back of the neck, and the feet. These areas may be just as prone to UV damage as more exposed areas. With this in mind, getting all the exposed skin coated equates to complete protection. Also, applying lip balm or sunscreen designed for the lips can prevent sunburn in this sensitive part of the body. Choosing a sunscreen that can cater to individual skin types—oily, dry, or sensitive—is also crucial in ensuring skin well-being. When consumers experience negative responses to organic components of sunscreens, they will avoid protection; hence, the use of superior inorganic sunscreens that offer broad-spectrum protection can reduce such issues without interfering with photoprotection (Maier & Korting, 2005). As chemical sunscreens work by absorbing radiation from ultraviolet light, physical sunscreens achieve that by reflection, resulting in different application methods. It is important to inform people of the advantages and drawbacks of both kinds to make the right decision. Chemical sunscreens need to be applied accurately, as they take time to be absorbed and create a barrier, whereas physical sunscreens have immediate protection upon application. In addition, knowledge of layering sunscreen under other skin care products or makeup can enhance effectiveness. A properly thought-out skincare routine, involving frequent exfoliation and moisturizing, may maximize skin barrier function and ultimately enhance the effects of sunscreen. All these measures together create an improved photoprotection strategy that, in the end, prevents skin cancer and photoaging due to exposure of the skin without protection (Figure 4.13).

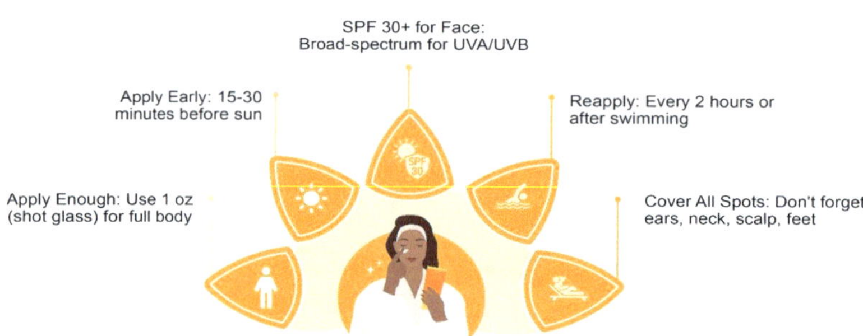

Figure 4.13. Sunscreen tips for sun protection.

Source: https://www.manipalhospitals.com/uploads/image_gallery/tips-for-sun-protection.jpg.

4.5.2. Frequency of Reapplication

Frequency of reapplication is a critical element of effective photoprotection, as much research has shown that most users apply sunscreen too infrequently or not at all to provide maximum protection. For instance, studies have proven that sunscreen's protective effects fade after a few hours, particularly if one gets wet or sweats, with popular recommendations suggesting reapplication every two hours, or if one swims or heavily sweats. Such a requirement is particularly strong in such regions as Brazil, where high levels of sun and UV radiation exposure are the norm due to geographic and climatic conditions (Schalka et al., 2014). Consequently, public health campaigns aimed at the reduction of skin cancer incidence should include education regarding the use of sunscreen, notably the requirement for frequency. Despite clear guidelines on the reapplication of sunscreen, data seem to reflect a disconnect between knowledge and behavior in the general public as well as workers outdoors. Empirical evidence points towards less than optimal sun protection behavior, including reapplication of sunscreen, and that, in most cases, sunscreen is applied before exposure to the sun, while daylong reapplications are not initiated. For example, a systematic review highlighted that the prevalence of sunburn among outdoor workers highlights the need to have specialized education programs with a focus on the reapplication need and general sun safety practices (Reinau et al., 2015). These activities are critical not just for the awareness of photoprotection principles but also for encouraging correct and consistent usage of sun protection measures to reduce skin cancer cases effectively. Besides, the reapplication frequency misconception is supplemented by the misconception about the application of sunscreen on cloudy days or during winter months, which negatively impacts skin health. It is disclosed through studies that UV rays are able to penetrate cloud cover and bounce off surfaces such as snow or water and thus increase exposure despite the sun being hidden by cover-up. Therefore, encouraging individuals to form a habit of regular sunscreen application, regardless of whether it is sunny or overcast, would make a great contribution to advancing photoprotection. Incorporation of reminders for reapplication, possibly through mobile apps or public health campaigns, might help to establish regular usage as a habit, finally altering culture in attitude towards sun protection and reducing the hazards of skin cancer related to inadequate sun protection behavior (Schalka et al., 2014) (Figure 4.14).

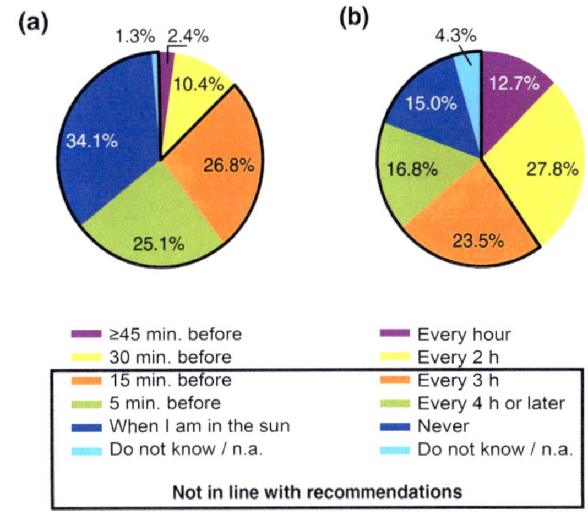

Figure 4.14. Timing of sunscreen application and reapplication. (a) Timing of sunscreen application before going out on a sunny summer day; and (b). Timing of sunscreen reapplication.

Source: https://www.researchgate.net/publication/337393282/figure/fig1/AS:1023350939865091@1620997285918/Timing-of-sunscreen-application-and-reapplication-a-Timing-of-sunscreen-application.png.

4.5.3. Considerations for Different Skin Types and Conditions

Skin heterogeneity necessitates an individualized approach to photoprotection, particularly in the application and formulation of sunscreens. Individuals with oily skin or acne prefer oil-free, non-comedogenic products as they don't wish to aggravate their condition. The adoption of light-texture formulations, i.e., gel-type or matte-finish sunscreens, can enhance compliance while ensuring sufficient UV protection. Conversely, the dry- or sensitive-skinned individual may need cream-based formulations supplemented with moisturizing agents, such as hyaluronic acid or glycerin, to counter irritation. Finally, supplementation with antioxidant compounds, such as mycosporines and mycosporine-like amino acids, provides an extra boost of photoprotection since they are capable of absorbing UV radiation and are antioxidants, which are suitable for a wide range of skin types that look for overall protection against UV-induced damage (Geraldes et al., 2021). Apart from skin type, there are some specific skin conditions that require individual consideration when choosing sunscreens. In patients suffering from conditions such as psoriasis and eczema, the risk of being irritated by conventional sunscreens makes one consider careful selection. Mineral sunscreens using zinc oxide or titanium dioxide are generally preferred since they have fewer chances of causing reactions. These products create a physical barrier against UV rays but are generally more gentle on inflamed skin. It is also necessary for individuals with such afflictions to undergo patch tests and take guidance from dermatologists in order to assess their compatibility with the treatment process and avoid negative impacts on underlying skin conditions. Precautions against the sun, such as the application of broad-spectrum sunscreen, are essential, especially considering that more than 80,000 people get skin cancer annually in Canada, with high predictability with UV exposure (Sander et al., 2020). In addition to skin type and conditions, external factors also must direct sun protection via sunscreen application. People who spend a lot of time out-of-doors, particularly during periods when the sun is producing maximum UV radiation, need to apply broad-spectrum sunscreens with higher values of SPF to protect against cumulative damage from extended sun exposure. Location is also an important factor in UV exposure, such that individuals living in locations of high altitude or nearer the equator are exposed to increased risks of intense UV radiation. Therefore, users need to reapply sunscreen every two hours or more often if swimming or perspiring. Individualizing photoprotection measures based on these factors is crucial for maximizing sun safety practices among different populations, ultimately helping to prevent skin cancer and protect skin health in different settings (Figure 4.15).

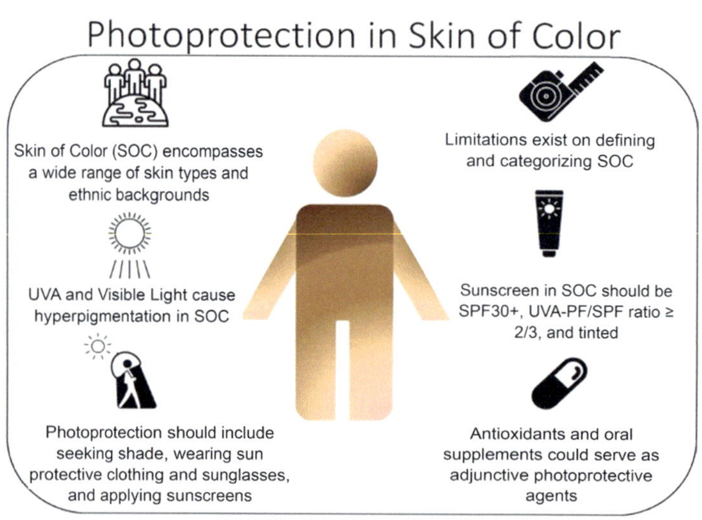

Figure 4.15. Photoprotection in skin of color.

Source: https://media.springernature.com/lw685/springer-static/image/art%3A10.1007%2Fs43630-022-00314-z/MediaObjects/43630_2022_314_Figa_HTML.png?as=webp.

Test Your Knowledge

1. What is the recommended amount of sunscreen to apply for effective coverage of the entire body in adults?
2. Why is reapplication important?

4.6. Controversies and Misconceptions

Learning Outcome

1. Discuss the myths surrounding sunscreen use
2. Deal with environmental concerns related to sunscreen ingredients
3. Focus on the debate over sunscreen safety and efficacy

The debate surrounding photoprotection and sunscreens is accompanied by myths and misconceptions whose origins are often due to inadequate knowledge of the complexities of the sun and skin well-being. Among such myths is that all sun exposure is bad, leading individuals to avoid sunlight altogether. This perspective neglects the essential role of UVB radiation in synthesizing vitamin D3, which is crucial for various bodily functions and overall health. While excessive UVB exposure does pose risks, including skin carcinogenesis, moderate sun exposure is necessary for promoting optimal vitamin D levels in the body, thereby fostering a balance between beneficial and detrimental effects of sunlight. This tacit perception matters because it always determines public perception and governs the application of sunscreens in terms not so much in tune with developing evidence in science regarding vitamin D production and its attendant health effects (Nazlı et al., 2025). The second large myth concerns the efficiency and safety of sunscreens. Some believe that applying sunscreen gives complete protection from any type of sun damage, and this leads to dangerous behavior: the longer a person spends in the sun without renewal. Different methods employed in the production of a sunscreen can result in different protective effects, which can contribute to creating misunderstandings regarding the effectiveness of a sunscreen. Adding to these issues, there are claims that some chemical ingredients of sunscreens may cause adverse effects, such as hormonal imbalance and dermal sensitization, raising concerns about their safety. While it is of interest to investigate the safe levels of the active components of sunscreens, there is a consensus that when used correctly, sunscreens reduce all risks of skin cancer and other UV-induced diseases (Neonilli et al., 2025).

Awareness of these subtleties is crucial in designing sun protection decisions. Finally, misconceptions about vitamin D and its interactions with skin health confuse attempts to discuss sunscreen efficacy. Some people argue that this use of sunscreen leads to a deficiency in vitamin D levels, hence neglecting the problems that would later arise from deficient vitamin D levels. But scientific research suggests that the majority of the world's population is already deficient in this vital vitamin, as it is synthesized endogenously in large quantities and not provided exogenously through food. The ambivalence entailed by the function performed by UVB radiation, in making it possible for vitamin D to be synthesized, yet increasing the risk of skin cancer, must be acknowledged. This ambivalence emphasizes maintaining appropriate levels of vitamin D for overall health, in addition to taking adequate photoprotective strategies. Lastly, empowering the balanced view of these myths and controversies will allow humans to handle the complexity of photoprotection and sun protection in a more realistic way (Nazlı et al., 2025; Neonilli et al., 2025).

4.6.1. Myths Surrounding Sunscreen Use

Myths regarding the use of sunscreen have a tendency to promote damaging myths about sun protection and skin care. One of the popular myths is that sunscreen is not required on a cloudy day or during winter. Such a myth is grounded on the belief that UV rays have an effect only in direct sunlight. However, studies have shown that up to 80% of UV light can penetrate through clouds, so individuals remain vulnerable to skin injury and long-term illness such as skin cancer even if the sun is obscured. Education is central to countering these myths; healthcare providers need to present correct information about the significance of regular sunscreen use, irrespective of weather conditions, to promote knowledge of effective photoprotection methods (Thompson et al., 2016). A further prevalent misconception is that an increase in SPF confers linear rises in protection and eliminates reapplication. This convinces most people that SPF 50 is twice as protective as SPF 25, which is not the case. The reality is that SPF 30 actually covers about 97% of the UVB rays, but SPF 50 covers around 98%. This slight difference can lead to a sense of security and cause prolonged sun exposure without reapplication. Its regular reapplication every two hours or immediately after swimming or sweating is necessary in order to maintain sufficient protection. Such information is crucial for people in order to effectively reduce their risk of skin cancer, and its dissemination is greatly needed in order to change these harmful misconceptions (Framil et al., 2021). Misconceptions surrounding the application of sunscreen can also discourage proper sun protection behavior. For instance, the majority of people wrongly believe that they should put sunscreen on every day in the morning. This wrong belief disregards the fact that sunscreen degrades over time, especially with the effect of sweat, water, or friction from clothing. Additionally, individuals apply less sunscreen than recommended, exposing skin that is not covered to harmful sun rays. Health care professionals are also a key in dispelling these myths by promoting education on the correct amount of sunscreen to apply—approximately one ounce for body coverage, and that frequent use is a necessary part of an integrated approach to sun protection. Through dissemination of information and providing clear guidance, health care professionals can greatly improve public understanding of effective methods of photoprotection (Thompson et al., 2016) (Figure 4.16).

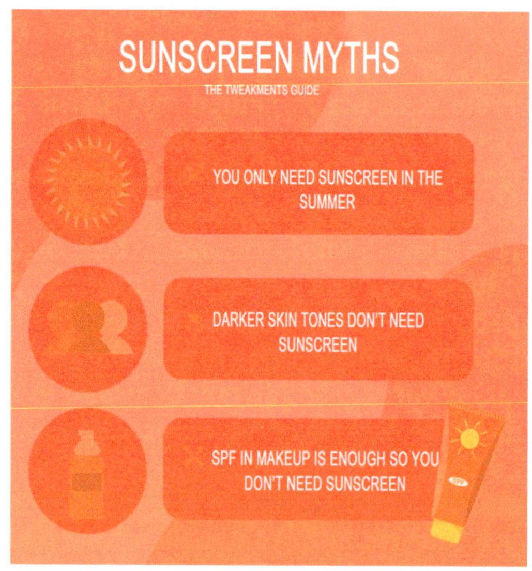
SUNSCREEN MYTHS
THE TWEAKMENTS GUIDE
YOU ONLY NEED SUNSCREEN IN THE SUMMER
DARKER SKIN TONES DON'T NEED SUNSCREEN
SPF IN MAKEUP IS ENOUGH SO YOU DON'T NEED SUNSCREEN

Figure 4.16. Sunscreen myths.

Source: https://thetweakmentsguide.com/wp-content/uploads/2022/02/The-Tweakments-Guide-Sunscreen-Myths-1.jpg.

4.6.2. Environmental Concerns Related to Sunscreen Ingredients

The growing consciousness of the detrimental impacts of UV radiation has considerably driven the utilization of sunscreens as a shield, but this surge has led to an escalating concern over their environmental impact. Oxybenzone and octinoxate are two chemical filters routinely used in sunscreen products, which have been recognized as being detrimental to marine life. Studies have shown that these substances have the tendency to build up in water environments, leading to coral bleaching that harms biodiversity and oceanic environments' overall health. Bioaccumulation of these substances not only harms marine ecosystems but also risks human health via seafood consumption. With environmentalists demanding more rigorous controls, manufacturers are confronted with increasingly pressing challenges to reconsider the composition of their products and confront an open conflict between conservation and protection in debates over whether or not to use sunscreen (Just-Sarobé, 2025). Aside from immediate impacts on marine ecosystems, there are also substantive concerns regarding the safety of some sunscreen chemicals and the long-term effects of their usage on wildlife and human populations. The systemic absorption of certain UV filters used by humans raises questions regarding endocrine disruption and other adverse health effects, further contributing to the complexity in environmental evaluations. Among these instances, inorganic filters like titanium dioxide (TiO_2) and zinc oxide (ZnO) can theoretically serve as an alternative source because both are generally considered safer by environmental and health regulations. However, concerns remain about the nanoparticle forms of these minerals, particularly their potential to generate ROS when exposed to sunlight. This duality highlights a critical need for comprehensive safety evaluations of all sunscreen ingredients, as the quest for effective photoprotection must not overshadow the necessity for ecological safety (Araki et al., 2025). New solutions are being created in the market for sunscreens, demonstrating an increasing allegiance to eco-friendly products. The development of the synthesis of organic UV filters and novel integration of bioactive compounds is opening doors for more environmentally friendly products. The new products not only target minimizing ecological damage but also strive to make customers safer by limiting the potential for skin reactions and systemic absorption. Innovations in the sunscreen industry highlight the potential for research-driven solutions that balance efficacy with environmental stewardship. As consumers become increasingly informed about the potential impacts of their choices, manufacturers are compelled to adopt greener practices and ingredient transparency. This shift indicates a promising trend towards harmonizing the need for effective photoprotection with a commitment to safeguarding our natural ecosystems, suggesting a path forward for responsible sunscreen use and development (Araki et al., 2025; Just-Sarobé, 2025) (Figure 4.17).

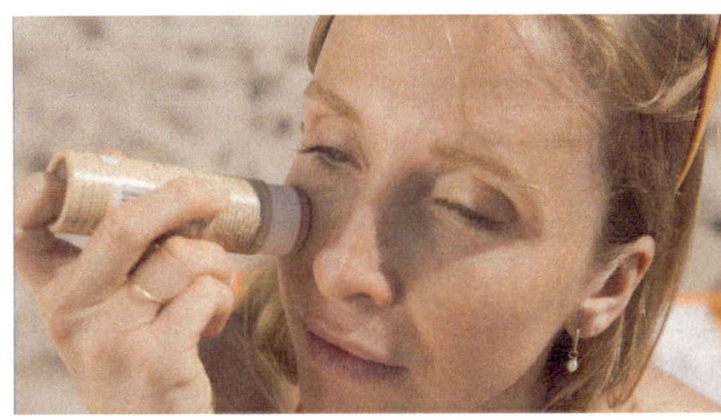

Figure 4.17. A woman applying stick sunscreen to her face at the beach, highlighting the importance of convenient and effective sun protection for maintaining skin health during outdoor activities.

Source: https://cdn.shopify.com/s/files/1/0785/4509/2921/articles/Blogue-ingredients-guide-BANNIERE.jpg?v=1702385611&width=1500&height=800&crop=center.

4.6.3. The Debate Over Sunscreen Safety and Efficacy

The argument concerning the safety and efficacy of sunscreens is pivotal to grasping their role in photoprotection and public health.

Sunscreens have been a standard component in skincare regimens for decades, intended to reverse the harmful effects of UV radiation, a known carcinogen. Although used well, the effectiveness of sunscreens has been doubted, particularly claims concerning the prevention of skin cancers and photoaging. Interestingly, the evolution of sunscreen formulations has resulted from regulatory variations across different regions, notably between the United States and Europe. While the U.S. Food and Drug Administration (FDA) regulates sunscreens as drugs, which necessitates compliance with stringent guidelines, the European Union permits a broader range of active ingredients. Such regulatory differences could impact consumer attitudes and the market, thus creating issues concerning the sufficiency of the protection provided by existing products (Mohiuddin, 2020). There is an increasing focus on distinguishing various types of UV radiation and the risks accompanying them. Sunscreens have in the past been designed to defend against UVB radiation, which is most often the cause of sunburns, but recent research has underlined the necessity of total protection against UVA rays that penetrate more deeply into the skin and initiate the development of skin cancer. The SPF therefore, might no longer be the only measure of the effectiveness of a sunscreen. Interestingly, the efficacy of active ingredients such as titanium dioxide and zinc oxide, as well as chemical filters such as avobenzone and octinoxate, has been investigated regarding their protective properties. Stability of such chemical filters to UV light is a basic subject of study since instability tends to reduce the protective nature of a product, therefore reviving controversy around the safety and efficacy of chemical compared to physical sunscreens (Serpone, 2021). In addition, the debate on the safety of sunscreens involves issues related to systemic absorption and possible hazards to human health from some chemical ingredients. Studies showing that chemicals such as oxybenzone can be absorbed into the blood have brought increased attention to their long-term impacts on human health. Although consensus on the application of sunscreens to prevent skin cancers and damage exists, research continues to evaluate the effects of long-term use. Complexity also stems from issues regarding possible endocrine interference and allergic contact dermatitis. A weighing of the advantages and disadvantages by the consumer requires the balancing of the requirement for efficient photoprotection against guarantees of safety. Ongoing innovations and regulatory reforms could open the way for more dependable sunscreen products that tackle both efficacy and health issues, ultimately boosting public confidence in protective products (Serpone, 2021).

Test Your Knowledge

1. What are environmental concerns related to sunscreen ingredients?
2. What do you understand by SPF?

SUMMARY

The importance of proper photoprotection cannot be overemphasized in today's world, with the increasing incidence of skin cancer and other solar-related disorders. While there is significant concern regarding the health hazards of excessive sun exposure, as reflected in a survey showing that 93% of Canadians are aware of such health risks, the application of this awareness into regular protective practice is minimal. The research points out that while 81% of the people apply some kind of protection from the sun, a mere 10% follow all the measures advised. This inconsistency reflects an immediate need for focused educational programs to fill the gap between information and action, especially among younger populations and those with more pigmented skin, who are less likely to appreciate the dangers of sun exposure or understand the limitations of traditional sun protection measures (Passeron et al., 2025). Investigating new photoprotective agents also helps us better understand the best ways to protect against the sun. Recent research has found that dyestuffs such as sunset yellow (SY) have shown good photostability and ROS quenching capabilities, which are implicated in skin damage and aging. Importantly, the results unveil SY as a new tool in the development of broad-spectrum sunscreens, thus increasing the toolbox of compounds for sun protection. Its efficacy towards the toxic effects of phototoxicants lends further value to the use of new agents in sunscreen products, thereby increasing user compliance and overall protection of skin health. Utilizing such innovations, we can enhance consumer trust in sunscreen products, towards which greater levels of consistent usage could be observed (Singh et al., 2024). In conclusion, in conjunction with the development of innovative photoprotective agents, enhanced education on sun protection measures is a complete approach to battling multifaceted challenges posed by sun exposure. Public education on the limitations of current practices of sunscreens and the introduction of appealing, technologically advanced product forms may help popularize safe sun habits. Furthermore, collaboration between healthcare professionals, researchers, and consumers is essential to foster a culture of proactive skin health. In the future, it will be crucial to prioritize these criteria in minimizing sun exposure risks and ensuring greater protection against skin cancer and other related diseases, ultimately leading to improved public health in photoprotection and sunscreens (Singh et al., 2024; Passeron et al., 2025).

The increasing threat of skin cancer caused by UV radiation has put sunscreens in the limelight for photoprotection strategies. With decades of scientific research bringing the risks of UV exposure into light, the importance of adequate sun protection became essential. Especially noteworthy is the fact that traditional sunscreens are designed to screen out only a limited amount of the UVB rays responsible for causing sunburn and underpinning skin cancers. However, studies in the recent past show that these products may not be enough to save human skin from UVA, which has a deeper penetration into the skin and is therefore credited with photoaging and malignant transformations. This misconception questions the effectiveness of most commercial sunscreens in the market today, raising further questions in the light of the active ingredients used and their actual shielding powers against both types of damaging radiation. The toxicity of traditional sunscreen chemicals has raised interest among consumers and researchers. Most chemical sunscreens, including octinoxate and avobenzone, were observed to be unstable under sunlight exposure and possibly reduce their efficacy against photoprotection while raising safety concerns about using them (Verma et al., 2023). In addition, the long-term impact of these compounds on the environment and human health must be ascertained. Natural phytochemicals, which have been discovered to be effective in enhancing photoprotection as alternative agents, differ from the discussed compounds. Not only are these compounds good absorbers of UV light, but they also have antioxidants that can prevent skin damage caused by oxidative stress. With the increasing demand for safer options, the investigation of these natural compounds might just transform the future of sun protection formulations (Verma et al., 2023). In conclusion, the entire conversation around photoprotection and sunscreens encompasses an entire range of efficacy, safety, and innovation. First and foremost, it would seem that any effective sunscreen should have all-around protection against both UVA and UVB sources of radiation and not be toxic to the skin. The findings call for effective regulatory measures and consumer care in the selection of sun protectants. Further, advances in the development of stable, non-toxic sun filters, whether conventional or novel phytochemical-based, hold the key to ensuring sunscreens' role in serving skin health. Finally, safety and effectiveness in sunscreens would be critical for public health, thus demanding constant surveillance and development in photoprotection (Verma et al., 2023).

KEY TERMS FROM THIS CHAPTER

- Compromised skin
- Environmental stressors
- Exposed skin
- Human health
- Melanocytes
- Photoaging
- Physical sunblocks
- Reactive oxygen species (ROS)
- Skin rejuvenation
- Ultraviolet (UV)
- Environmental aggressors
- Epidemiological data
- Harmful effects
- Keratinocytes
- Misconceptions
- Photoprotection practices
- Protective mechanisms
- Repair mechanisms
- Sunscreen
- Ultraviolet radiation

CRITICAL THINKING QUESTIONS

1. **What is the primary function of sunscreens?**
   a. To hydrate the skin
   b. To block or absorb UV radiation
   c. To remove dead skin cells
   d. To improve skin tone
2. **Which type of ultraviolet (UV) radiation is most responsible for causing sunburns?**
   a. UVA
   b. UVC
   c. UVD
   d. UVB
3. **What does SPF (Sun Protection Factor) indicate on a sunscreen product?**
   a. The length of time the sunscreen lasts
   b. The degree of water resistance
   c. The level of UV protection the sunscreen provides
   d. The percentage of ingredients in the formula
4. **Which of the following ingredients in sunscreens offers protection against UVA rays?**
   a. Zinc oxide
   b. Avobenzone
   c. Octinoxate
   d. All of the above
5. **What is the difference between physical and chemical sunscreens?**
   a. Physical sunscreens absorb UV radiation, while chemical sunscreens reflect UV radiation
   b. Chemical sunscreens absorb UV radiation, while physical sunscreens reflect UV radiation
   c. Chemical sunscreens provide more water resistance than physical sunscreens
   d. There is no difference between the two

Short Answer Questions

1. Explain the concept of SPF (Sun Protection Factor) and how it relates to the protection against UVB radiation.
2. What is the role of UVA and UVB radiation in skin damage, and how do sunscreens protect against each?
3. How does broad-spectrum protection in sunscreens differ from regular protection, and why is it important?
4. What is the recommended amount of sunscreen to apply to ensure adequate protection, and how often should it be reapplied?
5. What are some common ingredients found in sunscreens, and how do they work to block or absorb UV radiation?
6. Why is it important to use sunscreens year-round, even when it's cloudy or during the winter months?

Answer to Critical Thinking Questions

1. (b); 2. (d); 3. (c); 4. (d); 5.(b)

REFERENCES

1. Schalka, S., Steiner, D., Ravelli, F. N., Steiner, T., Terena, A. C., Marçon, C. R., Ayres, E. L., Addor, F. A., Miot, H. A., Ponzio, H., Duarte, I., Neffá, J., Cunha, J. A., Boza, J. C., Samorano, L.deP., Corrêa, M.deP., Maia, M., Nasser, N., Leite, O. M., Lopes, O. S., ... Brazilian Society of Dermatology (2014). Brazilian consensus on photoprotection. *Anais brasileiros de dermatologia*, *89*(6 Suppl 1), 1–74. https://doi.org/10.1590/abd1806-4841.20143971 (accessed on 11th June 2025).
2. Aguilera, J., Gilaberte, Y., & Gracia-Cazaña, T. (2023). New developments in sunscreens. https://core.ac.uk/download/589239532.pdf (accessed on 11th June 2025).
3. T. Maier, H.C. Korting; Sunscreens – Which and What for?. Skin Pharmacol Physiol 1 December 2005; 18 (6): 253–262. https://doi.org/10.1159/000087606(accessed on 11th June 2025).
4. Araki, S. M., & Baby, A. (2025). New perspectives on titanium dioxide and zinc oxide as inorganic UV filters: Advances, safety, challenges, and environmental considerations. *Cosmetics.* https://www.semanticscholar.org/paper/75af2fa35274fc013e5ecffe553881c9f5507593 (accessed on 11th June 2025).
5. Brar, G., Dhaliwal, A., Brar, A. S., Sreedevi, M., Ahmadi, Y., Irfan, M., Golbari, R., et al. (2025). A comprehensive review of the role of UV radiation in photoaging processes between different types of skin. *Cureus, 17.* https://www.semanticscholar.org/paper/0c844030d2f06d149ed94105da269ea6f5fae35d (accessed on 11th June 2025).
6. Cazenave, A., Dubois, E. L., Fisher, A. A., Freund, H., Fuhs, E., Messer, G., Garzon, R., et al. (1997). *Photo Testing and Photoprotection in LE.* https://core.ac.uk/download/12175365.pdf (accessed on 11th June 2025).
7. Chiou, W. L. (2024). Advancing new views on the causes and prevention of skin cancer and aging of the skin. *Medical Research Archives.* https://www.semanticscholar.org/paper/1931f0974cf011801a4dc6a076cfbc18d01f03d8 (accessed on 11th June 2025).
8. Cowden, A. M., Losantos, R., Whittock, A., Peñín, B., Sampedro, D., & Stavros, V. (2023). Ring buckling and C=N isomerization pathways for efficient photoprotection in two nature-inspired UVA sunscreens revealed through ultrafast dynamics and high-level calculations. *Photochemistry and Photobiology, 100*, 298–313. https://www.semanticscholar.org/paper/d48255f3cd5ba434c915f36f1f4f6e5a1423ed11 (accessed on 11th June 2025).
9. Ferrari, M., & Rocha-Filho, P. A. (2011). *Multiple Emulsions Containing Amazon Oil: Açaí Oil (Euterpe oleracea).* https://core.ac.uk/download/pdf/37448079.pdf (accessed on 11th June 2025).
10. Fonseca, M., Rehman, M., Soares, R., & Fonte, P. (2023). The impact of flavonoid-loaded nanoparticles in the UV protection and safety profile of topical sunscreens. *Biomolecules, 13*, 493–493. https://doi.org/10.3390/biom13030493 (accessed on 11th June 2025).
11. Framil, C. V., & Palumbo, A. J. (2021). *Evaluation of an Educational Intervention Regarding the Importance of Practicing Sun Protective Behaviors Among Racially Diverse College Students: A Quality Improvement Project.* https://core.ac.uk/download/484355991.pdf (accessed on 11th June 2025).
12. Freitas, J. V., Junqueira, H. C., Martins, W. K., Baptista, M. S., & Gaspar, L. R. (2018). Antioxidant role on the protection of melanocytes against visible light-induced photodamage. *Free Radical Biology and Medicine, 131*, 399–407. https://doi.org/10.1016/j.freeradbiomed.2018.12.028 (accessed on 11th June 2025).

13. Gabbanini, S., Ngwa Neba, J., Matera, R., & Valgimigli, L. (2024). Photochemical and oxidative degradation of chamazulene contained in *Artemisia*, *Matricaria* and *Achillea* essential oils and setup of protection strategies. *Molecules, 29.* https://www.semanticscholar.org/paper/7df97e72f481a7cec91e077b4066e1066ce8f58c (accessed on 11th June 2025).

14. Geraldes, V., & Pinto, E. (2021). Mycosporine-like amino acids (MAAs): Biology, chemistry and identification features. *Pharmaceuticals, 14*, 63–63. https://doi.org/10.3390/ph14010063 (accessed on 11th June 2025).

15. González, S., Aguilera, J., Berman, B., Calzavara-Pinton, P., Gilaberte, Y., Goh, C.-L., Lim, H. W., et al. (2022). Expert recommendations on the evaluation of sunscreen efficacy and the beneficial role of non-filtering ingredients. *Frontiers in Medicine, 9.* https://doi.org/10.3389/fmed.2022.790207 (accessed on 11th June 2025).

16. Gupta, A., Singh, A. P., Singh, V., Singh, P., Jaiswal, J., Kumari, N., Upadhye, V., et al. (2023). Natural sun-screening compounds and DNA-repair enzymes: Photoprotection and photoaging. *Catalysts, 13*, 745–745. https://doi.org/10.3390/catal13040745 (accessed on 11th June 2025).

17. Just-Sarobé, M. (2025). Sunscreens and their impact on human health and the environment: A review. *International Journal of Dermatology.* https://www.semanticscholar.org/paper/da5f9eeafd47fe8b24c12bb9e6e91e4e64159f4e (accessed on 11th June 2025).

18. Kotowicz, Z., Madoń, M., Orzeł, A., Pich-Czekierda, K., et al. (2024). *Ultraviolet-Protective Clothing and Sunscreen: Sun-Protection for Healthy Skin.* https://core.ac.uk/download/613193102.pdf (accessed on 11th June 2025).

19. Krutmann, J., Bouloc, A., Sore, G., Bernard, B., & Passeron, T. (2016). The skin aging exposome. *Journal of Dermatological Science, 85*, 152–161. https://doi.org/10.1016/j.jdermsci.2016.09.015 (accessed on 11th June 2025).

20. Krutmann, J., Schalka, S., Watson, R., Liu, W., & Morita, A. (2021). Daily photoprotection to prevent photoaging. *Photo Dermatology Photo Immunology & Photomedicine, 37*, 482–489. https://doi.org/10.1111/phpp.12688 (accessed on 11th June 2025).

21. Martinez, J. (2023). *Comparison of Oral Carotene Supplementation and Oral Polypodium Leucotomies in Preventing Photodamage.* https://core.ac.uk/download/604290671.pdf (accessed on 11th June 2025).

22. Mohiuddin, A. K. (2020). *An Extensive Review on Sunscreen and Suntan Preparations.* https://core.ac.uk/download/482242155.pdf (accessed on 11th June 2025).

23. Murase, J., & Trivedi, M. (2017). *Titanium Dioxide in Sunscreen.* https://core.ac.uk/download/322430979.pdf (accessed on 11th June 2025).

24. Papadopoulou, S. N. A., Anastasiou, E. A., Adamantidi, T., Ofrydopoulou, A., Letsiou, S., & Τσούπρας, A. (2025). A comprehensive review on the beneficial roles of vitamin D in skin health as a bio-functional ingredient in nutricosmetic, cosmeceutical, and cosmetic applications. *Applied Sciences, 15*, 796–796. https://doi.org/10.3390/app15020796 (accessed on 11th June 2025).

25. Passeron, T., Lim, H. W., Krutmann, J., Dréno, B., Abdulla, S., Ting, P., Li, M., et al. (2025). Here comes the sun! A study on sun exposure and associated risks in the Canadian population. *Journal of Cutaneous Medicine and Surgery.* https://www.semanticscholar.org/paper/0e892d47e0ee02701e28786bea20cc4b730dbe1a (accessed on 11th June 2025).

26. Reinau, D. (2015). *A Multifaceted Perspective on Skin Cancer Prevention.* https://core.ac.uk/download/33301463.pdf (accessed on 11th June 2025).

27. Rodrigues, N. D. N., & Stavros, V. G. (2018). *From Fundamental Science to Product: A Bottom-Up Approach to Sunscreen Development.* https://core.ac.uk/download/157788336.pdf (accessed on 11th June 2025).

28. Sainsbury, K., Walburn, J., Araújo-Soares, V., & Weinman, J. (2017). Challenges and proposed solutions for formative research to inform systematic intervention development in rare and unstudied conditions: The case example of Xeroderma Pigmentosum. *British Journal of Health Psychology, 23*, 229–237. https://doi.org/10.1111/bjhp.12287 (accessed on 11th June 2025).

29. Sander, M., Sander, M., Burbidge, T., & Beecker, J. (2020). The efficacy and safety of sunscreen use for the prevention of skin cancer. *Canadian Medical Association Journal, 192*, E1802 E1808. https://doi.org/10.1503/cmaj.201085 (accessed on 11th June 2025).

30. Serpone, N. (2021). *Sunscreens and Their Usefulness: Have We Made Any Progress in The Last Two Decades?* https://core.ac.uk/download/589948057.pdf (accessed on 11th June 2025).

31. Sharma, M. (2024). Understanding the impact of UV radiation on skin health: Mechanisms, risks, and photoprotection strategies. *Indian Journal of Health Care Medical & Pharmacy Practice.* https://www.semanticscholar.org/paper/3c59e22ad8990adecbb8e3271e6da314a74b6868 (accessed on 11th June 2025).

32. Singh, S., Mourya, D., Patel, S. K., Shukla, S., Kumar, V., Kotian, S. Y., Yadav, A., et al. (2024). Photoprotective efficacy of Sunset Yellow via inhibition of type-I and type-II pathway under exposure of sunlight. *Photochemistry and Photobiology.* https://www.semanticscholar.org/paper/31cc80d2cc9a2ba6ac9e0dc07b6197f9560f544c (accessed on 11th June 2025).

33. Sjerobabski Masnec, I., Kotrulja, L., Šitum, M., & Poduje, S. (2010). *New Option in Photoprotection.* https://core.ac.uk/download/14422811.pdf (accessed on 11th June 2025).

34. Škařupová, D., Vostálová, J., & Rajnochová Svobodová, A. (2020). Ultraviolet A protective potential of plant extracts and phytochemicals. *Biomedical Papers, 164*, 1–22. https://doi.org/10.5507/bp.2020.010 (accessed on 11th June 2025).

35. Tewari, A., Schuch, A. P., Schuch, A. P., Schuch, A. P., Schuch, A. P., Young, A. R., COLIPA, C., et al. (2012). DNA dosimetry assessment for sunscreen genotoxic photoprotection. https://core.ac.uk/download/pdf/8745669.pdf (accessed on 11th June 2025).

36. Thompson, A. R., & Van Onselen, J. (2016). *A Summary of New Nice Guidance on Sunlight Exposure: Encouraging Behavioral Change in Photoprotection.* https://core.ac.uk/download/83941756.pdf (accessed on 11th June 2025).

37. Tortini, G., Ziosi, P., Cesa, E., Molesini, S., Baldini, E., De Lucia, D., Rossi, C., et al. (2022). Criticisms in the development of high-protection and broad-spectrum "natural/organic" certifiable sunscreen. *Cosmetics, 9*, 56–56. https://doi.org/10.3390/cosmetics9030056 (accessed on 11th June 2025).

38. Tuchayi, S. M., Wang, Z., Yan, J., Garibyan, L., Bai, X., & Gilchrest, B. A. (2023). Sunscreens: Misconceptions and misinformation. *Journal of Investigative Dermatology, 143*, 1406–1411. https://doi.org/10.1016/j.jid.2023.03.1677 (accessed on 11th June 2025).

39. Uçar, N., & Holick, M. F. (2025). Illuminating the connection: Cutaneous vitamin D3 synthesis and its role in skin cancer prevention. *Nutrients, 17*, 386–386. https://doi.org/10.3390/nu17030386 (accessed on 11th June 2025).

40. Walburn, J., Foster, L., Araújo-Soares, V., Sarkany, R., Weinman, J., Sainsbury, K., & Morgan, M. (2023). Acceptability and influence of a complex personalized intervention on changes in photoprotection behaviors among people with xeroderma pigmentosum. *British Journal of Health Psychology, 28*, 1113–1131. https://doi.org/10.1111/bjhp.12675 (accessed on 11th June 2025).

41. Verma, A., Zanoletti, A., Kareem, K.Y. *et al.* Skin protection from solar ultraviolet radiation using natural compounds: a review. *Environ Chem Lett* **22**, 273–295 (2024). https://doi.org/10.1007/s10311-023-01649-4 (accessed on 11th June 2025).

42. Zduńska, K., Dana, A., Kołodziejczak, A., & Rotsztejn, H. (2018). Antioxidant properties of ferulic acid and its possible application. *Skin Pharmacology and Physiology, 31*, 332–336. https://doi.org/10.1159/000491755 (accessed on 11th June 2025).

CHEMICAL PEELS: SUPERFICIAL TO DEEP

5

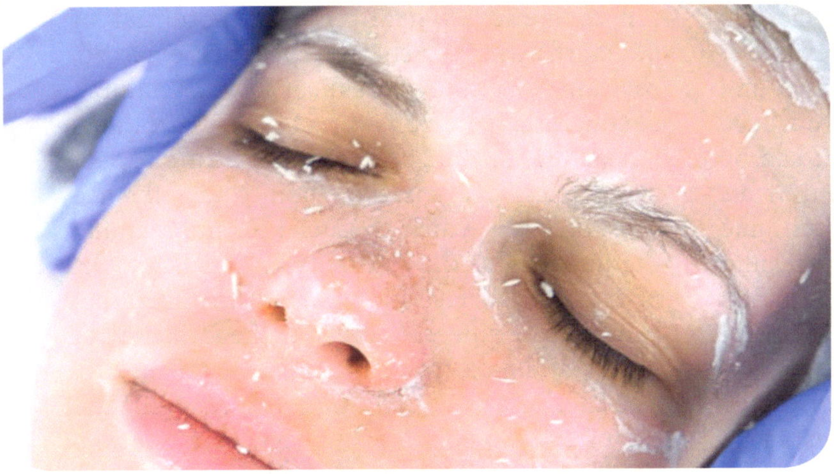

LEARNING OBJECTIVES

After studying this chapter, you will be able to:

1. Explain the types of chemical peels
2. Discuss about indications for chemical peels
3. Describe the chemical peel procedure
4. Understand the benefits of chemical peels
5. Define risks and side effects of chemical peels
6. Compare chemical peels with other skin treatments

Introduction

Chemical peels are a large and active area in aesthetic dermatology practice, of great interest as they can make the skin beautiful and treat various skin concerns. In tremendous quantities being used in cosmetic clinics, chemical peels constitute the process of using specific chemical solutions to the exfoliate of the outer skin layers, which results in cellular turnover and triggers the process of new, healthier, whiter skin replacement. Greater popularity among these treatments can be explained due to their effectiveness in treating issues such as acne, hyperpigmentation, and the visibility of aging, thus making them a multi-purpose treatment in the era of minimally invasive aesthetic treatments. In addition, as awareness of aesthetic dermatology improves, so does the need for in-depth knowledge of the available procedural options, including chemical peels, which form a key part of (Madnani et al., 2022). With the benefits of chemical peels being well recognized, there is a critical need for practitioners to have in-depth knowledge of the complexities involved in their use. The procedure is not risk-free, and providers and patients alike will have to navigate around the risk of complications that occur due to misuse or uninformed treatment with chemical agents. For this reason, clinicians need to ensure that they have a firm grasp of knowledge about the kinds of peels that are available, i.e., from superficial to deep peels, as well as the pre-and post-procedure care needed. The engagement of patients' concerns in an inclusive manner not only helps with patient safety but also enhances trust and satisfaction with aesthetic results. It requires collaboration of the best advice and evidence-based practice to augment procedure safety and efficacy so that each patient can be given a customized approach (Madnani et al., 2022). Trends in aesthetic dermatology continue to shift with improvements in technology and a greater number of treatments being made accessible to consumers. In terms of chemical peels, education, regulation, and responsible practice remain paramount. However, since aesthetic treatments are usually requested by patients for psychological, social, or health issues, the practitioner must put foremost an ethical and informed treatment approach. This concept then becomes part of the larger scope of improving healthcare processes and patient results, thus helping patients to achieve their aesthetic goals with greater safety and efficiency. The more this discussion on chemical peels evolves, the importance of knowledge about their scientific and practical concepts, which in turn makes sense for practitioners and patients alike to continuously learn about the treatment under this ever-changing landscape.

Definition of Chemical Peels

This term broadly encompasses a number of dermatological procedures that are aimed at improving the texture and appearance of the skin by topically applying acidic chemicals. These chemical agents, that may be either naturally derived or synthesized compounds, remove the topmost layers of the skin to allow for easier cell turnover and thus fresher, healthier-looking skin. Based on the level of application, chemical peels are divided into superficial, medium, and deep peels, each addressing various skin issues, for instance, fine lines, pigmentation, and acne scars. Efficacy and safety of the chemical peels are primarily determined by the active ingredients selected, concentration of acids employed, and patients skin condition and type. As formulators explore new ingredients for cosmetic applications, the potential of botanical extracts in chemical peels has emerged, revealing a path towards incorporating natural, sustainable solutions in skincare products (Guzm et al., 2021). One significant aspect of chemical peels is their ability to influence the skin's pH, which is crucial for maintaining the integrity of the skin barrier. The acidic pH of the skin surface is important in regulating keratinocyte differentiation and the formation of protective lipids, thus ensuring peak skin health. The chemical peels are efficient at changing the pH of the skin for healing and rejuvenation. This action resonates with evidence proving that topical usage products in the pH range of 4–6 improve the barrier function and overall health of skin. As such, understanding the mechanisms by which chemical peels interact with skin acidity can aid in designing more effective formulations that not only exfoliate but also maintain or restore healthy skin dynamics (Luki et al., 2021). Furthermore, the practice of administering chemical peels requires careful consideration of the patient's individual skin characteristics and desired outcomes. While peels are widely accepted in both medical and cosmetic dermatology, treatments must be tailored to be safe as well as effective by providers. Types of skin, sensitivity, as well as underlying conditions, must be evaluated in order to prevent potential negative reactions such as irritation or dyschromia. Chemical peels have also seen an increase in the inclusion of essential oils and botanical extracts, thereby ensuring their natural properties can be employed, while the risk of irritation is reduced to a bare minimum. With such sensitive selection of ingredients, chemical peels become very appealing as not only therapeutic treatments but as soothing and moisturizing treatments that promote a holistic skincare strategy for today's aesthetic environment (Guzm et al., 2021) (Figure 5.1).

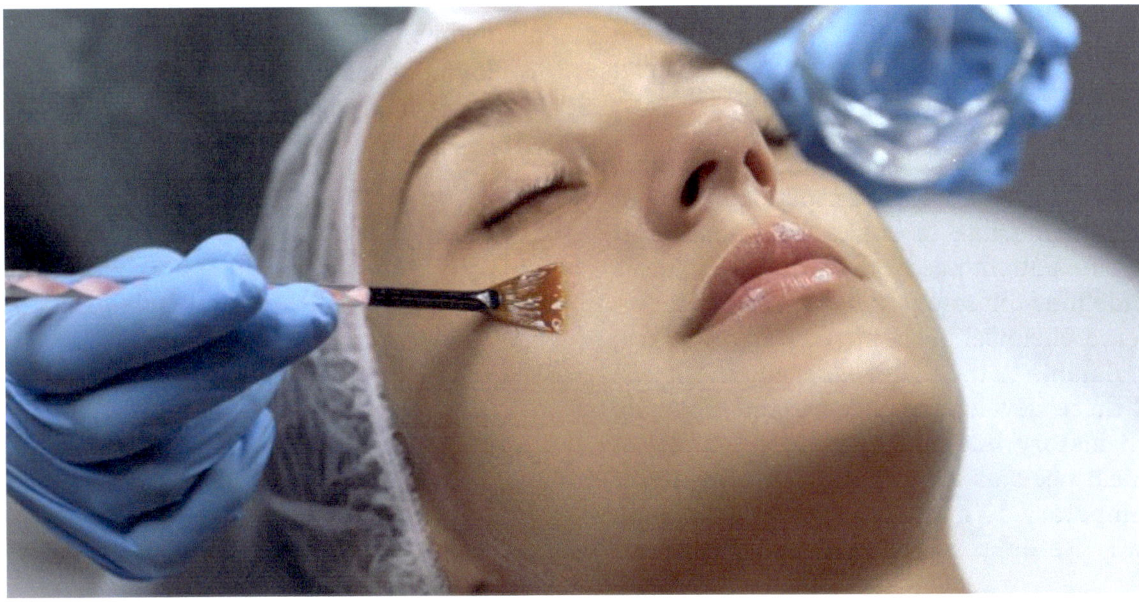

Figure 5.1. A chemical peel treatment.

Source: https://www.olivaclinic.com/wp-content/uploads/2021/01/Chemical-Peel.jpg.

Brief History of Chemical Peels

The evolution of chemical peels is characterized by a steady progression that mirrors advances in dermatological understanding and technological development. Chemical agents were first used for rejuvenation of the skin in ancient Egypt, where plant oils and sour milk were used to change the appearance of the skin. This process was continued throughout the centuries with increased scientific basis arriving only with the emergence of modern dermatology in the 19th century. By the 1920s, certain acids like phenol and trichloroacetic acid (TCA) started appearing in clinics. However, these chemicals paved the way for more advanced chemical peel treatments based on individual skin problems like pigmentation and texture irregularities. Further realization that exfoliation using chemicals could encourage healthier skin revolutionized dermatology practices, opening the way for modern uses of chemical peels. The mid-20th century also saw cultural popularity for chemical peels, riding a broader cultural tide to treat for appearance and health. Dermatologists and surgeons started refining procedures, differentiating between superficial, medium, and deep peels based on the agents used and intended depth of exfoliation. Over these years, chemicals like glycolic acid, an alpha hydroxy acid (AHA), entered practice, paving the way for peels to be established as a norm in general cosmetic use. In addition, clinical studies began to reveal chemical exfoliation mechanisms, demonstrating not just short-term cosmetic benefits but also long-term improvement of skin health. This scientific endorsement helped to legitimize chemical peels as standard dermatological procedures, allowing practitioners to improve their client skin quality. With the advancement of the field into the early 21st century, it also became more prevalent to incorporate chemical peels into general dermatological treatment schemes. Formulation and delivery system innovations enabled targeted treatments of appropriate scope for different skin types and issues, ultimately contributing to the wider application of peels in medical and aesthetic procedures. The development of new generations of peeling agents, such as Jessner's solution and mixtures of several acids, provided dermatologists with an armamentarium to create treatments that fit specific patient needs. In addition, advances in guidelines for safety and patient education rendered chemical peels increasingly practical and palatable to the public. The culmination of all of these developments represents not only a rich history but also ongoing evolution of chemical peels as fundamental implements of contemporary dermatology, effectively shaping the way we approach skin beauty and health today.

Importance of Chemical Peels in Dermatology

The relevance of chemical peels in dermatology is underscored by their wide range of uses from aesthetic enhancement to therapeutic purposes. Chemical peels are designed to eliminate the outermost layers of the skin, thereby stimulating cellular turnover and improving the quality of the skin. Clinically, chemical peels are also used to treat an array of skin concerns such as acne scars, hyperpigmentation, and signs of aging. It has been well-established by multiple studies that these treatments are safe and effective; chemical peels done appropriately really do offer substantial improvements in skin appearance and health.

Nevertheless, the practitioners need to possess a clear understanding of the chemical agents used and the specific skin conditions they are working on to maintain complications at a low level and achieve optimum results in their patients' skin health and appearance (Madnani et al., 2022). Increased popularity of non-surgical facial aesthetic treatments, such as chemical peels, is evidence of an even broader movement in dermatology towards minimally invasive procedures. The continuous development in technology increases versatility and effectiveness in the chemical peeling range that has made it very popular. That becomes the signal of increased interest in preventive care and early treatment of dermatological disorders. An agent of beauty for most patients, chemical peels is generally essential for the proper care of the skin.

As highlighted in recent reviews, a lack of understanding of the pre- and post-procedure care can undermine the overall efficacy of such aesthetic treatments. Thus, an educated practice of chemical peels, bringing both clinical skill and aesthetic demand together, has become increasingly crucial in modern dermatological practice (Madnani et al., 2022). Moreover, training and education in the application of chemical peels cannot be overemphasized. With aesthetic clinicians and dermatologists trying to remain in accordance with evolving industry standards, there is a requirement to advance the educational environment regarding such treatments.

There is significant evidence of a skills gap in the use of chemical peels for practitioners, particularly in the context of a rising beauty and aesthetics sector. This difference underscores that the training must be much more formalized, taking on more of an aesthetic education that will prepare the practitioner for appropriate and safe treatments. The continued discussion over aesthetics being included in the somatology training indicates a shift of considerable proportions, needing a blend of medical knowledge and aesthetic sensibility for better patient care in this discipline.

5.1. Types of Chemical Peels

Learning Outcome

1. Describe superficial peels
2. Understand medium-depth peels
3. Define deep peels

Chemical peels are classically classified into three general categories, consisting of superficial, medium, and deep peels to address various skin ailments. Superficial peels, most commonly utilizing AHAs such as glycolic and lactic acids, primarily influence the outermost epidermal layer. Peels with this level of concentration of alpha-hydroxy acids are quite mild and induce very little downtime; they are applied for a lighter degree of exfoliation to improve skin appearance in the areas of texture and brightness overall. As explained in recent research, AHAs enhance skin turnover, trigger apoptosis in the skin cells, and enhance collagen and elastin synthesis, thereby aiding conditions such as acne and photoaging (Almeman, 2024). Individuals with sensitive skin or chemical exfoliation-naive patients will appreciate the superficial peels the most, providing a foundation for more intense treatments in the future. Medium peels include the use of TCA or the use of a mixture of AHAs and TCA to penetrate deeper facial skin. Medium peels are performed to fix more severe issues, including moderate sun spots, fine lines, and pigmentation anomalies. Healing from a medium peel typically takes a few days, with the patient peeling and maybe having some redness while the facial skin heals. Of importance, medium peels strike a balance between efficacy and safety, with noticeable results and few side effects. Citing the dermatology literature, the precise TCA concentration involved is the key to guaranteeing the treatment outcomes and avoiding potential irritation, thereby necessitating professional advice in undertaking such procedures (Almeman, 2024). This conservative technique enables patients to enjoy the skin-enhancing benefit of medium peels but with fewer complications. Deep peels are the most invasive technique of chemical peeling, using agents such as phenol that penetrate into the lower dermal layers.

Deep peels tend to be reserved for those patients with severe skin problems, including deep wrinkles, severe photoaging, and extensive scarring. Recovery time with a deep peel is much longer, typically several weeks to fully recover, with patients needing to comply with closely monitored aftercare. Despite the longer recovery time, results with deep peels have been absolutely outstanding, with a more even, more youthful appearance. With cosmeceuticals becoming increasingly popular in treatments for the skin, the combination of new formulations with deep peeling treatments has experienced increasing interest as an effective means of optimizing outcomes. With the awareness of the particular skin type and concerns, practitioners can effectively customize deep peel regimens for a highly individualized treatment that weighs safety against effectiveness (Figure 5.2).

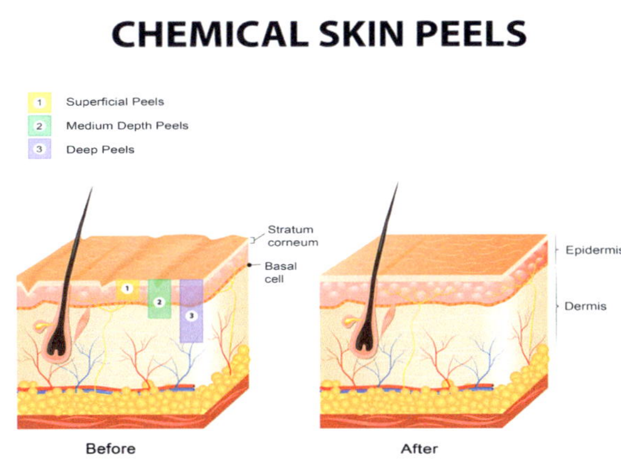

Figure 5.2. Chemical peels.

Source: https://www.hushla.net/wp-content/uploads/2022/07/Chemical-peels-Los-Anglese.jpg.

5.1.1. Superficial Peels

Superficial peels are one of the common varieties under the broader category of chemical peels, that is especially designed to peel the epidermal layers of the skin. They are the process of using lighter acids such as glycolic or lactic acid to achieve the rejuvenation of the skin without causing deep damage to the inner layers. Most suitable for patients looking to correct minor skin imperfections like fine lines, textured skin, and superficial pigmentation, superficial peels are effective yet non-invasive. Research has shown that these peels can improve skin luminescence and texture and are gaining popularity among dermatology and aesthetical clinics. Besides, the reparative effect of superficial peels is usually cumulative, encouraging patients to make them an integral component of skincare regimens in order to achieve a well-looked complexion and support the overall well-being of the skin. A second significant characteristic distinguishing superficial peels from other peeling techniques is the safety profile. Because they address the external layer of skin, the danger of severe side effects, such as scarring and prolonged erythema, is negligible. Patients typically experience mild discomfort and some temporary redness following the procedure, but this is only short-term to allow minimal downtime. This convenience can be transferred into a better patient experience because many are worried about more invasive procedures due to potential recovery time. Thus, superficial peels present an appealing alternative, with effectiveness in combination with convenience. The overall good acceptance of superficial peels is due to ongoing studies that vindicate their use in promoting the health of the skin and lowering cosmetic procedure risks. Apart from their cosmetic application, superficial peels have been identified for their therapeutic value when it comes to managing various types of skin disorders. For instance, superficial peels can be employed as adjuvant therapy for chronic acne, melasma, and photoaging to reinforce the effectiveness of concomitant therapies. Secondly, the application of superficial peels can increase penetration of topically applied drugs, which results in accelerated healing and reconstitution of the skin. As skin physiology becomes better, the use of superficial peels as part of an overall plan of treatment for skin is on the rise. Their application to dermatological practice is demonstrated by studies proving their capacity for inducing cellular turnover and improving skin barrier function, and thereby being beneficial to complete skin health management programs. Such a multidisciplinary strategy in good faith positions superficial peels at a center position of significance in both therapeutic and aesthetic dermatology (Figure 5.3).

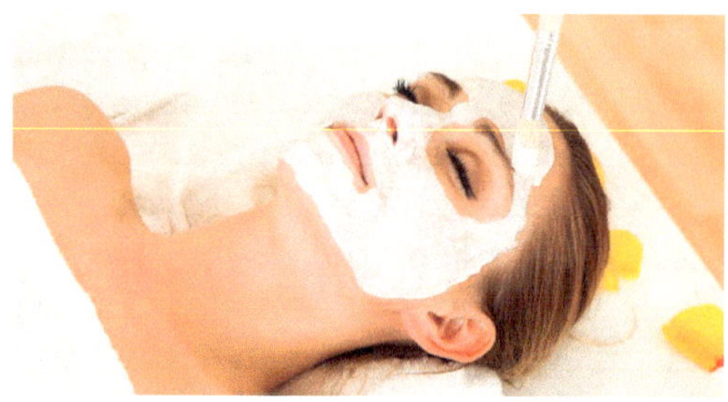

Figure 5.3. Using superficial peels.

Source: https://www.essential-derm.com/wp-content/uploads/2024/11/superficial-peels-needham-ma.jpg.

5.1.2. Medium-Depth Peels

An important advancement in dermatologic aesthetics is the medium-depth chemical peels, with an intermediary between the superficial and deep peels. It utilizes TCA concentrations of 20% to 35% to take effect in penetrating the epidermis and the upper dermis in effectively producing exfoliation of the impaired skin layers. This depth of the peel provides treatment of more prominent skin problems, such as moderate acne scars, fine lines, and pigmentation imperfections. By treating these specific issues, medium-depth peels enable deep rejuvenation of the skin with enhancement of the overall skin tone and texture. Moreover, since patients are in search of less invasive yet significant effects with minimal time out of it, medium-depth peels emerged as the focus of aesthetic practice, being advantageous to medical and cosmetic dermatology patients in need of functional solutions to their skin problems. Clinically, medium-depth peels may present with strong benefits but are not free of inherent risks related to their level of invasiveness. Erythema, peeling, and risk of PIH are frequent side effects, particularly in darker-skinned patients. It is essential for practitioners to take diligent patient assessments to identify skin type, past history of hyperpigmentation, and other pertinent factors before treatment. Moreover, post-peeling care is also needed to achieve maximum healing and outcomes, typically comprising sun protection regimens and emolliating agents to safeguard newly exposed skin. In this regard, medium-depth peels are not just cosmetic treatments but also a means of addressing underlying dermatoses, thus demonstrating their dual role of aesthetic enhancement and therapeutic advantage. Another region in which the application of medium-depth peels and the management of acne vulgaris and actinic keratoses can overlap involves conditions that are encountered by dermatology practitioners in managing these diseases. As above-described, acne vulgaris is very common, and treatment options usually include a combination of topical therapy and aesthetic procedures. Medium-depth peels make good adjunctive therapies since they improve texture of the skin and reduce acne scarring, and therefore mitigate psychologic distress of this common disorder of the skin (Bińczyk et al., 2024). In management of actinic keratoses also, medium-depth peels can be good adjuncts to field-directed therapy since they successfully treat sun damage lesions and simultaneously enhance the skin's appearance (Ferara et al., 2024). Hence, the use of medium-depth peels will further complement the overall therapeutic treatment of these frequent dermatological conditions in asserting their place within contemporary skin treatment routines (Figure 5.4).

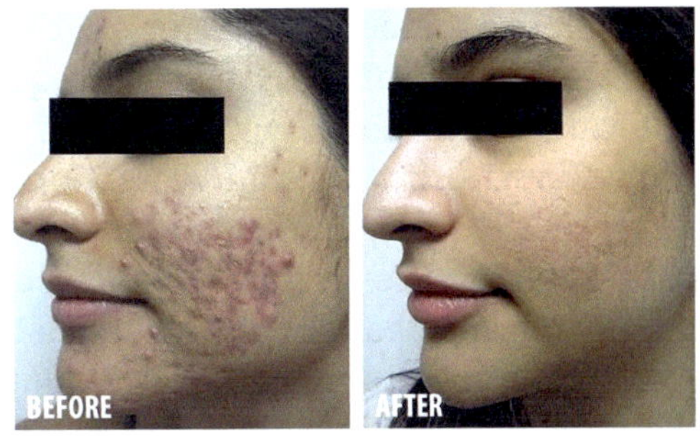

Figure 5.4. Patient treated with medium-depth peels.

Source: https://cdcssl.ibsrv.net/ibimg/smb/1400x850_80/webmgr/1n/5/p/propeel2.jpg.webp?57e6fdbc30d10b885d9b65ba735d00bd.

5.1.3. Deep Peels

Deep chemical peels are highly advanced forms of chemical exfoliation that apply strong agents, such as phenol or TCA, which work deeply to reach into the dermal layers of the skin. Where superficial and medium-depth peels work on the epidermis as a whole, deep peels are used to work on more intrinsic problems of the skin, such as extreme photoaging, deep wrinkles, and significant scarring. The technique requires careful preparation and follow-up care because the risks of complications, including scarring or pigmentation, are severely increased with deeper penetration of chemical solutions. The results of deep peeling are often dramatic and can provide long-lasting rejuvenation with better texture and tone of the skin. Therefore, these procedures require a thorough understanding of specific patient factors to provide a safe and effective result with minimal risk of adverse effects. Preparation for deep peeling is most important and involves pre-treatment orders as well as post-treatment care that has a significant impact on the result. Practitioners need to assess a patient's skin type and overall health because some diseases can rule out deeper peels. Pre-treatment may involve the administration of topical retinoids or other medications to induce skin resistance and maximize overall peel efficiency. Post-procedural care requires diligent adherence to a regimen that may encompass moisturization, sun protection, and possibly the use of specialized ointments to facilitate healing. The literature underscores that a well-informed patient undergoing a deep peel will often experience reduced downtime and a more favorable aesthetic result. Thus, pre- and post-care can contribute significantly towards optimizing patient satisfaction and long-term treatment benefits. This is consistent with recent evidence from cosmetic dermatology clinics (Madnani et al., 2022). A clear advantage of deep peels over other less aggressive treatments is for conditions that are not responsive to these. For instance, recent research has concentrated on the effectiveness of some peels in the management of melasma as well as other pigmentary conditions. The tretinoin peel is a superficial peel, and it has been studied for application and efficacy, particularly in the Brazilian population. But deeper peels provide more changes, particularly for photodamage and deep scars. With constant advances in dermatologic treatments, there is an immediate need for well-planned and controlled comparisons of synergy between various peels and adjunct treatments. These studies must concentrate on variables like vehicle, regimen, and concentration, which are paramount to maximizing benefits in differing dermatoses (Bagatin et al., 2017). Therefore, an integrated strategy for chemical peels, particularly deep forms, will be the future of aesthetic dermatology and patient treatment (Figure 5.5).

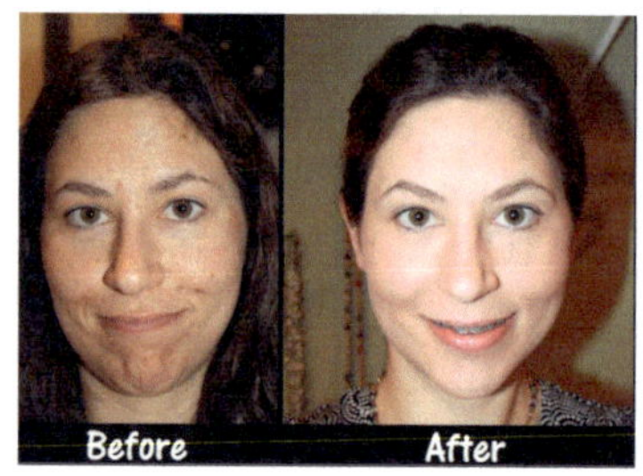

Figure 5.5. Deep peel before and after.

Source: https://blogger.googleusercontent.com/img/b/R29vZ2xl/AVvXsEhB7 Y8LclyhnWKYwu F7RieJHeK1aYt 9gpZ8hm8O tfhMsZIPVkM4zQ m5TVq0SBLp uV6cyGwpx PTeDvuZyG8RPhAp8 h23CMGY 0YMw8G4UPqDI3nOUIU fEFiSnPFW3yg7G zBYMK8b3CJ ZuKE/s640-rw/Chemical+ Peel+Before+ and+After+2.jpg.

Test Your Knowledge

1. What is the difference between superficial, medium, and deep chemical peels, and how do they affect the skin?
2. What are the key ingredients used in chemical peels, and how do they vary across different types

5.2. Indications for Chemical Peels

Learning Outcome

1. Describe acne and acne scars
2. Define the term hyperpigmentation
3. Understand fine lines and wrinkles

Determining the proper indications of chemical peels necessitates a thorough understanding of the condition of the skin and expectations from the treatment. Chemical peels are primarily indicated for individuals with many dermatological conditions, such as hyperpigmentation, post-acne scars, and signs of aging like fine lines and wrinkles. Practitioners may select the most suitable chemical agents according to thorough assessment of the skin type and specific concerns of the patient. It is also important to take necessary considerations regarding any contraindications, such as skin hypersensitivities or concurrent skin dermatoses, since these aspects can affect the efficacy of the peel as well as the safety of the treatment. An educated treatment plan ensures individualized approaches that not only accomplish the patient's aesthetic outcomes but also reduce the possible complications, hence increasing satisfaction with chemical peeling procedure results (Madnani et al., 2022). The therapeutic uses of chemical peels even go beyond cosmetic enhancements since they are also used to manage some medical skin conditions. Indications for chemical peels are the management of actinic keratosis and some types of acne, in which the exfoliating effect lowers the clogged pores and enhances skin texture. In addition, peels are useful in preparing the skin for follow-up dermatological treatments, like laser treatments or dermal fillers, in that they maximize skin health before these interventions. This utility of peels in such discrete indications renders the treatment an invaluable resource in the broader landscape of dermatology, permitting the practitioner to take a holistic approach to the health and appearance of the skin. Appreciation of these disparate indications not only increases the value of peels but also attests to their use in general dermatologic treatment (Mallia, 2003). The post-procedural care also plays an equally crucial role in both the recovery time and the final cosmetic outcome of chemical peel, hence the patient must be educated as to what they must do after the procedure, such as avoiding the sun, using only sensitive skincare products, and moisturizing during the recovery period. This focus on patient education is critical because improper aftercare can cause negative effects and spoil the advantage of the procedure. Also, continuous evaluations of the skin's reaction to the peel can serve to guide subsequent treatments or modifications in the cosmetic plan. Finally, successful results also depend not just on the treatment itself but on the active involvement of the patients during the aftercare, further emphasizing the value of educated participation in aesthetic dermatology (Madnani et al., 2022).

5.2.1. Acne and Acne Scars

The prevalence of acne is a worldwide affliction in most populations, occurring in the young during adolescence and later. Acne is primarily a chronic inflammatory disease of the sebaceous glands, producing lesions and, in some instances, permanent scarring. The scars can be atrophic and hypertrophic and are at times a psychological impediment, producing diminished self-esteem and social embarrassment. The typical form of atrophic scars usually displays a sunken appearance, which often becomes evident when the skin fails to renew itself after episodes of inflammatory acne. Because of this type of nature for acne scars, treatments that not only restore the appearance of skin but also eliminate the cause of acne itself, opened the gates to new approaches such as chemical peels (Gkouvi et al., 2025). Chemical peels have become a valid choice in the array of therapies for acne and acne scars. It is a non-surgical approach towards skin rejuvenation of the texture and prevention of scarring effects. The mode of action is also dependent on the use of chemical agents to further remove the top-most layers of the skin and further boost cellular turnover, thereby further facilitating the growth of healthy skin. Chemical peels may be divided into superficial, medium, and deep modalities, each ranging in depth of penetration and effect. Superficial peels usually involve the use of AHAs to correct mild scarring, and more intensive peels involving TCA or phenol for more significant acne scarring. The diversity of chemical peels allows dermatologists to tailor treatment protocols to meet specific requirements, enhancing their general efficacy in scar revision and skin regeneration (Gkouvi et al., 2025).

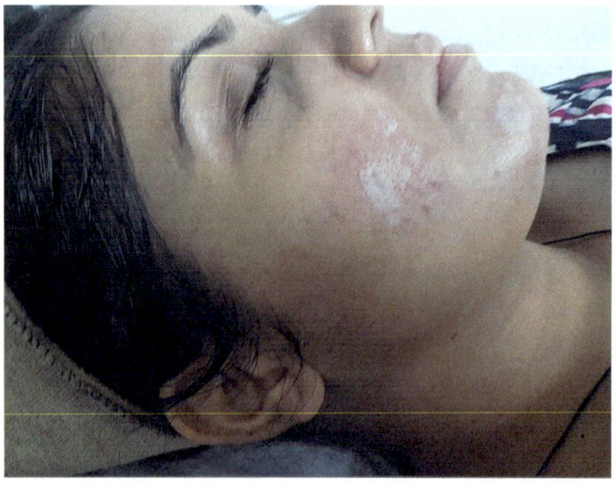

Figure 5.6. Salicylic acid is used for the treatment of acne.

Source: https://upload.wikimedia.org/wikipedia/commons/thumb/9/93/Salicylic_acid_for_treatment_of_acne.jpg/800px-Salicylic_acid_for_treatment_of_acne.jpg.

Fresh studies prioritize the efficacy of chemical peels as part of a complete therapeutic regimen for scarring acne. For instance, chemical peels improve not only skin smoothness but are also combined with other treatments such as laser or microneedling in order to provide better results. A combination of treatments may lead to synergistic effects that significantly minimize scar visibility and induce collagen production. Moreover, most patients are extremely satisfied with the outcome after treatment, as reflected by improvement scores gathered in clinical studies. These results support the belief that chemical peels, as a component of a comprehensive treatment plan, have the capability to measurably improve the acne scars and enhance the overall quality of life for those suffering from them (Lin et al., 2021) (Figure 5.6).

5.2.2. Hyperpigmentation

Hyperpigmentation is a ubiquitous dermatologic disorder that characterizes an over-production of melanin within the skin, resulting in darkened patches or spots. It can occur due to many etiologic causes, including exposure to the sun, endocrinologic changes, and skin injury in the form of acne, which is later followed by post-inflammatory pigmentary changes. For the individual who experiences hyperpigmentation, the cosmetic impact is more often than not significant, impacting self-esteem and leading to a search for effective treatment modalities. Though there are numerous treatments for hyperpigmentation, one of the most popular therapies now is indeed chemical peels as they work by exfoliating the skin and turning over cells to diminish darkened tones of the skin. Its success is also enhanced in that later topical treatments are rendered more absorptive, allowing a healthier appearance and state of the skin. When it comes to controlling hyperpigmentation, the choice of right chemical peels is paramount. Various peels, e.g., glycolic acid, salicylic acid, and TCA, have different effects based on their formulation and depth of penetration into the skin. Glycolic acid, for instance, targets primarily the surface of the skin and therefore finds application in mild hyperpigmentation, while TCA is employed for more deep-seated pigmentation issues because of its penetration. Salicylic acid, being comedolytic in action, can also be employed, particularly for post-acne hyperpigmentation. Recent studies show that salicylic acid enhances not only lesional but also hyperpigmented areas that result from acne vulgaris, which makes this agent useful in an approach toward multifaceted treatment of hyperpigmentation (Nafila et al., 2024). It is crucial, however, to use these peels only when tailored, since efficacy will actually depend on the condition of the hyperpigmentations treated and the patient's skin type. Besides these outcomes, mixing chemical peels with the use of other modalities may potentiate the results for people suffering from hyperpigmentation. Addition of photoprotection and brightening creams applied as well as laser therapies may create an effect potentiated by an additive sum greater than an isolated treatment.

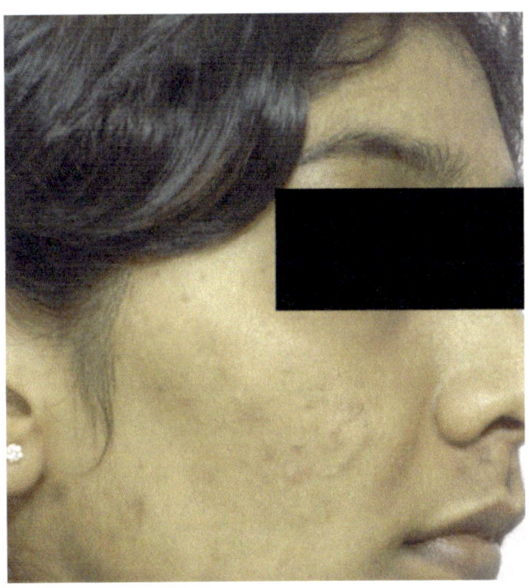

Figure 5.7. Post-inflammatory hyperpigmentation before glycolic acid peel.

Source: https://www.researchgate.net/publication/259628237/figure/fig7/AS:667197705822209@1536083737239/Postinflammatory-hyperpigmentation-before-glycolic-acid-peel.ppm.

It must be pointed out that while there are several benefits of chemical peels, patients should also be made aware of side effects such as irritation and redness and, in some cases, aggravation of pigmentation if not managed well. Therefore, the holistic management of hyperpigmentation not only encompasses the selection of the most suitable chemical peels but also the inclusion of an intense skincare regimen that focuses on photoprotection since insufficient protection may result in the recurrence of pigmentation (Halim et al., 2016). By following such protocols, clinicians are better positioned to manage hyperpigmentation, ultimately enhancing patient satisfaction and skin health outcomes (Figure 5.7).

5.2.3. Fine Lines and Wrinkles

Appearance of wrinkles and fine lines is a natural phenomenon of aging, usually caused by external factors as well as lifestyle issues. When the skin ages, its internal elasticity is compromised due to decreased collagen and elastin production, leading to outward textural and visual changes. A number of solutions have been invented to address these signs of aging, one of the strongest being chemical peels. These peels induce a controlled exfoliation of the skin, which enables the removal of damaged outer layers while inducing deeper regeneration of the skin, which will significantly improve the aesthetic appearance of fine lines and wrinkles. With these effects, patients usually report enhanced skin tone and texture, illustrating the potential of chemical peels to rejuvenate senescent skin in a non-surgical manner. The efficacy of chemical peels depends on the depth of the peels to treat fine lines and wrinkles. Superficial peels only treat the epidermis, producing minimal effects on the texture of the skin, whereas medium and deep peels penetrate down to deeper structures to bring about better results. The ability to reduce medium wrinkles, correct abnormalities in pigmentation, and improve the total homogeneity of the skin makes medium peels particularly remarkable. Recent research has indicated that chemical peels cause enhanced collagen production. This is the key to healthy and firm skin. Enhanced collagen formation gives a gradual plumping effect. As such, it is effective in minimizing the appearance of fine lines and allows the rejuvenation of the skin's appearance eventually, according to Manjula (2023). Therefore, for individuals who aim to reduce aging signs, these peel treatments are an option. In addition to the immediate cosmetic improvement, chemical peels can also create long-term healthy skin by enhancing cellular turnover. This increased process of eliminating dead skin cells can result in a more youthful complexion and reduction of fine lines and wrinkles because the skin is constantly resurfacing. Moreover, chemical peels also improve the texture and tone of the skin. They erase hyperpigmentation and uneven patches that add to the general ageing effect. The addition of blue light treatments as adjunct therapies will further add to the enhanced effects of chemical peels, affecting sebaceous glands and ultimately reducing oil production, which leads to curbing the tendency of their development, which leads to forming typical characteristics of aging skin, as indicated in Kamal et al. (2024). In short, chemical peels not only serve as a great remedy against wrinkles and fine lines but also contribute to long-term vitality and shine of the skin (Figure 5.8).

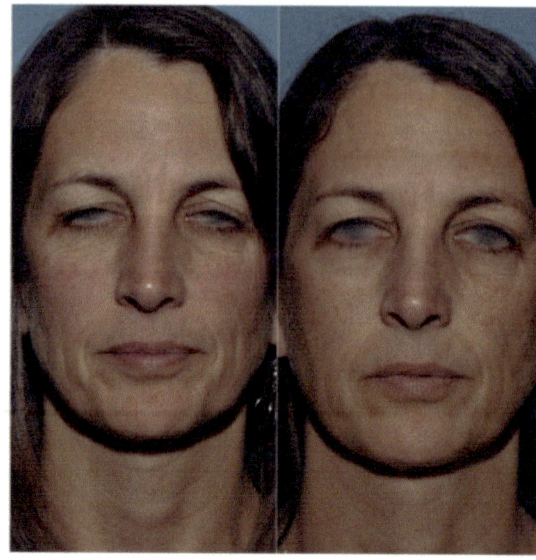

Figure 5.8. Subject treated with combination (onaBTX-A + chemical peel) at baseline (left) and at 10 weeks (right).

Source: https://www.researchgate.net/publication/292642531/figure/fig1/AS:344981618348033@1459261435160/Subject-treated-with-combination-onaBTX-A-chemical-peel-at-baseline-left-and-at-10.png.

Test Your Knowledge

1. What are the primary skin conditions that chemical peels are commonly used to treat, such as acne, hyperpigmentation, or fine lines?
2. How effective are chemical peels in treating acne scars, and which type of peel is most commonly recommended for this condition?

5.3. The Chemical Peel Procedure

Learning Outcome

1. Discuss pre-treatment consultation
2. Understand the application process of chemical peels
3. Explain how post-treatment care following chemical peels is crucial

Chemical peel treatment is a general dermatological procedure for enhancing the fine appearance of the skin by shedding its upper surface layers. A chemical solution is applied to the skin in the form of treatment, inducing intentional exfoliation that reveals healthier and less damaged skin beneath. Various types of chemical peels exist, and they are classified as superficial, medium, and deep peels, each of which addresses specific skin problems and varies in strength as well as recovery time. Superficial peels typically use weak acids, which include AHAs, to address subtle skin problems such as dryness or irregular texture. Deeper peels, on the other hand, use stronger chemicals, like TCA, to remove more prominent signs of aging, hyperpigmentation, and acne scarring, making it crucial for patients to seek consultations from healthcare experts to address the most appropriate method for their skin type and ailment. Patient selection is paramount to the success of chemical peel treatment, requiring careful pre-treatment evaluation. Skin type, medical history, and underlying skin conditions are assessed to provide the best outcomes and prevent possible adverse effects. During consultation, clinicians also educate patients on different types of peels, outcomes, and post-treatment procedures, including adherence to pre- and post-treatment directives for maximizing healing and results. Sensitive skin patients, for example, are treated with lighter organic peels containing natural substances like pumpkin enzyme extracts, which are known for skin renewal functions, as highlighted in current research studies. These natural substitutes demonstrated the therapeutic worth with a decrease in risks associated with more invasive chemical treatments, which again resulted in patient satisfaction and improved overall treatment results being seen (Rayer et al., 2024). Healing after chemical peels was significantly variable based on the depth of peels and individual dermatological responses. Most patients have only mild redness and irritation, similar to mild sunburn, after a superficial peel, but this usually resolves within a few days. Medium and deep peels can cause greater peeling and longer recovery time. The value of proper aftercare cannot be overemphasized; patients are told to stay out of the sun, use mild cleansers, and apply moisturizers to facilitate healing. Also, information on the peel science can enhance patient compliance and care compliance. Research on new agents, such as plant-derived coagulants to be employed in dermal formulations and their uses reflects the shifting trend in dermatological interventions that patients receive to select and prioritize based on their issues with efficacy and safety: examples such as natural coagulants (Rayer et al., 2024).

5.3.1. Pre-Treatment Consultation

The significance of a pre-treatment consultation before undergoing a chemical peel can never be overlooked. This is the initial step in the process that allows practitioners to treat patients type of skin type, medical background, and beauty objectives. Dermatologists routinely perform an extensive consultation where they determine any contradictions or dangers involved with chemical peels. A tailored strategy is of the utmost significance since skin sensitivity or pre-existing medical conditions may impact the choice of peel strength and type. Moreover, describing hoped-for outcomes and possible side effects informs patients, increases confidence levels, and ensures informed consent. Hence, the pre-treatment consultation is fundamental for creating realistic expectations and developing patient satisfaction through personalized care. In addition to medical assessment, pre-treatment consultation is an opportunity to educate patients regarding the chemical peel process. Familiarity with the varieties of peel solutions—superficial to deep peels—equips patients to choose their desired outcome for the skin. Practitioners may present information regarding the specific benefits of each type, such as the capacity to reduce hyperpigmentation or texture enhancement. It also presents an opportunity to address the significance of post-treatment, which is key to maximum recovery and outcomes. For example, patients will be required to change their skincare routines or stay away from exposure to the sun prior to and after the treatment.

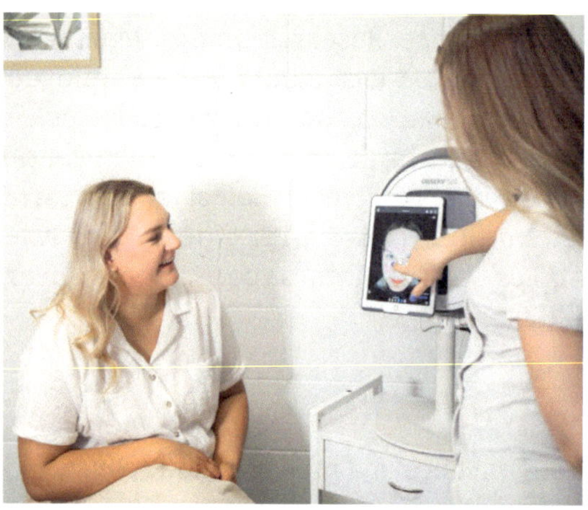

Figure 5.9. Skin Analysis for treatment.

Source: https://www.soulskin.com.au/wp-content/uploads/2015/04/LR-soul-skin-68-1000x700.jpg.

Therefore, a properly organized consultation serves to demystify the procedure and make patients adequately ready for what lies ahead. Pre-treatment consultation also ensures patients' psychological preparation for chemical peel treatment. Psychology can significantly affect the results, too, since anxiety or unmet expectations might give undesired results. Open communication can, therefore, allay fears and create an amicable relationship with clients, which is mostly what makes an encounter successful. In addition, discussing previous treatments and results is important in managing patient motivations and preferences. Having remedies to enhance comfort, such as discussing anesthesia choices when needed, can also reduce anxiety among patients. Lastly, the pre-treatment consultation not only focuses on skin health but also on the psychological realm of undergoing aesthetic treatments, leading to a comprehensive strategy for patient care (Figure 5.9).

5.3.2. Application Process

The application of chemical peeling is a sophisticated procedure with the involvement of careful consideration of various factors to achieve the best possible benefits. The applicants are first submitted to a full skin analysis by a skilled practitioner, where individual concerns and skin type are examined. This step is critical as it helps determine the selection of the chemical solution to be used, tailoring the treatment to individual needs. Following this analysis, the area of concern is properly cleaned in order to remove oil, grime, and makeup such that the peel can penetrate the skin. The first cleaning process serves as the basis for the final application, where the chemicals in the peel are provided with effectively with the skin layers and can cause the desired effect. Following skin preparation, application of the chemical solution begins, most often with either a brush or gauze to achieve an even layer. The depth of peel, superficial, medium, or deep, dramatically influences the duration of the application and the overall concentration of chemical applied. Superficial peels generally utilize less strong acids such as AHAs, while medium and deep peels tend to utilize TCA or phenol to achieve more dramatic results. Practitioners should carefully watch the skin's reaction to the application as reaction times differ. For instance, if a deeper peel is administered, timing is essential so as not to incur any adverse reaction, and therefore, the practitioner's technique is important at this level of treatment. Post-application care is also important so as to ensure that the chemical peel works effectively while limiting potential side effects.

Following the treatment, redness or sensitivity of the skin can be temporary; therefore, practitioners generally recommend a strict aftercare regimen. This may include the application of calming agents and instructing the patient to apply broad-spectrum sunscreen to prevent UV damage while the skin heals. Additionally, the patient is normally instructed not to apply exfoliating products for a certain period of time in order to allow the skin to heal. The discussion regarding the application process highlights the importance of both theory and practice, reflecting the complexity of achieving successful outcomes in chemical peel treatments, as observed in research regarding materials and preparation techniques within the corresponding fields (Ropes et al., 1987; Bowyer et al., 2018) (Figure 5.10).

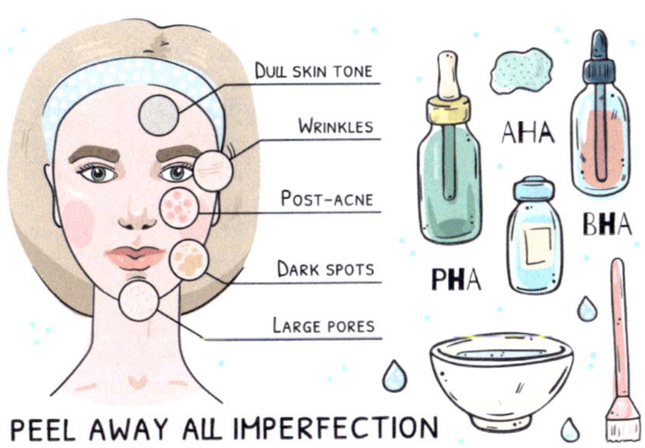

Figure 5.10. Suitable chemical peels for skin: AHA, BHA, PHA.

Source: https://ensoulclinic.b-cdn.net/wp-content/uploads/2022/01/AHA-BHA-PHA.png.

5.3.3. Post-Treatment Care

Post-peel care is required to optimize effects and prevent complications following chemical peels. Patients may experience a range of redness, swelling, and peeling depending on the depth of the peel that has been done. Simple post-care is begun by gently cleansing the treated area with a mild cleanser without employing aggressive scrubs or exfoliants that could exacerbate irritation. Besides, the use of a suitable moisturizer should be recommended to soothe the skin and retain moisture. At the time of skin renewal, educating patients on the peeling process, which tends to resolve within a week, is fundamental to reduce concern regarding appearance and also to standardize recovery expectations. In addition to topical care, protection from the sun forms a fundamental aspect of post-procedure management. Ultraviolet light exposure can contribute significantly to compromising the healing process and inducing unwanted pigmentation changes. Therefore, the patient is to be directed to wear a broad-spectrum sunscreen with a high SPF daily, irrespective of the fact that they might be indoors. Protective clothing and shade covering the most intense sunlight periods form a secondary line of protection. By making sun protection a foremost priority, patients are more efficiently able to optimize the effectiveness of the chemical peel and provide optimal healing, reducing the possibility of side effects such as post-inflammatory hyperpigmentation (PIH), an area of particular concern in darker skin tones. Furthermore, the use of newer-generation skincare products can also augment post-procedure care. Adding agents such as hyaluronic acid or antioxidants can boost skin hydration and repair, providing the best possible climate in which to heal. Professional consultation in the selection of a product cannot be stressed highly enough, with certain ingredients having deleterious interaction with healing skin. Proper education in such considerations is required, and evidence points to that compliance with post-treatment guidance evidences significantly improved outcomes and satisfaction rates for patients. Therefore, practitioners must ensure patients understand the importance of following detailed post-treatment care instructions to achieve the desired results from their chemical peel experience (Ambrosio et al., 2018; Abla et al., 2013) (Figure 5.11).

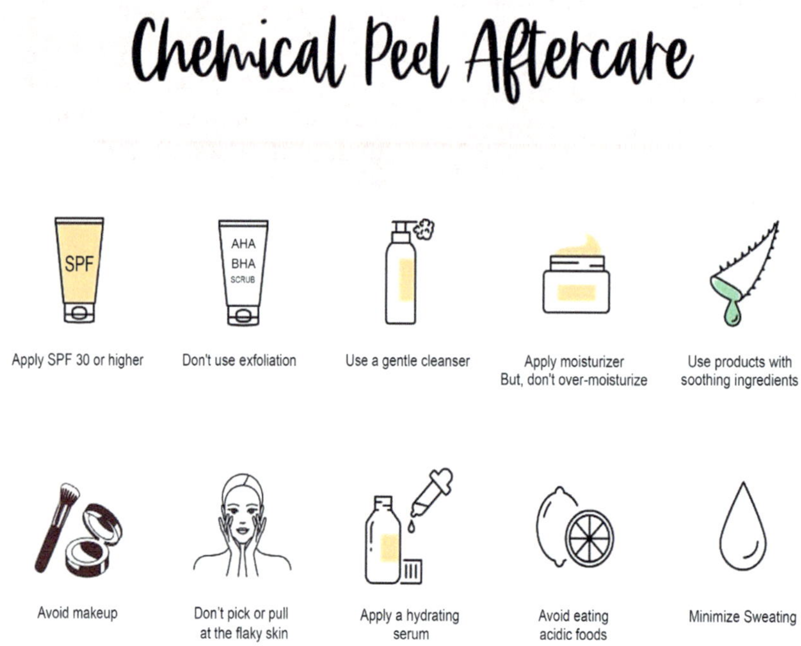
Chemical Peel Aftercare
SPF
Apply SPF 30 or higher
AHA
BHA
SCRUB
Don't use exfoliation
Use a gentle cleanser
Apply moisturizer
But, don't over-moisturize
Use products with
soothing ingredients
Avoid makeup
Don't pick or pull
at the flaky skin
Apply a hydrating
serum
Avoid eating
acidic foods
Minimize Sweating

Figure 5.11. Chemical peel aftercare.

Source: https://images.squarespace-cdn.com/content/v1/55db4cd3e4b0300a610091bb/13369062-5ca1-4988-9181-569ea1f7ba05/Chemical-peel-aftercare-instructions.jpg.

Test Your Knowledge

1. What steps are involved in the chemical peel procedure, and how long does the treatment typically take?
2. How does the preparation for a chemical peel (such as discontinuing certain skincare products) impact the outcome of the procedure?

5.4. Benefits of Chemical Peels

Learning Outcome

1. Discuss skin rejuvenation through chemical peels
2. Explain how to improve skin texture with chemical peels
3. Understand the phenomenon of enhanced product absorption

Chemical peels have been associated with having a higher level of popularity in dermatology since they allow for a dramatic rejuvenation of skin textures and tones. It is accomplished through applying chemical solutions to the skin that hasten exfoliation, thereby assisting in eliminating dead cells and stimulating new cell growth. This treatment not only exposes a new layer of skin but also triggers collagen synthesis, which is essential to help keep the skin firm and minimize the visibility of lines. In addition, chemical peels are able to address numerous skin issues, including acne, sun damage, and discoloration, thereby making them a highly effective treatment for skin patients looking to improve their complexion. The advances in chemical peel formulations have made them a safer and more effective treatment, making them more attractive in aesthetic practice, according to Mathur et al. (2024). Other than the cosmetic benefits that come with using chemical peels, one can also use them as a preventive measure against skincare concerns. When incorporated into a regular skincare routine, one may reduce one's chances of developing deeper lines, wrinkles, and other signs of aging. The process can assist with the maintenance of healthier, clearer skin through lessening such problems as pore clogs and acne flare-ups. With the changing world of dermatological procedures, the combination of chemical peels with complementary therapies has proven to maximize patient satisfaction and results. For example, the fusion of chemical peels with other treatments such as microneedling or laser treatment might be used to optimize the benefits and reduce downtime, and thus provide a more comprehensive skincare solution (Fabi et al., 2024). Further, the new technologies have led to more sophisticated chemical peeling options that can now address a wider range of skin issues and types. Patients today are able to enjoy personalized treatments that consider their individual skin conditions, tolerance levels, and desired outcomes. These developments not only maximize the effectiveness of chemical peels but also make the experience more comfortable for consumers. As a result, the popularity of these procedures continues to increase as more people learn about the long-term advantages that come with regular peels. The psychological benefit of enhanced skin texture and appearance cannot be overstated; individuals typically report increased confidence and satisfaction after the treatment, further establishing the multiple benefits of chemical peels within the field of aesthetic dermatology (Fabi et al., 2024).

5.4.1. Skin Rejuvenation

In recent times, the need for chemical peeling in skin rejuvenation has become very popular in clinical and cosmetic dermatology. Chemical peels, especially involving AHAs, induce programmed exfoliation of the skin and thus stimulate cellular turnover. Such a process not only cures surface imperfections such as fine lines and patchy pigmentation but also improves deeper dermal properties by inducing collagen synthesis. According to current studies, new products containing biostimulating acidic phytocompounds (ABAPs) can penetrate the skin's barrier effectively, synergizing with the effectiveness of traditional chemical peels. Focusing on the general appearance and texture of the skin, these new finds bode very well for non-surgical skin rejuvenation procedures that meet the needs of patients seeking overall improvement in the appearance of their skin (Iglesia et al., 2025). In assessing the effectiveness of chemical peels, it is important to look not only at the surface results but also at the changes taking place at a deeper level within the skin. A comparison study on 15% TCA peels showed that combining TCA peels with other rejuvenating therapies, like NCTF®135HA injections, was more effective. The synergistic action of such combination treatments greatly improved hydration of the skin, enhanced homogeneity, and reduced the appearance of aging more than the use of TCA peels alone. These results highlight the promise of combination strategies in skin rejuvenation and imply that the multi-aspectual nature of skin aging demands multi-faceted treatment programs that address both the epidermis and dermis (Smit, 2024).

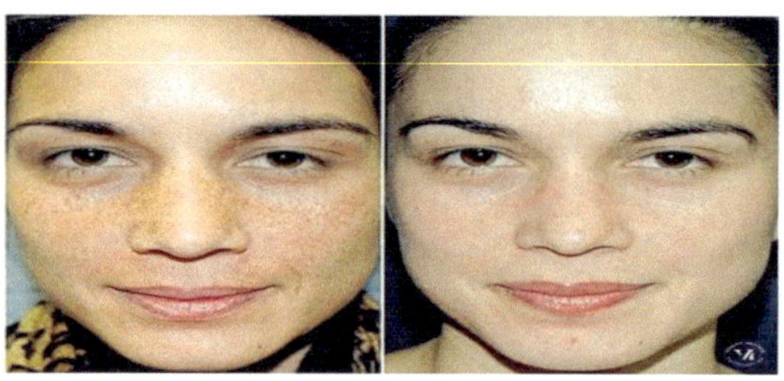

Figure 5.12. Clinical effect of Chemical peel on Sun damage.

Source: https://www.researchgate.net/publication/386032349_Revitalize_Your_Skin_A_Comprehensive_Review_of_Chemical_peel/fulltext/6740475427661f7ae6621813/Revitalize-Your-Skin-A-Comprehensive-Review-of-Chemical-peel.pdf?_tp=eyJjb250ZXh0Ijp7Im ZpcnN0UGFnZSI6Il9kaXJlY3QiLC wYWdlIjoicHVi bGljYXRpb24ifX0.

With patients increasingly seeking non-invasive methods for rejuvenating skin, the role of chemical peels in aesthetic treatment cannot be overemphasized. Educative campaigns about the safety and efficacy of various types of chemical peels empower practitioners and patients alike with the information necessary to make the right decisions regarding their treatment of the skin. Technologies, such as those concerning ABAP technology, continue to refine the peeling process so that more delivery mechanisms are available to aid therapeutic efficacy. This evolution toward increasingly advanced treatments not only enhances patient satisfaction but also establishes chemical peels as a cornerstone of modern cosmetic dermatology. With ongoing research uncovering new formulations and approaches, the field of skin rejuvenation is on the cusp of change, with potential to create breakthroughs further maximizing the body's natural healing processes (Iglesia et al., 2025) (Figure 5.12).

5.4.2. Improved Skin Texture

The desire for improved texture of the skin tends to send patients in search of a variety of dermatological treatments, among which chemical peeling has joined the mainstream. Chemical peels induce selective removal of dead skin cells through shedding of the top layers. Not only does this provide the skin's surface with a better appearance, but it also stimulates the growth of new healthy skin underneath. Patients often report after treatment a significant improvement in skin smoothness and overall glow. Also, with increasingly smoother skin, issues such as coarseness, uneven tone, and minor scarring will potentially be reduced, leaving a smoother and fresher complexion. The efficacy of chemical peels can typically be attributed to the specific acids used, which vary in intensity and formulation—each tailored to target specific skin concerns. Additionally, the overall benefit of chemical peels extends far beyond superficial exfoliation. According to recent studies, the interventions enable eminent improvement in elasticity and hydration of the skin, critical factors toward attaining optimum skin texture. The combination of home treatments with outpatient procedures ensures optimal overall outcomes, as is seen from considerable advances reported in interventions encompassing both procedures (Caruso et al., 2020). An individually customized treatment protocol, formulated by thorough clinical evaluation, allows for precise results, treating unique issues presented by different skin types and conditions. Throughout the repair process of the skin post-peel, issues such as hyperpigmentation and large pores can also see noteworthy improvement, leading to a generally better looks and feel of the skin. Besides this, chemical peel usage for treating certain skin concerns has seen widespread documentation. Particularly, methods of treating lightening of hyperpigmented lesions reflect the way chemical peeling will soften the color and texture of the skin through dermal clearance of pigmented lesions and lowering of skin blemishes (Halim et al., 2016).

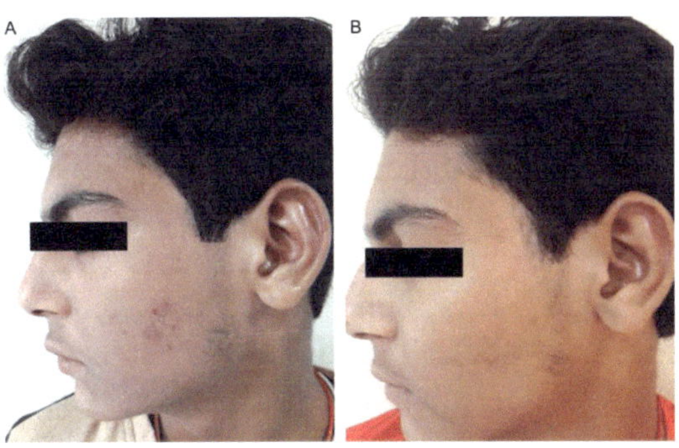

Figure 5.13. Images (A) and (B) show the baseline and 12-week results with phytic acid peel combination.

Source: https://www.researchgate.net/publication/335982535/figure/fig2/AS:820845953941507@1572716334921/mages-A-and-B-show-the-baseline-and-12-week-results-with-phytic-acid-peel-combination.ppm.

Not only docs this personalized method enhance the user experience, but it also ensures the optimal treatment for a patient's condition. It is important to pair chemical peels, however, with appropriate skin protection and adjunctive therapies to ensure the skin's new smoothness and clarity. Consequently, patients reap the rewards of a full spectrum of skin care that advances long-term improvement in skin texture, further reinforcing their confidence and level of satisfaction with cosmetic treatment (Figure 5.13).

5.4.3. Enhanced Product Absorption

Increased product penetration is a critical process behind chemical peel efficacy. Chemical peels work by exfoliating the surface of the skin, allowing for improved delivery of active ingredients in topical treatments. Such higher penetration is instrumental to the achievement of desired skin outcomes, such as improved texture, tone, and overall appearance. Augmentation methods involve the application of specific exfoliating agents that eliminate dead cells but also facilitate the permeability of the subsequent topical treatment. The incorporation of natural antioxidants, which can be obtained from by-products of food or unutilized plant species, has also been viewed as a novel method to enhance the protective effects of chemical peels, thereby enhancing the absorption of the product and overall skin health (Alves et al., 2019). Furthermore, the synergy of chemical peels with topicals can be optimized by supplementing them with bioactive constituents that are known to be synergistic on the skin. One such example is the utilization of phytochemicals from pomegranate, such as anthocyanins and hydrolyzable tannins, a form of antioxidant that may help topicals penetrate more when applied post-peeling. Not only do they offer protective benefits, but they may also interact positively with skin physiology to generate greater product efficacy. The way these antioxidants act may influence the absorption mechanisms, which is why variability in structure and function of such natural agents needs to be known when utilized in chemical peels (Wu & Tian, 2017). In addition to the chemical makeup of peel products, the application method and pH adjustment can affect the absorption of a product to a considerable degree. By controlling these factors, practitioners are able to create conditions to further increase the diffusion of active compounds into the skin layers. The role of pH is even more significant in that some components are in their optimal condition at a particular pH, thus enhancing their permeability. This nuanced understanding of how various elements interact together not only enhances the results of chemical peels but also optimizes the absorption of future treatments. With increased insight into the intricacies of skin physiology enabled by new studies, the potential to access advanced absorption will be kept at the forefront of dermatological advancement and skincare effectiveness.

Test Your Knowledge

1. How do chemical peels stimulate collagen production and contribute to overall skin rejuvenation?
2. How do chemical peels improve skin texture and tone, and what visible changes can a patient expect after treatment?

5.5. Risks and Side Effects

Learning Outcome

1. Discuss about common side effects of chemical peels
2. Explain rare complications by using chemical peels
3. Understand contraindications for certain individuals

The employment of chemical peels has several aesthetic benefits, but it is also necessary to consider the risks and side effects that arise from these procedures. Irritation of the skin is one of the most common side effects and manifests as redness, peeling, or burning following the procedure. Mild chemical peels tend to cause pain for a short duration, while deeper peels may cause more severe reactions, including swelling and prolonged erythema. The clinicians performing these procedures should have extensive knowledge of the chemical substances employed, as the level and composition of the acid used can greatly affect the result. Also, those with sensitive skin or pre-existing dermatological diseases should exercise extreme caution when undergoing chemical peels, as they are likely to be further affected by a more vigorous skin reaction. Therefore, patient education and educated decision-making are the primary requirements to minimize risks and attain successful outcomes among patients who opt for chemical peels (Madnani et al., 2022). Infection is another serious risk of chemical peels. When the skin's protective layer gets compromised in the process of a peel, the skin becomes liable to bacterial, viral, or fungal infections. The risk is greater if the post-procedure care is inadequate or if the procedure has been performed in non-sterile conditions. Moreover, patients with a history of herpes simplex virus or any other autoimmune condition are at higher risk of infections following peeling. It is crucial that medical care providers screen the patient for these conditions and advise him or her on correct post-procedure care to reduce the risk of infections. Furthermore, sun avoidance and sun exposure are discouraged in patients, and play with the treated area is avoided in order to further reduce complications. Anticipatory measures towards managing these risks are critical towards increasing patient safety and satisfaction within chemical peeling procedures

(Kamlenga et al., 2024). Pigmentation changes and scarring are additional possible risks implicated in chemical peels, particularly in darker skin types of patients. Hypopigmentation and hyperpigmentation are risks associated with the peel, resulting in skin tone that is not even and dissatisfaction with the cosmetic outcomes. This is of particular concern in the patient who has melasma or a comparable condition, as he or she may view increased discoloration after treatment. To reduce these risks, providers tend to suggest that the patch test be done before a full peel, enabling the clinician to assess the patient's skin reaction. Also, the application of pre and post-care protocols could minimize the potential for side effects. Due to the intricacies involved in chemical peeling treatments, it is important that practitioners have a critical perception of the benefits and limitations and render patient-specific interventions that are concerned with safeguarding patient safety as well as aesthetic demand (Madnani et al., 2022).

5.5.1. Common Side Effects

Chemical peels, while beneficial for initiating skin rejuvenation, can result in a range of normal side effects that need to be explained to patients before they receive the treatment. Redness, peeling, and skin irritation are among the most frequent side effects reported, and these tend to occur as the top layer of skin is shed. These side effects are typically mild and unavoidable, as they show that the chemical solution is effective in promoting cell turnover and healing. Redness can look similar to a sunburn and normally fades in a few days, but in some instances, people may have persistent irritation or sensitivity, especially if they have hypersensitive skin or pre-existing skin conditions. Knowledge of these side effects will enable patients to form realistic expectations and properly prepare for post-peel treatment. In addition to redness and inflammation, post-peel pigmentation alterations are to be anticipated, especially in darker skin types. PIH is an entity in which areas of the skin become darker due to inflammation secondary to the peel. This side effect is transitory but could be inconvenient to the patients, particularly those anticipating seeing quick and consistent results. Alternatively, some individuals may experience hypopigmentation in which the lightening takes place in spots.

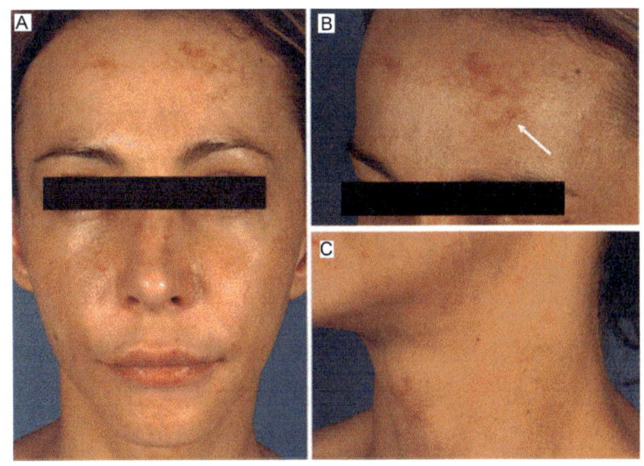

Figure 5.14. Persistence of long-term adverse effects 2 months post chemical peeling. (A) Persistent facial hyperpigmentation 2 months after initiation of therapy; (B) Long-term adverse reaction, including scarring (indicated by arrow); and (C) Nearly complete resolution of the hyperpigmentation on the neck after 2 months of therapy.

Source: https://www.researchgate.net/publication/267932469/figure/fig1/AS:272609279475731@1442006525148/Persistence-of-long-term-adverse-effects-2months-post-chemical-peeling-A-Persistent.png.

These changes do justify the significance of pre-treatment sessions where one assesses the patients' skin type as well as advises them as necessary. Informing patients about potential changes assists in the alleviation of worry about unplanned outcomes and prevents nonadherence to aftercare. Lastly, while uncommon, more severe side effects such as scarring or infection may occur, particularly if strict adherence to post-peel aftercare is not maintained. Proper aftercare is critical because it minimizes the risk of complications and promotes healing. Patients are usually advised to stay out of the sun and to use mild skincare products after a peel. In addition, side effects in the form of excessive dryness or rash can occur because of the skin's healing process, necessitating individualized strategies for moisturizing replenishment. Through a thorough management of these typical side effects and stressing the importance of aftercare commitment, chemical peel treatments can be both safe and effective for individuals desiring successful skin rejuvenation (Figure 5.14).

5.5.2. Rare Complications

The application of chemical peels as a routine cosmetic procedure holds the potential for brilliant rejuvenation and, conversely, rare complications. With the numerous benefits that include removing hurt surface layers and blanching pigmentation, some may have unexpected side effects. The most commonly reported unusual complications are hypertrophic scarring, PIH, and in a few cases even atrophic scarring. While the complications of these types are uncommon, they can tremendously affect patient satisfaction and long-term results. Being aware of the risk factors involved, e.g., the skin type and the solution used, can assist practitioners in lessening the potential risks and managing patient expectations in case of having chemical peels (Timraz et al., 2025). Awareness is paramount in a clinical environment where enhancing the look of the skin must be balanced against the ethical implications of patient safety. Considering the variety of complications with chemical peels, the role of practitioner experience and training as a factor in preventing adverse results emerges as the major determinant. A retrospective evaluation of complicated patients indicates that even experienced practitioners can experience unforeseen complications during the treatment. The complexity of chemical peel procedures requires critical understanding and experience, particularly in selecting the specific patient parameters and level of susceptibility to complications (Murray et al., 2024). Even non-invasive procedures, while generally held to be safer than traditional surgery, do have limitations. Accordingly, it is essential that providers are appropriately trained in the detection and management of complications that may arise so that they are able to manage situations that would lead to permanently adverse outcomes for patients. Additionally, an active approach towards complication management is vital in an effort to enhance patient safety and outcomes in chemical peel therapies.

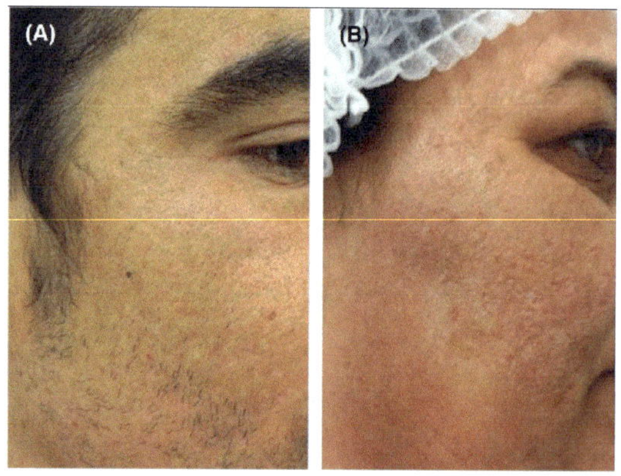

Figure 5.15. Complications seen with the use of 90% TCA: (A) the patient with hypopigmentation; and (B) the patient's scar became wider.

Source: https://www.researchgate.net/profile/Ana-Paula-Manzoni/publication/293015449/figure/fig5/AS:446803221979140@1483537597188/Complications-seen-with-the-use-of-90-TCA-A-the-patient-with-hypopigmentation-and.png.

Continuous training on new methods and innovation in chemical peels can also assist practitioners in acquiring expertise. Despite the rising popularity of non-surgical cosmetic treatments, there exists a growing risk of complications, and therefore there must be an in-depth system for standardized training amongst the providers (Murray et al., 2024).

The risk of unusual complications must also be explained to patients such that they can make appropriate decisions regarding their treatment. Ultimately, fostering an environment focused on patient education and practitioner competency will enhance the overall efficacy of chemical peels while minimizing the risk of enduring complications. This holistic approach is crucial in promoting not only aesthetic satisfaction but also long-term trust between patients and their healthcare providers (Figure 5.15).

5.5.3. Contraindications for Certain Individuals

When making preparations for chemical peels to rejuvenate the skin, contraindications should be considered to exclude patients from such treatments to avoid any harm. Patients with a history of severe allergies or hypersensitivity, particularly to the active ingredients used in chemical peels, should exercise care. Moreover, patients with conditions like eczema, psoriasis, or dermatitis need to be assessed with utmost care, as these conditions tend to worsen post-peel complications and can cause reactions. Also, patients with active infections, such as herpes simplex or bacterial infection, are not recommended a chemical peel until the infections are completely cleared to avoid further irritation or infection spread. Pregnant and nursing mothers are yet another group that is warned to avoid chemical peels since systemic absorption of the chemicals can occur and their effect on the fetus or baby is unclear. Even if milder peels are deemed safe, it is advisable to err on the side of caution. Furthermore, those with a keloid or hypertrophic tendency to scar have a greater tendency to develop these side effects from a peel. This is particularly true for darker skin types since they are apt to suffer from PIH. It is, therefore, critical that consultation and patient history are taken meticulously to check the patient's eligibility for chemical peels. Some medications are contraindicated for chemical peels, which require careful patient assessment. Patients on systemic isotretinoin or similar medications should be warned against chemical peeling for at least one year following therapy due to the extreme influence such drugs have on skin sensitivity and healing responses. The scenario of multiple therapeutic options for skin diseases, as depicted in the acne treatment consensus document, shows the need to plan treatment in an integrative manner (Arsiwala et al., 2022). Being aware of the advantages and disadvantages of chemical peels is important. While professionals work towards providing effective skin care, patient safety can be ensured only by identifying such contraindications (Molina, 2004).

Test Your Knowledge

1. What are the most common side effects following a chemical peel, and how long do they usually last?
2. What are the potential risks of deeper chemical peels, such as scarring or changes in skin pigmentation?

5.6. Comparison with Other Skin Treatments

Learning Outcome

1. Differentiate between chemical peels and microdermabrasion
2. Compare Chemical peels and laser treatments
3. Distinguish between chemical peels and topical treatments

Chemical peels are increasingly recognized for their efficacy and favorable safety profile when compared to various skin treatments, such as laser therapies and microdermabrasion. For instance, while laser treatments can achieve significant results for conditions like melasma and acne scars, they often require longer recovery times and can present risks such as hyperpigmentation or burns. In contrast, chemical peels utilize a variety of agents to exfoliate the skin and promote cell turnover, resulting in improved texture and appearance. The versatility of chemical peels, from superficial to deep formulations, enables practitioners to tailor treatments to diverse skin types, effectively addressing issues ranging from fine lines to hyperpigmentation without the extensive downtime typically associated with more invasive procedures (Gentili et al., 2022). In addition, research has established that more recent formulations, including those containing the patent-pending blend of next-generation acids like ELPA25™, provide better tolerance for sensitive skin. Ideally, these developments are particularly significant compared to historical ingredient treatments, like mandelic acid serums, which can be less comfortable and less effective for some patients. Studies have proven that Miamo Renewal Peel Serum has the potential for causing terrific improvements in the softness and elastin content of the skin, thus showing its supremacy over other surface treatments (Gentili et al., 2022). Therefore, chemical peels are a reality for those looking to revitalize and invigorate their complexion accordingly, primarily when other methods are less feasible or inconceivable. Apart from their direct benefits, chemical peels have found acceptance in part because of the relative safety they offer when compared to dietary supplements commercially available for skin health. The increasing prevalence of supplement reliance for skin betterment often results in undesired side effects and imbalances in nutrition, especially among athletes and health-conscious consumers seeking unproven products. Chemical peels, on the other hand, offer a scientifically-proven treatment option with controlled and predictable results that remove the risk of untested and unpredictable side effects from dietary supplements. In the end, by offering a scientifically-proven treatment option compared to the unstable landscape of dietary supplements, chemical peels can produce aesthetic results as well as confidence in safety and effectiveness, demonstrating them as the better option among dermatological treatments.

5.6.1. Chemical Peels vs. Microdermabrasion

The contrast between chemical peels and microdermabrasion highlights two different methods of skin rejuvenation, each with its respective advantages and limitations. Chemical peels are achieved by applying a chemical solution to the skin, which stimulates controlled exfoliation, resulting in the removal of the topmost layers. The procedure effectively treats a host of different skin issues, such as acne scars, hyperpigmentation, and fine lines. In contrast, microdermabrasion utilizes a physical exfoliation method, applying abrasive crystals or a diamond wand to strip away dead skin cells from the skin's surface. Although both processes provide subtle enhancements to skin texture and tone, chemical peels tend to penetrate more deeply into the skin, which makes them a better choice for people who want to address more serious dermatological concerns. As a result, the decision between these two alternatives typically hinges on the patient's skin type and the outcomes that the client desires. In practice, chemical peels and microdermabrasion have entirely different safety and efficacy profiles. Chemical peels range from superficial to deep peels, deep peels having more recovery time and more dramatic consequences. For example, superficial peels may be done in an outpatient department with minimal down time, whereas deeper peels may require extensive aftercare. By contrast, microdermabrasion is often regarded as less invasive with almost no down time, and the patient may return to normal activities instantly. It should, however, be noted that although microdermabrasion provides a lighter level of peeling, it does not necessarily deliver the same degree of change as deeper chemical peels (Ambrosio et al., 2018).

Therefore, the treatment selection has to match patients' individual skin problems and tolerance for post-procedure recovery. Additionally, professional experience and patient education are decisive in identifying the appropriate treatment method for skin problems. Advanced aesthetic techniques are being brought more into the realm of beauty therapy education, with the focus being on the need for therapists to be current with the newest techniques, skills, and safety procedures used in these treatments (Ambrosio et al., 2018). Dermatological clinicians often prescribe chemical peels, especially for patients with chronic conditions such as acne, where deeper exfoliation is more beneficial than microdermabrasion. Given the potential for bacterial resistance in acne treatment, incorporating a variety of non-antimicrobial therapies, including chemical peels, can be essential for optimal patient outcomes. Ultimately, understanding the nuances of both chemical peels and microdermabrasion will empower patients to make informed decisions suited to their individual skin care goals (Figure 5.16).

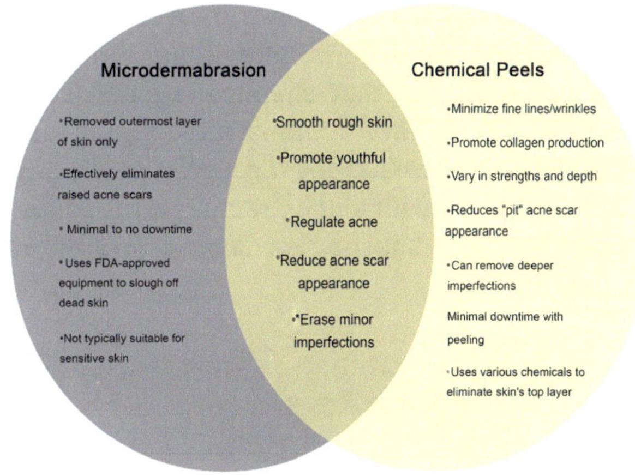

Figure 5.16. Microdermabrasion and chemical peels.

Source: https://www.atlaserlights.com/wp-content/uploads/2013/11/microderm-vs-chemical-peels.png.

5.6.2. Chemical Peels vs. Laser Treatments

Chemical peels and laser treatment are two well-respected procedures used in dermatology to enhance skin texture and treat many skin conditions. While both are aimed at resurfacing the skin and reducing such issues as acne, blemishes, and lines, they do so through very different approaches. Chemical peels encompass a solution of acids that remove the outermost layers of the skin, thus permitting cellular turnover and promoting growth of new skin. This type of treatment can range from superficial to deeper treatments based on the patient's needs, typically leading to noticeable improvements in skin tone and texture. Laser treatments, however, employ focused light energy to target dermal tissues selectively, inducing repair and producing collagen over a course of time. Recognition of these differences, and their implication and results, is essential to make the correct decisions both for practitioner decision-making and for patients' treatment decisions. One of the most important strengths regarding chemical peels is that they are available and easy to apply for overall mild-to-moderate conditions like acne vulgaris. Research indicates that chemical agents, such as salicylic acid, have demonstrated significant efficacy in acne treatment through penetrating the stratum corneum and extracting comedones, thus preventing subsequent lesions (Nafila et al., 2024).

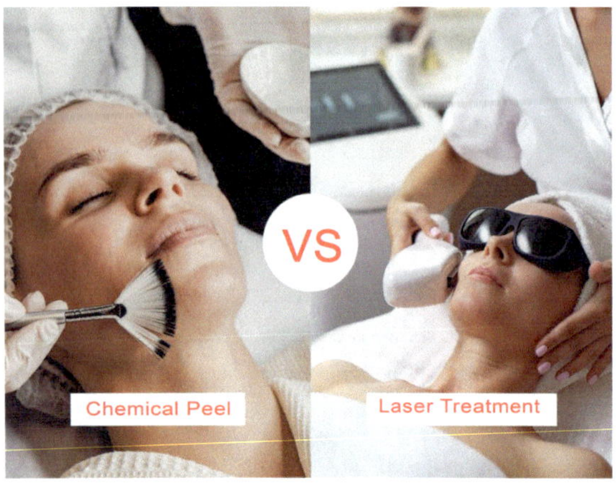

Figure 5.17. Chemical peel vs. laser treatment.

Source: https://skinnfit.in/wp-content/uploads/2024/06/Chemical-Peel-vs-Laser-Treatment.jpg.

Such a feature renders chemical peels a fundamental first-line therapy for acne that can be adapted to different skin conditions and types. In addition, downtime for chemical peeling procedures is generally shorter than for laser procedures, so patients may get back to their regular activities sooner. However, it is important that dermatologists assess the risks of PIH, particularly in darker-skinned patients, to maximize outcomes and patient satisfaction. On the other hand, laser treatments are sometimes used because they are accurate and go deeper into skin layers, potentially causing radical changes in skin firmness and texture. To fix severe acne and scarring, laser treatments can create incredible results that perhaps no chemical peel alone would be able to achieve. Studies have emphasized the efficacy of combination therapy, involving both laser and topical agents to augment overall effects (Whitney & Ditre, 2011). But the patient must be briefed on the fact that there will be a longer healing time because laser treatments tend to cause more intense redness and swelling immediately following treatment. Hence, a decision between chemical peels and laser treatment needs to consider the specific skin issues to be addressed, the preferred recovery of the patient, and the cosmetic outcomes desired, to make it necessary for healthcare providers to tailor both therapy recommendations and patient education accordingly (Figure 5.17).

5.6.3. Chemical Peels vs. Topical Treatments

The dichotomy that exists between chemical peels and topical treatments shows quite different approaches to dermatological problems. Chemical peels, where a chemical solution is applied to peel off the outermost skin layers, are famous for their depth of penetration over topical treatments. This deeper penetration comes along with more cellular turnover, which is why chemical peels are fantastic treatments for hyperpigmentation, acne scarring, and fine lines. Lactic acid exemplifies these benefits in being a dual action exfoliant and hydrator of the skin, as it shows some antibacterial efficacy and heals, thus it's widely used in cosmetic dermatology (Chen et al., 2024). As a non-surgical intervention, chemical peels typically have little down time, offering a more attractive option than the length of some topical solutions. Topical treatments include creams, lotions, and serums that typically come with wide formulations of products aimed at taking care of specific skin issues. Treatments typically contain active ingredients like retinoids, antioxidants, and peptides that may help improve the texture of the skin while reducing its age lines. However, topical treatments cannot compare to chemical peels because they are less invasive in terms of penetrating into the skin. With continued use, though, topical treatments can indeed be effective. The appeal of the topical products is in their accessibility and simplicity of integration into everyday skincare regimens. Studies show that such products, particularly those infused with bioactive components, could exhibit strong dermatological advantages, such as skin renewal and sun protection, thus increasing their attractiveness as continuous maintenance treatments (Naser et al., 2021). Such topical treatments are a vital partner to chemical treatments for an integrated skincare program. By observing the combination of chemical peels and topical treatments, a synergistic method emerges as the most viable to achieve optimal skin well-being. Chemical peels for occasional intensive maintenance will indeed redefine the skin while the topical treatments would be keeping up with, or even enhancing the outcome obtained through the peels. In this combined method, not only is the treatment of present issues in the skin, but long-term care maintenance in the skin is also achieved. Using the sequential combination of chemical peels with subsequent proper topical treatments can be tailored to respond to the individual skin types and issues, enabling tailored skincare regimes. Each modality of treatment has its strengths, and it would promote patients to view their skin health as a journey and not as distinct interventions, ensuring that both the chemical peels and topical treatments would be optimized in producing luminous skin.

Test Your Knowledge

1. How does the depth and effectiveness of chemical peels compare to microdermabrasion in treating skin texture and pigmentation?
2. What are the main differences between chemical peels and laser treatments in terms of precision, recovery time, and results?

SUMMARY

The controversy surrounding chemical peels has illuminated their multiple benefits as well as possible side effects and consequently fostered a clearer comprehension of their use in dermatology. As reiterated throughout the chapter, chemical peels can address skin problems ranging from acne scars and abnormal pigmentation to fine lines and age signs. Nonetheless, their effectiveness is often dependent on the particular peel applied, the skin type of the patient, and the particular conditions to be treated. Both patients and practitioners must be thoroughly informed regarding the various chemical agents utilized, in addition to the methods used in the treatment to maximize results. This information provides a climate for decision-making that is concerned with safety and is consonant with the patient's skin health goals, hence maximizing the therapeutic potential of chemical peels. Further, the evolution of chemical peel treatments attests to the progress of dermatologic procedures in response to patient needs and technological advancement. New products and techniques have been formulated to significantly reduce recovery time and minimize side effects. This shift is part of a larger trend in contemporary medicine, where patient comfort and safety are prioritized equally to aesthetic results. Furthermore, greater public education regarding skin care and scientific developments has allowed patients to play an active role in determining their treatment options. This shift in more educated consumers adds strength to the importance of practitioners providing explicit and comprehensive information on alternatives, potential risks, and expected outcomes of multiple chemical peels. Ultimately, this communication between healthcare providers and patients can yield more pleasing results and higher treatment success rates. As a whole, this in-depth review of chemical peels does prove that they are a useful tool in cosmetic dermatology. With constant research and advancements in technology, there's always the possibility of perfecting such procedures. This is added by incorporating patient education into the treatment process, as this educates people on making the right decision for their skin. Since the public discourse surrounding dermatological procedures grows, there will be a need to respond to any arising concerns that might influence people's perceptions of such procedures. As the dynamics of skin care evolve, so does the dialogue between patient and practitioner to ensure that benefits from chemical peels are achieved without being followed by side effects. Thus, it is expected that an education platform combined with discourse will be a pathway to increased trust and better health outcomes with chemical peels.

Chemical peels have become widely utilized in dermatology as they help enhance the look of skin by removing dead outer layers. They are classified into three categories: superficial, medium, and deep, each differing depending on depth of penetration and type of agent. Superficial peels are generally accomplished with AHAs and work best for minor imperfections of the skin. Middle peels, typically accomplished with TCA, correct more pronounced dermal defects such as fine lines and mild acne scars. Deep peels accomplished with phenol actually penetrate down to the dermis, and are therefore used for more extreme destruction of the skin for deep rejuvenation and longer recoveries. Such differences highlight the significance of choosing the right peel depending on skin type and desired therapeutic outcome. Besides cosmeceutic benefits, chemical peels can potentially provide ancillary therapeutic advantages that are increasingly being recognized in the medical community. Studies have revealed that certain chemical agents have antioxidant activity and can scavenge deleterious free radicals, implying other health benefits beyond the level of the skin. For instance, the phenolics derivable from sweet potato peels (SPP) have been reported to play a positive role in the health of skin through their radical-scavenging activity, and innovation of formulation is a likelihood. In addition, comparative analyses of various extraction methods, as embodied in RSM and ANN studies, mirror growing scientific interest in optimizing the activity and safety of ingredients used in chemical peels. This vow of improved formulations is one that coincides with current debates over the integration of more natural ingredients in cosmetic treatments. The changing state of chemical peels also raises issues of safety and long-term effects on the skin. Although chemical peels may produce dramatic aesthetic results, they are not risk-free, with the possibility of allergic reactions or chemical burns if applied incorrectly. Dermatologists emphasize the need for thorough patient examination before the treatment for personalized approaches based on skin condition and type. Further, the higher use of less invasive peels indicates a shift towards emphasizing sequential, more natural means of improvement. As awareness picks up among consumers, the trends in the application of chemical peels may begin shifting towards utilizing biocompatible and gentle-to-skin care materials, therefore addressing concerns on both effectiveness and safety to the patient. This crossroads of innovation and safety is at the center of the debate about the future of chemical peels in aesthetic and therapeutic dermatology.

KEY TERMS FROM THIS CHAPTER

- Acidic chemicals
- Aggressive treatments
- Collagen formation
- Elastin production
- Exposed skin
- Patient safety
- Plastic surgery
- Skin texture
- Therapeutic treatment
- Trichloroacetic acid (TCA)
- Aesthetic treatments
- Alpha hydroxy acid (AHA)
- Cosmetic dermatology
- Exfoliants
- Facial rejuvenation
- Photoaging
- Potential side effects
- Superficial pigmentation
- Traditional surgery

CRITICAL THINKING QUESTIONS

1. **Which of the following acids is most commonly used for superficial chemical peels?**
   a. Trichloroacetic acid (TCA) 35%
   b. Phenol
   c. Glycolic acid 30–50%
   d. Salicylic acid 70%
2. **What is the primary indication for a medium-depth chemical peel?**
   a. Deep wrinkles and severe acne scars
   b. Mild pigmentation and dullness
   c. Tattoo removal
   d. Actinic keratoses and moderate photoaging
3. **Which of the following best describes a deep chemical peel?**
   a. Removes only the stratum corneum
   b. Penetrates into the reticular dermis
   c. Has no downtime and is safe for all skin types
   d. Usually performed weekly for optimal results
4. **Which patient is not a good candidate for deep chemical peels?**
   a. A fair-skinned patient with deep facial wrinkles
   b. A patient with Fitzpatrick Skin Type VI
   c. A patient with actinic keratosis
   d. A patient with perioral rhytides
5. **Which statement about post-peel care is true?**
   a. Sunscreen is optional after superficial peels
   b. Retinoids should be restarted immediately after any peel
   c. Occlusive ointments are recommended after deep peels
   d. Chemical peels eliminate the need for other skincare

Short Answer Questions

1. 2Name at least two agents commonly used in superficial chemical peels and describe their typical indications.
2. What are the main risks and complications associated with medium-depth peels like trichloroacetic acid (TCA) 35%?
3. For which skin types are deep chemical peels generally contraindicated, and why?
4. How does phenol differ from other peeling agents in terms of mechanism of action and systemic risks?
5. What pre-treatment protocols are typically recommended before performing a medium or deep chemical peel?
6. Compare the expected outcomes and indications for a glycolic acid peel versus a phenol peel.

Answer to Critical Thinking Questions

1. (c); 2. (d); 3. (b); 4. (b); 5. (c)

REFERENCES

1. Abla, L. E. F., Atzingen, D. A. N. C. V., Cardoso, L. L. F., et al. (2013). *Unripe Musa Sapientum Peel in The Healing of Surgical Wounds in Rats.* https://core.ac.uk/download/37710856.pdf (accessed on 11th June 2025).
2. Almeman, A. (2024). Evaluating the efficacy and safety of alpha-hydroxy acids in dermatological practice: A comprehensive clinical and legal review. *Clinical, Cosmetic and Investigational Dermatology, 17*, 1661–1685. https://www.semanticscholar.org/paper/bfadf3486711fff7cd4a3dd51877f2186f5eb139 (accessed on 11th June 2025).
3. Alves, V. D., Lourenço, S. C., & Moldao-Martins, M. (2019). *Antioxidants of Natural Plant Origins: From Sources to Food Industry Applications.* https://core.ac.uk/download/250590170.pdf (accessed on 11th June 2025).
4. Ambrosio, D. V. (2018). *Incidence and Need of Advanced Aesthetic Somatology in South Africa.* https://core.ac.uk/download/222968033.pdf (accessed on 11th June 2025).
5. Anástacio, A., Carvalho, I. S. de, & Silva, R. (2016). *Phenolics Extraction from Sweet Potato Peels: Modelling and Optimization by Response Surface Modelling and Artificial neural Network.* https://core.ac.uk/download/160795614.pdf (accessed on 11th June 2025).
6. Ariyanti, D., Purbasari, A., Kusumayanti, H., & Handayani, N. A. (2019). Penentuan proses pretreatment untuk pemanfaatan limbah kulit singkong sebagai bahan baku bioetanol melalui hidrolisa enzimatis menggunakan *Aspergillus* spp. *METANA.* https://www.semanticscholar.org/paper/7920c1145f01d98b3ce00d28696ba63cd7967842 (accessed on 11th June 2025).
7. Arsiwala, S., Dhawan, S., Girdhar, M., et al. (2022). *Expert Consensus on The Management of Acne in India.* https://core.ac.uk/download/539910243.pdf (accessed on 11th June 2025).
8. Aziz, Z., Keshavarz, T., et al. (2020). *Recycling and the Environment: A Comparative Review Between Mineral-Based Plastics and Bioplastics.* https://core.ac.uk/download/305119262.pdf (accessed on 11th June 2025).
9. Bagatin, E., Leonardi, G. R., & Sumita, J. M. (2017). *Tretinoin Peel: A Critical View.* https://core.ac.uk/download/328364457.pdf (accessed on 11th June 2025).
10. Bińczyk, W., Dróżdż, O., Lissak, K., et al. (2024). *Topical Treatment and Aesthetic Procedures in Management of Acne Vulgaris.* https://core.ac.uk/download/613694708.pdf (accessed on 11th June 2025).
11. Blatt, M. R., Garia-Mata, C., Papanatsiou, M., et al. (2015). *Hydrogen Sulphide Regulates Inward-Rectifying K^+ Channels in Conjunction with Stomatal Closure.* https://core.ac.uk/download/42361239.pdf (accessed on 11th June 2025).
12. Bowyer, M. C., Golding, J. B., Hasperué, J. H., et al. (2018). *Pretreatment of Citrus By-Products Affects Polyphenol Recovery: A Review.* https://core.ac.uk/download/228178304.pdf (accessed on 11th June 2025).
13. Burgos, N., Garrigós, M. del C., Jiménez, A., et al. (2015). *Natural Pectin Polysaccharides as Edible Coatings.* https://core.ac.uk/download/32325601.pdf (accessed on 11th June 2025).
14. Caruso, D., Lo Faro, C., Melfa, F., et al. (2020). *At-Home Cosmeceutical Application and Outpatient Treatments: A 3D Stepwise Facial Rejuvenation Approach.* https://core.ac.uk/download/359939375.pdf (accessed on 11th June 2025).

15. Chandan, M. S. (2023). The role of chemical peels in trauma patients: Accelerating skin healing and restoring confidence. *International Journal of Science and Research (IJSR).* https://www.semanticscholar.org/paper/92f8d82021690dacf6634178b098156336cf4f85 (accessed on 11th June 2025).

16. Chen, Y., Feng, X., Gu, Z., Liu, Y., Luo, X., & Shang, J. (2024). *Lactic Acid Chemical Peeling in Skin Disorders.* https://core.ac.uk/download/615005519.pdf (accessed on 11th June 2025).

17. Dhananjaya, B. L., Beulah, C., Devi, A. T., F., et al. (2015). *Phyto-Antiquorumones: An Herbal Approach for Blocking Bacterial Trafficking and Pathogenesis.* https://core.ac.uk/download/482239696.pdf (accessed on 11th June 2025).

18. Madnani, N., Vedmurthy, M., Parthasarthi, A., Dhawan, S., Kandhari, R., Pillai, R., & Nischal, K. C. (2022). Expert opinion on pre and post procedure care in aesthetic dermatology. *International Journal of Research in Medical Sciences, 10*(4), 991–1000. https://doi.org/10.18203/2320-6012.ijrms20220999 (accessed on 11th June 2025).

19. Whitney, K. M., & Ditre, C. M. (2011). Management strategies for acne vulgaris. *Clinical, cosmetic and investigational dermatology, 4*, 41–53. https://doi.org/10.2147/CCID.S10817(accessed on 11th June 2025).

20. Dogiparthi, S. N., Mohan, S., Bala, A., & Jenson, J. (2023). Effectiveness of various organic peels in facial rejuvenation and treatment of sensitive skin. *Journal of Medical and Scientific Research.* https://www.semanticscholar.org/paper/8e84d36b745c5299300b19c65c9bef27d3804058 (accessed on 11th June 2025).

21. Ehiobu, J., & Ogu, G. (2018). Phytochemical content and *in vitro* antimycelial efficacy of *Colocasia esculenta* (L), *Manihot esculenta* (Crantz) and *Dioscorea rotundata* (Poir) leaf extracts on *Aspergillus niger* and *Botryodiplodia theobromae. 1*, 9–18. https://www.semanticscholar.org/paper/6df330b581388b5a3bdb85519bb3330924524b1c (accessed on 11th June 2025).

22. Elewski, B. E., Chen, E., & Canavan, T. N. (2016). Optimizing non-antibiotic treatments for patients with acne: A review. https://link.springer.com/content/pdf/10.1007%2Fs13555-016-0138-1.pdf (accessed on 11th June 2025).

23. Fabi, S., Boen, M., Weinstein Velez, M., Woodward, J. A., Austin, A. H., & Dayan, S. (2024). Expert roundtable on skin care integration after aesthetic procedures: Consensus recommendations. *Journal of Drugs in Dermatology: JDD, 24*(1), 47–53. https://www.semanticscholar.org/paper/ac2c330163fd8948432db9fe23a198403b551230 (accessed on 11th June 2025).

24. Ferara, N., Franceschi, N., Šitum Čeprnja, Z., et al. (2024). *Treatment of Actinic Keratoses and Field Cancerization–Croatian Perspective.* https://core.ac.uk/download/620817167.pdf (accessed on 11th June 2025).

25. Gentili, G., Perugini, P., Bugliaro, S., & D'Antonio, C. (2022). Efficacy and safety of a new peeling formulated with a pool of PHAs for the treatment of all skin types, even sensitive. *Journal of Cosmetic Dermatology, 22*, 517–528. https://doi.org/10.1111/jocd.15215 (accessed on 11th June 2025).

26. Gkouvi, A., Tsiogka, A., Corbo, A., Tsimpidakis, A., & Gregoriou, S. (2025). Efficacy of heterologous type I collagen injections in treating atrophic acne scars: A prospective study. *Skin Appendage Disorders.* https://www.semanticscholar.org/paper/6df904d6d9ccdc0122b709ca555973c80b9a3b75 (accessed on 11th June 2025).

27. Guzmán, E., & Lucía, A. (2021). Essential oils and their individual components in cosmetic products. *Cosmetics, 8*, 114–114. https://doi.org/10.3390/cosmetics8040114 (accessed on 11th June 2025).

28. Halim, A. S., & Yan, T. K. (2016). *Treatment Modalities for Hyperpigmented Skin Lesions: A Brief Overview.* https://core.ac.uk/download/132566787.pdf (accessed on 11th June 2025).

29. Iglesia, S., Jiang, L. I., Kononov, T., & Zahr, A. (2025). Effective skin rejuvenation by a novel antioxidant bio stimulating treatment. *Journal of Cosmetic Dermatology, 24.* https://www.semanticscholar.org/paper/557d957da814c9274a3068178995563cc5a5338c (accessed on 11th June 2025).

30. Kamal, A., Kamal, M., Mehboob, B., Naz, T., Zafar, S., & Hussain, S. M. (2024). Blue light therapy: A skin treatment mask using blue light to cure skin disorders. *Sukkur IBA Journal of Emerging Technologies.* https://www.semanticscholar.org/paper/e29041749ee9a9c3af29ebe4e94495969def30f7 (accessed on 11th June 2025).

31. Kamlenga, M., Murhunzi, B., Ojukwu, C., & Olukanni, et al. (2024). *Application of Cassava-Peels and Palm-Oil-Sludge Digestate on Bean Crop for Sustainable Growth.* https://core.ac.uk/download/622435193.pdf (accessed on 11th June 2025).

32. Kotsias, K. (2018). *The Evolution of Trade Policy on GMOs in Europe.* https://core.ac.uk/download/160283126.pdf (accessed on 11th June 2025).

33. Lin, L., Liao, G., Chen, J., & Chen, X. (2021). A systematic review and meta-analysis on the effects of the ultra-pulse CO_2 fractional laser in the treatment of depressed acne scars. *Annals of Palliative Medicine, 11*(2), 743–755. https://www.semanticscholar.org/paper/a70fb0a5fe401b30e8afdcac8a045ceeab870b99 (accessed on 11th June 2025).

34. Lukić, M., Pantelić, I., & Savić, S. (2021). Towards optimal pH of the skin and topical formulations: From the current state of the art to tailored products. *Cosmetics, 8*, 69–69. https://doi.org/10.3390/cosmetics8030069 (accessed on 11th June 2025).

35. Mallia, A. (2003). *Dermal Fillers.* https://core.ac.uk/download/46604550.pdf (accessed on 11th June 2025).

36. Mathur, T., Jain, N., Garg, U., & Pandey, M. (2024). The remarkable role of nano-Phyto cosmeceuticals for elevating skincare in facial hyperpigmentation. *Nanoscience & Nanotechnology-Asia.* https://www.semanticscholar.org/paper/1524e19269b3c20df2c169dacff83dbe5b49246f (accessed on 11th June 2025).

37. Maughan, R. J., Burke, L. M., Dvořák, J., Larson-Meyer, D. E., Peeling, P., Phillips, S. M., Rawson, E. S., et al. (2018). IOC consensus statement: Dietary supplements and the high-performance athlete. *British Journal of Sports Medicine, 52*, 439–455. https://doi.org/10.1136/bjsports-2018-099027 (accessed on 11th June 2025).

38. Molina, R. M. (2004). *Curriculum Manual for The Esthetician Course at Fullerton College.* https://core.ac.uk/download/160477585.pdf (accessed on 11th June 2025).

39. Murray, T., Lohray, R., Schultz, K. P., Boutros, S., & Friedman, P. M. (2024). Complications of chemical peels, lasers, and energy-based device procedures performed by core cosmetic physicians: A retrospective analysis. *Lasers in Surgery and Medicine.* https://www.semanticscholar.org/paper/80b3dc69c427ddc9d9535bd4092f9d7097e6d3b4 (accessed on 11th June 2025).

40. Nafila, A., Nursanto, D., Pramuningtyas, R., et al. (2024). *The Effectiveness of Salicylic Acid Therapy in Mild and Moderate Acne Vulgaris.* https://core.ac.uk/download/599140274.pdf (accessed on 11th June 2025).

41. Naser, W. (2021). *The Cosmetic Effects of Various Natural Bio Functional Ingredients Against Skin Aging: A Review.* https://core.ac.uk/download/482243766.pdf (accessed on 11th June 2025).

42. Pokharkar, K. K., Delvadia, D. V., Jadhav, P., & Bhor. (2017). Effect of pre-treatments and drying methods on moisture percentage of dried tomato slices. *1*, 024–026. https://www.semanticscholar.org/paper/c1e209451f34b7d048f6701608d3126d70d5fdee (accessed on 11th June 2025).

43. Esther Jebarani Rayer, Mimi Suliza Muhamad, Najeeha Mohd Apandi, Norshuhaila Mohamed Sunar, & Roslinda Ali. (2024). Combined Effects of Banana Peels and Pith as Dual Natural Plant-Based Coagulants for Turbidity Removal. *Journal of Advanced Research in Applied Mechanics, 116*(1), 75–87. https://doi.org/10.37934/aram.116.1.7587(accessed on 11th June 2025).

44. Ropes, J. W. (1987). *Preparation of Acetate Peels of Valves from The Ocean Quahog, Arctica Islandica, For Age Determinations.* https://core.ac.uk/download/11018483.pdf (accessed on 11th June 2025).

45. Singh, S., Singh, V., & Patel, S. (2024). Cosmeceuticals; the fusion of cosmetics and pharmaceuticals. Feb–Mar 2024. https://www.semanticscholar.org/paper/24c5e610a535706a8d2ead98f92580eefd7e5169 (accessed on 11th June 2025).

46. Sivakumar, P., Manoharan, A. P., & Muthusamy, D. (2024). Effect on some physicochemical qualities of the minced chicken meat cutlet mixed with raw banana peel powder. *Journal of Environment and Bio-Science.* https://www.semanticscholar.org/paper/0bea024224be6adb6bae859162a695e62ab808d0 (accessed on 11th June 2025).

47. Smit, R. (2024). Evaluation of the efficacy of a TCA medium peeling procedure combined with skin bio revitalization in face rejuvenation: A case series. *Journal of Dermatology & Cosmetology.* https://www.semanticscholar.org/paper/6cbb630056ae075ebf4b26283dc5f3c52fd22763 (accessed on 11th June 2025).

48. Wu, S., & Tian, L. (2017). Diverse Phytochemicals and Bioactivities in the Ancient Fruit and Modern Functional Food Pomegranate (Punica granatum). *Molecules (Basel, Switzerland), 22*(10), 1606. https://doi.org/10.3390/molecules22101606 (accessed on 11th June 2025).

49. Timraz, J., Bakour, H. A., Samman, R. R., Alawi, K. M., Bava, F. S. M., Alkhdaidi, F. A., Alghorab, M. A., et al. (2025). Advancements in non-invasive plastic surgery techniques: Evaluating efficacy, safety, patient outcomes and potential complications. *South Eastern European Journal of Public Health.* https://www.semanticscholar.org/paper/806bda9dd733843545f1a64dad22f242c2e2a678 (accessed on 11th June 2025).

50. Wu, B., Qiu, P., Shi, S., Zhang, Y., Huang, X., & Nie, Z. (2023). Study on anti-corrosion performance and applicability of self-healing coating for tubulars in CO_2 /H_2S environment. *Day 3 Thu, May 25, 2023.* https://www.semanticscholar.org/paper/6c65343493adb3fa5da87843e7dd685738247b3d (accessed on 11th June 2025).

51. Yang, Y., Zhang, J., Zhou, Z., Zhang, Z., Park, M., Yu, Q., Li, Z., et al. (2021). Recent development of chemically complex metallic glasses: From accelerated compositional design, additive manufacturing to novel applications. *Materials Futures, 1.* https://www.semanticscholar.org/paper/070cb23f93bd9ece4566110c8aa1f10dcad95efb (accessed on 11th June 2025).

COLLAGEN INDUCTION THERAPY

6

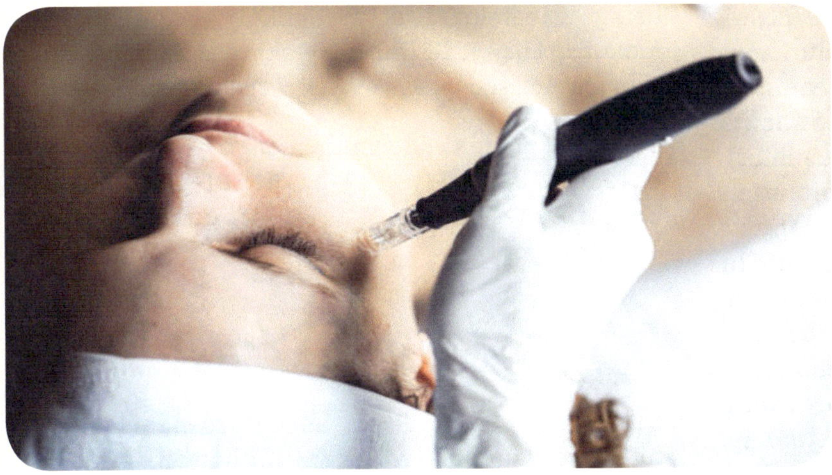

LEARNING OBJECTIVES

After studying this chapter, you will be able to:

1. Understand mechanism of action of collagen induction therapy (CIT)
2. Explain the types of collagen induction therapy
3. Discuss about indications for use
4. Define the benefits of collagen induction therapy
5. Describe risks and side effects
6. Focus on patient considerations in collagen induction therapy

Introduction

Collagen induction therapy (CIT), or microneedling, is a revolutionary therapeutic intervention in aesthetic medicine and dermatology. This novel treatment involves the process of using a group of very thin needles to create small injuries to the skin that subsequently trigger the body's own repair system. In this process, collagen and elastin are highly amplified, which the skin uses for rejuvenation, remodeling of scars, and improving a number of skin diseases. Given the growing popularity of non-surgical cosmetic treatments, CIT presents a viable alternative option since it not only produces a fresher appearance but also supports the general health of the skin. Its effects resonate with broader biological mechanisms, particularly with the processes relating to getting older, where long-term inflammation may be a hindrance to effective healing and initiator of several dermatological issues, as indicated in recent research on aging and inflammation (Li et al., 2023). Other benefits of the therapeutic effects of CIT go beyond just aesthetic improvements. They cut across wound healing and tissue regeneration, and the mechanism by which CIT works mimics the body's natural wound healing response-it triggers a series of biological reactions that enhance the synthesis of collagen and also improve texture and elasticity of the skin. The treatment has shown promise in addressing chronic wounds that are often resistant to traditional interventions. Chronic wounds, as previously stated, are problems of great challenge in clinical practice, both for the quality of patients and for healthcare costs. Therefore, CIT offers a potential new solution in the broader context of chronic wound treatment, in accordance with the need for treatments that can efficiently battle the multidisciplinary character of healing wounds. This exploration of CIT within the wound healing context further enforces relevance and necessity in contemporary medical practice, as outlined by Kolimi et al. (2022). Importantly, besides the physical benefits, CIT indeed entails more critical questions from the patient regarding patient satisfaction and emotional wellbeing. Visual improvements from CIT facilitate both self-esteem and self-confidence, making the procedure a desirable option for individuals to enhance their looks. In addition, as consumers seek minimally invasive procedures rather than surgeries, the capability of CITs to deliver with minimal downtime makes it superior in the market. If one examines the psychosocial aspects of aesthetic treatments besides their immediate physical effects, they seem to reflect a whole healthcare concept, thereby attending to the body and mind at one go. With continued advances in research, the safety and effectiveness of CIT will most likely be further aided by technological advancements as well as tailored protocols that can accommodate the different needs of patients, further establishing it in the future of cosmetic and therapeutic dermatology (Figure 6.1).

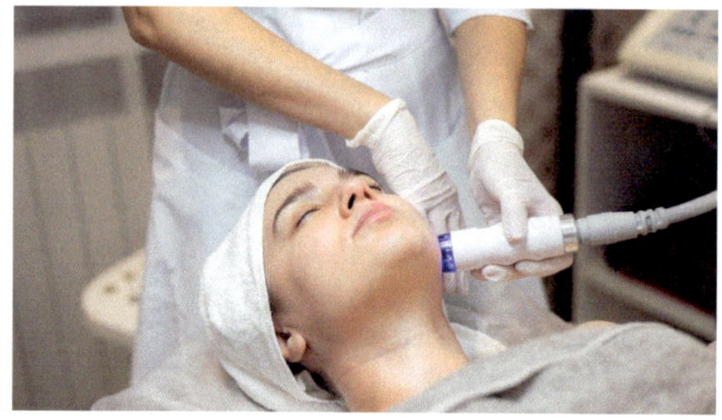

Figure 6.1. A patient receiving a facial treatment using a handheld device, likely employing radiofrequency or LED therapy, aimed at improving skin tone, elasticity, and overall facial rejuvenation.

Source: https://dermalyn.in/wp-content/uploads/2023/03/young-beautiful-girl-lies-beautician-s-table-receives-procedures-1-1200x675.jpg.

Definition of Collagen Induction Therapy

CIT, also referred to as micro-needling or percutaneous collagen induction, is a revitalization process that seeks to work with the skin texture and heal it by stimulating the formation of greater amounts of collagen in the skin. The basic theory behind CIT is that tiny needles cause controlled micro-injuries in the dermis that stimulate the body to activate normal processes of wound healing. Since the healing process takes place in the skin, a peak in collagen and elastin production leads to increased skin elasticity and youthfulness. CIT is used to correct some issues of the skin, including scars, wrinkles, and general laxity of the skin. The efficacy of CIT is ensured by its minimal invasiveness and rapid recovery times after treatment (Dębiec et al., 2024). The procedural aspect of CIT is significant in that it can be adapted to fit the specific needs and conditions of an individual patient. During a session, one can use a topical anesthetic to alleviate pain initially and then treat with a microneedling device that pierces the skin at variable depths. This adaptability allows practitioners to treat specific dermatological issues effectively. New technologies have also introduced adjunctive treatments such as platelet-rich plasma (PRP) to treat and improve the healing and outcome. Research indicates that CIT not only smooths the surface of the skin but also positively affects dermal architecture below, paving the way towards healthier skin and restoration (Benati et al., 2020). Hence, CIT has emerged as an effective therapeutic intervention in clinical as well as cosmetic dermatology. As non-invasive skin treatments gain popularity, the esthetic benefits of CIT are only a start. Research continually elucidates tissue remodeling biomechanics to CIT and its ability to cure other cutaneous defects and improve overall skin condition. The treatment initiates fibroblasts to construct collagen and, thereby, increases skin density and texture over time. Also, the minimal downtime of the procedure allows it to be integrated into the overall skin care regimen without extreme disruptions in daily activity. As therapy agents become more advanced, CIT is at the forefront, offering a comprehensive approach to skin rejuvenation with an emphasis on collagen as the key to maintaining fresh, healthy-looking skin. Continued investigation of CITs application and effects further solidifies its position as a practice-altering variable in dermatology (Figure 6.2).

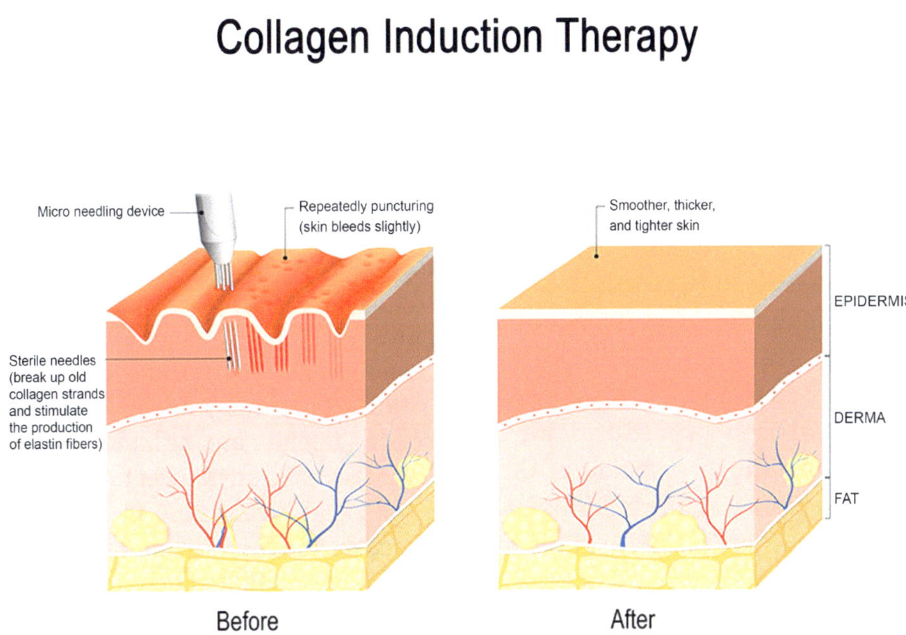

Figure 6.2. Collagen induction therapy (CIT).

Source: https://images.squarespace-cdn.com/content/v1/5cdb875dfb22a539095ca9e5/1576119048504-79UTZN9TEQNYWIMG6IFI/Collagen+Induction+Therapy+Skin+Needling+Sydney.jpg.

Historical Background and Development

The history of CIT is rooted in a new understanding of the physiology of skin and wound healing. The past processes involved in rejuvenating the skin have ranged from chemical peels to more invasive surgery. However, in the quest for less invasive treatments, CIT became an alternative that uses microneedling to stimulate the production of dermal collagen. This technique was first described in the 1990s when dermatologists began to realize the benefits of needling in the treatment of various skin concerns, such as scars, striae, and skin texture overall. The hype for CIT arose from the possibility of making beneficial aesthetic alterations with minimal downtime, compared to traditional surgery that usually takes a long time to recover from and has more chances of complications. Technological advancements in medical technology and dermatological science in the late 20th and early 21st century were what fueled the development of CIT. Automated microneedling devices were invented, allowing for controlled penetrating depth to the skin, thus raising the effectiveness of the procedure.

In this respect, scientific studies in dermatology explained the process undertaken in collagen synthesis – it identified controlled injury as the cause of evoking a healing response to the skin. These studies provided the foundation for optimizing CIT protocols, integrating it successfully with other treatments in order to maximize outcomes. Of particular interest, integrating CIT with topical agents, including hyaluronic acid and growth factors, has been found to enhance the therapeutic outcomes, allowing practitioners to better adapt treatments to patient requirements and conditions. Evidence-based procedures have also positioned the evolutionary course of CIT firmly under the verandas of dermatological therapy. Clinical evidence increasingly validated the efficacy of CIT in the management of acne scarring, hyperpigmentation, and fine lines, establishing it as a proven entity of aesthetic treatments. Patient satisfaction and the great safety profile of microneedling positioned it as an inclusion in the cosmetic armamentarium. As in the areas dealt with, the incorporation of novel modalities such as radiofrequency (RF) and laser technology continues to be a driving force in the advancement of CIT techniques. The studies now in progress regarding the immunologic response to collagen production will further elucidate the best outcomes and ultimately result in better protocols and wider applications of collagen induction therapies in dermatology and many other fields (Yani et al., 2024; Wang et al., 2024).

Importance of Collagen in Skin Health

The role of collagen in the health of the skin cannot be exaggerated, as collagen is a vital structural protein that imparts strength and elasticity to dermal layers. The fibrous protein is secreted by fibroblasts and constitutes 70–80% of the dry weight of the skin. With progressive aging, the manufacture of collagen decreases with advancing age and, thus, signs of aging become visible in the shape of wrinkles, loss of skin tightness, and lack of elasticity. This decrease in collagen levels can even lead to impaired wound healing as well as an overall weakening of skin. With such attempts, the restoration of collagen, particularly with therapies such as CIT, has gained significant importance due to the prospects of restoring the appearance of young skin as well as better conditions for the whole skin. Therapeutic modulation of the synthesis of collagen may be a promising strategy for alleviating dermal aging-related decline and enhancing aesthetic results. Apart from its structural function, collagen plays a very significant role in several physiological processes in the skin, and thus it plays a central role in maintaining general skin health. Collagen helps maintain hydration by creating a scaffold on which water is retained, necessary for skin firmness and elasticity. The interaction with the other extracellular matrix proteins also underscores the importance; it has an interaction with elastin and glycosaminoglycans to facilitate the capacity of the skin to oppose stretching forces and compressive forces. Recent findings have shown that effective strategies for the enhancement of collagen synthesis have effects on the texture and appearance of the skin, providing a compelling rationale for the use of CIT. This treatment not only aims to stimulate the body's own collagen production but also yields a therapy consideration that addresses a number of parameters of skin health, from moisturizing retention to stability. New studies continue to explore novel modalities of collagen augmentation, with special emphasis placed upon the accomplishments in CIT. By employing treatments such as microneedling, practitioners are capable of creating micro-injuries that stimulate the body's repair mechanism, resulting in increased collagen production in the addressed tissues. This process of healing is not only beneficial to treating alterations due to aging, but a plethora of dermatologic disorders such as scarring and melanin variation. Further, studies of adjunct treatments with CIT-like peptides and isothiocyanate compounds show additional mechanisms of stimulating the production of collagen, such as studies on compounds like sulforaphane, which have shown remarkable effects on proliferation and migration of cells (Arlt et al., 2014). Thus, the context of these new treatments highlights the pivotal role of collagen not just as a structural component of the skin but also as a working player in the facilitation of the best skin health and beauty.

6.1. Mechanism of Action

Learning Outcome

1. Discuss how collagen induction therapy (CIT) stimulates collagen production
2. Explain the role of micro-needling in the process
3. Describe the biological response to skin injury

The mechanism of action of CIT, or microneedling, is based on the process of controlled micro-injury to the skin, stimulating the body's inherent healing processes. The treatment is achieved by the creation of microchannels in the dermis with the help of very fine needles, stimulating a cascade of physiological processes. Through the process, fibroblasts are triggered, resulting in increased production of collagen and elastin, which are critical elements of skin structure and elasticity. The boosted collagen eventually results in improved texture within the skin, reduces scars, and enhances the general look of the skin. Moreover, induction of such healing processes is also characterized by the release of growth factors that facilitate tissue repair and regeneration, highlighting the multi-faceted capability of CIT to facilitate skin health and repair. Beyond its primary mechanisms, microneedling also can enhance the penetration and efficacy of agents applied topically post-procedure. The needles facilitate microchannels for increased penetration of therapeutic agents, like hyaluronic acid or growth factor-enriched serums, thus producing a more effective treatment outcome. This combination of microneedling and topical therapies may provide improved results in such indications as aging and acne scars. A targeted delivery of active ingredients by virtue of enhanced delivery enablement allows for the treatment of specific skin issues while producing the utmost in therapeutic benefit from CIT. Research shows that combining microneedling with other modalities, such as low-level laser treatment, can likely maximize these effects further, highlighting the therapeutic flexibility and aesthetic application of this treatment in cosmetic dermatology (Sukarnadi et al., 2023). The role played by inflammatory processes in the mechanism of action of CIT cannot be overlooked either. The controlled damage induced by microneedling not only stimulates collagen but also induces a local inflammatory reaction. Crucial to tissue repair, inflammatory cytokines are secreted and orchestrate the process of healing by recruiting immune cells into the site of injury. This effect is especially crucial for the management of morphea, where the therapeutic modality targets the control of inflammation and healing by stimulating collagen deposition. Evidence has demonstrated that treatments with these inflammatory components present impressive clinical improvements, as evidenced by diminished scores on the instruments used in practice (Nopriyati et al., 2024). It is because of this that understanding the intricate interaction between injury, inflammation, and healing is fundamental in the attainment of optimal benefits of CIT (Figure 6.3).

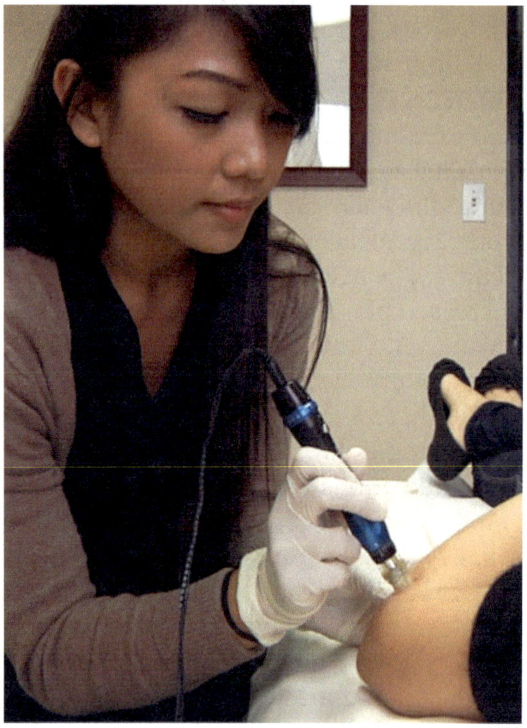

Figure 6.3. Nurse performing collagen induction therapy for scar reduction using a microneedle stamping device.

Source: https://upload.wikimedia.org/wikipedia/commons/6/66/LVN_Collagen_Induction_Therapy_AMAskincare.jpg.

6.1.1. How Collagen Induction Therapy Stimulates Collagen Production

CIT exploits the body's natural mechanisms of repair to induce collagen production through micro-injury. CIT uses controlled micro-needles to cause minute lesions in the skin that trigger the body's inflammatory response. The ensuing healing cascade precipitates an inflow of growth factors to the treated area, such as epidermal growth factor, a major cog in collagen development. The resulting activation of fibroblasts increases levels of different collagen types, mainly type I and type III, required for skin elasticity and strength. With time, these changes bring an evident correction in skin texture and appearance, which proves the effectiveness of CIT as a non-invasive rejuvenation method to stimulate the production of collagen and improve skin health. Thus, CIT is the premier dermatological treatment that capitalizes on the body's own capabilities for beauty enhancement. Systemic delivery of CIT not only induces collagen but is also renowned for its versatility in treating almost any skin condition. Acne scarring, stretch marks, and general laxity of the skin are some of the conditions that derive much advantage from this therapy. Because the micro-needling technique enables the agents to penetrate deeper, patients are able to experience higher absorption and a synergistic effect when combined with collagen boosters or growth factors. Micro-injury, which activates fibroblasts, results in increased deposition and remodeling of collagen, which repairs damaged skin and results in a more youthful appearance. Therefore, the overall benefits of CIT are bestowed upon other dermatological conditions and hence become a desirable option for contemporary skincare regimens, which aim to restore and rejuvenate the integrity of skin. It is revealed in research that the biological mechanisms associated with CIT are closely associated with growth factor release and cellular mechanisms encompassing tissue repair and remodeling. For instance, fibroblast proliferation is typically stimulated by growth factors in the skin, whose vital functions include collagen production. The study pointed out the correlation between the intervention and the upregulation of cytokines responsible for stimulating cell signaling processes involved in the synthesis of collagen (Shahrajabian et al., 2023). In addition, the chronic development of inflammatory mediators may initiate a cycle towards additional collagen synthesis and remodeling and thus indicate a continuous and effective response of the body to CIT. Overall, the interaction of the collagen induction process with cellular dynamics leads to effective collagen production, validating CIT as a dynamic remedy for enhancing skin quality and integrity (Brenda et al., 2023) (Figure 6.4).

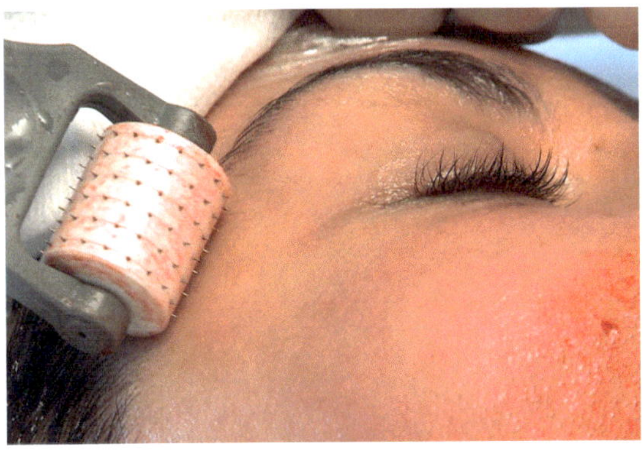

Figure 6.4. Stimulating collagen production.

Source: https://www.environskincare.com/za/wp-content/uploads/2019/07/700x466_1.png.

6.1.2. Role of Micro-Needling in the Process

Because of its stimulation of the body's natural wound healing mechanisms, micro-needling is of extremely significant use in collagen induction treatment since it helps improve the elasticity and texture of the skin. The treatment would basically involve the use of fine needles to puncture very small holes in the dermis, thereby stimulating a reaction of physiological demands. The micro-injuries will release proteins such as elastin and collagen, which basically give firmness and elasticity to the skin. More than just elevating the collagen levels, the therapy of micro-needling allows for better absorption of topical products; thus, the skincare products applied subsequently after the treatment become even more effective. This is the reason why most patients who undergo this particular procedure tend to benefit from better outcomes on almost every dermatological issue, such as wrinkles, fine lines, and even acne scars. This new method of skin rejuvenation emphasizes the therapeutic potential of micro-needling as a component of the overall application of CIT. Micro-needling can also be supplemented with other techniques, such as nanofat grafting, which utilizes stem cells and growth factors to enhance overall skin rejuvenation. Nanofat collected from autologous fat is transformed into a biologically active agent possessing regenerative properties and hence, a great complement to micro-needling treatments. The synergistic treatment optimizes the action of CIT by not only stimulating enhanced production of collagen but also providing healing and restoration-promoting nutrients. Micro-needling with incorporation of nanofat can cure a multitude of skin concerns, expanding the range of procedures that can be performed on patients requiring cosmetic improvement. With the combination of these methods, practitioners can have a more extensive and enriching treatment regimen, which in turn leads to better patient satisfaction and outcomes. Although the combined treatment of micro-needling and nanofat has potential, it is important to explore the safety and long-term efficacy of such techniques. The interaction between various biomaterials in biological matrices raises pertinent issues regarding the toxicity and side effects of the delivery of foreign objects. As literature implies, nanoparticles' performance and behavior can vary significantly based on their physicochemical properties, such as size, surface charge, and chemical structure, making caution of utmost importance when used clinically (Abbasi et al., 2023). Additional research on the mechanism of treatment and potential complications associated with micro-needling and nanofat therapy is needed to establish optimal practices in skin rejuvenation therapy. Understanding these factors will facilitate appropriate and well-informed use of CIT in dermatology and aesthetic clinics to guarantee that patient well-being and health are always the utmost concern (Figure 6.5).

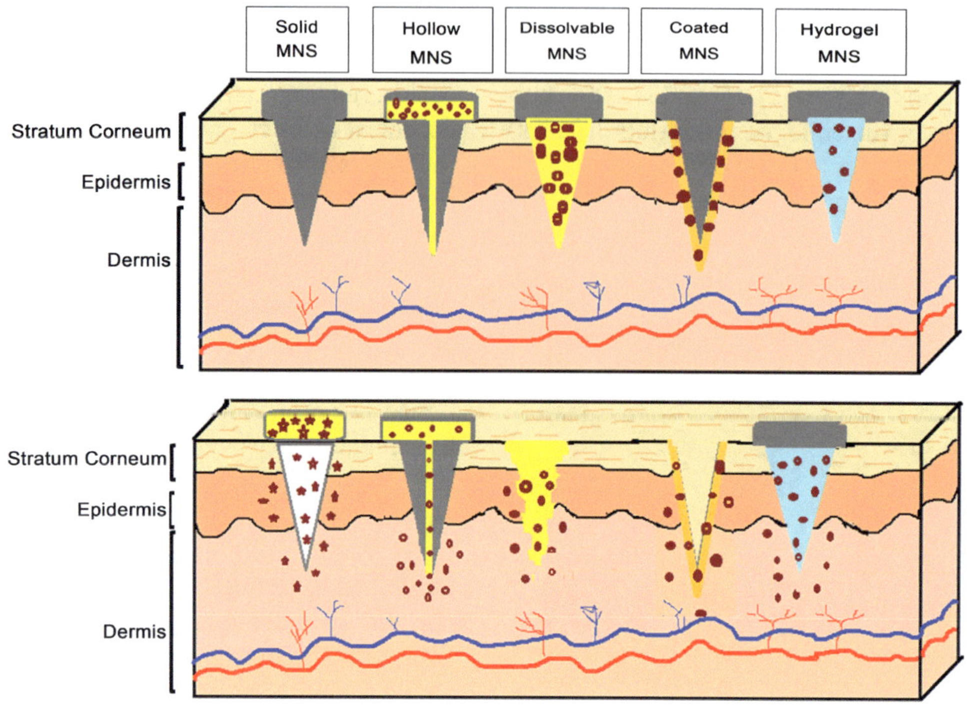

Figure 6.5. Types of microneedles (solid, hollow, dissolvable, coated, and hydrogel MNs).

Source: Hamed R, Abu Nahia BJ, Alkilani AZ, Al-Adhami Y, Obaidat R. Recent Advances in Microneedling-Assisted Cosmetic Applications. Cosmetics. 2024; 11(2):51. https://doi.org/10.3390/cosmetics11020051

6.1.3. Biological Response to Skin Injury

The cellular and molecular pathways of the biological response to cutaneous injury are intricate, well-orchestrated events crucial for optimal wound healing. When injured, the body evokes a series of events beginning with hemostasis, followed in quick succession by inflammatory, proliferation, and remodeling stages. The acute inflammatory reaction is provoked primarily by pro-inflammatory cytokines, which play a pivotal role in the recruitment of immune cells to the site of injury. For instance, tumor necrosis factor alpha (TNFα) and interleukin-1 beta (IL-1β) have been recognized as key initiators of the initial inflammatory response, facilitating hemostasis to inflammation transition and cellular involvement in healing processes. These cytokines not only support the maintenance of inflammatory cell migration but also engage in various growth factors involved in tissue repair, providing a platform for the ensuing regenerative process. As the inflammatory stage continues to progress, cell-to-cell communication is essential, with notable involvement by signaling molecules like interleukins (ILs). For instance, interleukin-10 (IL-10) plays a critical role in regulating the inflammatory process, supporting anti-inflammatory signals in bridging the wound from the inflammatory to the proliferation stage. It was observed in preclinical studies that while IL-10 induces the deactivation of monocytes and macrophages to inhibit inflammation, its therapeutic potential in chronic inflammatory disease is compromised by its complex pro-inflammatory properties (Mühl et al., 2013). In contrast, interleukin-22 (IL-22) has been discovered to significantly contribute to the maintenance of epithelial tissue integrity, enhancing cellular proliferation and survival in the site of injury. Such intricate interactions highlight the delicate balance of inflammatory mediators that are needed for optimal skin repair, where pro-inflammatory and regulatory signals have to coordinate sufficiently. Tissue remodeling and the synthesis of extracellular matrix molecules, most notably collagen, follow later on in the wound healing process, which is essential to restore the function and integrity of the skin. CIT exploits the body's own repair mechanisms by deliberately inducing micro-injuries, resulting in a physiological response that provokes increased collagen synthesis. Treatments with this aim have the intention of exploiting the body's own biological processes, tapping into the wound healing processes started by growth factors and cytokines. Animal models have demonstrated that cytokines like TNFα and IL-1β play a vital role in osseous and soft tissue wound healing, highlighting the central function of inflammation during early recovery from trauma (Gillen et al., 2002). Therefore, understanding the biological response to cutaneous injury not only illuminates effective treatment approaches like CIT but also highlights the importance of finely modulating inflammatory responses to optimize overall outcomes of healing.

Test Your Knowledge

1. How does microneedling stimulate collagen production in the skin?
2. What role do fibroblasts play in CIT?

6.2. Types of Collagen Induction Therapy

Learning Outcome

1. Understand the concept of traditional micro-needling
2. Describe automated micro-needling devices
3. Discuss about combination therapies with other treatments

CIT refers to a group of approaches to stimulating collagen formation and elasticity of the skin, primarily by provoking the body's own repair processes. Microneedling is such an approach that has gained more popularity because its process is rather non-invasive. Microneedling is the creation of microscopic injury in the skin using thin needles, which makes the body react with a response similar to wound healing. Thus, the production of elastin and collagen is enhanced, which gives an individual a younger appearance. Microneedling is also versatile as it is applicable on different skin conditions and types, such as acne scars, striae, and general skin rejuvenation, thereby indicating its efficacy and universal use in cosmetic dermatology. The second CIT response to laser therapy is a combination of microneedling and PRP. The new treatment adds an extra dimension to the laser therapy by leveraging the patient's own growth factors and platelets to trigger further collagen production. Following microneedling, the targeted area is saturated with PRP. Studies have indicated that this combination not only accelerates skin recovery but also enhances overall results, leading to improved elasticity and texture of the skin. Importantly, adding PRP minimizes the risk of side effects and is more customized because it acts in conjunction with the patient's own biological material, thus making it an exciting option for numerous patients seeking effective CIT treatments. The other method of this type of collagen induction is chemical peels, which significantly differ from microneedling and PRP treatments. It uses different types of acid, which strip away the top layers to provide fresh, very young-looking skin. With this, chemical peeling can also induce cellular turnover that shows increasing deeper layers of the skin, leading to increased collagen production.

While numerous acids exist, i.e., glycolic and salicylic acid, the choice depends upon the skin type as well as the desired effects of treatment. Synergy of chemical peeling with other modalities such as microneedling or PRP would further enhance the collagen-evoking effects, which ultimately culminate in maximum rejuvenation of the skin. These multi-pronged approaches mirror the new thrust areas that are being researched in CIT and highlight the importance of personalized treatments to achieve desired aesthetic outcomes in patients.

6.2.1. Traditional Micro-Needling

The use of conventional micro-needling, or the use of CIT, has been in the spotlight for its effectiveness in making the skin more texturally appealing and for treating several dermal conditions. This procedure involves the use of tiny needles to produce controlled micro-injuries in the skin, triggering the body's own wound healing process. Due to this, the production of collagen and elastin is triggered, which is essential for keeping the skin firm and elastic. Classical micro-needling heals minimally invasively, thus providing a relatively short duration of downtime, which the patient highly values if the restoration is cosmetic and the recovery time is minimal. Besides aesthetic enhancement, it also has the benefit of a potential increase in the absorption of the topical treatments given subsequent to the procedure, thereby potentially enhancing their effect and speeding the healing process (Annunziata et al., 2010; Sivaranjani, 2019). One key application of the classical micro-needling is its impact on the treatment of atrophic acne scars, which are common in a high percentage of the population. Acne scars have a deep psychological effect on people, inducing social embarrassment and low self-esteem. Classical micro-needling treats these scars by triggering a controlled injury that evokes remodeling of the scar tissue through triggering collagen production. Research findings show that patients report excellent improvement in the appearance of scars, and therefore experience better quality of life and satisfaction with their skin (Annunziata et al., 2010).

Besides making the scarring visually pleasing, this treatment also helps rejuvenate the skin, resulting in smoother, more resistant skin. With the integration of traditional micro-needling in symptomatic treatment protocols, dermatologists are now in a position to offer effective interventions for the management of acne scar psychosomatic load (Sivaranjani, 2019). The versatility of traditional micro-needling also extends its applications to other skin issues, excluding scarring. Other skin issues, such as enlarged pores, stretch marks, and uneven skin tone, are some of the other issues that can be treated using this groundbreaking technology. Through the increase of collagen and elastin, normal micro-needling can lead to dramatic improvements in skin texture and overall appearance. In addition, the treatment is well-tolerated by patients with any skin type and tone, adding to its status as a valuable treatment modality in dermatology. Treatment regimens can be tailored to the specific needs of individual patients by practitioners, adjusting the depth and frequency of needle penetration to achieve the best results. On being conferred these advantages, classical micro-needling is a fundamental component of contemporary practices in CIT, which proves to be appealing to diverse groups of patients interested in advancing their skin condition and appearance (Annunziata et al., 2010; Sivaranjani, 2019) (Figure 6.6).

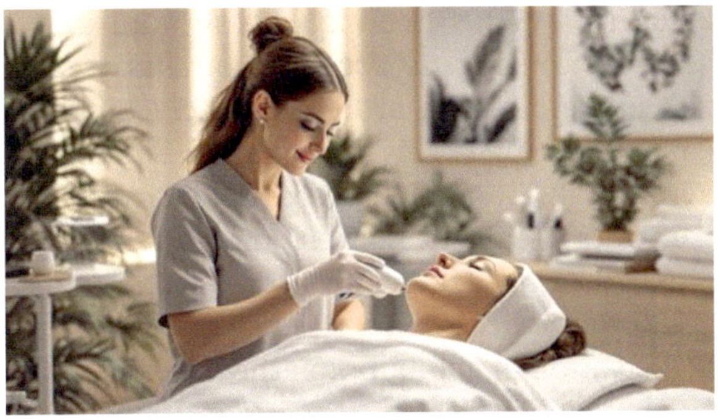

Figure 6.6. Traditional micro-needling.

Source: https://external-content.duckduckgo.com/iu/?u=https%3A%2F%2Ftse4.explicit.bing.net%2Fth%3Fid%3DOIP.uuvnlmkUroQQruDwa1k PdAHaEI%26pid%3DApi&f=1&ipt=88a90e5ec4bf31f508 48 4b91a0409e9162c538a6324d19d8b6bf7f9458b4011a.

6.2.2. Automated Micro-Needling Devices

With the innovation of automated micro-needling devices, CIT has become less painful and more efficient, allowing practitioners to achieve better results with less patient discomfort. The device does this by inflicting micro-injury to the skin using fine needles, which triggers a healing process that leads to collagen and elastin production. Their precision and varying needle depths enable practitioners to customize treatments according to the specific needs of individual patients, treating particular skin concerns like acne scarring, stretch marks, and general skin rejuvenation. Automated micro-needling can yield more uniform results compared to conventional manual procedures, thus leading to improved patient satisfaction. Moreover, the technologies promote a cleaner treatment environment by minimizing the risk of infection because the devices are usually furnished with single-use cartridges, hence ensuring optimal processes of hygiene. Apart from providing superior results, micro-needling devices have simplified the incorporation of adjunctive treatments, including the application of autologous platelet concentrates (APCs), which is now a point of discussion among recent clinical literature. These growth factor-dense concentrates have been increasingly used in aesthetic medicine and have been successful in complementing CIT. Through combined automated micro-needling and APCs, practitioners can provide more comprehensive treatment with multiple skin ailments being addressed simultaneously.

This complementary approach highlights the importance of the use of evidence-based therapies and technologies, as pointed out in Davies & Miron (2025), which focuses on the great potential of APCs in aesthetic treatment. With the integration of these modalities, there is a promising pathway in improving skin quality and appearance, thus relieving the growing demand for effective minimally invasive treatments. Treatment with automated micro-needling devices also necessitates high awareness of healing processes and scar management, as described in current texts committed to wound care. Upon the use of the devices by practitioners within treatment protocols, consideration of the factors that will influence healing outcomes must be done, including skin type, penetration depth of the needles, and post-treatment. The development of scar management strategies, such as those discussed in Téot et al. (2021), is seen as the use of evidence-based best practices when trying to harness innovative technologies in aesthetic medicine. As science continues to advance, probably more investigations will clarify what the best modalities are for integrating automated micro-needling and with what other treatments to enable healthcare professionals to deliver high-quality and safe treatments for different populations of patients seeking successful measures of skin rejuvenation (Figure 6.7).

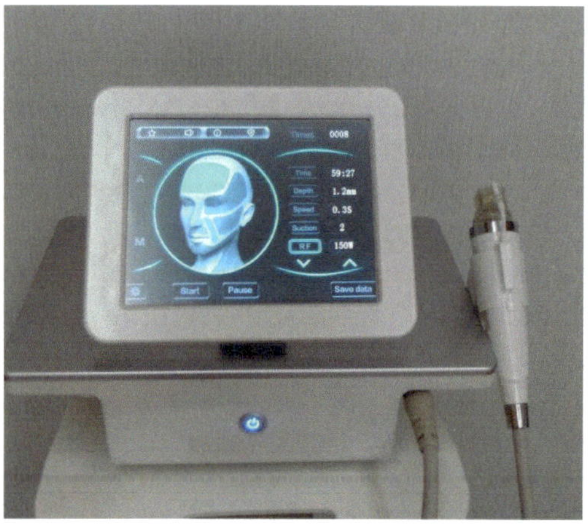

Figure 6.7. Fully automatic micro-needling RF machine.

Source: https://5.imimg.com/data5/FB/PT/FC/ANDROID-36838030/product-jpeg.jpg.

6.2.3. Combination Therapies with Other Treatments

The study of combination therapy in CIT points to the potential for enhanced clinical outcomes through a synergistic effect with other treatments. By administering CIT in combination with medical treatments such as growth factors or lasers, practitioners are experiencing remarkable improvement in scar reduction and skin rejuvenation. For instance, when combined with local agents such as growth factors, CIT not only promotes collagen production but also enhances dermal repair, producing greater aesthetic results. Interactive therapy can similarly decrease treatment downtime and maximize patient satisfaction, as the positive patient response to skin texture and elasticity enhancement attests. Moreover, the combination of CIT with other treatments, such as PRP therapy, is one instance of complementary treatment that augments the regenerative effects on the skin. PRP is derived from the patient's blood and comprises many growth factors that, when applied after CIT, can optimize tissue regeneration and redistribute skin volume. Early studies show that more therapeutic efficacy, including quicker wound healing and better facial contouring, is seen in patients treated with a combination of CIT and PRP compared to monotherapies. This combination is becoming increasingly popular in aesthetic dermatology due to its ability to harness the patient's own natural healing factors to increase the impact of CIT with little side effects. In cancer, the investigation of combination therapies with CIT has also been increasing, particularly in cosmetic and reconstructive procedures following cancer therapy. Combination with drugs such as venetoclax or gilteritinib is a vision to extend improving patient outcomes to addressing not only the aesthetic effects of treatment, but also the pathophysiological issues underlying skin expressions of cancer. The therapeutic potency of venetoclax in overcoming resistance in acute myeloid leukemia (AML) may be teachable in therapies where CIT enhances the quality of tissues in treatment-induced skin changes in patients. Similarly, investigating the role of gilteritinibs in this respect can reveal the possible routes for integrating CIT with targeted therapy to provide multi-level care that can effectively address physical appearance as well as health outcomes (Pratz et al., 2023; Mila et al., 2022) (Figure 6.8).

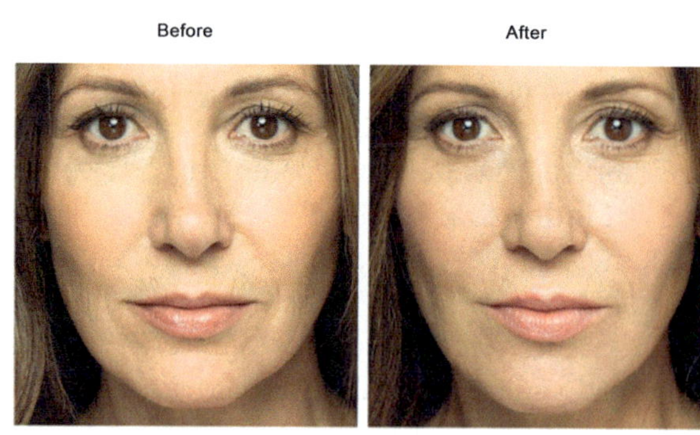

Figure 6.8. Before and after combination therapy.

Source: https://www.isaacluxe.co/wp-content/uploads/2021/09/Collagen-Induction-Therapy-1.png.

Test Your Knowledge

1. What are the main types of devices used in CIT?
2. How does automated microneedling (dermapen) differ from manual dermarolling?

6.3. Indications for Use

Learning Outcome

1. Understand the treatment of acne scars by CIT
2. Focus on the reduction of fine lines and wrinkles
3. Deal with the improvement of skin texture and tone

CIT, also known as microneedling, has been in the limelight for its diverse therapeutic applications in dermatology. Its primary indications include the treatment of cosmetic problems such as facial acne scars, fine lines, and wrinkles. It enhances the look of the skin by triggering collagen production and stimulating skin remodeling. Further, more recent evidence suggests that CIT is effective in patients with all types of scars other than traditional acne. For instance, efficacy in managing hypertrophic scars and scars from surgery has been documented, thus becoming even more relevant in aesthetic and reconstructive dermatology. Furthermore, anecdotal evidence increases its possible capacity to improve skin texture and tone even for stretch marks, indicating a broader array of applications in skin rejuvenation procedures. Beyond its cosmetic application, CIT has also shown promise in the treatment of some medical conditions due to chronic wounds. The therapeutic response observed with CIT is particularly noted when coupled with newer wound procedures, such as negative pressure wound therapy (NPWT). Promising results lead to clinical practice wherein clinicians are starting to use silver collagen oxidized regenerated cellulose dressings along with NPWT. With a general consensus regarding the use of such treatments by medical professionals, uses have been broadened to higher-level wound types like diabetic ulcers, venous leg ulcers, and pressure ulcers. Such versatility of CIT further testifies to its growing impact towards the treatment of wound care that is aimed at accelerating healing as well as improving patient outcomes in outpatient and inpatient settings (Robert et al., 2024). Apart from the therapeutic aspect of CIT is its use is in inflammation and hyperpigmentation disorders. The therapy has the potential to cause good effects in melasma and post-inflammatory hyperpigmentation (PIH), where the process of remodeling collagen leads to a more even skin tone. This means that CIT is not simply rejuvenation but is also correction of skin irregularities caused by other conditions, showing a broad-angle approach to dermal interventions. With more and more evidence mounting in support of these new applications for CIT, it only becomes clearer that CIT can be a cornerstone in full-skincare regimens. This adaptability shows that with evolving dermatological science, the integration of these treatment modalities will be required for the best patient care (Parkin et al., 2024).

6.3.1. Treatment of Acne Scars

Acne scarring has been a big focus of the last few years because of its potential for inducing psychological and cosmetic pain. There are numerous techniques that comprise laser treatments, dermabrasion, and chemical peels; however, these have large amounts of downtime and the potential for unwanted side effects.

Among the more recent developments, CIT, including microneedling, has become popular for being a less invasive process with fewer complications. Through the induction of dermal collagen production, microneedling stimulates repair and rejuvenation of the skin, effectively filling in the structural deficiencies present in atrophic scars. In addition, research has shown that microneedling not only enhances the texture of scars but also reduces the potential for complications associated with traditional treatments, making it a desirable option for patients looking to improve the appearance of their skin while keeping recovery time to a minimum. Demonstrating its efficacy, recent research supports the benefits of microneedling in treating atrophic acne scars. In a study with Fitzpatrick skin type IV to V patients, treatment with a dermaroller showed promising outcomes. Patients underwent multiple sessions of microneedling one month apart, which led to a significant reduction in scar severity, which was measured with Goodman and Baron's qualitative grading system. Of the patients initially scored with severe acne scarring, an impressive 88.90% demonstrated a decrease to a significantly less severe state. The data confirms that microneedling can cause effective aesthetic change with minimal downtime in comparison to other procedures, hence enhancing patient satisfaction and quality of life in acne scarring patients (Mistry et al., 2023). The mechanisms by which microneedling improves scars set it apart from other cosmetic treatments. Unlike traditional ablative therapies which induce severe skin wounding, microneedlings stimulate the process of healing by less intense inflammatory responses. This triggers collagen remodeling without inducing a prolonged convalescence period typical of more intrusive interventions. The procedure invokes the classical phases of wound healing that include inflammation, proliferation, and remodeling, but in a bracketed manner that does not lead to the creation of scar tissue (Kloth et al., 2012). The micro-injuries induced by the dermaroller stimulate the body's natural repair mechanisms and allow increased collagen deposition and skin texture enhancement. Therefore, the results are reflected in the appearance of a more even, smoother-looking skin, validating microneedling as a viable treatment for the correction of acne-scarring skin (Figure 6.9).

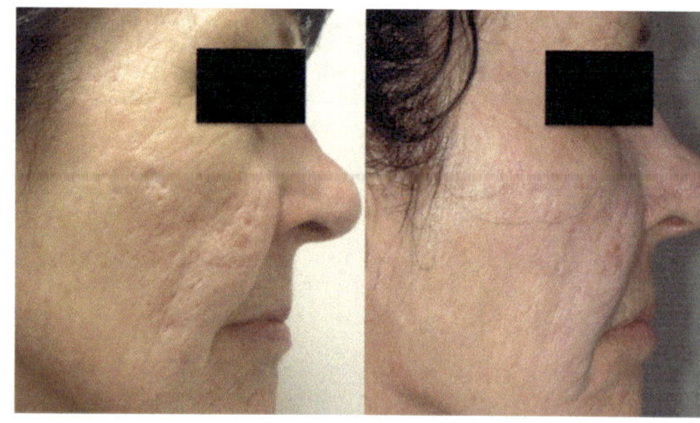

Figure 6.9. An improvement in acne scarring and photodamage in a patient treated with one session of skin needling.

Source: https://www.researchgate.net/publication/277928046_Skin_needling_as_a_treatment_for_acne_scarring_An_up-to-date_review_of_the_literature/link/55e05d6e 08ae2fac471b490 9/download?_tp=eyJjb250ZXh0Ijp7ImZpcnN0UGFnZSI6Il9kaXJlY3QiLCJwYWdlIjoicHVibGlj YXRpb24ifX0.

6.3.2. Reduction of Fine Lines and Wrinkles

Reduction of wrinkles and fine lines is of utmost importance in dermatological beauty, particularly in the application form of CIT. The natural production of collagen by the skin diminishes with aging, causing fine lines and lowered elasticity. CIT, also simply known as microneedling, triggers the body's natural healing processes by creating controlled minor injuries on the skin surface. This stimulates collagen and elastin resynthesis, eventually leading to improved skin texture and firmness. These kinds of therapeutic measures are essential not just for beauty improvement but also for enhancing general skin health since impaired skin is more prone to oxidative stress as well as other external stimuli that contribute to aging manifestations. Consequently, adoption of CIT has grown and empirical studies have validated its effectiveness in rejuvenating aging skin and reversing the signs of aging. Furthermore, the efficacy of CIT in reducing fine wrinkles can further be improved by incorporating natural products into the treatment regimen. Recent studies have shown that antioxidant and anti-inflammatory compounds, such as polyphenols and fatty acids, play a role in enhancing the resistance of skin to external influences, the culprit behind premature aging. With the incorporation of these bioactive compounds in post-treatment skin care, the potential for achieving complete healing and regeneration is greatly improved. For instance, natural compounds can modulate immune reactions in the skin by inducing tissue repair and reducing inflammation, thereby improving overall results of CIT. The synergistic process not only addresses the surface manifestations of aging but also, at a cellular level, enhances the strength of the skin and homeostasis, hence the causative factors of fine lines and wrinkles (Andreia et al., 2023). As the global cosmetics industry continues to evolve, naturally, there is a move towards the natural use of ingredients as a result of consumer awareness of the effects on skin care of man-made chemicals. In this, the demand for effective anti-wrinkle treatments has spurred innovation to develop solutions that bring together natural products with CIT. The growing popularity of holistic skin care treatments drives additional study into the advantages of such synergistic combinations, which have the potential to provide multi-action benefits for rejuvenating skin. The combination of CIT with products from diverse biological origins not only underscores a dedication to safety and efficacy in cosmetic procedures but also responds to consumer demands for transparency and performance in skin care. By building upon this trend, the cosmetics industry can enhance the provision of anti-aging products that combat the loss of fine lines and wrinkles through creative, nature-inspired formulations (Ji-Liu, 2022) (Figure 6.10).

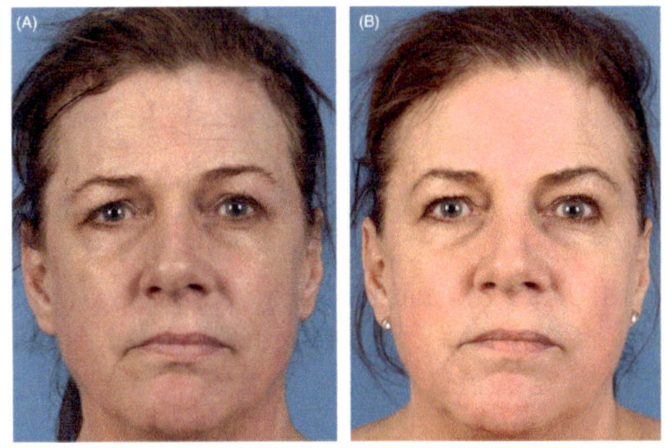

Figure 6.10. (A) 57-year-old female baseline photographs; and (B) 57-year-old female post microneedling procedure.

Source: https://www.researchgate.net/publication/359879876/figure/fig3/AS:11431281180391388@1691588551490/A-57-year-old-female-baseline-photographs-B-57-year-old-female-post-microneedling.png.

6.3.3. Improvement of Skin Texture and Tone

Improvement of skin tone and texture is one of the main benefits of CIT, especially for people choosing better overall skin well-being. This process allows the creation of collagen and elastin, two important components bearing the responsibility of skin elasticity and tightness. Microneedling is just one of the most popular treatments in this category, which consists of fine needles applied to cause minimal controlled injuries in the skin, triggering the body's natural healing process. This micro-trauma induces cell turnover and regeneration, and with this, over a period of time, it gives visibly softer skin texture. While stimulating the dermis, CIT does not just reduce the appearance of fine lines and wrinkles but also induces an even skin tone, thereby fighting concerns such as coarseness and dullness that are typically present in most skin types. Besides the effectiveness of CIT in improving skin tone quality, studies have demonstrated that it improves skin hydration and pigmentation significantly. Induction of micro-injuries throughout the process results in an increase in vascularity and the delivery of nutrients to the skin, rendering it healthier. Also, the application of APCs, as illustrated in the literature, enhances the effect of the therapy. These concentrates provide growth factors that facilitate cellular repair and regeneration, therefore maximizing outcomes in pigmented and uneven-toned areas such as melasma and PIH. Consequently, patients experience enhanced overall skin quality, proving that CIT is not a superficial treatment but a deep-rooted method of enhancing skin vitality and look in the long term (Davies & Miron, 2025). Besides, the procedural aspect of CIT, particularly microneedling, is characterized by its flexibility and minimal downtime, making it a popular treatment option for individuals with varied forms of skin problems. Its effectiveness in treating atrophic scars, acne, and other conditions has been identified through research. As an example, microneedling has proven to be very promising in the case of treating acne scars, with patients noticing an undeniable improvement in scarring as well as overall skin texture, achieving smoother and more defined skin surfaces (Sivaranjani, 2019). The fact that treatment plans can be highly customized based on the special requirements of the skin ensures that the patients get specifically targeted therapy, achieving higher satisfaction and efficacy. Therefore, with the addition of CIT into their skin regimen, people can expect to have their overall skin texture and tone improved, resulting in greater confidence in their appearance.

Test Your Knowledge

1. What are the primary dermatological conditions treated with CIT?
2. Is CIT suitable for all skin types, including darker skin tones? Why or why not?

6.4. Benefits of Collagen Induction Therapy

Learning Outcome

1. Discuss about non-surgical nature of the procedure
2. Explain the advantages of CIT in the realm of minimal downtime and recovery
3. Focus on long-lasting results of CIT compared to other treatments

CIT is one of the new, exciting aesthetic treatments offered for many of the everyday issues plaguing the skin, providing dramatic improvements for those who desire a brighter, more youthful look. Its foundation stems from its power to induce natural collagenesis, an essential protein responsible for keeping the skin elastic and taut. Through the use of microneedling, CIT produces minor injuries that initiate the body's healing process, resulting in improved collagen and elastin production. After a period, the patients can experience astoundingly better skin texture, tone, and elasticity, so CIT is a desirable solution for those who want to fight against wrinkles and loose skin. This intrinsic healing is not just highly effective but also quite safe, considering it avoids causing more destructive procedures. Aside from its cosmetic benefits, CIT also presents therapeutic uses within the field of scar management and dermatology. The stimulation of collagen synthesis through CIT has proven to diminish the visibility of acne scars, surgical scars, and other forms of scarring, rendering it an effective treatment for those with a history of skin injury. The treatment improves the skin's rejuvenating potential by stimulating a healthy extracellular matrix, important for efficient tissue repair. Additionally, research indicates that CIT can be used adjunctively in combination with other modalities, including fat-derived exosome treatments, to enhance outcomes in the prevention and healing of scars. The many-aspect nature of CIT facilitates individualized treatment approaches to manage diverse skin issues effectively. With CIT, less invasive treatments are chosen with priority for comfort and quicker recovery for the patient. Conventional cosmetic interventions-for example, facelifts and chemical peels-require a lot of downtime and pose a greater risk of complications. CIT therefore, is an alternative that is less invasive and shorter in duration for recovery times.

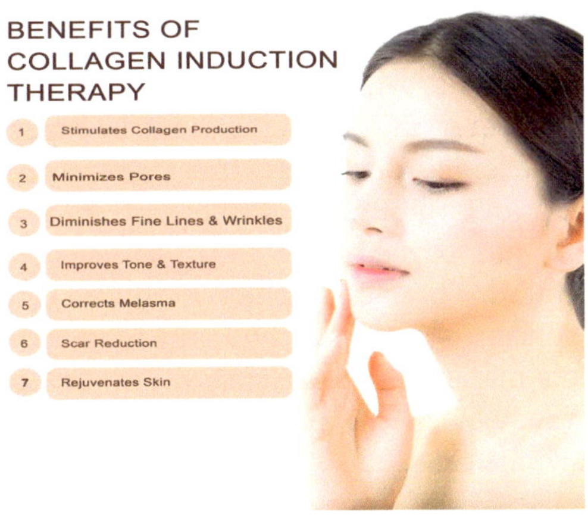
BENEFITS OF
COLLAGEN INDUCTION
THERAPY
1 Stimulates Collagen Production
2 Minimizes Pores
3 Diminishes Fine Lines & Wrinkles
4 Improves Tone & Texture
5 Corrects Melasma
6 Scar Reduction
7 Rejuvenates Skin

Figure 6.11. Collagen induction therapy benefits.

Source: https://encrypted-tbn0.gstatic.com/images?q=tbn:ANd9GcQS7rzCBppTYPSMA7EjdenuQteoiPKSH8eV-Q&s.

The patient can return to his or her daily routines within a short period after undergoing the treatment. This ease, along with inherent biocompatibility induced by the therapy, particularly a grand success of different grafts in regenerative therapy, such as Fascia Lata in periodontal therapy and its promise in soft tissue regeneration, sets off the impression of increasing use of CIT in everyday practice. Both immediate and long-term consequences have hence been pushing the celebrity use of CIT in order to treat as well as maximize skin well-being and appearance in individuals (Figure 6.11).

6.4.1. Non-Surgical Nature of the Procedure

CIT, also known as microneedling, has garnered significant attention for its effectiveness in rejuvenating the skin while maintaining a non-surgical approach. The procedure involves using a device equipped with fine needles to create controlled micro-injuries to the skin's surface, which stimulates the natural healing process and promotes collagen production. Compared to traditional surgical processes, CIT does not involve any cuts or extensive recovery times and is therefore a favored process for those who desire aesthetic enhancement without surgery's risks. The procedure is non-surgical and hence induces minimal pain and faster recovery, demonstrating the compatibility of the process with the low-risk and less invasive trend in cosmetic treatment. The fact that CIT is non-surgical also adds to its convenience and accessibility across a wider population. As patients frequently look for alternatives to surgery because of issues with anesthesia, scarring, and extended downtime, CIT provides a suitable alternative. Furthermore, the technique is easily adjustable according to different skin types and issues, such as acne marks, fine lines, and improvement of general skin texture. Patients may experience several sessions in a clinical facility or even at home, based on the device applied and their individual preferences. Such flexibility represents a large move toward more patient-oriented care in dermatological therapy, maximizing the effectiveness of the procedure while being sensitive to personal comfort levels. Moreover, the non-surgical procedures align with current trends emphasizing non-invasive aesthetic treatments, which are continuously gaining traction in the healthcare market. As there is a growing inclination toward minimally invasive solutions, CIT represents an important advancement in regenerative dermatology, balancing efficiency with patient safety. Studies have demonstrated that CIT can achieve results comparable to more invasive procedures without incurring the associated complications or extended recovery periods. This feature is highly significant in terms of the potential for non-surgical treatments to confer major advantages with minimal exposure of patients to the psychological and physical stresses usually associated with surgical treatments, opening the door to innovation and more widespread adoption within standard aesthetic medicine (Figure 6.12).

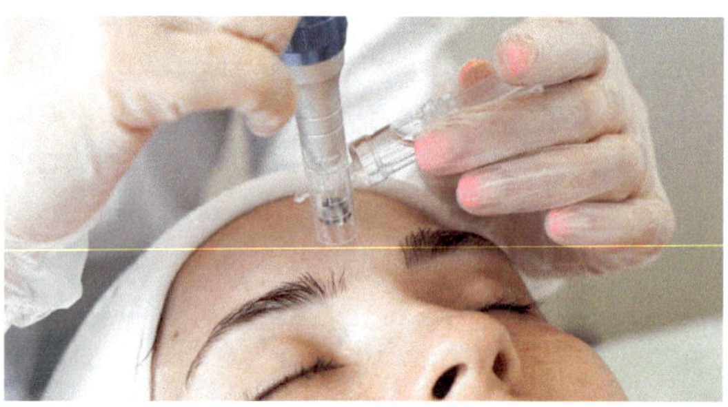

Figure 6.12. A close-up of a microneedling procedure being performed on a patient's forehead, demonstrating the use of fine needles to create controlled micro-injuries that stimulate collagen production and skin regeneration.

Source: https://laserclub.co.uk/wp-content/uploads/2024/02/image001.png.

6.4.2. Minimal Downtime and Recovery

The benefits of CIT span far into the arena of minimal recovery time. The treatment, also commonly known as microneedling or percutaneous CIT, stimulates the body's natural healing mechanisms by creating micro-wounds within the skin. Stimulating this way actually facilitates the production of collagen, which enhances the texture and look of the skin. Crucially, this technique is renowned for its relatively short recovery time relative to more aggressive treatments. Patients feel only minimal discomfort, usually manageable with topical anesthetics, and the majority can return to routine activities within 24 to 48 hours after treatment. This characteristic of minimal downtime is a distinguishing factor that has made CIT highly popular among individuals opting for aesthetic enhancement without the prolonged recovery time involved with conventional surgical procedures (Lakshmi et al., 2020). Further emphasizing the benefits of minimal downtime, CIT has been shown to yield significant improvements in various skin conditions with limited negative impact on daily life. Following the procedure, it is common for patients to experience mild redness or a sunburn-like sensation that generally subsides quickly. This temporary response permits a smooth integration of treatment in a patient's lifestyle since, for most, the therapy is done during lunch hours or working hours, so their social and professional commitments are not disrupted. The fact that CIT is able to improve the condition of skin without any long-term side effects makes it a promising alternative option for those who fear more invasive procedures (Lakshmi et al., 2020). This excellent combination of efficacy and convenience is still expanding its patient base. The long-term result with the least amount of downtime in CIT also promotes compliant treatment programs. Patients who suffer less disruption in their routine are likely to continue with follow-up sessions, which are essential for optimal outcomes. In most instances, practitioners prescribe a course of treatments to yield the desired skin rejuvenating effects, and the flexibility of recovery intervals makes such compliance feasible. In addition, the additive benefit of cumulative treatments can produce improved texture, increased scar diminishment, and overall skin improvement over time, making it possible for the patient to continue commitments while treating concerns aesthetically. The consistency of this treatment, coupled with the minimal recovery requirements, highlights the attractiveness of CIT as an innovative approach to dermatological treatment in contemporary practice (Lakshmi et al., 2020).

6.4.3. Long-Lasting Results Compared to Other Treatments

Then, CIT is the second most important aesthetic treatment since it creates lasting effects in terms of the rejuvenation and healing of the skin. Typically, such conventions like chemical peeling, lasers, among others, only provide a short-term aesthetic effect without persistence over time. CIT, however, triggers the natural body healing response to initiate collagen production through microneedling. This produces more enduring skin that has become more elastic and aesthetically enhanced. Some research findings have indicated that the collagen matrix formed by this process can last for months or even years as a solid base for sustaining skin health. This regenerative potential is what sets CIT apart from more temporary alternatives, which, to continue their effects, might need repeated treatments performed regularly. With consumers ever more looking for something that will last, the enduring effect of collagen induction is an appealing feature for those contemplating aesthetic treatments. In terms of the importance of long-term outcomes, the relative safety profile also must be considered for CIT compared with other treatments. Most cosmetic treatments, particularly the invasive ones, also carry a number of risks, including side effects such as scarring and protracted recovery periods. CIT, on the other hand, is minimally invasive, leading to less downtime and fewer unwanted effects. Such a safety advantage not only encourages compliance among patients but also illustrates why CIT can prove so enticing to patients who worry about the side effects of more invasive therapies. Most importantly, the long-term advantages, with reduced complications, make CIT an amazing option for patients looking for effective and safe skin rejuvenation procedures, further solidifying its position in aesthetic medicine. The new findings in CIT indicate the efficacy of this treatment, which, similar to many other new treatments in medicine, possibly delivers more durable results. For instance, there are some immunosuppressive methods that, at least in the example of converted donor cells in kidney transplantation, ensured a long-term advantage through the induction of donor-specific unresponsiveness and non-toxic titers at very low levels (Morath et al., 2022). It is also possible to see the same principles with CIT, wherein the induction of natural healing processes may have more long-term consequences rather than adverse side effects associated with unnatural interventions. Additionally, studies are being released that inject other modalities with CIT to enhance its overall result and produce even longer-lasting results. Therefore, the continuous research into synergistic treatments highlights the significance of comprehending long-term effects in the wider setting of patient satisfaction and treatment adherence, reiterating the relevance of CIT in aesthetic medicine and more broadly.

Test Your Knowledge

1. What is the primary aesthetic benefit of CIT?
2. How does CIT improve the appearance of acne scars and other skin irregularities?

6.5. Risks and Side Effects

Learning Outcome

1. Understand common side effects post-treatment
2. Discuss potential complications and how to mitigate them
3. Explain the importance of professional administration

The landscape of CIT is not devoid of potential risks and side effects, which warrant careful consideration by both practitioners and patients. As a minimally invasive technique aimed at promoting skin rejuvenation and healing, it carries the possibility of adverse reactions. Common side effects include post-procedure redness, swelling, and bruising, which typically resolve within a few days. However, in some cases, patients may experience more serious complications of infection, scarring, or allergy to the topically used anesthetics. Moreover, the effectiveness of therapy may be lost if previous skin disease or improper aftercare is not adequately resolved, thereby making proper full patient evaluation and adherence to post-treatment advice crucial. Furthermore, the biological mechanisms underlying CIT can also establish a dichotomy of action where low dosing is pro-healing, while higher dosing may initiate more issues. For instance, as with the biphasic effect of isothiocyanates on some cellular responses, stimulation of collagen production may vary in effectiveness based on context and dosing applied. This interaction demands strict control and individualized treatment protocols to avoid dangers of oversaturation of collagen production. Patients should be made aware of their individual dermatological needs and possible side effects and the necessity of designer treatment to maximize the effect without sacrificing security. Besides these short-term physical effects, the psychological effect of CIT is yet another aspect that deserves consideration. Patients tend to have exaggerated expectations regarding the outcomes of the treatment, which may result in discontentment if the outcomes are not as perceived. This situation tends to impact a patient's mental health and result in emotional distress, particularly in social scenarios where appearance is significant. Practitioners should thus undertake thorough pre-treatment consultations for the purpose of setting realistic expectations regarding outcomes and dispelling any myths surrounding the therapy. Open discussion regarding the risks and safe side effects stimulates the doctors to work harder in terms of patient satisfaction and hence trust, resulting in a more optimistic treatment outcome.

6.5.1. Common Side Effects Post-Treatment

Post-treatment, patients of CIT can present with several common side effects of varying degrees and durations. The side effects are generally mild to moderate in nature and are largely due to a reaction in the skin, considering the fact that the therapy is by micro-needling to induce collagen production. Common immediate reactions are erythema and edema of the treated sites, which are akin to a sunburn. These responses are an immediate response to the healing process of the skin, i.e., the body's reaction to treatment. According to expert analysis, inflammation can stimulate collagen production, which contributes to the overall success of the therapy while temporarily increasing pain levels for the patients. These side effects are, therefore, important to understand since they help the patient in giving guidance about staying optimistic during the recovery period after the treatment. The long-term effects appear during the time the skin continues healing, in addition to the immediate results. Among them is PIH which will be more apparent in darker skin tones. This pigmentation change can also be due to the inflammatory reaction of the skin and will settle over time. There can also be scarring or allergic reactions to the treatment through micro-needling that occur when improper techniques or less-than-optimal post-treatment care are employed. Although these side effects do not occur in all patients, they need to be remembered while teaching the patient regarding post-treatment care. The aim shall be to keep the skin appropriately hydrated and protected against the sun to reduce the risks of PIH. These possible side effects, as well as their management, must, therefore, be discussed in a thorough pre-treatment consultation. Finally, psychological factors can also contribute to the perceived side effects post-CIT. Because patients invest time, money, and emotional capital in their skin rejuvenation treatments, expectations for results can amplify any annoyance experienced after treatment. For example, concern about rehabilitation or dissatisfaction with the immediate result might amplify the physical side effects experienced. Reducing invasive practices, such as the use of soothing serums and check-ins with skilled practitioners, can help reduce some of these emotional stressors. Lastly, acknowledgment of the universal side effects, whether physical or psychological, is extremely important for the improvement of patient outcomes and satisfaction from CIT. In fact, as the clinical findings attest, an integrated approach can be instrumental for improving both the therapeutic experience and the result (Jimenez et al., 2012; Forrester et al., 2016).

6.5.2. Potential Complications and How to Mitigate Them

The application of CIT, though with many aesthetic and therapeutic benefits, is not free of possible complications that need to be managed by practitioners. These complications include post-treatment inflammation, scarring of tissues, and infection risk. Inflammatory response may appear as redness and swelling, which though usually mild, may discourage patients from seeking further sessions. To avoid such issues, the practitioners can educate patients on good pre- and post-treatment care, such as the application of cooling treatments immediately following the therapy to alleviate pain and let them know the healing time to expect. Also, sterile environments cannot be overstressed since this is critical in the avoidance of infections that can be caused by micro-trauma resulting from the procedure. Strict hygiene procedures must be implemented in clinical practice to minimize the risk of adverse events during and after treatment. More serious complications of CIT do exist, though, and require attention, especially related to fibrotic reactions and structural integrity of the tissue. As reviewed in the case of other medical complications, including those caused by radiation injury, treatments like Pirfenidone have proven to be effective in the prevention of such side effects by inhibiting inflammatory and fibrotic activity in tissues. For example, employing agents that block these pathways has been proven to greatly enhance outcomes by acting to maintain the function of treated tissue and avoid unnecessary scarring. During CIT, practitioners may incorporate some additional therapies based on inflammatory markers or apply biological therapies, like growth factors, in combination with conventional collagen induction for further maximizing the regeneration of tissues and reducing fibrosis. In addition, having an extensive follow-up protocol is crucial for minimizing the complications arising from CIT successfully. Regular monitoring of patient recovery ensures detection of complications such as extended periods of discomfort, adverse reactions, or scar patterns that are not within the normal range. Perioperative post-procedure assessment is part of the overall plan to assist practitioners in making appropriate protocol adjustments early on. Informed patients about signs of complications and enhance their active participation in the recovery process and encourage them to communicate openly with their physician concerning their own needs. Such an active approach, accompanied by efficient interventions against inflammatory responses as shown by research conducted on anti-inflammatory drugs, demonstrates how to prevent complications and maximize results for patients who receive CIT, with the end result being safer and more satisfactory outcomes (Gouveia et al., 2025; Scripcariu et al., 2025) (Figure 6.13).

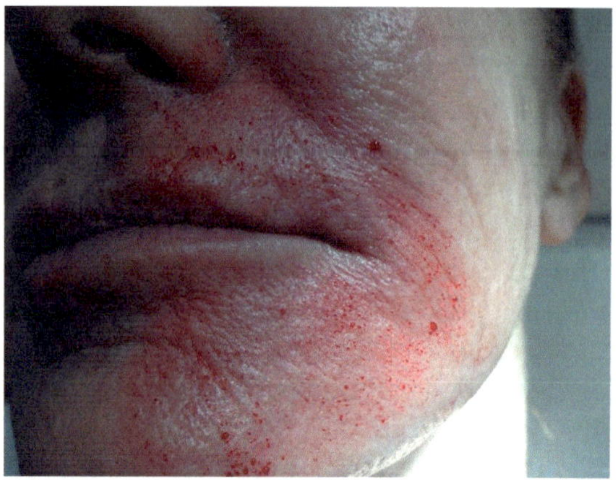

Figure 6.13. Pinpoint bleeding serves as a guide to indicate the treatment end point.

Source: https://www.researchgate.net/profile/Paul-Graham-10/publication/318997589/figure/fig4/AS:667793183744000@1536225710019/Pinpoint-bleeding-serves-as-a-guide-to-indicate-treatment-end-point.jpg.

6.5.3. Importance of Professional Administration

Of course, professional administration in the case of CIT cannot be overemphasized. CIT, involving controlled induction of collagen formation by micro-needling, is increasingly becoming popular in dermatology and aesthetic procedures. However, the success of CIT depends on the professional competence of the practitioner who is performing the procedure. Adequate knowledge of skin anatomy, correct technique of micro-needling, and awareness of personal needs of each patient are crucial in minimizing complications and maximizing outcome. Properly trained personnel not only ensures safety and effectiveness of the treatment but also enhances patient satisfaction by maintaining good communication and management of expectations. Scientific administration itself is a platform on which therapeutic success of CIT is built. Professional management of CIT is important for regulatory compliance and guidelines. Because aesthetic procedures are constantly changing, proper practices should be followed by medical and dermatological associations. Professionals can deal with the intricacies of regulatory matters so that the treatments will take place in well-equipped facilities with protocol-based sterile procedures. This is more so in light of the fact that poor management can result in complications, including infection and scarring. Professionalism and accountability would make practitioners part of the efforts towards fortifying the basis of trust between patients and the general medical world. As CIT continues to evolve, it is also being added into more and more treatment practices, which means the more that the competence of administering is called for. This means that professional management is not just required to achieve results but also to propel forward the development of research and knowledge base on CIT. Educated and trained providers are better placed to enter into clinical research and assist in providing evidence to guide best practices. For example, application of biomarkers such as E-selectin in evaluating the efficacy of therapy in similar inflammatory disorders shows how learned clinicians can apply scientific advances to achieve greatest benefits for patients (Gompels et al., 2010). Learning from research can lead to improved techniques or methods that eventually enhance aesthetic medicine practice. The applicability of professional management, therefore, extends beyond the local clinic environment, and evidence of a wider commitment to continuing education, innovation, and excellence in CIT.

Test Your Knowledge

1. What are the most common short-term side effects of CIT?
2. What are the potential risks if CIT is not performed under sterile conditions?

6.6. Patient Considerations

Learning Outcome

1. Describe ideal candidates for CIT
2. Discuss pre-treatment consultation and assessment
3. Deal with post-treatment care and maintenance

One of the key points in patient considerations for CIT is awareness of the patient's individual medical history and condition. For instance, patients who have undergone previous treatments like chemotherapy may respond differently to CIT because of immune system change. Studies have indicated that chemotherapy alters the infiltrative pattern of immune cells in tumors and this may affect healing after treatment. In particular, the presence of substantial CD45+ immune cell density adjacent to E-selectin expressing inflamed vessels in chemotherapy-treated tumors suggests that prior treatments may complicate skin regeneration. Thus, careful evaluation of such factors is vital to develop a tailored approach for each patient to optimize treatment efficacy and minimize adverse effects, as variations in immune response could affect the success of therapy significantly (Chervoneva et al., 2020). Patient demographics, age, and underlying chronic illness must be observed during CIT. An older patient or one suffering from chronic illness responds biologically in a way that is different from younger individuals. This variability calls for greater care, since an older patient might respond slowly to regenerative treatments and develop infections. Furthermore, diseases like idiopathic pulmonary fibrosis will change the overall health and responsiveness of a patient. Physiologic changes in patients with IPF, for instance, over-expression of serotonin receptors, may further overlap with body repair processes and influence the response to CIT. Evaluation of these variables is able to enable optimal planning and effective delivery of protocols suited to each patient that would thus result in improved outcomes with less complication in treatment (Amarie et al., 2010). Another vital aspect of successful CIT is a requirement to educate the patient and, of course, obtain appropriate informed consent. It is necessary that patients have proper enlightenment about possible benefits and risks of treatment and plausible recovery and skin enhancement expectations. Having a conversation with them about treatment plans can build trust and guide people to follow their post-procedure care. For example, psychological factors, such as anxiety about aesthetic outcome, may also be one in determining treatment methods or choice of therapy settings. This aspect calls for the taking care of these emotional and psychological factors so that maximal compliance and satisfaction for the patient are assured. This, in turn, will help professionals to achieve better psychological as well as physical results among patients by emphasizing patient education and involvement in the therapeutic process (Amarie et al., 2010; Chervoneva et al., 2020).

6.6.1. Ideal Candidates for Collagen Induction Therapy

In selecting the best candidates for CIT, it is important to assess the individual's skin condition and issues. This treatment works well for those who want to treat aged or sun-damaged skin because it can induce collagen and improve the elasticity of the skin. Patients with superficial scarring, like scarring due to injury or acne, will benefit immensely from the treatment since the therapy is in contact with skin texture and minimizes the visibility of scarring. Individuals who have melasma or any other skin pigmentation issue will be apt to undergo collagen induction treatment, which smoothes the complexion and initiates its own anti-aging processes. Worth of note is that the treatment has been often well accepted and may be individually tailored to meet the specific needs of an individual patient, thereby the intervention being exceedingly flexible in aesthetic dermatology. There is also an evaluation of the patient's general health and medical history. The ideal candidates should neither have conditions that would result in complicated healing nor raise the risk of side effects such as uncontrolled diabetes, autoimmune disease, or previous history of keloid scarring. Secondly, pregnant women or those already on anticoagulants are not usually advised on CIT to avoid any possible complications. A proper pre-procedure consultation covering these issues is critical in patient safety and best results. The decision-making process has a very important role from the end of the healthcare provider by considering the factor of appropriateness in patients as well as the presently established guidelines for CIT. As stated in the ESC Guidelines, clinicians should exercise careful clinical judgment when determining appropriate therapeutic strategies to align with each patient's specific health conditions and needs (Glikson et al., 2021). Lastly, psychological readiness of the candidates also determines the success of CIT. Candidates seeking this kind of treatment normally have internal elements of self-concept and self-esteem levels. Therefore, people seeking therapy with realistic expectations are normally best treated with positive outcome and experience. It is necessary that medical providers have open discussion with patients regarding the expectation and recovery in terms of outcome, reminding them that even though CIT will improve the appearance greatly of the skin, it is not a one-size-fits-all kind of treatment. Such discussion is helpful in establishing informed consent and patient-provider relationship. Lastly, a successful patient is one who not only meets the medical requirements of the process but also has an appropriate understanding and acceptance of the process, thus more likely to be satisfied with the outcome (Glikson et al., 2021) (Figure 6.14).

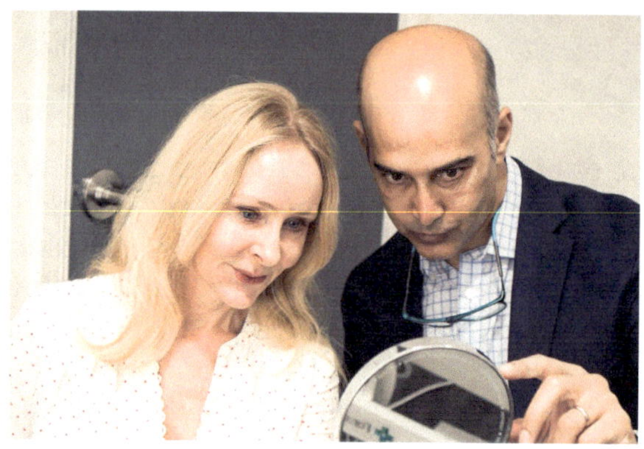

Figure 6.14. A patient consulting with a dermatologist to evaluate candidacy for microneedling treatment, emphasizing the importance of professional assessment in determining appropriate skin rejuvenation procedures.

Source: https://www.thedoc.com.au/wp-content/uploads/2025/03/who-is-a-good-candidate-for-skin-needling-microneedling-treatment-img.jpg.

6.6.2. Pre-Treatment Consultation and Assessment

In the realm of CIT, pre-treatment consultation and assessment emerge as vital components in ensuring optimal patient outcomes. This initial phase is crucial for establishing a comprehensive understanding of the patient's medical history, skin type, and specific concerns. During the consultation, practitioners should engage in thorough discussions that address the patient's objectives and expectations, thereby fostering a more tailored treatment plan. The individual characteristics of each patient significantly impact the choice of techniques and devices employed in CIT. Not only does this personalized approach enhance the efficacy of the treatment, but it also mitigates potential risks associated with the procedure, ensuring that the patient is fully informed and prepared for the upcoming interventions. Furthermore, a detailed assessment during the pre-treatment phase involves evaluating skin conditions that may influence treatment effectiveness. Factors such as existing scars, pigmentation issues, and overall skin elasticity must be considered. This evaluation helps practitioners to identify any contraindications and to make informed decisions about potential adjunctive therapies that could enhance results. Additionally, it offers an opportunity for clinicians to educate patients about the science behind CIT, including the mechanisms of skin regeneration and healing in response to micro-needling. By equipping patients with knowledge, practitioners can foster trust and collaboration, essential elements for a successful therapeutic relationship and improved satisfaction with the treatment outcomes. Lastly, ethical considerations also play a pivotal role in the pre-treatment consultation and assessment process. Health professionals have to ensure that potential patients are aware of what is involved in and expected from CIT. Informed consent dictates this requirement, especially since most of the patients who approach such health providers will be different in background and health status. All healthcare providers have to style their communication so that patients at all levels of health literacy understand what will happen to them in treatment, potential side effects, and after-care needs. Additionally, it is vital to adhere to established guidelines that champion equal access to quality care, as underscored by organizations like the Thalassemia International Federation (TIF) (Farmakis et al., 2022) and outlined within professional medical frameworks (Glikson et al., 2021). These guidelines provide a structured approach, promoting best practices that enhance the safety and effectiveness of the CIT experience (Figure 6.15).

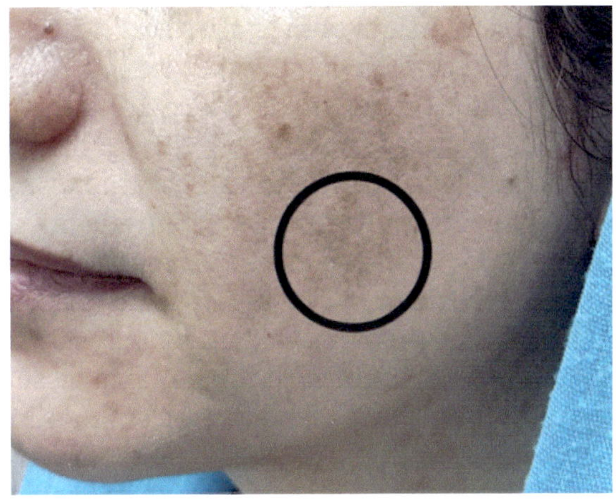

Figure 6.15. A pre-treatment photograph of a patient from the B2 group undergoing microneedling combined with 10% tranexamic acid (TA) and the modified Kligman formula, illustrating baseline melasma severity.

Source: https://www.researchgate.net/publication/382326983/figure/fig5/AS:11431281287522129@1730263786181/Panel-A-shows-a-pre-treatment-photograph-of-a-patient-from-the-B2-group-undergoing.png

6.6.3. Post-Treatment Care and Maintenance

Post-treatment care and maintenance following CIT are crucial to optimal results. Patients need to be instructed on the importance of adhering to post-procedure instructions by preventing complications and ensuring healing. The instructions can include staying indoors and using high-SPF sunscreen as protective measures for the skin, which is sensitive after the treatment. Moisturizing the treated skin with proper topical agents following treatment is also of the highest priority to optimize hydration of the skin for recovery and healing. An adequate posttreatment regimen speeds healing, facilitates the achievement of even, aesthetically acceptable results, and addresses the usual concerns about compromised skin integrity in the first days following treatment. The success of CIT might rely to a large extent on the general health of the patients and certain post-treatment care habits. For example, the use of serums that include growth factors or hyaluronic acid may contribute further to the healing process. In addition, patients are sometimes asked to abstain from strenuous exercise and heat exposure during the week after the procedure. These recommendations will lower the risk of inflammation and provide optimal healing conditions for the skin tissue. Such therapeutic care enhances the stimulation of collagen synthesis to better structure the extracellular matrix, thus potentially improving the skin's texture and quality overall. Like the acute phase of CIT, long-term follow-up is equally critical to maintain the benefits to be gained over further sessions. Patients are educated to schedule regular maintenance appointments to prolong the benefits of their treatment. Depending on individual skin types and objectives, 6–12-month treatments may be recommended. Furthermore, an antioxidant and peptide-based balanced skincare regimen may benefit the patient's skin in its ability to better withstand the signs of aging. Research indicates that a proactive approach in skin maintenance can significantly improve patient satisfaction and long-term outcomes in scenarios where collagen production is critical for skin health, as noted in studies that discuss the implications of understanding growth factor activity (Allen et al., 2001) and hormone influence on treatment outcomes (Meyer et al., 2014) (Figure 6.16).

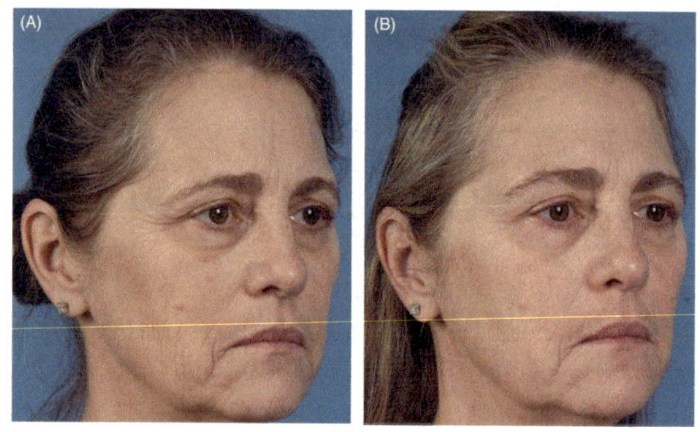

Figure 6.16. (A) 54-year-old female baseline photographs; and (B) 54-year-old female 3 months post last microneedling procedure.

Source: https://www.researchgate.net/publication/359879876/figure/fig1/AS:11431281180391353@1691588530145/A-54-year-old-female-baseline-photographs-B-54-year-old-female-3months-post-last.png.

Test Your Knowledge

1. What skin concerns make someone an ideal candidate for CIT?
2. What key factors should be evaluated during a pre-treatment consultation for CIT?

SUMMARY

CIT is a major breakthrough in the field of cosmetic and dermatological treatments that is minimally invasive and provides a means to rejuvenate the skin without invasive procedures while treating several conditions like scarring and aging. Its effectiveness is based on the fact that it triggers the body's own collagen production by causing controlled micro-injuries to the dermis. This treatment not only restores the texture and appearance of the skin but also facilitates the healing of wounds, providing a tightened and younger face. The ease of CIT, combined with its affordability and lower rate of side effects when compared to other treatments, is why it becomes a very popular choice for clients who are seeking good alternatives for skin rejuvenation. Moreover, recent studies indicate that CIT may also be practiced in conjunction with other treatments to enhance the effectiveness of the treatment against a vast range of dermatological issues. The incorporation of new technologies and equipment into CIT has created improved patient results in patients with diverse needs and conditions, from scar issues from acne and other ailments to hair transplantation. Synergistic treatments may supplement the microneedling process, allowing for tailoring of therapies to individual patient profiles, which optimizes the results. This kind of adaptability further asserts the status of CITs as pivotal techniques of modern dermatology and cosmetic practice, thus catering to an increasing demand for personalized, effective care (Fisher et al., 2024). Additionally, as new studies emerge and techniques evolve, the future of CIT is poised for further advancements and refinements. The exploration of outcomes related to immune responses, such as the induction of regulatory T cells and inflammatory mediators, may pave the way for enhanced therapeutic frameworks. For example, knowledge gained from concomitant immunological research, for example, on dendritic cells, can provide guidelines on best practices in combining immune modulation with conventional CIT techniques (Fisher et al., 2024). As scientists explore further the complex mechanisms of collagen synthesis and their therapeutic potential, there is a promising outlook for broadening the indications and effectiveness of this novel technique, ultimately enhancing patient treatment in aesthetic medicine.

Microneedling, or CIT, has been the focus of a lot of attention as a minimally invasive treatment for a variety of skin issues, including wrinkles, scarring, and overall skin revitalization. Essentially, the treatment involves the use of microneedles to create micro-injuries in the skin, which subsequently stimulates the body's inherent healing response and increases collagen synthesis. This is particularly relevant in the instance of regenerative medicine, seeking new treatment modalities for tissue regeneration and renewal. By stimulating the production of collagen, CIT not only addresses surface skin imperfections but also intradermal issues, promoting more comprehensive skin rejuvenation. For this reason, the treatment represents a multi-dimensional remedy for cosmetic therapy, sought after by both patients and practitioners for maximum, long-lasting results. Studies have pointed to the value of CIT, especially in its application in scar healing, like acne or surgery scars. The process works through not only collagen formation but the remodeling of fibers that are already present, making the skin tighter and more elastic. With clinical trials further confirming its safety and effectiveness, practitioners are now more and more adopting this process into practice. Particularly, patient outcomes are frequently quite variable based on individual variables like age, skin type, and previous therapies. The need, therefore, for individualized treatment protocols tailored to the individual patient becomes evident. Secondly, cumulative series of treatment effects demonstrate that ongoing treatment protocols can optimize outcomes, further solidifying collagen induction therapies place in modern dermatology. Moreover, combination of CIT with other treatments such as topical serums or laser therapy can enhance its effectiveness, and a synergistic effect on the rejuvenation of the skin can be realized. As continuous technological development polishes the precision and effectiveness of microneedling, combining statistical data from various studies plays a crucial role in establishing standardized treatment protocols. The role of CIT in evidence-based aesthetic medicine is ever better established, with clinicians emphasizing the importance of clinical guidelines to maximize patient safety and satisfaction. Given the parallels between this therapy and new cellular therapies, such as those detailed in regenerative medicine literature, there lies potential for further exploration of combined strategies in both aesthetic and medical fields, addressing broader questions of optimal treatment implementation and patient care in regenerative health (Kyryk, 2024; Othman et al., 2024).

KEY TERMS FROM THIS CHAPTER

- Acute myeloid leukemia (AML)
- Anti-inflammatory compounds
- Clinical practice
- Dissatisfaction
- Healing process
- Homeostasis
- Micro-injury
- Natural healing process
- Proliferation
- Repair mechanisms
- Aesthetic treatments
- Autologous platelet concentrates (APCs)
- Dermatological conditions
- Elastin production
- Healthcare professionals
- Inflammatory responses
- Microneedling devices
- Primary mechanisms
- Radiofrequency (RF)
- Surgical procedures

CRITICAL THINKING QUESTIONS

1. **What is the primary mechanism of action in CIT?**
   a. Stimulating sebaceous glands for oil production
   b. Inducing controlled skin injury to promote collagen production
   c. Increasing blood circulation in the skin
   d. Reducing pigmentation by inhibiting melanin production
2. **Which of the following is commonly used in CIT?**
   a. Botox injections
   b. Chemical peels
   c. Laser resurfacing
   d. Microneedling
3. **What is a common benefit of CIT?**
   a. Permanent hair removal
   b. Increased collagen and elastin production leading to skin tightening
   c. Immediate elimination of wrinkles
   d. Permanent removal of acne scars
4. **Which of the following is a potential side effect of CIT?**
   a. Post-procedure redness and swelling
   b. Hyperpigmentation
   c. Excessive hair growth
   d. Complete skin necrosis
5. **How long does it typically take to see results from CIT?**
   a. 1–2 days
   b. 1–2 weeks
   c. 2–3 months
   d. 6 months

Short Answer Questions

1. What is CIT and how does it work?
2. What are the primary skin concerns that CIT is used to treat?
3. How does the depth of needle penetration affect the treatment outcome in CIT?
4. What are some contraindications for CIT?
5. What post-treatment care is recommended after a CIT session?
6. How many CIT sessions are generally needed to see visible results?
7. What are the possible side effects or risks associated with CIT?
8. How does CIT compare to other skin rejuvenation techniques like chemical peels or laser resurfacing?

Answer to Critical Thinking Questions

1. (b); 2. (d); 3. (b); 4. (a); 5. (c)

REFERENCES

1. Abbasi, R., Shineh, G., Mobaraki, M., Doughty, S., & Tayebi, L. (2023). Structural parameters of nanoparticles affecting their toxicity for biomedical applications: A review. *Journal of Nanoparticle Research, 25.* https://doi.org/10.1007/s11051-023-05690-w (accessed on 11th June 2025).
2. Ajimizu, H., & Sakamori, Y. (2024). Narrative review of indication and management of induction therapy for thymic epithelial tumors. *Mediastinum, 8.* https://www.semanticscholar.org/paper/9b66b585238846a4a8ab137c732b0ac6710085fa (accessed on 11th June 2025).
3. Allen, J. T., & Spiteri, M. A. (2001). *Growth Factors in Idiopathic Pulmonary Fibrosis: Relative Roles.* https://core.ac.uk/download/104302.pdf (accessed on 11th June 2025).
4. Amarie, O. V., Dumitrascu, R., Eickelberg, O., Grimminger, F., et al. (2010). *Increased Expression of 5-Hydroxytryptamine(2A/B) Receptors in Idiopathic Pulmonary Fibrosis: A Rationale for Therapeutic Intervention.* https://core.ac.uk/download/19450584.pdf (accessed on 11th June 2025).
5. Angelini, F., Barretta, A., Biondi Zoccai, G., Cavarretta, E., et al. (2016). *B-Blockers Treatment of Cardiac Surgery Patients Enhances Isolation and Improves Phenotype of Cardio Sphere-Derived Cells.* https://core.ac.uk/download/74319313.pdf (accessed on 11th June 2025).
6. Annunziata, M. C., D'Arco, V., De Vita, V., Fabbrocini, G., et al. (2010). *Acne Scars: Pathogenesis, Classification and Treatment.* https://core.ac.uk/download/pdf/8465034.pdf (accessed on 11th June 2025).
7. Antoniac, I., Bellin, G., Bressan, E., Ferroni, L., et al. (2018). *Graphene-Based Nanomaterials for Tissue Engineering in The Dental Field.* https://core.ac.uk/download/168405329.pdf (accessed on 11th June 2025).
8. Arlt, A., Giudice, A., Herman-Antosiewicz, A., Lau, A., Lister, A., Melchini, A., Speciale, A., et al. (2014). *Benefits and Risks of The Hermetic Effects of Dietary Isothiocyanates on Cancer Prevention.* https://core.ac.uk/download/29110797.pdf (accessed on 11th June 2025).
9. Barrett, J. H., Bowman, S. J., Conaghan, P. G., Cooper, C., et al. (2005). *Association of FCGR3A and FCGR3B Haplotypes with Rheumatoid Arthritis and Primary Sjögren's Syndrome [POSTER PRESENTATION].* https://core.ac.uk/download/57870.pdf (accessed on 11th June 2025).
10. Beitz, J. T. (2020). *The Effects of Exosomes on The Regeneration of Rat Calvaria.* https://core.ac.uk/download/322936747.pdf (accessed on 11th June 2025).
11. Benati, D., Bernardi, P., Borojevic, R., Carias, A., et al. (2020). *Photoaging Skin Therapy with PRP and ADSC: A Comparative Study.* https://core.ac.uk/download/346628001.pdf (accessed on 11th June 2025).
12. Cheng, X., Dong, H., Li, Y., Yu, S., Yue, G., & Wang, X. (2025). Cell-free therapy based on adipose stem cell-derived exosomes to inhibit scar formation proactively: Mechanisms and clinical targeting applications. *Journal of Biomedical Research & Environmental Sciences.* https://www.semanticscholar.org/paper/cbe2445486ef8b3f9595275c5018e277451566cf (accessed on 11th June 2025).
13. Chervoneva, I., Davis, R., Gorenstein, D. G., Hasan, T., et al. (2020). *Functional Blockade of E-Selectin in Tumor-Associated Vessels Enhances Anti-Tumor Effect of Doxorubicin in Breast cancer.* https://core.ac.uk/download/299811593.pdf (accessed on 11th June 2025).

14. Meyer, D. M., Eastwood, J. A., Compton, M. P., Gylys, K., & Zivin, J. A. (2014). rLOAD: does sex mediate the effect of acute antiplatelet loading on stroke outcome. *Biology of sex differences, 5*, 9. https://doi.org/10.1186/2042-6410-5-9 (accessed on 11th June 2025).

15. Davies, C., & Miron, R. J. (2025). Autolougous platelet concentrates in esthetic medicine. *Periodontology 2000, 97*(1), 363–419. https://doi.org/10.1111/prd.12582 (accessed on 11th June 2025).

16. Dębiec, P., Gondko, D., Pietrzak, N., Roman, M., et al. (2024). *Clinical Applications of Phototherapy in Treating Skin Disorders.* https://core.ac.uk/download/613193124.pdf (accessed on 11th June 2025).

17. Farmakis, D., Porter, J. B., Taher, A., Cappellini, M. D., Angastiniotis, M., & Eleftheriou, A. (2022). 2021 Thalassaemia International Federation Guidelines for the management of transfusion-dependent thalassemia. *HemaSphere, 6*, e732–e732. https://doi.org/10.1097/hs9.0000000000000732 (accessed on 11th June 2025).

18. Fernandes, A. S., Rodrigues, P., Pintado, M., & Tavaria, F. K. (2023). A systematic review of natural products for skin applications: Targeting inflammation, wound healing, and photo-aging. *Phytomedicine, 115*, 154824–154824. https://doi.org/10.1016/j.phymed.2023.154824 (accessed on 11th June 2025).

19. Fisher, M., Kurilin, V., Bulygin, A. S., Shevchenko, J., Philippova, J., Taranov, O., Ivleva, E. K., et al. (2024). Dendritic cells transfected with DNA constructs encoding CCR9, IL-10, and type II collagen demonstrate induction of immunological tolerance in an arthritis model. *Frontiers in Immunology, 15.* https://www.semanticscholar.org/paper/95c5af1ccf6c5fb6c8858091342fb55088523980 (accessed on 11th June 2025).

20. Forrester, J. V., Griffith, M., Kuffová, L., Rajendran, P., et al. (2016). *High-Risk Corneal Allografts: A Therapeutic Challenge.* https://core.ac.uk/download/42130548.pdf (accessed on 11th June 2025).

21. Téot L, Mustoe TA, Middelkoop E, et al., editors. Textbook on Scar Management: State of the Art Management and Emerging Technologies [Internet]. Cham (CH): Springer; 2020. Available from: https://www.ncbi.nlm.nih.gov/books/NBK586066/ doi: 10.1007/978-3-030-44766-3(accessed on 11th June 2025).

22. Gillen, T. (2002). *The Effects of Tumor Necrosis Factor and Interleukin 1 On Osseous and Soft Tissue Wound Healing.* https://open.bu.edu/bitstream/2144/35611/1/Gillen_Thomas_2002_web.pdf (accessed on 11th June 2025).

23. Glikson, M., Nielsen, J. C., Kronborg, M. B., Michowitz, Y., Auricchio, A., Barbash, I. M., Barrabés, J. A., et al. (2021). 2021 ESC Guidelines on cardiac pacing and cardiac resynchronization therapy. *European Heart Journal, 42*, 3427–3520. https://doi.org/10.1093/eurheartj/ehab364 (accessed on 11th June 2025).

24. Glikson, M., Nielsen, J. C., Kronborg, M. B., Michowitz, Y., Auricchio, A., Barbash, I. M., Barrabés, J. A., et al. (2022). 2021 ESC Guidelines on cardiac pacing and cardiac resynchronization therapy. *EP Europace, 24*, 71–164. https://doi.org/10.1093/europace/euab232 (accessed on 11th June 2025).

25. Gompels, L. (2010). *In Vivo Fluorescence Imaging Of E-Selectin: Quantitative Detection of Endothelial Activation in Arthritis.* https://core.ac.uk/download/1589084.pdf (accessed on 11th June 2025).

26. Gouveia, P. Q., Fanelli, C., Ornellas, F. M., Garnica, M. R., Francini, A. L., Murata, G. M., Matheus, L. H. G., et al. (2025). Adipose tissue stem cells (ASCs) and ASC-derived extracellular vesicles prevent the development of experimental peritoneal fibrosis. *Cells, 14.* https://www.semanticscholar.org/paper/91e82b9ea033c7bd5dcd0387b9716af7aa714f94 (accessed on 11th June 2025).

27. Griffioen, M. S., de Leeuw, D. D., Janssen, J., & Smit, L. (2022). Targeting acute myeloid leukemia with Veneto lax; biomarkers for sensitivity and rationale for Veneto lax-based combination therapies. *Cancers, 14.* https://www.semanticscholar.org/paper/f4f821ed8777c082c4511a7e523647b023fb9bfd (accessed on 11th June 2025).

28. Jimenez, S. A., Lee, J. B., Mendoza, M. D., et al. (2012). *A prospective Observational Study of Mycophenolate Mofetil Treatment in Progressive Diffuse Cutaneous Systemic Sclerosis of Recent Onset.* https://core.ac.uk/download/129190941.pdf (accessed on 11th June 2025).

29. Jimenez, S. A., Mendoza, M. D., Fabian, A., & Rosenbloom, J. (2013). *Strategies for Anti-Fibrotic Therapies.* https://core.ac.uk/download/83049954.pdf (accessed on 11th June 2025).

30. Klein, R. J., Desvigne, M. N., Greenstein, E., Napolitano, R. J., Milne, C., Speyrer, M. S., & Weir, D. (2024). Use of silver collagen oxidized regenerated cellulose dressings in conjunction with negative pressure wound therapy: Expert panel consensus recommendations. *Wounds: A Compendium of Clinical Research and Practice, 36(8)*, 263–273. https://www.semanticscholar.org/paper/c2ae0a19d3a6262bba5f2d3b12dcc73fdbcec0f9 (accessed on 11th June 2025).

31. Kloth, L. C., & Liebl, H. (2012). *Skin Cell Proliferation Stimulated by Microneedles.* https://core.ac.uk/download/213061324.pdf (accessed on 11th June 2025).

32. Kolimi, P., Narala, S., Nyavanandi, D., Youssef, A. A. A., & Dudhipala, N. (2022). Innovative treatment strategies to accelerate wound healing: Trajectory and recent advancements. *Cells, 11*, 2439–2439. https://doi.org/10.3390/cells11152439 (accessed on 11th June 2025).

33. Kyryk, V. (2024). Stem cell therapy for cardiac regeneration: Key points. *Cell and Organ Transplantology.* https://www.semanticscholar.org/paper/6a1b536f3691ad0d162e4187a4a2e2ffd1507b5f (accessed on 11th June 2025).

34. La Padula, S., Ponzo, M., Lombardi, M., Iazzetta, V., Errico, C., Polverino, G., Russo, F., et al. (2023). Nanofat in plastic reconstructive, regenerative, and aesthetic surgery: A review of advancements in face-focused applications. *Journal of Clinical Medicine, 12*, 4351–4351. https://doi.org/10.3390/jcm12134351 (accessed on 11th June 2025).

35. Lakshmi, Y. V., Reddy, L. S., Devi, K. N. N., Kumar, K. P., Karthik, G. G., Chakravarthy, P. S., & Rao, K. N. (2020). Evaluation of microneedling therapy in management of facial scars. *Journal of Craniofacial Surgery.* https://www.semanticscholar.org/paper/c4d70386959373e003b07e531697d9e1892e0faa (accessed on 11th June 2025).

36. Li, X., Li, C., Zhang, W., Wang, Y., Qian, P., & Huang, H. (2023). Inflammation and aging: Signaling pathways and intervention therapies. *Signal Transduction and Targeted Therapy, 8.* https://doi.org/10.1038/s41392-023-01502-8 (accessed on 11th June 2025).

37. Liu, J. K. (2022). Natural products in cosmetics. *Natural Products and Bioprospecting, 12.* https://doi.org/10.1007/s13659-022-00363-y (accessed on 11th June 2025).

38. Mistry, A., Vaishnani, B., Momin, M., Bosamiya, S., et al. (2023). *Effect of Microneedling by Dermaroller on Acne Scars: An Observational Study at Tertiary Care Hospital.* https://core.ac.uk/download/553557942.pdf (accessed on 11th June 2025).

39. Morath, C., Schaier, M., Ibrahim, E., Wang, L., Kleist, C., Opelz, G., Süsal, C., et al. (2022). Induction of long-lasting regulatory B lymphocytes by modified immune cells in kidney transplant recipients. *Journal of the American Society of Nephrology, 34*, 160–174. https://www.semanticscholar.org/paper/950300b47f4240e08ab8ed64e8b47db506407de2 (accessed on 11th June 2025).

40. Mühl, H. (2013). Pro-inflammatory signaling by IL-10 and IL-22: Bad habit stirred up by interferons? https://core.ac.uk/download/14528354.pdf (accessed on 11th June 2025).

41. Nair, P., & Tandel, J. (2021). Microneedling: A means of collagen induction therapy. *Journal of Dermatology and Dermatologic Surgery, 25*, 49–53. https://www.semanticscholar.org/paper/73aaca83ef777cd055840a3506e92abc5c6029ea (accessed on 11th June 2025).

42. Nopriyati, Yusuf, H., & Suherman, A. (2024). Effect of autologous serum therapy (AST) as adjuvant management in morphea: A pilot study. *Journal RSMH Palembang.* https://www.semanticscholar.org/paper/9ac2763d62b3fb134dc1157638d0c218174a49d9 (accessed on 11th June 2025).

43. Othman, J., Hwang, A., Brodermann, M. H., Abdallah, I., McCloskey, K., Gallipoli, P., Clarke, G., et al. (2024). Outcomes with single-agent glitterati for relapsed or refractory FLT3-mutant AML after contemporary induction therapy. *Blood Advances, 8*, 5590–5597. https://www.semanticscholar.org/paper/06780430a91a4a5bb5cd15f076e07488b4ca6bd1 (accessed on 11th June 2025).

44. Parkin, B., Escobar, C., Patel, R., Smith, T., Browning, A., Pancari, P. A., Gayle, A. A., et al. (2024). Omission of venetoclax ramp-up dosing during induction therapy for acute myeloid leukemia in combination with DNA hypomethylating agents is safe and well-tolerated. *Blood.* https://www.semanticscholar.org/paper/1b8c0d9baa63d59adfe52b837d695aa96e300156 (accessed on 11th June 2025).

45. Pratz, K., Cherry, M., Altman, J., Cooper, B., Podoltsev, N., Cruz, J., Lin, T. L., et al. (2023). Gilteritinib in combination with induction and consolidation chemotherapy and as maintenance therapy: A Phase IB study in patients with newly diagnosed AML. *Journal of Clinical Oncology, 41*, 4236–4246. https://www.semanticscholar.org/paper/7a0a425b7710487136aeccc57300cee8341a90f2 (accessed on 11th June 2025).

46. Rosas López Portillo, F., González Jiménez, M. V., Reyna Solís, C. L., Soberanes Galindo, M. L., Rocha López, A., Guzmán Celaya, G. E., Olivas Velázquez, A. K., et al. (2025). Fascia lata: Utilization and applications in dental therapy: A comprehensive review. *International Surgery Journal.* https://www.semanticscholar.org/paper/03322376db500b868b3887e5e9b2e1895322b670 (accessed on 11th June 2025).

47. Scripcariu, D., Caratașu, C. C., Ciorpac, M., Alexa-Stratulat, T., Szilagyi, A., Buga, C. R., Dobrovat, B., et al. (2025). Comparative efficacy of Pirfenidone and Meloxicam on early radiotherapy-induced anal sphincter dysfunction in rats. *Frontiers in Pharmacology, 16.* https://www.semanticscholar.org/paper/195d044f059de3a15d289f9138fa84050ff52307 (accessed on 11th June 2025).

48. Seymour, B. J., Trent, B., Allen, B. E., Berlinberg, A. J., Tangchittsumran, J., Jubair, W., Chriswell, M. E., et al. (2023). Microbiota-dependent indole production stimulates the development of collagen-induced arthritis in mice. *The Journal of Clinical Investigation, 134.* https://www.semanticscholar.org/paper/0ff5cdfffdb70d942a7dabeebeacbba3ae235635 (accessed on 11th June 2025).

49. Shahrajabian, M. H., & Sun, W. (2023). Mechanism of action of collagen and epidermal growth factor: A review on theory and research methods. *Mini Reviews in Medicinal Chemistry.* https://www.semanticscholar.org/paper/c0392ee33194559c2d9839b8b46e19b9c5e8426f (accessed on 11th June 2025).

50. Silkenstedt, E., & Dreyling, M. (2024). To consolidate or not to consolidate: The role of autologous stem cell transplantation in MCL. *Hematology. American Society of Hematology. Education Program, 2024(1)*, 42–47. https://www.semanticscholar.org/paper/2391bedca47e53dc63e1f404de283c8672dd5e68 (accessed on 11th June 2025).

51. Sivaranjani, J. *Percutaneous Collagen Induction in the Treatment of Atrophic Acne Scars using an Automated Microneedling Device: A Novel Approach.* Diss. Stanley Medical College, Chennai, 2019.(accessed on 11th June 2025).

52. Suber, Y. B., Doshi, B. S., French, R., Merricks, E., Nichols, T. C., & Samelson-Jones, B. J. (2024). Success of immune tolerance induction after AAV gene therapy in high-responding inhibitor hemophilia A dogs may be F8 genotype dependent. *Blood.* https://www.semanticscholar.org/paper/96676bf3b6f5ae2f533c2b8cc449a5d59f28950c (accessed on 11th June 2025).

53. Sukarnadi, M., & Hidayat, S. (2023). Efficacy of low-level laser therapy combined with scalp microneedling using clobetasol propionate 0.05% solution for the management of androgenetic alopecia. *Journal of Medical and Health Studies.* https://www.semanticscholar.org/paper/f3ae66a584f365a288cbcec0a70560d004563838 (accessed on 11th June 2025).

54. Wang, Y., & Su, S. (2024). Alleviating lung injury and pulmonary fibrosis in radiotherapy-immunotherapy combination: The role of low-dose radiation therapy. *Journal of Clinical Oncology.* https://www.semanticscholar.org/paper/e87a731ee54fff121a71988f4bbf9dde08492274 (accessed on 11th June 2025).

55. Zwaan, C., Kolb, E., Mires, D., Vigliotti, M., Xie, J., Downs, P., DeCillis, A., et al. (2019). A phase 1/2 study of quizartinib (Q) in combination with re-induction chemotherapy and as single-agent continuation therapy in pediatric and young adult patients with relapsed/refractory (R/R) FLT3-ITD acute myeloid leukemia (AML). *Blood.* https://www.semanticscholar.org/paper/62a64b908ceecf25fcd819fb5e182338a216866e (accessed on 11th June 2025).

LASER AND LIGHT-BASED THERAPIES

7

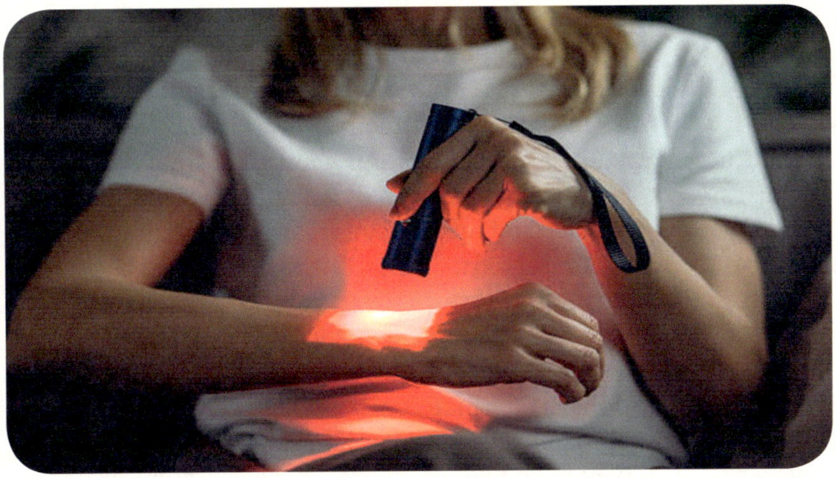

LEARNING OBJECTIVES

After studying this chapter, you will be able to:

1. Understand the mechanisms of action underlying laser and light-based therapies in cosmetic dermatology
2. Explain the types of laser therapies
3. Describe light-based therapies
4. Focus on applications of laser and light-based therapies in cosmetic dermatology
5. Discuss risks and side effects
6. Deal with advances in the technology of laser and light-based therapies

Introduction

Cosmetic dermatology has been revolutionized in the past few years through the development of laser and light-based treatments. These new technologies have become critical modalities for the treatment of a range of skin disorders, such as but not limited to pigmentation, acne scarring, and vascular lesions. The appeal of these therapies is not only in their minimally invasive nature, but also in the capability to achieve significant improvements in the aesthetic appearance of the skin. Given the patient's need to opt for less invasive procedures with minimal recovery time, the role of lasers and light therapy in cosmetic procedures is becoming essential. Further, all the growing evidence in the clinical setting that emphasizes the effectiveness and safety of these methods underlines the significance of these techniques as important to the practice of modern dermatology in ushering in a new age of skin care and treatment. Further emphasis is given by manifold technological advancements in lasers, including ablative and non-ablative lasers. Ablative lasers like CO_2 and erbium: YAG work by peeling the outer layers of skin, promoting new skin formation and texture. Non-ablative lasers dive deeper into the skin without damaging the surface, stimulating collagen formation and enhancing skin elasticity. The use of these treatments with others like microneedling and pharmacologic therapies constitutes a more holistic treatment of patients. These combinations try to maximize the therapeutic result of treatment with a reduction of the hazards of scarring and pigmentary alterations, particularly for darker-complexioned patients at greater risk for complications. The possibility for innovation lies in the very nature of the current research and clinical studies in new uses and advancements within existing technology. Additionally, photoacoustic imaging introduces a thrilling new frontier to the field of laser technologies with special benefits in accuracy and precision for dermatology. Photoacoustic imaging takes advantage of the phenomenon of light-to-sound conversion, thus generating high-contrast images capable of identifying different tissue types without the destructive ionizing radiation effects. Applications range from functional imaging of dermatological lesions to surgical guidance; it promises to refine not only the diagnostic potential but the therapeutic potential as well in dermatology. Since laser and light-based treatment integration is constantly under development, it's clear that practitioners should remain current with new techniques and recent research findings. The optimization of patient satisfaction and treatment outcome underscores the necessity of continuous education and adaptation in the ever-evolving specialty of cosmetic dermatology (Steinberg et al., 2019; Nast et al., 2020).

Definition of Laser and Light-Based Therapies

Definition of laser and light-based treatments includes the application in cosmetic dermatology of a number of techniques with the purpose of rejuvenating skin, addressing several conditions of the skin, and helping achieve an optimum result. These treatments apply specific wavelengths of light and heat for tissue targeting and produce localized tissue effects that enhance the texture, tone, and appearance of the skin. The laser treatment provides intense light energy on a specific skin layer in order to stimulate the production of collagen and speed up the renewal of the skin. These advanced technologies have changed the face of cosmetic treatment to enable much less intrusive procedures, yielding faster recovery with remarkable outcomes for patients. Also, because the demand for non-surgical treatments is increasing very fast, there is every reason why laser and light-based treatments must have this fundamental role as they have for ages in cosmetic dermatology. Variety also follows laser and light-based technologies insofar as this can be used to provide various treatment options for dermatological issues spanning from photodamage to vascular lesions. The modalities, however, consist of fractional laser resurfacing, pulsed dye lasers, and intense pulsed light (IPL). Every modality is set in place to correct different types of conditions and aesthetic goals. For instance, fractional lasers utilize the light from a beam to stimulate micro-injuries that are beneficial for the body to heal on its own, and pulsed dye lasers focus their attention on vessels filled with blood to diminish redness and skin tone. These targeted treatments elevate the safety and efficacy profile of therapy because practitioners can target treatment to precise areas without damaging the rest of the tissue. This precision highlights the significance of grasping the basis of the technologies employed in such procedures, which are still advancing and refining the outcome for patients. Most importantly, the concept of PDT is a model for a new application of light-based treatment in a clinic: from beauty treatment to cancer. A process used in PDT involves intravenous delivery of a photosensitizer followed by local illumination with light that leads to a photochemical reaction, forming reactive oxygen species (ROS) that destroy target cells. PDT has been proven to be clinically effective in the treatment of a few cancers with remarkable therapeutic effectiveness. Despite its effectiveness, PDT is not a common practice; therefore, there is a need for greater awareness and training in its application in the practice of cosmetic dermatology and related specialties. This further underlines the dynamic nature of laser and light-based treatments, which offer more than just cosmetic improvement and have yet more possibilities in the line of therapy in treating many conditions of the skin, as has reportedly been seen in this topic (Demian et al., 2017) (Figure 7.1).

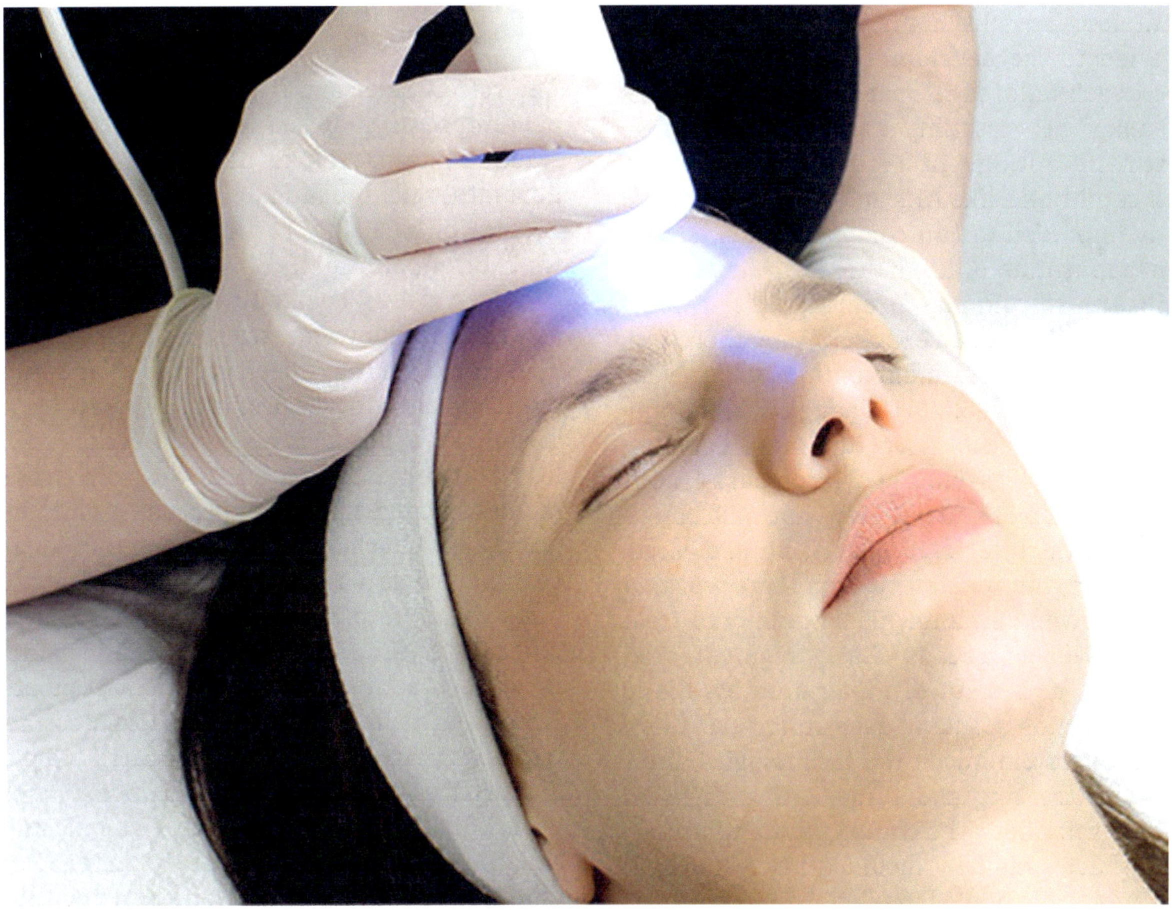

Figure 7.1. A patient undergoing a laser treatment for melasma or pigmentation removal, showcasing the use of targeted light therapy in cosmetic dermatology to address uneven skin tone and hyperpigmentation.

Source: https://www.khromdermatology.com/wp-content/uploads/2021/03/melasma-and-pigment-laser-removal-brooklyn-ny.jpg.

Historical Context of Their Use in Dermatology

The history of laser and light therapies in dermatology plots a dramatic evolution in modes of treatment for the cure of various skin conditions. The initial dermatological therapies were essentially pharmacological or surgical in nature, with limited exposure to advanced technologies. The big breakthrough came in the 1960s with the pioneering work of Maiman, who developed the first ruby laser, opening up avenues for further studies on lasers in medical applications. This advancement marked the beginning of a new era where targeted light therapies could selectively impact skin tissues. Over time, continuous advancements in laser technology have led to the development of various laser types, each tailored to specific skin conditions, revealing the versatility and efficacy of these treatment options in modern dermatology. Such conditions, like AKs and photoaging, have vastly improved the outcomes of patients with their application of laser therapy. AKs are one of the most common premalignant lesions, caused by chronic sun exposure, and, therefore, require proper treatment options to prevent SCC (Ferara et al., 2024). Though cryotherapy and surgical excision were the more common treatments, there emerged laser-based non-surgical therapies; indeed, they were much more precise with fewer side effects. By and large, with lasers, the possibility for a large working range allowed dermatologists not only to treat AK but even correct issues of pigmentation, erythema, and textural abnormalities, really revolutionizing cosmetic dermatology. As more practitioners embraced the technologies, their places in treating and rejuvenating the skin became solidified. The training in dermatology has, in fact, gradually included laser and light treatments due to the latter's usefulness in both clinical and cosmetic practice. The fact that there is no systematic training emphasizes a deficiency in postgraduate training, which must be strict to help prepare the dermatology resident for the role he or she is to take on (Kumar, 2021). Recent efforts have focused on creating evidence-based educational frameworks that ensure emerging dermatologists are proficient in utilizing these therapies effectively. As the field continues to advance, the historical context of lasers and light therapies serves as a crucial reference point, guiding future innovations and enhancing understanding of their strategic implementation within dermatologic practice. This continuous development highlights the importance of combining technological advancements with structured training for the best patient care in cosmetic dermatology.

Importance of These Therapies in Modern Cosmetic Practices

The role of laser and light therapies cannot be overemphasized in modern cosmetic surgery since it has proven to be a breakthrough in dermatological beauty. The procedure has revolutionized the art of skin procedures that offer minimally invasive methods to correct various cosmetic imperfections such as pigmentation, acne scars, and aging marks. These therapies have been very popular because the safety and efficacy profile allow practitioners to deliver a broad array of procedures with less downtime compared to the conventional method. For example, laser procedures including fractional resurfacing and intense pulsed light therapy are now routine procedures that yield outstanding improvement in skin texture and color with fewer side effects. This made it possible to address a growing client population who are in need of speedy and efficient cosmetic treatment, which further consolidated the place for such treatments in routine practice (Madnani et al., 2022). Other than their use in applications, timeliness in laser and light treatments also emerges from their desirable sociocultural meaning. With the growing awareness of the public for cosmetic treatments, consumers want faster alternatives that will satisfy their desire for flawless skin. The conditions, such as post-inflammatory erythema or hyperpigmentation, which can greatly affect self-esteem, are now being treated by targeted laser treatments with promise and outcomes for many patients. Moreover, as access to such treatments becomes higher globally, even in regions where these kinds of treatments were not available before, ever more patients are realizing their full potential. The raised access not only enhances psychological well-being in individuals but also develops a culture of well-educated decision-making towards skin care. It promotes behavior change towards greater acceptance and respect for active cosmetic treatment (Madnani et al., 2022). The final integration of laser and light treatments into clinical practices highlights the importance of constant education among practitioners. Though the technology has seen remarkable strides, proper practice of these therapies is observed in a sound understanding of pre- and post-procedure care for different treatments. As highlighted by recent research, there exists an educational gap among clinicians on the nuances of aesthetic treatments that could lead to suboptimal results if not addressed (Madnani et al., 2022). Only by way of these ongoing professional education and training on such complicated modalities do practitioners ensure safe and effective treatment with optimization of patient satisfaction. Therefore, the worth of such treatments in contemporary cosmetic procedures far exceeds technology itself, to the genuine critical function that well-educated and talented practitioners can exert in optimizing both patient treatment and outcome.

7.1. Mechanisms of Action

Learning Outcome

1. Discuss how lasers interact with skin tissues
2. Explain the types of light used in therapies
3. Understand biological responses triggered by laser treatments

The mechanisms of action underlying laser and light-based therapies in cosmetic dermatology are multifaceted and vary across different treatment modalities. Primarily, these therapies leverage the principles of photobiomodulation, where specific wavelengths of light penetrate the skin to target dermal structures. For instance, in laser skin resurfacing, focused light energy is directed at the epidermis, promoting ablation of damaged skin while stimulating collagen production in the underlying dermis. This healing process results in a decrease in skin texture, tone, and elasticity, which suggests the efficacy of lasers as ablating and non-ablating agents. Furthermore, the particular aim of these treatments reduces surrounding tissue destruction, facilitating faster recovery times and fewer opportunities for complications, essential factors when considering cosmetic treatments in dermatology, addressed by recent advances within the discipline (Boffa, 2004). In addition, certain wavelengths of light have been found to exert therapeutic effects by modifying biological reactions at the cellular level. An example is blue light treatment, which is very effective in the treatment of acne vulgaris because it can target and kill the bacteria *Propionibacterium acnes* (*P. acnes*) by PDT. This process activates a chemical reaction that yields ROS, leading to damage to the infection and suppression of inflammation. The selective absorption of light by the acne lesion makes this treatment a non-invasive procedure in the sense that surrounding healthy skin suffers as little damage as possible and, thus, maximizes patient satisfaction with the aesthetic outcome. Such mechanisms not only improve the instantaneous effects of aesthetics but also result in a critical long-term control of skin diseases; the greatest leap in curative dermatology (Cantisani et al., 2014). The last point is regarding the functions of laser and light treatments for managing skin cancers, particularly nonmelanoma skin cancers (NMSC). Their comprehension is thus crucial. Photodynamic therapy (PDT) is unique because it can cause selective death in cancer cells and spare normal tissue. When the procedure is done, a photosensitizing agent is placed on the lesion and activated by certain wavelengths of light. The photosensitizing agent's activation triggers a sequence of events that ends with the apoptotic death of cancer cells. One of the key benefits of this method is its very good cosmetic results, particularly in its use within the initial phases of treatment for skin cancer. The nature of being able to control disease without excessive aesthetic compromise not only improves the physical well-being of patients but also their psychological health, and thus such therapies play a central role in the changing world of cosmetics and dermatologic health (Cantisani et al., 2014).

7.1.1. How Lasers Interact with Skin Tissues

The interaction of lasers with skin tissues comprises intricate energy transfer mechanisms that can be very beneficial in cosmetic dermatology. When a laser produces a certain wavelength of light, it is taken up by chromophores on the skin in the form of melanin and hemoglobin. Upon absorption, it causes photothermal effects that may cause cellular injury, tissue remodeling, and ultimately, aesthetic enhancement. For example, in the removal of skin lesions or unsightly pigmentation, the laser energy that is targeted selectively damages the pigmented cells without harming surrounding tissues. This level of precision is particularly important to avoid side effects and ensure maximum healing, for lasers to be an optimum instrument for many applications in dermatology. Also, ongoing studies of different laser wavelengths and their individual interactions with skin tissues further enhance our understanding of how to achieve desired effects safely and effectively in skin treatment. In addition to the correction of pigmentation, lasers play an important role in the management of skin fibrosis and postoperative scars. Research indicated that LED-red light (LED-RL) had the ability to modulate major cellular processes implicated in skin fibrosis, suppressing overproduction of collagen and fibroblast activity. The outcomes of two phase I clinical trials indicated that LED-RL was tolerable and safe, but of significant promise in a broad range of clinical applications for therapeutic use against scars. Aided by precise dosing and timing following surgery, LEDs may potentially enhance wound healing as well as avoid the formation of abnormal scars. This treatment confirms the hypothesis that laser therapy can provide both aesthetic and functional outcomes in skin healing by promoting controlled interactions with underlying tissue and paving the way for new treatment paradigms in dermatology (Heilman et al., 2019). Another significant application of laser technology in cosmetic dermatology is for PDT in the treatment of non-melanoma skin cancer. PDT essentially employs a photosensitizer in conjunction with specific light wavelengths, creating a photochemical reaction in targeted tissues that will selectively kill malignant cells.

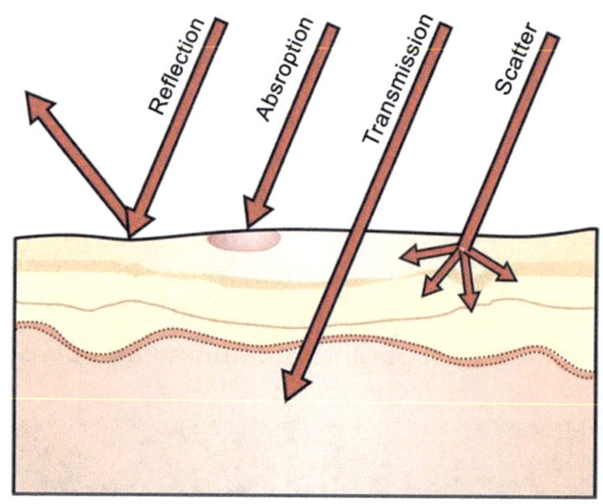

Figure 7.2. Laser tissue surface interactions.

Source: https://www.findlight.net/blog/wp-content/uploads/2018/12/image006324.jpeg.

This modality finds application in actinic keratosis, basal cell carcinoma, and other similar pre-cancerous lesions via the use of intrinsic absorption of particular wavelengths by photosensitizers. Interestingly, the combination of PDT with other therapeutic modalities, like cryotherapy or surgical procedures, has proven increased efficacy along with better patient outcomes. While new targeted delivery systems and photosensitizers continue to emerge, the future for PDT to become even more integrated within the treatment paradigm in dermatology continues to grow, illustrating the revolution caused by lasers for skin cancer treatment (Löhr et al., 2017) (Figure 7.2).

7.1.2. Types of Light Used in Therapies (e.g., LED, IPL)

The era of cosmetic dermatology has also seen a sea change with the assistance of several light treatments against tens of dermatological ailments and aesthetic issues. Among the most sought-after non-invasive treatments now is that of LED, whose different wavelengths target several skin issues at their root. Blue, for instance, has been shown to be highly effective at healing acne by attacking the development of Propionibacterium acnes, and red light stimulates collagen production to significantly reduce fine lines and wrinkles and leave the skin feeling smoother. This heterogeneity is proof that the indications for the use of LED therapy in dermato-clinical practice are broad, with the benefit of being an effective treatment that improves the appearance of a patient without downtime compared to other, more aggressive treatments. Another important breakthrough in phototherapies is intense pulsed light (IPL) therapy. In contrast to other lasers, which produce a single wavelength of light, IPL uses a wide spectrum of light, which can be filtered to treat specific skin issues like hyperpigmentation, vascular lesions, and general skin rejuvenation. Because of its flexibility, IPL can have settings modified according to individual patient requirements, making it safer and more effective. Interestingly, the ultraviolet radiation damage-reflecting issues are best addressed by IPL and thus represent an excellent treatment for patients who have clear-cut signs of sun damage and photoaging. That the treatment is non-invasive, and IPL simultaneously addresses a variety of different skin problems in one session, has contributed to its popularity among dermatologists and aesthetic practitioners. Among the strong applications of light in the curative treatment of numerous diseases, including precancerous lesions and NMSC, is PDT. It is outstanding in that it is highly unique and innovative. When undergoing PDT, there is a photosensitizer placed on the skin that reacts to a specific wavelength of light, generating a photochemical effect that destroys target cells. The method not only destroys the pathological cells but is also immunomodulatory, thus supplementing the skin's natural healing processes. It has been particularly good for PDT in the treatment of actinic keratosis and superficial basal cell carcinoma, as it resulted in satisfactory cosmetic outcomes when applied at the beginning stages of skin cancers. The minimally invasive character and effectiveness on larger and multiple lesions make this method an integral part of modern dermatological practice, the best example of the strong potential presented by light-based therapy in cosmetic dermatology (Cantisani et al., 2014; Lin et al., 2014) (Figure 7.3).

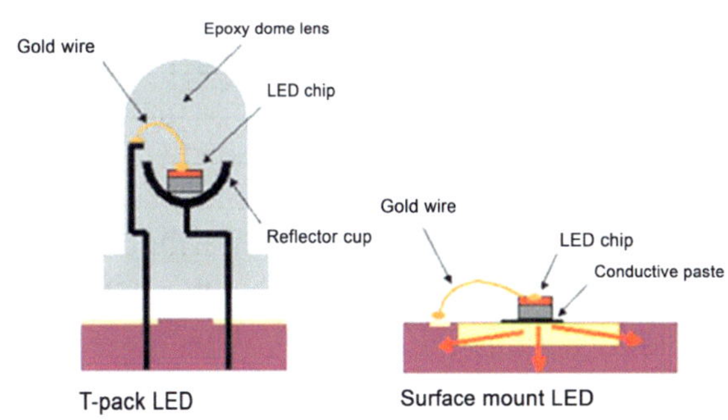

Figure 7.3. LED technology.

Source: https://www.researchgate.net/profile/Daniel-Barolet/publication/23797391_Light-Emitting_Diodes_LEDs_in_Dermatology/links/59e6902b0f7e9b13aca3cadf/Light-Emitting-Diodes-LEDs-in-Dermatology.pdf?_tp=eyJjb250ZXh0Ijp7ImZpcnN0UGFnZSI6Il9kaXJlY3QiLCJwYWdlIjoicHVibGljYXRpb24ifX0.

7.1.3. Biological Responses Triggered by Laser Treatments

The biological changes induced by laser treatments represent a complex interaction of cellular and molecular pathways necessary to repair and rejuvenate skin. The exposure of the lasers on the skin causes thermal injury at various depths, in which a cascading series of biological events will stimulate the healing mechanisms in the body. This phenomenon is particularly evident in ablative and non-ablative laser treatments, where laser-induced damage to the tissues intentionally promotes elastin and collagen production as a response to repair, endowing the skin with enhanced elasticity and texture. The resulting inflammatory process serves to recruit fibroblasts and other essential cells required to form the new tissue, demonstrating that treatment with lasers can effectively leverage the body's own repair processes to induce cosmetic change. Understanding these biological responses underscores the efficacy of laser therapies as non-invasive alternatives in professional dermatological practice aimed at restoring both the health and appearance of the skin. Additionally, immunomodulatory effects are crucial components of laser treatment in the effectiveness for most dermatological conditions. Laser therapy can selectively target and decrease hyperactivated immune responses associated with inflammatory dermatological conditions such as psoriasis and acne. By creating immunosuppression in a local area without compromising systemic immunity, laser applications can minimize the manifestations of these diseases while simultaneously provoking a normal skin environment. In addition to eradicating the pain associated with these disorders, this targeted therapy also enhances the efficacy of concurrent topical or systemic treatments. Laser therapy's capability to modulate immune responses makes it increasingly important in current dermatological practice, potentially opening doors to novel, multi-faceted treatment regimens that address both cosmetic and therapeutic goals in patient management. Moreover, as dermatology continues to become more sophisticated, the application of laser technology increasingly redefines our understanding of skin physiology and its reactions to stimuli. This new information in itself rests upon a more profound understanding of skin structure and function, plus the role of cellular biology in aesthetic and therapeutic results. Advances in laser wavelengths and delivery devices have improved specificity, allowing for less collateral injury with enhanced treatment effect. This can be seen in the ways through which new developments improve patient satisfaction and clinical outcomes, making laser therapy the core of non-invasive dermatologic practices. As the industry starts adopting these advancements, very vital research into the biology of the interactions that the laser triggers will continue to perfect the techniques and establish evidence-based practices, as necessary, to meet a diverse population of patients, which will further entrench lasers in modern cosmetic dermatology (Boffa, 2004; Cantisani et al., 2014Boffa, 2004) (Figure 7.4).

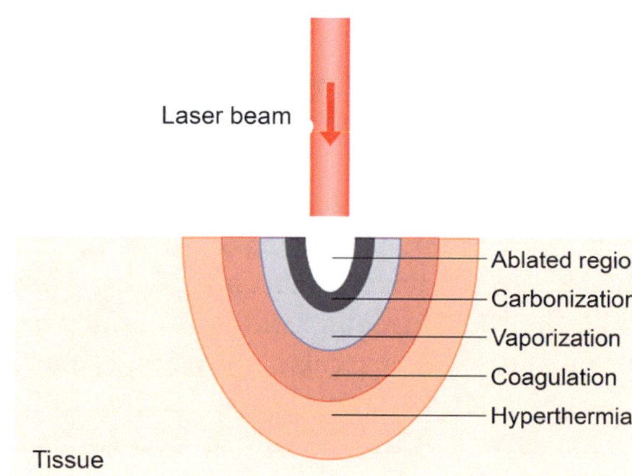

Figure 7.4. Laser-induced photothermal reactions in the biological tissue.

Source: https://www.researchgate.net/publication/370005348/figure/fig8/AS:11431281146001774@1681474586133/Laser-induced-photothermal-reactions-in-the-biological-tissue.png.

Test Your Knowledge

1. What is the interaction between laser and skin tissue?
2. What are the biophysical effects of laser therapy?

7.2. Types of Laser Therapies

Learning Outcome

1. Describe ablative and non-ablative lasers
2. Explain commonly used laser types
3. Focus on indications for different laser therapies

When exploring the various types of laser therapies in cosmetic dermatology, it is essential to understand the spectrum of applications and technological advancements that underpin this field. Among the most notable types is ablative laser therapy, which targets the outer layers of the skin, promoting the regeneration of tissues and significantly reducing imperfections, such as fine lines and scars. This method works by peeling off the damaged skin cells, revealing healthier skin underneath. The most effective laser technique for patients with photodamage, acne scars, and textural abnormalities, which yields enhanced skin tone and texture after treatment. Importantly, the success of the procedures often depends on the patient's skin type and the type of laser used, so a customized approach is desirable to achieve maximum results.

Another significant class of laser therapy includes non-ablative laser methods, which involve stimulating the production of collagen without harming the outer skin. This method provides a less invasive alternative for those who want to treat skin laxity, issues with pigmentation, and skin rejuvenation in general. Non-ablative lasers employ controlled energy to pass through the skin, triggering the body's own healing responses, thereby increasing skin elasticity and creating a smoother look. These treatments often require minimal downtime, making them appealing for patients with busy lifestyles. The versatility of non-ablative options means they can be tailored to cater to a variety of skin concerns, underscoring their relevance in the evolving landscape of cosmetic dermatology as demonstrated in clinical studies exploring their efficacy compared to traditional methods. PDT is a significant advance in laser treatment, particularly when its application in the control of disease states such as NMSC is taken into consideration. By the effect of specific wavelengths of light combined with photosensitizing agents, PDT selectively kills diseased tissue while causing little harm to surrounding tissues. Research has demonstrated that PDT is the best in cosmetic outcomes when applied in the treatment of skin cancers superficial to the skin, particularly in the early stages, hence enhancing patient quality of life and aesthetic satisfaction. The curative ability of treatment for multiple lesions simultaneously further establishes its position as a viable alternative to surgery. With the growing incidence of skin diseases, awareness and development of laser treatments such as PDT are essential to enhance therapeutic regimens of cosmetic dermatology, marking a turning point towards more modern and minimally invasive treatment methods (Bailey et al., 2010; Cantisani et al., 2014) (Figure 7.5).

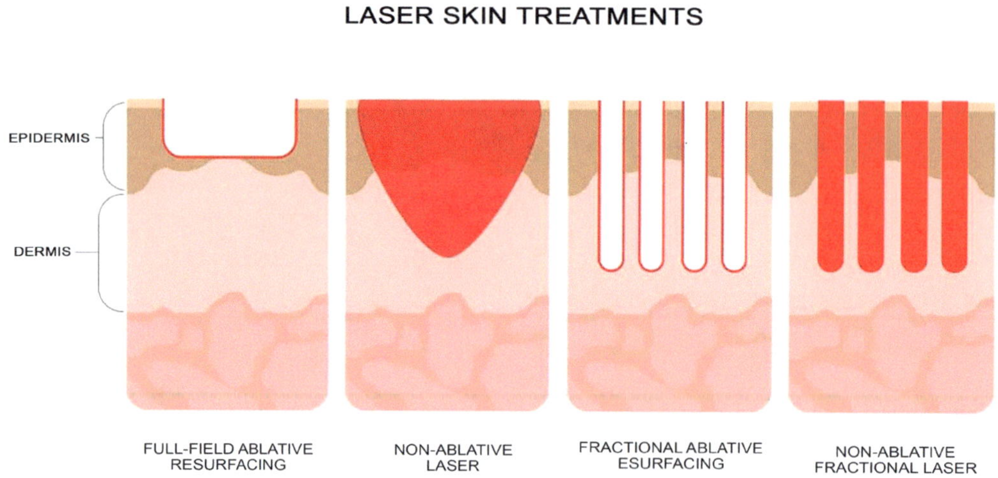

Figure 7.5. Laser skin treatment.

Source: https://ensoulclinic.b-cdn.net/wp-content/uploads/2022/12/fractional-laser-ablative-lasers-non-ablative-laser-ensoul-clinic.jpg.

7.2.1. Ablative vs. Non-Ablative Lasers

In cosmetic dermatology, ablative and non-ablative lasers are two separate modalities that treat various skin conditions and patient requirements. Ablative lasers, including carbon dioxide (CO_2) and erbium YAG lasers, destroy the top layers of the skin through vaporization, which leads to profound collagen remodeling and stimulates deep tissue repair. This invasive method is effective in treating deeper scarring, wrinkles, and photodamage, but requires a greater recovery time as a result of the damage caused to the skin. Patients usually have post-treatment redness, swelling, and peeling, lasting from a few days to several weeks. On the other hand, non-ablative lasers, employing wavelengths that are calculated to penetrate into the skin without damaging its top layer, stimulate collagen formation with minimal downtime. Practitioners, therefore, have to balance the benefits of faster recovery with more significant results achieved with ablative methods. Although ablative lasers have excellent outcomes in severe skin aging and damage, they are associated with higher risks and side effects. For example, the aggressive nature of ablative treatments may cause infection, scarring, as well as pigmentation changes, especially in patients with darker skin types. In contrast, non-ablative lasers, including IPL sources, are safer alternatives, suitable for a broader range of skin types, and less likely to produce adverse effects like PIH. According to a consensus by experts in pigment laser surgery, although non-ablative lasers are effective for treating conditions such as lentigos or dermal hypermelanocytosis, they may not be suitable for all hyperpigmented lesions, emphasizing the need for careful diagnosis before treatment (Passeron et al., 2019). Therefore, the selection between these lasers requires knowledge of the patient's skin type as well as an evaluation of the condition that is being treated. The second essential point in differentiating between ablative and non-ablative lasers is the general patient experience, especially in terms of comfort and satisfaction levels while undergoing the procedure. Patients commonly complain of discomfort related to ablative procedures, which can necessitate analgesia or cooling methods in order to make the experience bearable. Non-ablative treatments, on the other hand, typically cause minimal discomfort, rendering them the better option for patients who require a fast and effective fix with less interruption to their lifestyle. A European Dermatology Forum suggestion is that procedural comfort, safety, and efficacy should dictate the selection of laser therapy (Morton et al., 2019). In this scenario, thus aligning to both the clinical patient needs as well as the aesthetic goals, not to mention lifestyle considerations, would be decisions made in terms of using either an ablative or a non-ablative laser based on a treatment plan (Figure 7.6).

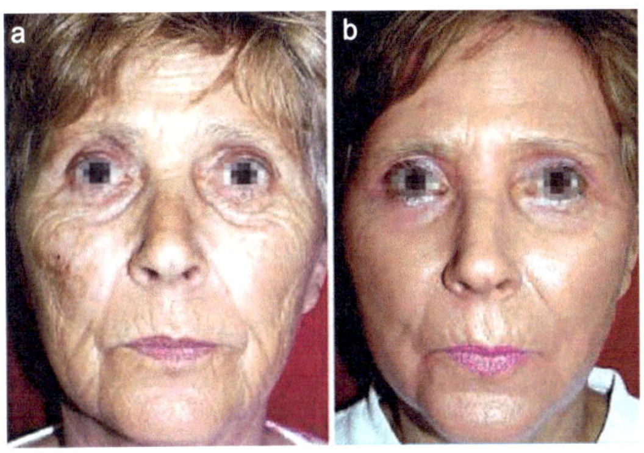

Figure 7.6. Full-face ablative laser resurfacing in a 58-year-old female plus post-procedural LED-LLLT. (a) Baseline findings showing severe photoageing with dyschromia, and deep lines and Wrinkles due to excessive solar exposure during skiing; and (b) Result only 6 weeks after Er: YAG/CO_2.

Source: https://www.researchgate.net/profile/R-Glen-Calderhead-2/publication/288856338/figure/fig8/AS:314795258597378@1452064446569/Full-face-ablative-laser-resurfacing-in-a-58-year-old-female-plus-post-procedural.png.

7.2.2. Commonly Used Laser Types (e.g., CO_2, Erbium)

The greater use of laser technology in cosmetic dermatology has caused several laser modalities to become popular, with the CO_2 and Erbium lasers being foundation modalities. The CO_2 laser is commonly utilized for ablative treatments and has been shown to be effective in the treatment of damaged skin by removing the outer layers of skin. This laser's precision enables dermatologists to target specific areas, facilitating significant improvements in conditions such as acne scars, photoaging, and wrinkles. The fractional CO_2 laser, a more advanced form of this technology, has garnered attention for its ability to promote healing while minimizing downtime, thus appealing to patients who seek effective yet less invasive options for skin rejuvenation. The efficiency achieved with CO_2 lasers has made it an effective gold standard in the treatment of various dermatological conditions, just as there is a general trend with increasing use of sophisticated laser treatments in cosmetic procedures (Murray et al., 2024). Of the two, Erbium lasers, which include Erbium: YAG and Erbium: Glass lasers, are more inclined for more superficial corrections in skin. These lasers primarily target water within the skin, allowing for precise removal of the epidermis and superficial dermis without excessive thermal damage to the surrounding tissue. Therefore, Erbium lasers are celebrated for more rapid recovery times and decreased postoperative discomfort compared to CO_2 lasers. They are particularly ideal for the correction of fine lines, wrinkles, and skin pigmentation disorders, meeting the cosmetic needs of the majority of patients. As studies in this field go on, evidence points to the fact that incorporating Erbium lasers in addition to adjunct therapies such as chemical peels or skin conditioning enhances results. Thus, the application versatility of Erbium lasers contributes to their ubiquitous and growing usage in cosmetic dermatological clinics (Wen et al., 2024). The aesthetic outcome desired, in turn, increasingly determines the type of laser selected. Technological advances have also increased the wavelengths of light that can be used, enabling specific treatments for different skin conditions and types. For example, the Nd: YAG laser has become a consistent choice for deeper treatments, while picosecond lasers offer up-to-the-minute advancements in treatment effectiveness and reduce patient downtime. As a result, clinicians are increasingly being encouraged to stay abreast of current developments in laser treatment. Continuing research into the safety and effectiveness of lasers and the integration of new information demonstrates the dynamic nature of laser applications within cosmetic dermatology. Ultimately, grasping the differences and uses of CO_2 and Erbium lasers is important to maximize patient care and improve aesthetic results through precise laser treatments (Murray et al., 2024) (Figure 7.7).

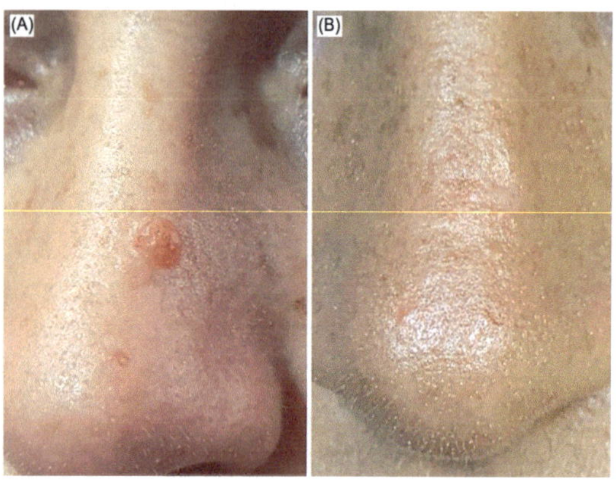

Figure 7.7. CO_2 laser treatment of dermal nevus; (A) before treatment; and (B) after treatment.

Source: https://www.researchgate.net/publication/347897097/figure/fig2/AS:11431281173844726@1689056643414/CO2-laser-treatment-of-dermal-nevus-A-before-treatment-B-after-treatment.png.

7.2.3. Indications for Different Laser Therapies

Cosmetic dermatology has been greatly revolutionized by the developments in the technology of lasers, enabling the management of a variety of skin diseases. Among the most well-known indications for the use of laser therapy is in the management of NMSCs. One of the most widely known types of laser treatment is PDT, which has proven to be a critical treatment option for superficial NMSC patients. The success of PDT is particularly significant when used in the early stages of the condition, whereby it demonstrates dramatic cosmetic outcomes in the healing of widespread and multiple lesions. Aside from this, PDT is a noninvasive procedure; thus it is an attractive alternative to more traditional surgical intervention that results in scarring and other adverse effects. The use of laser treatments in such cases is one example of a shift in practice paradigm toward less invasive therapy with more focus on efficacy and cosmetic results, with further development of the integral position of lasers in contemporary dermatologic practice (Cantisani et al., 2014). In addition to NMSC treatment, laser treatments are increasingly utilized for the treatment of disorders related to skin rejuvenation and restoration, e.g., photoaging and pigment disorders. Ablative lasers, including CO_2 and Erbium YAG lasers, provide targeted resurfacing of the skin, effectively improving texture, tone, and overall appearance. These lasers work by removing the outer layers of damaged skin while promoting new collagen production, which is critical for maintaining youthful skin. It is essential to consider the varying wavelengths and depths of penetration offered by different laser modalities to tailor treatments for individual patient needs. Such tailoring maximizes therapeutic benefits and reduces the chances of adverse effects. As the need for aesthetic augmentations remains on the increase, laser therapies certainly play a critical role in solving the varied issues related to aging as well as environmental damage, further cementing their position in cosmetic dermatology (Proietti et al., 2021). Additionally, the inclusion of laser treatments in postcancer therapy emphasizes their relevance to enhancing survivors' quality of life. Cancer treatments tend to create permanent alterations in the appearance of patients, hence negatively impacting their self-perception and body satisfaction. In this regard, laser therapies like fractional lasers can be helpful in managing scarring and other skin-related conditions resulting from surgical removal or radiotherapy. Laser treatment allows practitioners to adopt a holistic approach based on restoration at both the physical and psychological levels to assist cancer patients. Evaluating safety and effectiveness in practice and taking special precautions for the vulnerable population are essential. Through enabling cosmetic enhancements via laser treatments, medical practitioners can promote a more complete model of care that emphasizes the value of sustaining quality of life in cancer survivors, in demonstrating the complexity of benefits achievable with high-tech dermatological treatments (Cantisani et al., 2014; Proietti et al., 2021) (Figure 7.8).

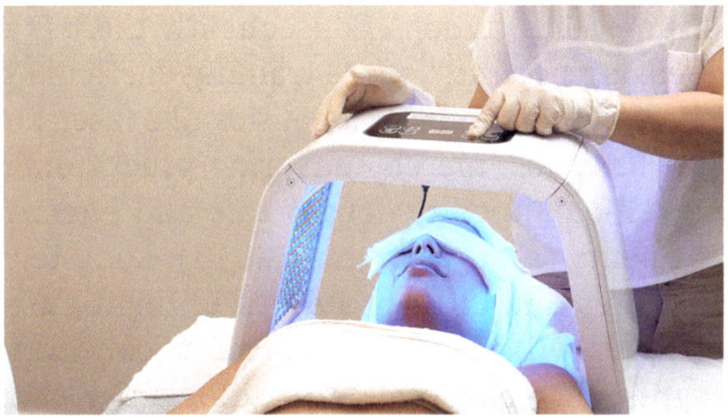

Figure 7.8. Photodynamic therapy (PDT).

Source: https://sjhdermatology.com/wp-content/uploads/2019/06/Services_Photodynamic.png.

Test Your Knowledge

1. Which is better, an ablative or non-ablative laser?
2. What type of laser is used in dermatology?

7.3. Light-Based Therapies

Learning Outcome

1. Understand the concept of intense pulsed light (IPL) therapy
2. Explain the benefits of LED light therapy
3. Differentiate between light-based therapies to laser treatments

Evolution of light-based therapies has dramatically changed the field of cosmetic dermatology by providing a variety of minimally invasive treatment options. Laser therapy, IPL, and PDT are the technologies that have risen to prominence for their ability to treat a myriad of skin issues, from disorders of pigmentation, vascular lesions, to acne scars. New developments in the field of skin biology have accelerated these therapies' efficacy and safety profiles. For example, as pointed out in research, such treatments use targeted wavelengths of light to reach deeper skin layers with less harm to surrounding tissue and induce improved healing responses. By continually advancing these methods, dermatologic practice is embracing more accurate and patient-focused techniques, expanding treatment possibilities and satisfying heterogeneous patient demands for aesthetic enhancement (Boffa, 2004). The popularity of aesthetic treatments has jumped internationally, leading to the incorporation of light-based therapy into routine dermatological practice. This phenomenon is particularly relevant in different global contexts, as beauty specialists increasingly pursue aesthetic training to expand services. With the decreasing distinctions between beauty and medical aesthetics, education and proficiency improvement in light-based treatments take on increasing importance. Qualified practitioners in the field of somatology have recognized the necessity to incorporate advanced aesthetic treatments within their practice scope to address evolving consumer expectations. Consequently, there is an increasing need to update training curricula to include contemporary modalities like laser and light therapies, thereby ensuring practitioners are well-equipped to deliver safe and effective treatments (Ambrosio et al., 2018). Long-term follow-ups and efficacy studies on light-based therapies will be important for continued progress in cosmetic dermatology. Different modalities have unique potential advantages and risks; therefore, there is a need for significant, robust clinical trials and additional follow-up research to ensure comprehensive guidelines for use. The mainstay of interdisciplinary collaboration between dermatologists and other medical professionals serves as an enhancement for greater patient safety and better outcomes. By instituting standardized procedures, practitioners are able to more easily manage the intricacies of integrating aesthetic therapies into medical practice. In the transition of the somatology profession towards an increasingly medically centered paradigm, the introduction of light-based therapy represents a demonstration of the changing landscape of skincare. It is in response to patient demand and recognition of the highly developing technological environment of dermatology (Boffa, 2004).

7.3.1. Overview of Intense Pulsed Light (IPL) Therapy

IPL therapy has emerged as a prominent modality in cosmetic dermatology, leveraging broad-spectrum light to address various skin concerns. This non-invasive treatment works by emitting pulses of light that are selectively absorbed by targeted chromophores in the skin, such as melanin and hemoglobin. As the light penetrates the skin, it generates heat, which can effectively diminish pigmented lesions, vascular lesions, and signs of photoaging. Research has established that IPL has the ability to drastically enhance skin texture and tone, as well as minimize the visibility of sun damage, acne scars, and age spots. The versatility of IPL, coupled with its minimal downtime, has made it a popular choice among patients and dermatologists alike, thereby making it a popular option in aesthetic treatments (Cantisani et al., 2014). In addition, IPL therapy provides a good and safer option over conventional laser therapy, which tends to employ a single wavelength of light. Based on its wide-spectrum nature, IPL therapy can be tailored to address the individual needs of patients, making it easier for practitioners to modify settings depending on skin type and conditions.

Notably, the treatment has been said to produce fewer side effects compared to other light therapies. This flexibility is one of the primary attractions of IPL, attracting patients who want to beautify themselves with minimal pain. In addition to this, IPL can be combined with other modalities, enhancing the patient's overall treatment experience as they treat multiple skin conditions at once (Lin et al., 2014). Even with all the advantages it poses, IPL therapy is not free from limitations, which therapists have to keep in mind while suggesting it to patients. One significant drawback is that results can vary greatly among individuals, often influenced by skin type, tone, and the specific condition being treated. Additionally, while IPL is effective for a range of concerns, it may not yield optimal results for deeper lesions or certain types of skin abnormalities. Practitioners should conduct thorough consultations to establish realistic expectations and determine whether IPL is the most suitable course of action. Overall, although IPL treatment is very useful in the field of cosmetic dermatology, it should be realized that such a procedure has its limitations must be fulfilled by the patients and practitioners for optimal results (Cantisani et al., 2014; Lin et al., 2014) (Figure 7.9).

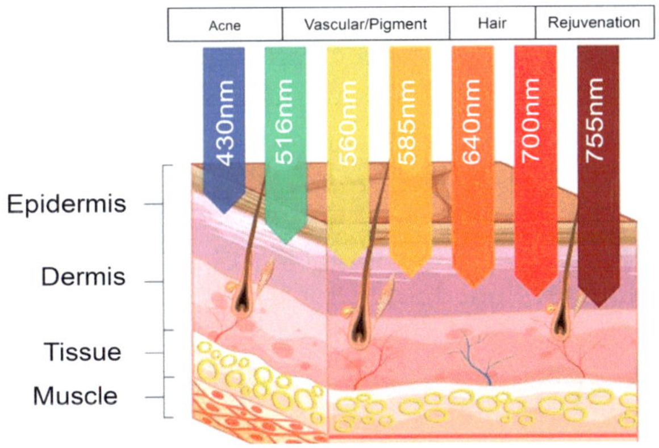

Figure 7.9. Intense pulse light therapy wavelengths with corresponding conditions treated.

Source: https://www.researchgate.net/publication/384104097/figure/fig1/AS:11431281278513869@1726656548769/Intense-pulse-light-therapy-wavelengths-with-corresponding-conditions-treated.png.

7.3.2. Benefits of LED Light Therapy

The emergence of LED light therapy in cosmetic dermatology has transformed the treatment landscape by offering non-invasive options for various skin concerns. Unlike traditional therapies, LED light therapy utilizes specific wavelengths of light to penetrate the skin and promote cellular processes. This therapy is acclaimed for its ability to stimulate collagen production, enhance skin rejuvenation, and reduce inflammation, making it an attractive option for individuals seeking to improve skin texture and reduce signs of aging. Research has shown that repeated sessions of LED light treatment can cause a noticeable decrease in wrinkles and increased skin elasticity, attributing this to fibroblast stimulation within the dermis responsible for producing proteins like collagen and elastin, ultimately giving rise to a more youthful complexion. Additionally, the malleability of LED light treatment in the case of the treatment of acne is a reflection of its increasing role in cosmetic dermatology. Studies have identified certain wavelengths, in particular blue light, as being able to selectively target and destroy acne-causing bacteria without harming surrounding tissue. This non-surgical process can be especially useful for inflammatory acne sufferers because it reduces scarring and post-inflammatory pigmentation that usually follows conventional treatments. Further, research has also reported the effective combination of LED light therapy with PDT to improve treatment outcomes among patients, proving that when combined, these treatments can maximize the diminishment of acne lesions, exhibiting a significant improvement in managing acne-prone skin (Bailey et al., 2010).

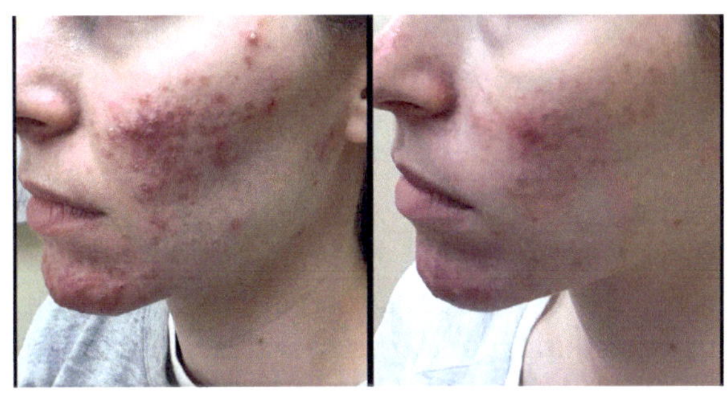

Figure 7.10. LED light therapy acne before and after.

Source: https://www.monadermatology.com/wp-content/uploads/2019/08/LEDLight_1.jpg.

The advantages of LED light therapy are not limited to acne and aging; it is also an important factor in general skin health and healing. The therapy has been described to enhance wound healing and diminish post-operative complications, and therefore serves as a useful adjunct to many dermatologic procedures. As suggested in recent literature, LED light therapy has the potential to stimulate the repair of tissue by improving blood flow and quelling inflammation, resulting in more efficient recovery times following dermatologic procedures (Lin et al., 2014). As evidence favoring the effectiveness of LED light therapy accumulates, its inclusion in standard skin care routines and clinical settings appears inevitable. Therefore, this treatment not only provides many cosmetic advantages but also encourages the overall well-being of the skin, representing a turning point toward more holistic practices in dermatology (Figure 7.10).

7.3.3. Comparison of Light-Based Therapies to Laser Treatments

The rapidly developing specialty of cosmetic dermatology is greatly impacted by the emergence of light-based treatments and laser procedures, both with specific advantages and disadvantages. The light-based treatments, including PDT, utilize photosensitizers that become activated when exposed to particular wavelengths of light, and then destroy abnormally formed skin cells. The non-invasive nature of this method proves to be very successful for the management of conditions such as precancerous cells and superficial NMSC. For example, research shows that PDT produces good cosmetic outcomes with little discomfort and downtime, rendering it an attractive option compared to more invasive treatments. Laser treatments, on the other hand, involve concentrated beams of light capable of penetrating deeper into the skin, facilitating specific changes in the texture and pigmentation of the skin. Although the two methods share rejuvenation and restoration of health as their fundamental goals, the mechanisms and clinical uses of the two are distinct in practice. For skin malignancy treatments, light-based treatments and laser treatments could be seen as potential options; nevertheless, their efficacy could be dramatically diverse for the particular condition. PDT is extensively documented to be effective in the treatment of superficial lesions and has had encouraging success with early NMSC, particularly when given in proper regimens (Cantisani et al., 2014). Its immunomodulatory activity also adds to patient success by fostering the body's own defense against residual pathological cells. Laser treatments, such as ablative lasers, on the other hand, treat more profound tissue layers and can treat a wider variety of dermatological conditions. Their potential to cause thermal damage while activating collagen synthesis makes them incredibly useful in anti-aging treatments, scar treatment, and pigmentation conditions. Hence, even as both technologies are progressively being developed, the choice tends to primarily depend upon the nature of the skin condition, the desired outcome, and specific patient-centric factors. Patient demand and specific clinical priorities indeed play an important role in the choice between light-based treatments and laser therapy. Numerous patients are attracted to the less invasive character of light treatments such as PDT, which calls for limited recuperation time and causes fewer side effects (Lin et al., 2014).

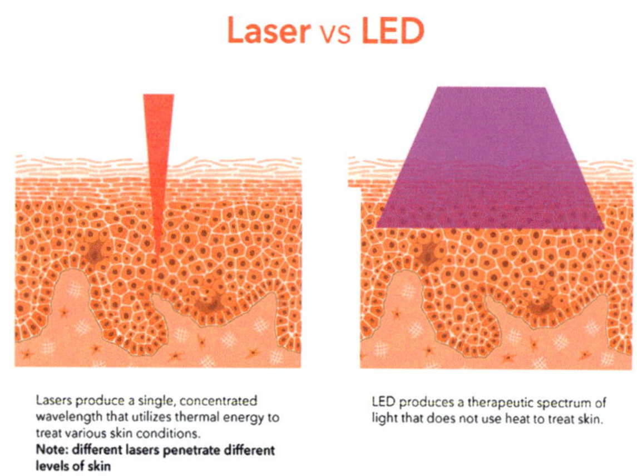

Figure 7.11. LED skincare light therapy vs laser facials.

Source: https://cdn.shopify.com/s/files/1/0565/0802/2940/files/LED_treatment_vs_laser_facials_graphic.png?v=1638396842.

Such ease makes patients seek such treatments for regular skin care and precancerous lesions. However, the more visible and quicker effects of laser therapy are beneficial for those with serious issues like deeper wrinkles or significant sun damage. In addition, decisions are made according to cost, sessions, and long-term success. As such, professionals will need to assess all of these factors to provide patients with a managed treatment plan based on their particular conditions and requirements. As both laser and light-based therapies continue to advance, the integration of these treatments into cosmetic dermatology will probably further improve treatment outcomes and patient satisfaction (Figure 7.11).

Test Your Knowledge

1. What are the key differences between lasers and non-laser light-based devices, such as IPL, in terms of their mechanism and clinical use?
2. How does IPL therapy treat multiple skin conditions, such as pigmentation, vascular lesions, and photoaging, in a single session?

7.4. Applications in Cosmetic Dermatology

Learning Outcome

1. Discuss about treatment of skin pigmentation issues by laser and light-based therapies
2. Describe laser hair removal techniques
3. Explain the use of laser and light-based therapies in skin rejuvenation and anti-aging

Advances in laser and light-based treatments have transformed cosmetic dermatology through innovative approaches that address almost every conceivable clinical condition. Ablative lasers, including CO_2 and Er:YAG, are commonplace treatments for various skin abnormalities, improving epidermal texture and facilitating greater skin flexibility, tone, and glow, all achieved through controlled thermal damage in the skin. Fractional laser therapy, specifically, makes safer treatments with low downtime possible because they do not disturb surrounding tissue, promoting faster healing and fewer side effects. As the operator gains more insight into laser parameters and their interaction with skin anatomy, treatment protocols improve, improving safety profiles and efficacy of these treatments (Alhallak, 2021). This continual advancement underscores the growing importance of such technologies in the repertoire of contemporary cosmetic dermatology. Beyond the treatment of surface irregularities, laser and light-based therapies also address more complex dermatological concerns such as hypertrophic scars and keloids. New recommendations indicate that a comprehensive strategy involving combinations of different modalities, such as laser therapy, can provide substantial improvements in flexibility, pigmentation, and pain related to these difficult skin lesions (Nast et al., 2020). Non-ablative treatments such as pulsed dye lasers have proven to be effective in cutting down vascular supply to scar tissue and thereby preventing its pathological characteristics. The incorporation of lasers into therapeutic treatment plans may also improve patient satisfaction since the cosmetic results often equate to enhanced quality of life. Laser treatments, therefore, not only beautify but also function to restore function and comfort, underlining their vital contribution to scar management. The application of laser and light therapies goes beyond correctional purposes to include preventive interventions in cosmetic dermatology. For instance, preventive laser treatments can help mitigate the formation of hypertrophic scars after surgical procedures by modulating the inflammatory response and fibroblast activity at the wound site. By employing low-energy pulsed dye lasers and other light therapies in the early postoperative stages, clinicians can effectively diminish the risk of abnormal scarring, providing a proactive approach to patient care. In addition, the use of laser treatments alongside new therapies like silicone gel sheeting or intralesional injection can contribute further to healing processes and maximize results in patients prone to scar development. This combined treatment model is indicative of how laser technology is not only a reactionary tool but can be effectively used for preventive protocols in cosmetic dermatology (Nast et al., 2020).

7.4.1. Treatment of Skin Pigmentation Issues

As awareness surrounding cosmetic dermatology continues to expand, the treatment of skin pigmentation issues has garnered significant attention from both patients and practitioners. Laser and light-based therapies stand at the forefront of this domain, providing effective solutions for conditions such as hyperpigmentation, melasma, and vitiligo. The various laser modalities used comprise fractional lasers and intense pulsed light therapy targeting melanin to break it down and promote a more equal complexion. Most importantly, these interventions have therapeutic purposes in addressing and treating patients who suffer from pigmentation disorders. A thorough understanding of the underlying conditions associated with pigmentation is vital for clinicians to tailor treatments that align with individual patient needs and expectations, thereby improving overall satisfaction with aesthetic outcomes. Moreover, the increasing prevalence of cosmetic procedures in dermatology underscores the need for informed decision-making surrounding treatment options. Nonsurgical or minimally invasive techniques, such as chemical peels and microdermabrasion, complement laser therapies in the holistic management of pigmentation issues. Understanding the diversity of available treatments, along with their associated risks and benefits, is essential for healthcare providers to guide patients effectively. Though laser and light therapies have demonstrated notable effectiveness, by following pre- and post-procedural care protocols, as articulated by experts (Madnani et al., 2022), clinicians can maximize patient outcomes and avoid complications. Such an overall approach validates the importance of patient-centric treatment, where not only is the plan specific to the particular pigmentation problem but also to the patient's skin type and general health. Lastly, the complexities of skin pigmentation treatments necessitate an ongoing dialogue between clinicians and patients to navigate individual experiences and expectations. For instance, in the case of vitiligo, patients often seek depigmentation therapy with the hope of achieving a more uniform skin tone.

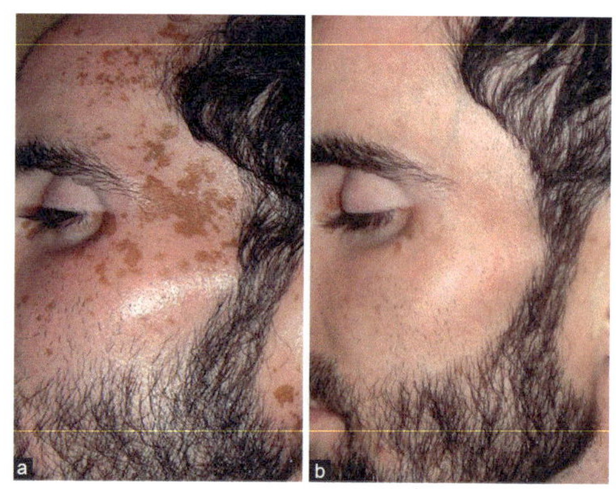

Figure 7.12. (a) Patchy residual pigmentation on face; and (b) after treatment with Q-switched Nd:YAG laser.

Source: https://www.researchgate.net/publication/256490696/figure/fig1/AS:202901088673794@1425386797338/a-Patchy-residual-pigmentation-on-face-b-after-treatment-with-Q-switched-NdYAG-laser.png.

The paradoxical desire for depigmentation among some patients, as noted in the literature (Madnani et al., 2022), highlights the emotional and psychological dimensions of cosmetic dermatology. Consequently, it is essential that practitioners adopt a sensitive approach while discussing treatment options, ensuring that patients are fully educated about the possible results and any side effects associated with their chosen therapies. In such a landscape of informed consent and shared decision-making, the role of laser and light-based treatments for pigmentation problems not only relates to clinical efficacy but spans deep down into clinical psychology and emotional effects related to cosmetic treatments (Figure 7.12).

7.4.2. Laser Hair Removal Techniques

The advent of laser hair reduction techniques has remarkably transformed the landscape of cosmetic dermatology, making hair reduction both effective and simple for a vast range of individuals. This technology deploys highly concentrated beams of light that aim for the melanin in the follicles of hair, killing them without damaging the surrounding tissue. Various laser types, including alexandrite, diode, and Nd:YAG lasers, present different wavelengths and fitting treatment options according to hair type and skin tone. As the procedure cannot guarantee permanent hair removal for everyone, it is often characterized as a long-term hair reduction solution that necessitates multiple sessions. As a result, patients seeking this treatment usually need to manage expectations and adhere to treatment protocols to achieve optimal results. Aside from the technology, patient comfort and safety throughout laser hair removal treatments continue to be of utmost importance. Pre-treatment consultations are important contact points where dermatologists evaluate skin types, color of hair, and medical history to ensure that risks are kept at a minimum. Furthermore, innovation in skin science has led to the incorporation of cooling technologies to desensitize pain brought about by the lasers. This shift toward prioritizing patient experience not only enhances comfort but also fosters a trusting environment, encouraging individuals to seek treatment. Furthermore, as the popularity of these procedures rises, educational programs for practitioner training become essential to ensure skillful administration and adherence to safety protocols, ultimately bridging the gap in somatology education as discussed in the context of somatology in aesthetic practice (Ambrosio et al., 2018).

Lastly, the landscape of laser hair removal techniques continues to evolve, showcasing promising advancements aligned with emerging skincare needs. Recent studies underscore the relationship between various skin rejuvenation methods and laser applications, enhancing the appeal of comprehensive aesthetic solutions. For instance, combined therapies that incorporate laser hair removal alongside treatments targeting facial pores have gained traction. Practitioners can provide a more holistic and effective approach to patient care by simultaneously addressing multiple skin concerns. This validation not only supports the growth of laser applications in cosmetic dermatology but also emphasizes the need for ongoing research to solidify the safety and efficacy of current technologies (El-Kholy et al., 2022). Ultimately, the evolution of laser hair removal reflects a dynamic intersection of client demand, technological advancement, and the necessity for continuous education in the field (Figure 7.13).

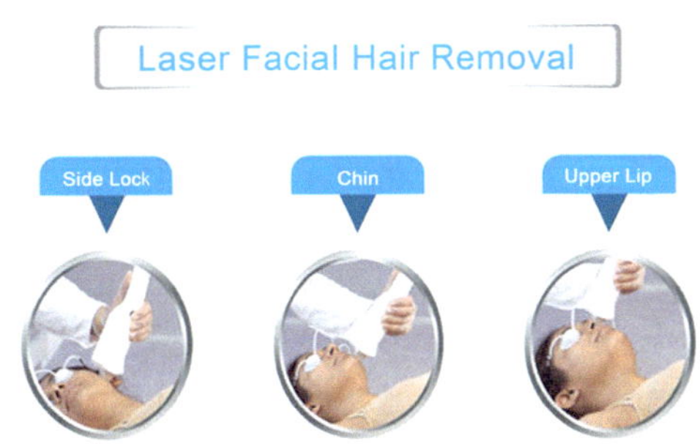

Figure 7.13. Laser facial hair removal.

Source: https://richfeel.com/wp-content/uploads/2020/01/laser-facial-hair-removal.jpg.

7.4.3. Use in Skin Rejuvenation and Anti-Aging

The role of laser and light-based therapies in skin rejuvenation and anti-aging has become increasingly prominent within cosmetic dermatology. These advanced modalities offer patients a non-invasive alternative to traditional surgical procedures, addressing various signs of skin aging, such as wrinkles, sagging, and pigmentation irregularities. Laser treatments work by delivering energy to the skin, stimulating collagen production and promoting cell turnover. This biological reaction is critical for reestablishing skin elasticity and texture. With the advancement of dermatological treatments, the combination of lasers with other non-surgical techniques has led to increasingly sophisticated means of cosmetic rejuvenation that support modern aesthetic ideals of natural-appearing results with minimal recovery time, which appeals to an increasingly diverse patient population that desires aesthetic enhancement without surgical complications (Portilla et al., 2024). Laser technology, particularly with fractional and ablative lasers, has revolutionized the dermatologist methods in skin rejuvenation. Fractions send energy in a grid pattern to the area to be targeted without harming the tissue surrounding it; healing becomes more immediate, and downtime is reduced. Such treatments are perfect for fine wrinkles and lines and other photoaging signs. In addition, the presence of non-ablative laser treatments further makes this industry function, which in an ideal world delivers optimum anti-aging outcomes with minimal unwanted side effects. Tailoring treatment to unique skin types and conditions further attests to a move toward individualized medicine in cosmetic dermatology, allowing practitioners to optimize results while reducing risk, a contention by Madnani et al. (2022). Besides laser procedures, various complementary processes like chemical peels and microneedling have become popular stable alternatives for skin renewal. They tend to exacerbate the impact of laser treatments through further stimulation of skin rejuvenation and texture refinement. For example, peels using chemicals exfoliate the superficial skin layer, thus correcting surface flaws and improving the general look of the skin when complemented with laser treatment. Also, microneedling causes collagen production through controlled micro-injuries in the skin that may also be partnered with laser treatments for increased rejuvenating effects. As the landscape of cosmetic dermatology continues to progress, the importance of understanding the synergistic effects of these techniques becomes critical for achieving optimal patient outcomes and fostering a comprehensive approach to anti-aging (Portilla et al., 2024) (Figure 7.14).

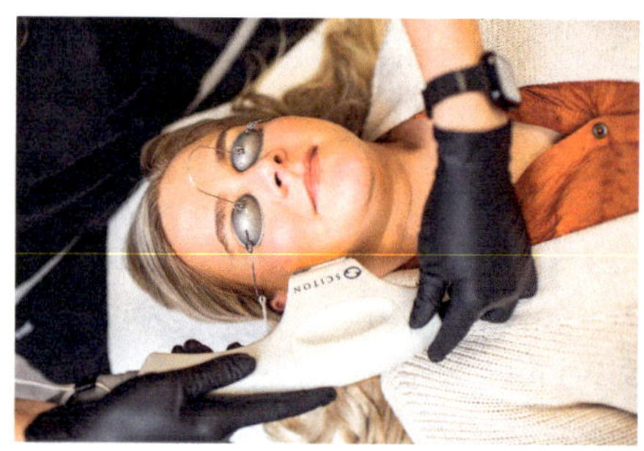

Figure 7.14. Laser therapy in skin rejuvenation.

Source: https://dermacarehr.com/wp-content/uploads/Laser-season-9-ways-lasers-and-light-based-treatments-can-improve-your-skin-this-fall-and-winter.jpg.

Test Your Knowledge

1. What is the best laser treatment for skin pigmentation?
2. Which laser treatment is best for aging skin?

7.5. Risks and Side Effects

Learning Outcome

1. Discuss about common side effects associated with laser treatments
2. Understand long-term risks of laser and light therapies
3. Explain the importance of patient selection and consultation

The use of laser and light treatments in cosmetic dermatology brings such miracles, such as skin rejuvenation and hair replacement. However, this invasive progression in aesthetic medicine also has associated risks and side effects to which everybody concerned, patients and practitioners alike, should be attentive. Side reactions may range from a minor erythema and swelling to more serious complications, including hyperpigmentation, hypopigmentation, or scarring. The incidence of these side effects also varies with variables like skin type, the treatment protocol used, and the proficiency of the practitioner. It is thus imperative that dermatologists are well informed about the risk factors and are capable of explaining to the patient what should be expected during and after procedures. Anticipatory communication is important in achieving optimal patient satisfaction and minimizing the occurrence of unwanted effects. In addition, even though numerous laser treatments are relatively safe, professionals experience difficulties that come with patient choice and pre-operative evaluation. Not all patients are suitable for these interventions, and sensitivity to individual medical conditions is important in lessening risks. For example, patients with keloid history or particular skin diseases may suffer aggravated side effects from laser treatments. Inadequate screening of candidates may lead not only to ineffective treatments but also to severe patient distress and dissatisfaction. Madnani et al. (2022) assert that most clinicians have limited knowledge about the advantages and risks of aesthetic interventions. This point highlights the need for extensive pre-treatment assessment and education of patients to facilitate informed choices. In addition, the long-term effects of various laser treatments are sparsely documented, particularly for special conditions like alopecia areata. There are currently many treatments with few strict, randomized, and controlled trials that demonstrate meaningful efficacy and safety profiles, and thus doubt follows in their administration. While some modalities, like topical immunotherapy, appear to hold promise, not having definitive, long-term treatment regimens may put patients at risk from inappropriate side effects or ineffectiveness. Patients should be told that, as Alsantali et al. (2011) posed, there is currently no agent with established curative effect, and therefore treatment choice needs to be addressed in a strategic way both in terms of effectiveness and safety. Detailed discussion of potential harm, along with continued patient follow-up, will enhance patient safety without discouraging the judicious use of laser and light technologies in cosmetic dermatology.

7.5.1. Common Side Effects Associated with Laser Treatments

Laser procedures in cosmetic dermatology have become extremely popular as they are able to address different skin issues. Their popularity does not, however, justify the signs and symptoms related to any laser procedure. Depending on the laser treatment used and the skin type of the patients, the impacts might not be completely identical. Among the most frequently seen side effects are erythema and edema, in which redness and swelling of the treated areas occur in patients. These events are generally transient, subsiding within hours to days following treatment. Although of minor severity, the appearance of erythema may be capable of producing patient discomfort, thus affecting their satisfaction with the procedure itself. Patient selection, therefore, becomes integral along with proper pre-treatment counseling in order to set realistic expectations as well as obtain informed consent. Sometimes PIH may occur, especially with darker skin, while side effects include erythema and swelling, but also other effects that are such as crusting or scarring, all of which depend upon the intensity of the lasers and the depths of penetration. Crusting is more probable with ablative laser therapy since the lasers will channel the energy more aggressively to the skin in order to induce collagen remodeling. Proper aftercare then becomes a requirement for healing and avoiding complications. Furthermore, patients will frequently report pain or discomfort during the procedure and immediately after the procedure, which is typically likened to the snapping of a rubber band on the skin. Such discomfort can typically be minimized with topical anesthetics applied before therapy. Knowledge about these side effects is critical for both patients and dermatologists to provide the best results and follow proper postoperative care, which in turn will increase the overall effectiveness of laser treatments (Cantisani et al., 2014). Apart from the localized side effects, a few patients might experience systemic reactions, though extremely uncommon, like fever or chills. The infection risk, in the case of laser treatments, is a special concern inasmuch as any skin-breaking treatment provides an entry port for microorganisms. Herein, practitioners must take best sterile procedures to undertake during treatments, and patients must be adequately informed to be aware of signs of infections as post-treatment. Additionally, there is recent research in dermatology that is emphasizing advances in laser technology to minimize side effects and achieve optimal therapeutic benefit. As noted, procedures such as PDT have good potential for the treatment of skin disease and cosmetic problems with excellent aesthetic outcomes and without the traditional side effects associated with more aggressive therapies (Boffa, 2004) (Figure 7.15).

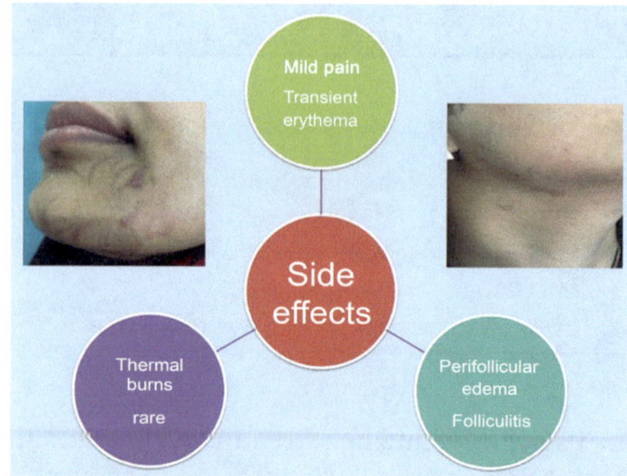

Figure 7.15. Side effects of laser hair removal.

Source: https://www.researchgate.net/profile/Yasmeen-Bhat-2/publication/340875098/figure/fig2/AS:883566615478273@1587670105481/Side-effects-of-laser-hair-removal.jpg.

7.5.2. Long-Term Risks of Laser and Light Therapies

Increased use of laser and light treatments in cosmetic dermatology has undoubtedly changed the mode of treatment for many skin diseases. But closer observation of the long-term side effects of these treatments reveals some serious issues that cannot be overlooked. One of the primary risks is the possibility of skin damage in the form of scarring and dermatological disorders, especially for darker-skinned individuals who will likely be more at risk for complications. Furthermore, the lack of a large series of randomized controlled trials that review long-term outcomes calls into question the safety and efficacy of these treatments in the long term. Hence, clinicians need to assess the individual's skin type and history with caution to limit possible complications and ensure safe application of these emerging technologies (Alsantali et al., 2011). Another vital consideration is the psychological implications that would result from long-term laser and light treatment. Even though many patients receive these treatments for aesthetic enhancement, they may have undesirable effects affecting their self-perception and psychological well-being. For example, individuals can create unrealistic expectations about the effectiveness of treatment so that they are dissatisfied and have a poor quality of life if results do not meet their expectations. Also, the ongoing requirement for financial investment in treatment maintenance can increase stress and feelings of inadequacy unless results are obtained repeatedly. This psychological load actually highlights the value of adequate patient education and realistically addressing what is to be expected and what the boundaries of laser and light therapy (Keri & Shiman, 2009) are.

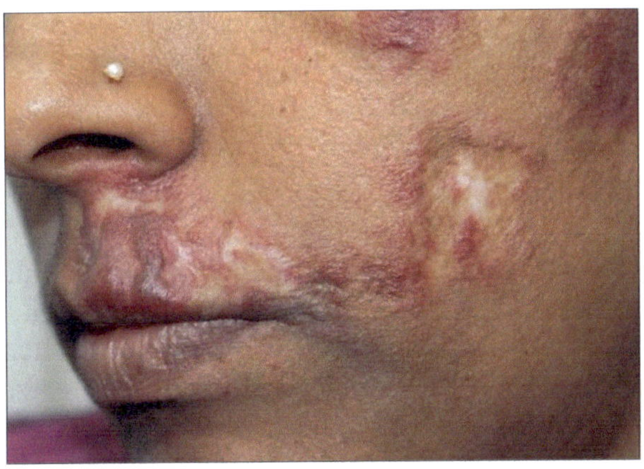

Figure 7.16. Laser imprint following intense pulse light.

Source: https://ijdvl.com/content/126/2019/85/1/Images/ijdvl_2019_85_1_24_247689_f9.jpg.

Furthermore, the long-term effect on skin integrity remains a question not entirely known, particularly with more recent technologies always emerging in scientific literature. The frequent, minute interventions made by practitioners create the need for sensitivity to the overall effect that such treatments might have on skin conditions to be developed. Frequent and more intense treatment can, for instance, drive skin aging and worsen some existing conditions. Long-term consequences, like the potential development of hypersensitivity and incompatibility with future dermatological treatments, must be researched further in order to develop comprehensive guidelines for safe practice. The dynamic character of cosmetic dermatology necessitates that providers and patients engage in continued dialogue about the long-term risks of laser and light therapy to prevent ill-informed choices and optimize skin health results (Alsantali et al., 2011) (Figure 7.16).

7.5.3. Importance of Patient Selection and Consultation

A critical component of the success of laser and light therapies in cosmetic dermatology is proper patient selection. This involves a evaluation of different factors like the medical history of a patient, skin type, and personal concerns to which they would rather approach a solution through treatment. Through thorough consultations, experts can determine not just whether such sophisticated interventions suit particular patients, but also their psychological preparedness for them. Interestingly, an understanding of patient expectations and their level of comprehension regarding probable outcomes and risks heavily affects satisfaction rates. As underscored by the increase in aesthetic dermatology procedures, proper patient selection can mitigate complications and enhance efficacy, ensuring that both the provider and patient are aligned in their treatment goals (Madnani et al., 2022). The significance of informed consultation cannot be overstated in the realm of cosmetic dermatology. Such discussions provide the opportunity for practitioners to educate patients about all the laser treatments that are available, as well as how a specific individual's needs and concerns will be met. By engaging in open conversation, practitioners can debunk myths, talk about possible side effects, and establish what, if any pre- and post-procedure care is necessary. Significantly, the preparation process institutes a relationship of trust and receptivity between patient and practitioner that heavily conditions the overall treatment experience. The consultation process itself is not ritualistic; it constitutes laying down the grounds for attainable outcomes of treatment and serves to define reasonable expectations in order to minimize the chances of post-treatment dissatisfaction (Madnani et al., 2022). In addition to this, the intricacies involved with individual skin disorders, like vitiligo, also highlight the importance of careful patient selection and consultation. In conditions where the irreversible treatment of alopecia areata is sought, knowledge of their respective situations becomes highly pertinent. Practitioners need to explain that the course of vitiligo cannot be predicted, nor can the effect of treatments on appearance. Such discussions not only help in informed decision-making but also establish preparation for emotional and aesthetic implications of patient choices. According to documented literature, a holistic dialogue regarding the risks and benefits of procedures can enhance patients' compliance and satisfaction, thereby offering a better therapeutic approach by respecting the autonomy of patients while protecting safety.

Test Your Knowledge

1. What are the side effects of laser skin treatment?
2. Does laser treatment have long-term side effects? Explain.

7.6. Advances in Technology

Learning Outcome

1. Focus on innovations in laser technology
2. Describe emerging light-based treatment modalities
3. Understand future trends in cosmetic dermatology

Evolution of laser and light treatments in aesthetic dermatology is a key breakthrough in the field, which has empowered practitioners to address an array of skin problems with precision and minimal intrusiveness. Advances in technology in recent years have facilitated our understanding of skin pathology and outcomes of treatment, so that dermatologists are now able to create individualized treatment programs specifically sensitive to patients' own needs. For example, the treatment of wrinkles, acne scars, and pigmentation problems has been much improved with fractional laser technologies. It provides less downtime, minimizes side effects, and is associated with excellent results. As noted by contemporary literature, such advances not only reflect an ongoing progress in the treatment modalities but also illustrate an improved comprehension of skin biology that thereby allows health care practitioners well-versed in it to treat intricate skin disorders more effectively (Boffa, 2004). Apart from lasers, other light treatments, such as IPL, have also become available, providing multi-functional treatments for disorders like rosacea and vascular lesions. The integration of these technologies has been extremely valuable in that they can be employed to specifically target chromophores in the skin to produce highly personalized rehabilitative treatments with minimal collateral damage to the surrounding tissue. These treatments have been maximized through the current innovations for improved delivery of fluence and have shown good safety profiles and acceptable results. Besides that, ongoing research into combination therapy is expanding the limits of how dermatologists rejuvenate and rebuild skin in ways in which treatment modalities not only work but are safe to apply on a long-term basis (Cantisani et al., 2014). The integration of new technologies also finds its place in the field of PDT, which has remained a leading adjunct to the treatment of NMSCs. PDT involves the use of photosensitizing substances in conjunction with certain light sources to destroy malignant cells, justifying the light's revolutionary role in therapeutic situations. Experiments have proven that, when used appropriately, this noninvasive method has good cosmetic results, especially for superficial lesions. Additionally, its ability to be employed in various regimens showcases its adaptability to patient needs. Given the rising incidence of skin cancers, particularly linked to UV exposure, harnessing such advancements in light-based therapies proves essential, not only for aesthetic benefits but also for cancer prevention strategies (Cantisani et al., 2014).

7.6.1. Innovations in Laser Technology

The advancement of laser technology has had a significant impact on the field of cosmetic dermatology, providing advanced methods for rejuvenating and repairing skin. Some of these advancements include the creation of fractional laser systems, which provide energy in small, pixelated areas, leaving untreated skin between targeted areas. This technique not only improves healing but also reduces downtime, allowing for easier incorporation into patients busy schedules. Fractional lasers work especially well in treating the concerns of photoaging, including pigmentation, fine lines, and irregularities in texture, improving the skin overall. Their inclusion reflects the dermatology discipline's emphasis on marrying effectiveness with patient comfort, evidencing an industry-wide trend towards less invasive yet highly effective treatments. These innovations align with newer strategies that advance non-invasive methods as effective alternatives to conventional surgical methods in the industry (Portilla et al., 2024). An important innovation of laser technology is the development of multiple wavelengths, allowing for customized treatment programs sensitive to the individual skin type and problems. Along with all these, such technologies as the 1064 nm Nd:YAG and the 585 nm pulsed dye laser have become available for directed treatment of conditions including vascular lesions, melasma, and others. These advances have, therefore, widened the breadth of laser treatment given for therapeutic purposes, ensuring clinicians achieve desired results while minimizing the risk of side effects. The ability to customize treatments based on precise assessments of intrinsic and extrinsic determinants of skin aging, as outlined by the most current research, highlights the importance of a customized strategy in managing skin disorders effectively (Fernández-Varela-Gómez et al., 2024). Adaptability not only provides patient satisfaction but also maintains the vital role of accepting novel laser modalities for the multifactoriality of skin aging. Furthermore, the interaction of laser technology with other treatments has created synergistic effects in cosmetic dermatology. The combination of modalities like resurfacing lasers with fillers or neurotoxin injections optimizes aesthetic outcomes and ensures longevity of the effects. Such a multi-dimensional approach recognizes that skin aging is multifactorial and must be addressed with an integrated approach, combining various interventions into one comprehensive treatment plan. The creation of combination treatments as a result of advancements in laser technology highlights the discipline's advancement toward improving both the effectiveness and safety of cosmetic treatments. Practitioners are increasingly recognizing opportunities to increase patient experience and levels of satisfaction through the utilization of the benefits offered by various modalities, thereby creating a more holistic model for cosmetic enhancement that is better aligned with modern dermatology (Portilla et al., 2024) (Figure 7.17).

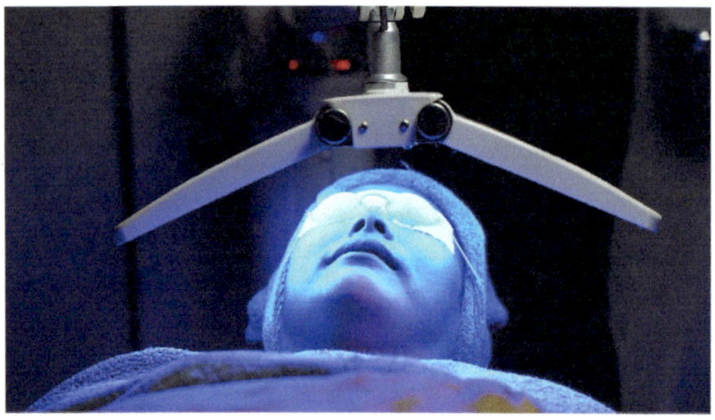

Figure 7.17. Innovations in laser technology.

Source: https://dynotech-solutions.com/blogs/wp-content/uploads/2024/06/New-Project-2024-06-05T114639.380.jpg.

7.6.2. Emerging Light-Based Treatment Modalities

With the progress of cosmetic dermatology, there are now more developed light-based treatment modalities with known LEDs that may be used in terms of treatment for various diseases such as pigmentation disorders and skin fibrosis. Through studies, LEDs such as red-light therapy have been proven to modulate important cellular processes that are concerned with scarring and collagen synthesis. In one recent trial, the efficacy of LED therapy was tested for its ability to limit post-surgical skin fibrosis, offering a non-invasive option that ensures optimal wound healing and discourages excessive scarring. These new therapies emphasize the urgent need for effective anti-scarring treatment options within dermatology, as attested to by fibrotic dermatoses rates and their stark impact on patients' quality of life (Heilman et al., 2019). Alongside the treatment of fibrotic disorders, light therapies have also become a treatment for pigmentation disorders and possess a double concern for depigmentation and therapeutic treatment. For instance, patients with diseases like vitiligo can pursue depigmentation therapy to achieve balanced skin pigmentation, which on some occasions causes paradoxical emotional reactions toward their skin's appearance. This is a reflection of the intricate interplay of therapeutic objectives and patient attitudes in cosmetic dermatology practice. Additionally, advancements in laser and chemical peels have enabled impressive improvements in skin color and texture, accompanied by global cosmetic enhancements. All these modalities contribute to cosmetic changes and broader mental health implications by correcting diseases that cause psychological morbidity among patients who suffer from such diseases (Boffa, 2004). The continuous research and clinical use of light treatments represent a paradigm shift in cosmetic dermatology. Not only do these modalities offer site-specific treatment choices for different skin issues, but they also prioritize the safety and tolerability aspect. As with the case of LED-RL therapy trials, such advances can revolutionize treatment benchmarks by allowing patients to incorporate safer, non-invasive options into their skincare regimen. Moreover, with the emergence of in-home light therapy devices, patients can have a sense of increased control over their treatment procedures, even more so, personalizing their dermatological treatment. The combination of these technologies will surely challenge current paradigms and stimulate future study focused on treating an even broader range of dermatological conditions, validating light-based treatments as a cornerstone component of contemporary cosmetic dermatological practices.

7.6.3. Future Trends in Cosmetic Dermatology

The cosmetic dermatology landscape is on the cusp of dramatic change, thanks to the growth in laser and light-based treatments. One of the most visible trends is the growing use of non-surgical methods, specifically lasers, that provide excellent results with limited downtime. With increasing demand for cosmetic treatments, practitioners are expanding their services to address a clientele that prioritizes safety and ease of access more and more.

Educational campaigns will form the pillar of this development, allowing practitioners to acquire skills to integrate the latest technology into practice. This is particularly relevant in regions such as South Africa, where the need for normalized training in aesthetic procedures is so significant, as highlighted by recent studies into the industry's need for advanced aesthetics education to bridge existing skills gaps among practitioners (Ambrosio et al., 2018). Another important trend is the integration of technology into treatment protocols, through enhancing diagnostic capabilities as well as treatment outcomes. Technology may be introduced in the form of modalities like optical coherence tomography (OCT) incorporated into laser therapies, making it easier for dermatologists to personalize treatment plans. For example, the application of OCT-guided 1064nm Nd:YAG laser therapy for basal cell carcinomas shows how combining diagnostic imaging with therapy can provide improved clearance rates and patient satisfaction. This combination of diagnostic and therapeutic procedures enables practitioners to closely observe treatment response and reduce protocols, thus generating increased safety and efficacy (Giral et al., 2023). With increasing research in the field rendering ever-deeper understanding, cosmetic dermatology is bound to witness a move toward more holistic strategies that value individualized patient care. Finally, the future of cosmetic dermatology will witness a strengthening focus on interdisciplinary collaboration between beauty experts, medical professionals, and cosmetologists. The overlap of these fields presents innumerable opportunities for development and enhancement of patient outcomes. Since research shows, medical doctors and aesthetic practitioners would value the fact that working alongside each other would do more to ensure treatment success and patient safety. Ideally, it would perhaps resemble combined training courses and cross-disciplinary approaches to aesthetic application, collectively becoming integral skincare alternatives. Moreover, with the cosmetic dermatology industry continuing to evolve, integration of advanced training and educational models will be necessary to respond to increased consumer demand for advanced aesthetic therapies, demonstrating the necessity for ongoing investment in professional development within the industry (Ambrosio et al., 2018).

Test Your Knowledge

1. What do you understand by photodynamic therapy (PDT)?
2. What is the best light therapy for skin conditions?

SUMMARY

The application of laser and light-based therapies in cosmetic dermatology represents a significant advancement in addressing various skin concerns, including scars, pigmentation, and vascular lesions. These modalities leverage specific wavelengths of light to achieve targeted treatments, resulting in precise interventions with minimal impact on surrounding tissues. However, the responses to these treatments depend much on the kind of condition and its severity under treatment, thus requiring case-by-case treatment protocols. Due to differences in response to treatment that depend on the patient's skin type and appearance of lesions, the practitioner will have to consider a well-rounded assessment and implement protocols in response to these to guarantee higher patient satisfaction and outcomes of treatment (Nast et al., 2020). In addition, incorporation of new imaging methods, including photoacoustic imaging, into laser treatment protocols is an exciting future direction for optimizing treatment accuracy and outcome evaluation. This new non-invasive technology enables clinicians to visualize deep skin structures and lesions with high resolution and facilitate improved diagnosis and treatment planning. As highlighted in the literature, progress in instrumentation and imaging agents has led to a vast potential for application of photoacoustic imaging in dermatology, which may transform the practice regarding many skin diseases by the practitioner (Steinberg et al., 2019). Further clinical work will be needed to validate and standardize protocols that incorporate such new technologies, while cosmetic dermatology is fast expanding with ever-increasing demand from patients. In conclusion, the landscape of laser and light-based therapies in cosmetic dermatology reflects a dynamic and rapidly evolving field that offers substantial benefits for patients seeking aesthetic and therapeutic improvements. The ability to customize treatments to individual needs, alongside the integration of advanced imaging techniques, promises enhanced outcomes and greater patient satisfaction. Nevertheless, challenges such as the variabilities in treatment responses and the need for continued research into long-term effects remain. By fostering an evidence-based approach and embracing innovation, cosmetic dermatologists can optimize treatment efficacy while promoting evidence-driven practices in the management of skin conditions, thereby significantly enhancing the quality of care provided to patients.

Cosmetic dermatology has spread widely, with major developments covering laser and light-based therapy for solving issues regarding the skin. With the numerous surges that these areas have undergone, the scope today encompasses non-invasive to almost minimally invasive means of treatment for the sophisticated demands of their high-end patients, who require signs of aging and skin deterioration to be abolished. At the heart of this debate is the movement away from conventional surgical methods, including facelifts and blepharoplasty, to more advanced techniques employing technologies such as ultrasound and lasers. As can be seen in this review of surgical and dermatological methods, such advances are not only effective but also advantageous in that they cut down on recovery time and the complications involved with more invasive methods (Portilla et al., 2024). This transformation highlights the importance of adapting treatments to offer safer alternatives while maintaining high efficacy in cosmetic outcomes. In addition to rejuvenation strategies, laser and light-based therapies are intricately connected to the management of pigmentation disorders. The therapeutic goals often center on depigmentation, which can be essential for conditions like vitiligo and other skin blemishes. Patients may look for laser treatments to attain a more even tone to the skin. This indicates that the solutions for both cosmetic needs and associated disorders should be present. These solutions can help the skin improve cosmetically; therefore, patient self-esteem as well as quality of life may be improved. As explained above, a variety of modalities-from lasers, chemical peels, and light therapy-is used to directly address pigmentation problems and thus is a highly desirable treatment in contemporary dermatologic care (Portilla et al., 2024). Such versatility underscores the significance of laser therapies in achieving comprehensive skin rejuvenation and correction. Furthermore, the effective use of laser and light therapies extends beyond simple cosmetic enhancements and into broader therapeutic realms. These technologies are useful not only for aesthetic purposes but also for the treatment of various dermatological conditions, which can fundamentally alter the patient experience positively. The role of lasers in treating conditions like scars, stretch marks, and active acne showcases their multifaceted applications within cosmetic dermatology. The exploration of minimally invasive techniques such as Ultherapy and thread lifts also emphasizes the growing preference for procedures that yield substantial results without extensive downtime (Portilla et al., 2024). The integration of laser and light-based therapies is holistic in its focus on cosmetic improvements and therapeutic resolutions, in line with the general idea that cosmetic dermatology is beauty as well as health.

KEY TERMS FROM THIS CHAPTER

Dermatological disorders
Dissatisfaction
Hypermelanocytosis
Non-invasive treatment
Non-surgical treatments
Photochemical effect
ost-treatment redness
Skin physiology
Superficial skin
Surgical procedures
Dermatology practice
Fibroblast activity
Microdermabrasion
Non-melanoma skin cancer
Patient management
Photodynamic therapy (PDT)
Skin elasticity
Skin problems
Surgical complications
Textural abnormalities

CRITICAL THINKING QUESTIONS

1. **Which of the following is the most commonly used laser for hair removal?**
   a. Carbon Dioxide (CO_2) Laser
   b. Alexandrite Laser
   c. Fractional Laser
   d. Nd:YAG Laser
2. **Which type of laser is commonly used for skin resurfacing and reducing wrinkles?**
   a. Diode Laser
   b. Erbium: YAG Laser
   c. Pulsed Dye Laser
   d. CO_2 Laser
3. **Which light-based therapy is commonly used for the treatment of acne vulgaris?**
   a. Blue Light Therapy
   b. Red Light Therapy
   c. Green Light Therapy
   d. Yellow Light Therapy
4. **Which of the following laser types is most effective for treating vascular lesions such as spider veins?**
   a. CO_2 Laser
   b. Pulsed Dye Laser
   c. Nd:YAG Laser
   d. Alexandrite Laser
5. **In laser skin resurfacing, what is the primary target chromophore for the CO_2 laser?**
   a. Melanin
   b. Water
   c. Hemoglobin
   d. Collagen

Short Answer Questions

1. What are the key differences between ablative and non-ablative lasers, and how do they affect the skin during cosmetic treatments?
2. Explain the mechanism of action of fractional lasers in treating skin conditions such as scars and wrinkles.
3. What are the primary indications for using intense pulsed light (IPL) therapy in cosmetic dermatology?
4. Describe the role of laser therapies in the treatment of hyperpigmentation disorders, such as melasma and sunspots.
5. How does laser hair removal work, and what are the potential side effects or complications associated with the procedure?
6. What are the different types of lasers commonly used for skin resurfacing, and what specific conditions do they treat?
7. Discuss the safety precautions and contraindications that need to be considered before performing laser treatments on patients with darker skin tones.
8. How do light-based therapies like photodynamic therapy (PDT) work in the treatment of acne, and what are the advantages over traditional treatments?

Answer to Critical Thinking Questions

1. (c); 2. (d); 3. (a); 4. (b); 5. (b)

REFERENCES

1. Alhallak, K. (2021). Skin, light and their interactions, an in-depth review for modern light-based skin therapies. *Clinical Dermatology & Therapy, 7*, 1–15. https://doi.org/10.24966/cdt-8771/100081 (accessed on 11th June 2025).
2. Alsantali, A. (2011). Alopecia areata: A new treatment plan. https://core.ac.uk/download/pdf/8602857.pdf (accessed on 11th June 2025).
3. Ambrosio, D. V. (2018). Incidence and need of advanced aesthetic somatology in South Africa. https://core.ac.uk/download/222968033.pdf (accessed on 11th June 2025).
4. Avram, M. M. (2021). Board certification in cosmetic surgery: An evaluation of training backgrounds and scope of practice. *Plastic & Reconstructive Surgery, 148*, 494e–496e. https://doi.org/10.1097/prs.0000000000008243 (accessed on 11th June 2025).
5. Bailey, E. C., Hamilton, T. A., Kang, S., Orringer, T., et al. (2010). Photodynamic therapy for acne vulgaris: A randomized, controlled, split-face clinical trial of topical aminolaevulinic acid and pulsed dye laser therapy. http://deepblue.lib.umich.edu/bitstream/2027.42/79403/1/j.1473-2165.2010.00483.x.pdf (accessed on 11th June 2025).
6. Boffa, M. J. (2004). *Dermatology.* https://core.ac.uk/download/46601884.pdf (accessed on 11th June 2025).
7. Portilla, A. S. P., Portilla, C. S. P., Palacios, G. S. G., Rodríguez, B. S. P., Castillo, S. G. A., Espin, N. E. P., & Pita, G. P. M. (2024). The integration of surgical and dermatological techniques in the treatment of cutaneous aging: multidisciplinary approaches and clinical outcomes - a comprehensive systematic review of current literature. *International Journal of Research in Medical Sciences, 12*(5), 1659–1667. https://doi.org/10.18203/2320-6012.ijrms20240943 (accessed on 11th June 2025).
8. Madnani, N., Vedmurthy, M., Parthasarthi, A., Dhawan, S., Kandhari, R., Pillai, R., & Nischal, K. C. (2022). Expert opinion on pre and post procedure care in aesthetic dermatology. *International Journal of Research in Medical Sciences, 10*(4), 991–1000. https://doi.org/10.18203/2320-6012.ijrms20220999(accessed on 11th June 2025).
9. El-Kholy, B. M., Kandil, A. H., & Nawwar, E. M. A. (2022). New insight in the treatment of wide facial pores: Review article. https://core.ac.uk/download/524771765.pdf (accessed on 11th June 2025).
10. Ferara, N., Franceschi, N., Šitum Čeprnja, Z., Šitum, M., et al. (2024). Treatment of actinic keratoses and field cancerization–Croatian perspective. https://core.ac.uk/download/620817167.pdf (accessed on 11th June 2025).
11. Fernández-Varela-Gómez, F., Sandoval-García, A., & Valeria Cabrera-Rios, K. (2024). Signs of skin aging: a review. *International Journal of Research in Medical Sciences, 12*(7), 2674–2679. https://doi.org/10.18203/2320-6012.ijrms20241935(accessed on 11th June 2025).
12. Heilman, E., Isseroff, R. R., Jagdeo, J. R., & Jakus, J., et al. (2019). A dose-ranging, parallel group, split-face, single-blind phase II study of light emitting diode-red light (LED-RL) for skin scarring prevention: Study protocol for a randomized controlled trial. https://core.ac.uk/download/323070347.pdf (accessed on 11th June 2025).

13. Keri, J., & Shiman, M. (2009). An update on the management of acne vulgaris. *Clinical, cosmetic and investigational dermatology, 2*, 105–110. https://doi.org/10.2147/ccid.s3630(accessed on 11th June 2025).
14. Kim, T. H. (2021). Depigmentation. https://core.ac.uk/download/478113284.pdf (accessed on 11th June 2025).
15. Kumar, N. (2021). Design, development and implementation framework for a postgraduate non-surgical aesthetics curriculum. https://core.ac.uk/download/480391006.pdf (accessed on 11th June 2025).
16. Lin, J. Y., & Wan, M. T. (2014). Current evidence and applications of photodynamic therapy in dermatology. https://core.ac.uk/download/28949556.pdf (accessed on 11th June 2025).
17. Löhr, F., Papakonstantinou, E., & Raap, U. (2017). Photodynamic therapy and skin cancer. https://core.ac.uk/download/322432943.pdf (accessed on 11th June 2025).
18. Proietti, I., Skroza, N., Mambrin, A., Marraffa, F., Tolino, E., Bernardini, N., Marchesiello, A., Rossi, G., Volpe, S., & Potenza, C. (2021). Aesthetic Treatments in Cancer Patients. *Clinical, cosmetic and investigational dermatology, 14*, 1831–1837. https://doi.org/10.2147/CCID.S342734 (accessed on 11th June 2025).
19. Mhatre, M., Mulekar, S., & Mulekar, S. (2019). Depigmentation therapies in vitiligo. https://core.ac.uk/download/322444965.pdf (accessed on 11th June 2025).
20. Morton, C. A., Szeimies, R.-M., Basset-Séguin, N., Calzavara-Pinton, P., Gilaberte, Y., Hædersdal, M., Hofbauer, G. F. L., et al. (2019). European Dermatology Forum guidelines on topical photodynamic therapy 2019 Part 1: Treatment delivery and established – actinic keratoses, Bowen's disease and basal cell carcinomas. *Journal of the European Academy of Dermatology and Venereology, 33*, 2225–2238. https://doi.org/10.1111/jdv.16017 (accessed on 11th June 2025).
21. Murray, T., Lohray, R., Schultz, K. P., Boutros, S., & Friedman, P. M. (2024). Complications of chemical peels, lasers, and energy-based device procedures performed by core cosmetic physicians: A retrospective analysis. *Lasers in Surgery and Medicine.* https://www.semanticscholar.org/paper/80b3dc69c427ddc9d9535bd4092f9d7097e6d3b4 (accessed on 11th June 2025).
22. Nast, A., Gauglitz, G. G., Lorenz, K., Metelmann, H.-R., Paasch, U., Strnad, V., Weidmann, M., et al. (2020). S2k guidelines for the therapy of pathological scars (hypertrophic scars and keloids)–Update 2020. *JDDG Journal der Deutscher Dermatologist Gesellschaft, 19*, 312–327. https://doi.org/10.1111/ddg.14279 (accessed on 11th June 2025).
23. Palacio Giral, A. (2023). Optical coherence tomography-assisted 1064nm Nd:YAG laser therapy of superficial and nodular basal cell carcinomas with ≤1mm tumor thickness. https://core.ac.uk/download/618185853.pdf (accessed on 11th June 2025).
24. Passeron, T., Genedy, R. M., Salah, L. A., Fusade, T., Kositratna, G., Laubach, H.-J., Marini, L., et al. (2019). Laser treatment of hyperpigmented lesions: Position statement of the European Society of Laser in Dermatology. *Journal of the European Academy of Dermatology and Venereology, 33*, 987–1005. https://doi.org/10.1111/jdv.15497 (accessed on 11th June 2025).
25. Steinberg, I., Huland, D. M., Vermesh, O., Frostig, H., Tummers, W. S., & Gambhir, S. S. (2019). Photoacoustic clinical imaging. *Photoacoustics, 14*, 77–98. https://doi.org/10.1016/j.pacs.2019.05.001 (accessed on 11th June 2025).

26. van Straten, D., Mashayekhi, V., de Bruijn, H., Oliveira, S., & Robinson, D. J. (2017). Oncologic photodynamic therapy: Basic principles, current clinical status and future directions. *Cancers, 9*, 19–19. https://doi.org/10.3390/cancers9020019 (accessed on 11th June 2025).

27. Yang, W., Cai, Y., Zhang, L., Li, L., Wang, J., Jiang, F., Sun, N., et al. (2024). Research situation, hotspots, and global trends in laser treatment of acne scars: A bibliometric analysis of related research from 2014 to 2024. *Journal of Cosmetic Dermatology, 24*. https://www.semanticscholar.org/paper/2e67f993c858cb2cadee09a0ae4b4a77cb5e9f1c (accessed on 11th June 2025).

NON-ABLATIVE SKIN REJUVENATION AND FRACTIONAL LASERS

8

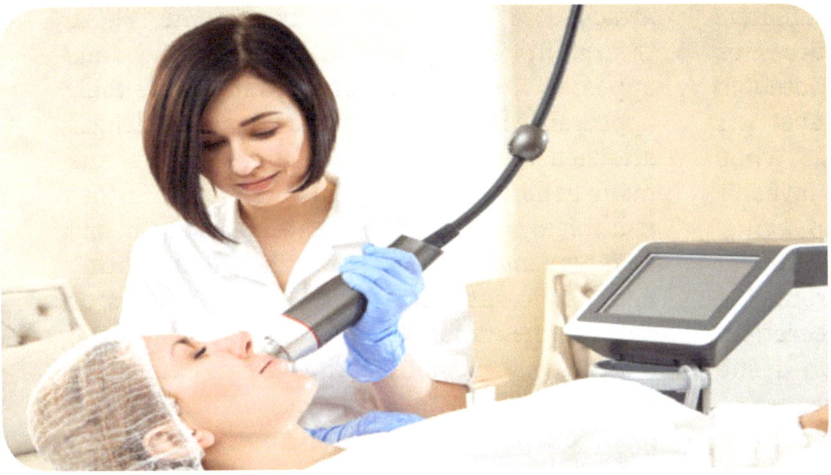

Introduction

In dermatology, the search for young, rejuvenated skin remains a major issue for both practitioners and patients. Technology has made it possible to create newer, non-surgical treatments designed to restore some of the most prevalent faults of aging, including fine lines, wrinkles, and other imperfections. Non-ablative skin rejuvenation uses technology that stimulates the formation of collagen without destroying the barrier of the skin, thereby being associated with a less harsh recovery compared to the recovery associated with traditional ablative treatment. Fractional lasers are one of the many forms of non-ablative technologies that have gained popularity due to their safety and effectiveness profiles for the treatment of various disorders in the skin. These lasers send finely targeted microbeams to the skin, allowing for gradual resurfacing while preventing the risk of side effects commonly found in more invasive treatments. In addition, non-ablative treatments have a crucial role in treating the signs of photoaging, an affliction that

LEARNING OBJECTIVES

After studying this chapter, you will be able to:

1. Understand the mechanism of action for non-ablative skin rejuvenation
2. Explain the types of non-ablative lasers
3. Discuss about indications for treatment with non-ablative fractional lasers
4. Define the benefits of non-ablative treatments
5. Describe potential risks and side effects
6. Focus on post-treatment care

is considerably advanced by ultraviolet radiation with the passage of time. Research shows that cumulative damage caused by UV is responsible for skin aging through collagen degradation and skin roughness. Therapeutic approaches like photodynamic therapy (PDT), which is a platform that bridges ablative and non-ablative techniques, have indicated promising results in rejuvenating photo-damaged skin by improving the skin texture and pigmentation (Masnec et al., 2014). In that regard, the practitioner integrates other treatments with non-ablative modalities to maximize patient outcomes since a treatment strategy is multifaceted in approach and will address at one level the dermatological and aesthetic concerns while minimizing risks associated with more invasive treatments. Besides treating signs of aging, non-ablative treatments are also important in improving the quality of the skin and reducing big pores and excessive sebaceous secretion. Small pores on the face become an issue among the majority of individuals because of the adverse cosmetic effect they contribute to, but particularly because they reduce one's self-esteem and lower their level of living. There are numerous treatment modalities available, ranging from topical agents to the sophisticated laser technologies, but these treatments still have continuing clinical evaluation studies for efficacy and safety (El-Kholy et al., 2022). The most promising non-ablative facial rejuvenation technology of them all is the fractional lasers, which could potentially enhance skin texture and possibly reduce pore size with a good side effect profile. Increasing evidence assures us of the trend of use of these technologies as part of routine dermatological practice as a paradigm shift towards less invasive but effective options in skin rejuvenation.

Definition of Non-Ablative Skin Rejuvenation

The cosmetic dermatological scene has changed since the advent of non-ablative skin rejuvenation methods. Unlike ablative treatment, which removes layers of the skin, non-ablative treatment works on the inner layers without damaging the skin surface. The procedure makes the skin texture smoother, tone better, and elasticity improved through stimulation of collagen production and encouragement of the body's natural healing processes. Non-ablative treatments would be laser therapy and RF. These are treatments where the modalities offer rejuvenation without the risks and downtime attached to more invasive treatments. These treatments cause little discomfort and thus appeal to clients who would want to have their appearance improved with the least of challenges attached to surgical interventions. One of the main benefits of non-ablative renewal is that it is highly versatile and can be used on any skin type and concern. It works well in treating minor concerns such as fine lines, large pores, or hyperpigmentation. The newer studies, however, indicate that the non-ablative treatments might be beneficial by closing off accessibility of facial enlarged pores that the majority of women possess on their faces. As discussed by studies, the problem is solved through the reduction and regulation of sebum by an alteration in follicle size. Non-ablative rejuvenation, thus, not only improves the esthetic feature of the skin but also contributes to overall skin health through the implementation of such methods as micro-needling and fractional laser technology that induce micro-injury, initiating channels for collagen stimulation and texture enhancement, providing progressive and safe outcomes to patients seeking cosmetic improvement (El-Kholy et al., 2022). Moreover, the advances in techniques and technology have driven the growth of non-ablative skin rejuvenation in facial plastic surgery. Fractional laser devices offer a new approach that brings energy to fractional parts of the skin, allowing selective therapy with sparing of nearby tissues. The method maximizes healing and rejuvenation to address patient needs for natural-looking results. Recent literature stresses that the method of facial plastic surgery continuously combines methods of dermatology and aesthetic medicine to maximize the effectiveness of non-ablative treatments. The cross-pollination enhances skin rejuvenation and also general aesthetic enhancement, allowing experts to expand their skill set and address the differing needs of patients (Barnes et al., 2016) (Figure 8.1).

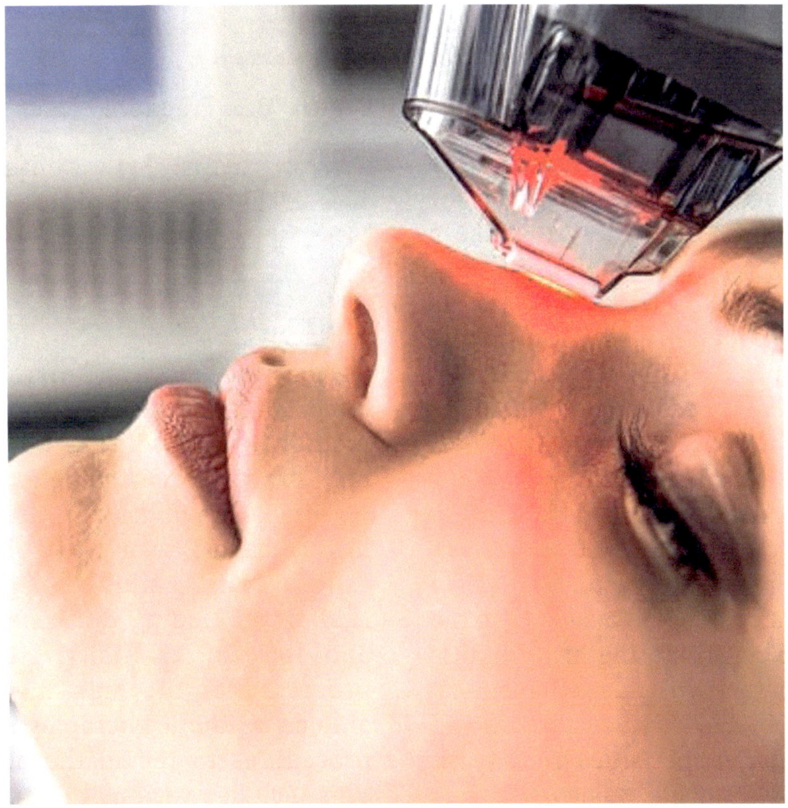

Figure 8.1. A close-up of a non-ablative laser treatment being performed on a patient's face, illustrating a dermatological procedure designed to stimulate collagen production and improve skin texture with minimal downtime.

Source: https://www.skinceuticals.com/dw/image/v2/AANG_PRD/on/demandware.static/-/Sites-skinc-us-Library/default/dw3711d61d/images/treatment-detail-page/23_1019_PRO_TREATMENT_PAGES_ARTICLE_DETAIL_HERO_BANNER_NON-ABLATIVE_LASERS_D.jpg?sw=400&sh=400&sm=cut&q=70.

Overview of Fractional Laser Technology

The intricacies of fractional laser technology present a transformative approach in the field of non-ablative skin rejuvenation. Unlike traditional laser therapies that operate on the principle of ablating the entire surface of the skin, fractional lasers deliver targeted beams that create micro-injuries within the skin, sparing the surrounding tissue. This method promotes rapid healing while simultaneously triggering the body's natural collagen production. By concentrating on specific areas of concern, fractional lasers can address various skin issues, including fine lines, wrinkles, and scar tissue, thereby enhancing skin texture and tone. Furthermore, the precision of fractional technology allows for versatile applications across different skin types, making it an attractive option for a broad patient demographic seeking cosmetic improvements. Additionally, the development of fractional laser technology has widened treatment options considerably, equipping practitioners with sophisticated instruments for monitoring and revising procedures. Of particular importance, non-invasive imaging modalities such as reflectance confocal microscopy (RCM) have proven to be useful adjuncts for laser treatments. With RCM, one can make a precise characterization of skin morphology, of special utility for evaluation of changes following treatment in regions such as the epidermis and dermis. Research shows that this monitoring ability improves results by enabling dermatologists to assess the efficacy of fractional lasers in real time, thus maximizing treatment regimens for vascular conditions and pigmentary problems (Amato et al., 2023). Consequently, RCM not only supports the customization of individual treatment courses but also adds to the mounting evidence regarding the effectiveness of fractional laser systems. The use of fractional lasers goes beyond rejuvenation of the skin and is interwoven with other specialties in cosmetic and reconstructive treatments. Being part of the general field of facial plastic surgery, fractional lasers are combined with other methods, such as injectable fillers and neural modulators, to achieve better aesthetic results (Barnes et al., 2016). This multi-disciplinary strategy mirrors the ever-changing environment of facial aesthetics, where pioneering technological innovations lie at the heart of enhancing the efficacy of treatment and patient satisfaction. Fractional laser technology is thus a key element in current cosmetic procedures, allowing clinicians to provide more discerning, individualized treatment while serving the needs of patients in skin rejuvenation. In general, the assimilation of fractional laser technology with any number of other cosmetic therapies places it as the bedrock of any nonablative rejuvenation therapies (Figure 8.2).

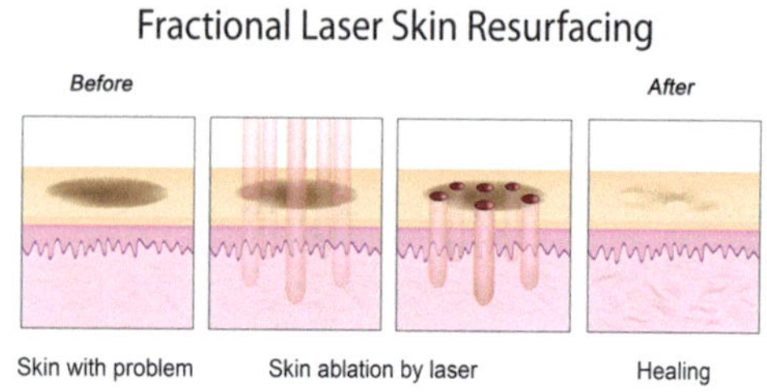

Figure 8.2. Fractional laser resurfacing.

Source: https://www.enfusemedspas.com/files/2017/01/pearl-pic.jpg.

Importance of Skin Rejuvenation in Dermatology

Dermatology more and more acknowledges the importance of skin rejuvenation as a worthwhile method to overcome aging signs, which not only improves the aesthetic value but also the general health of the skin. As people grow older, intrinsic and extrinsic causes like UV radiation exposure and pollution negatively affect the skin, often leading to wrinkles, discoloration, and lack of elasticity. Here, rejuvenation processes of the skin have developed not only as aesthetic therapies but also as crucial procedures to regain the beauty of the skin. This includes various therapies, from external medication to the most advanced technology in the form of laser beams, that all work together to recast skin texture, tone, and tautness, along with correcting inner biological alterations seen with aging. Therefore, awareness of the mechanisms and benefits of such rejuvenation procedures is essential for dermatologists in preparing perfect treatment protocols for patients. One of the major steps made in skin rejuvenation is the advent of non-ablative laser technologies, which have a number of benefits over traditional methods. Non-ablative lasers, unlike their ablative equivalents, attack the dermal layers underneath by stimulating them without eliminating the surface epidermis. This results in faster recovery and fewer side effects, thus making these technologies more appealing to patients seeking effective but minimally invasive treatments. Dermal fibroblasts' function and collagen synthesis induction are critical factors in this treatment. By causing thermal and biological responses, non-ablative lasers allow healthy regeneration of skin. In addition, laser technology development continues to be centered on optimizing outcomes, heralding a historic paradigm shift in the way dermatology is treating skin rejuvenation (Beigvand et al., 2020). The combination of both non-ablative and ablative methods has increased the range of possibilities for patients and dermatologists. Though ablative fractional CO_2 laser shows promising outcomes in treating extensive skin damage, such as deep folds and extreme photoaging, which come with additional side effects and a longer recovery time (Baldin et al., 2023). Non-ablative treatments, on the other hand, are more appropriate for those who want gentle changes with minimal time off. This approach would allow for individualization in treatment based on the trend of patient individualized care required by patients in the field of dermatology. Indeed, increased knowledge and utilization of such technologies point towards the need for constant research and development of clinical practice in the field so that rejuvenation treatment is safe, feasible, and effective for patients with a varying set of backgrounds and needs.

8.1. Mechanism of Action

Learning Outcome

1. Explain how non-ablative lasers work
2. Understand the role of fractional technology in skin treatment
3. Compare with ablative laser treatments

The action mechanism of non-ablative rejuvenation of the skin with the use of fractional lasers is based on therapeutic thermal injury to the dermal layer, which triggers a cascade of biological reactions. As opposed to ablative procedures, which strip the skin of its outer layer, non-ablative lasers like the Erbium:YAG and carbon dioxide lasers induce microscopic zones of heat in the skin, maintaining the epidermis. This selective targeting stimulates fibroblast activity, which is essential for collagen and elastin synthesis, leading to improved skin texture and elasticity. Furthermore, studies indicate that this laser-induced injury results in the reduction of matrix metalloproteinases (MMPs), which are responsible for extracellular matrix degradation, thereby enhancing dermal stability and resilience in treated areas (Beigvand et al., 2020). The improved remodeling of collagen maintains the structural integrity of skin over time and reduces the appearance of aging, making non-ablative techniques appealing to patients who are looking for rejuvenation without requiring significant downtime. Besides activation of fibroblasts, the healing response induced by nonablative fractional lasers stimulates keratinocyte proliferation in the epidermis, which contributes even more to skin rejuvenation. The targeted application of laser energy promotes the migration and differentiation of these cells, which are fundamental in restoring a healthy skin barrier and improving pigmentation irregularities associated with the aging process. It is through this mechanism that non-ablative lasers can effectively address a diverse range of skin conditions, including fine lines, sun damage, and uneven skin tone. While the skin heals, the new keratinocytes create a smoother and more even surface, improving the overall visual result (Dhillon et al., 2024). This multi-modal system differentiates non-ablative treatments as more desirable in aesthetic dermatology for individuals who want extensive rejuvenation with little pain and downtime. In addition, it is important to recognize the synergy between different treatment modalities to further improve the results of non-ablative skin rejuvenation. By combining energy-based devices, such as fractional lasers and radiofrequency (RF) treatments, practitioners can optimize results through synergistic effects. For instance, while laser treatment addresses dermal restructuring, complementary methods can enhance moisture levels and suppleness through the application of injectables like hyaluronic acid. Such integrative approaches not only expedite and amplify healing but also increase patient satisfaction. However, despite the promising outcomes, ongoing research is crucial to comprehensively evaluate the long-term safety and efficacy of these interventions, as well as to standardize treatment protocols (Dhillon et al., 2024). Thus, the evolution of non-ablative techniques is a dynamic area of study in dermatology, offering a roadmap for future innovations in skin rejuvenation.

8.1.1. How Non-Ablative Lasers Work

Non-ablative lasers are an advancement in dermatological treatments, primarily designed to rejuvenate the skin without causing as much thermal damage associated with ablative methods. Non-ablative lasers basically do not remove epidermal layers like traditional lasers do. Instead, they target the deeper layers of the skin, leaving the epidermis intact. This is achieved through mechanisms such as fractional photothermolysis, in which laser energy is concentrated in certain micro-zones within the skin. It is through this selective treatment that collagen and elastin production may be stimulated without requiring extended healing time; thus the procedure is less invasive and more available to a willing population seeking dermal rejuvenation or scar remodeling.

By concentrating on a fraction of the tissue, non-ablative lasers minimize the risk of complications and enhance recovery, aspects highly valued in cosmetic dermatology. The underlying principles of non-ablative laser technology hinge on the absorption of laser light by chromophores within the skin, primarily targeting water, hemoglobin, and melanin. With the conversion of laser energy into heat by these chromophores, the mechanism of controlled thermal injury confined to the dermis is excited. This mechanism effectively stimulates the activity of fibroblasts, leading to increased synthesis of collagen over time, thereby improving texture and smoothing out signs of aging or damage.

Additionally, the one-of-a-kind fractional technique, treating only a fraction of the skin, is designed to leave surrounding tissues unharmed, acting as a scaffold for rapid biological healing. Such a mechanism is critical for conditions like acne scars and periorbital wrinkles, where rejuvenation is desired with minimal downtime, demonstrating the practical applicability and popularity among patients seeking effective treatments without the extensive recovery associated with ablative lasers (Allemann & Kaufman, 2018). Clinical applications for non-ablative lasers are diverse, addressing various aesthetic concerns such as skin laxity, fine lines, textural irregularities, and vascular lesions. The U.S. Food and Drug Administration (FDA) has approved non-ablative fractional lasers for multiple indications, which include treatment of melasma and actinic keratoses, among others. Research continues to expand the understanding of how these lasers interact with skin physiology, particularly with the integration of imaging technologies like RCM to monitor treatment effects. RCM not only improves the assessment of dermal and epidermal structures before and after treatment but also helps in tailoring the protocols for different pathologies by visualizing the alterations in the epidermal and dermal structures. Thus, non-ablative lasers have been opening a new page toward tailoring treatment procedures, thereby becoming an essential part of modern-day dermatology practice (Amato et al., 2023) (Figure 8.3).

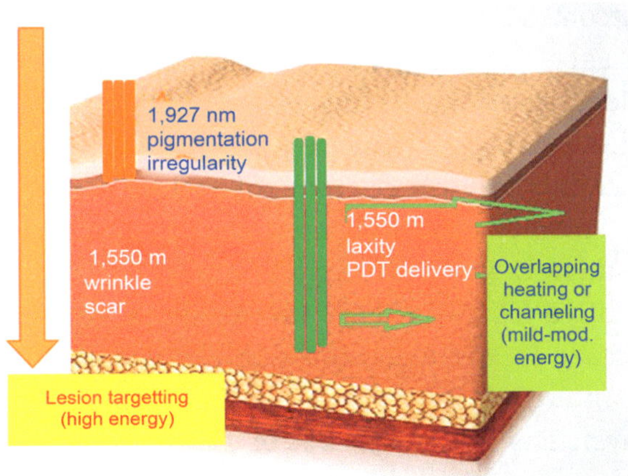

Figure 8.3. Schematic diagram of two treatment strategies for nonablative fractional dual laser. PDT, photodynamic therapy.

Source: https://www.researchgate.net/publication/348085478/figure/fig2/AS:976076851384321@1609726264390/Schematic-diagram-of-two-treatment-strategies-for-nonablative-fractional-dual-laser-PDT.png.

8.1.2. Role of Fractional Technology in Skin Treatment

Fractional technology has transformed the treatment of skin, particularly concerning non-ablative rejuvenation. Lasers provide energy to the whole surface, whereas fractional lasers provide energy in a grid, thereby creating microscopic zones of heat while leaving the tissue around it intact. A new way of doing this can potentially facilitate efficient skin remodeling with minimal recovery periods and side effects. Comfort of the patient and compliance with treatment plans are improved because the fractional method reduces downtime, presenting a desirable alternative for patients who want less destructive solutions to age-related problems of the skin, including wrinkles, pigmentation, and texture alterations. As exemplified by recent research, fractional laser technology opens up new avenues for treatments that can enhance skin quality without the side effects of more invasive ablative treatments (Baldin et al., 2023). Current investigations into the synergistic combination of fractional ablative and non-ablative lasers further emphasize the efficacy of fractional technology in treating the skin. By using these various laser wavelengths sequentially, practitioners are able to obtain excellent cosmetic results while drastically reducing patient downtime. For example, the cumulative effect of a fractional ablative CO_2 laser in combination with a non-ablative 1540 nm laser was found to enhance treatment efficacy and provide an added overall improvement in skin color and texture. The controlled delivery of energy, coupled with the preservation of surrounding skin structures, contributes to this technique's remarkable ability to stimulate collagen production and promote skin remodeling, demonstrating the versatility and effectiveness of fractional technologies in modern dermatological practice (Viviano et al., 2022). Additionally, the increasing versatility of fractional technologies has led to innovative treatment protocols that cater to individual skin types and conditions. The clinician can now tailor laser procedures to meet the particular patient requirements so that the wavelengths chosen, pulse forms, and levels of energy can be best suited to meet the specific dermatological needs for which treatment is being sought. Histological assessment of the effects of such treatments has now assumed a central importance, demonstrating the direct effect of the fractional laser at the cellular level. As evidence continues to accumulate for their efficacy, the incorporation of fractional technology into standard dermatologic practice is set to increase, solidifying its position as a pillar of non-ablative rejuvenation techniques. By adopting these cutting-edge methods, the discipline of dermatology can continue to innovate, offering patients the best possible means of achieving fresh, youthful-looking skin (Viviano et al., 2022; Baldin et al., 2023) (Figure 8.4).

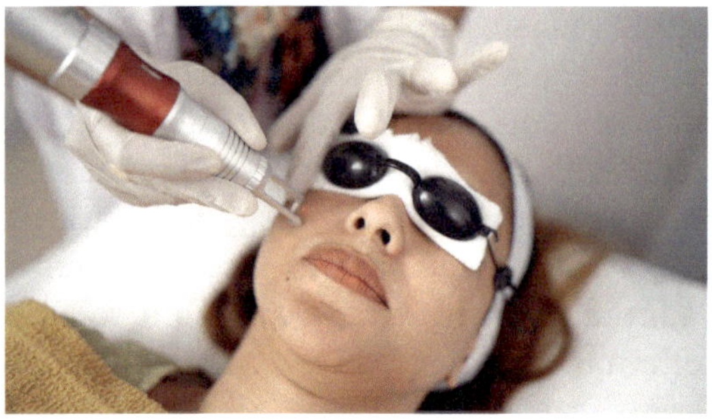

Figure 8.4. Fractional CO_2 laser resurfacing.

Source: https://dermavue.com/wp-content/uploads/2023/12/Fractional-CO2-Laser-Resurfacing-3.jpg.webp.

8.1.3. Comparison with Ablative Laser Treatments

The striking contrast between ablative and non-ablative laser treatments underlines contrasts in mechanisms and results in terms of skin rejuvenation. Ablative lasers, including fractional CO_2 lasers, ablate the outer layer of the skin, thus immediately making alterations in texture and color of the skin more apparent. It is for this reason, though, that this treatment can cause extended periods of downtime as the skin recovers, with redness, swelling, and pain common in patients after recovery. In contrast, non-ablative treatments, like those using fractional non-ablative lasers, destroy deep dermal layers without harming the epidermis, allowing for a faster recovery and less pain associated with it.

Consequently, although ablative procedures offer immediate outcomes, non-ablative treatments appeal to those wanting less aggressive treatment with minimal disruption to their lifestyles, and thus they are becoming more popular in modern dermatologic practice. Further, combined treatment regimens incorporating both ablative and non-ablative lasers are attracting attention in the field. Studies indicate that an approach synergistically combining both modalities can maximize outcomes by capitalizing on the benefits present in each modality. As an example, one study underscored the promise of a fractional ablative followed by non-ablative laser treatment as maximizing cosmetic benefits while reducing downtime that accompanies conventional ablative therapy. Through the use of fractional ablative lasers initially to create the required surface injury and then non-ablative therapy to induce more intense dermal remodeling, physicians can attain better skin quality with an easily tolerated healing process.

This novel technique demonstrates how mixing various laser technologies might represent a superior yet patient-friendly treatment for skin rejuvenation, as evidenced by recent preclinical results (Viviano et al., 2022). Contrarily, within the paradigm of skin renewal, the biological response to ablative compared to non-ablative laser is fundamentally different, thereby fundamentally altering the selection of therapy used upon specific need. Ablative laser treatment induces a wound healing response that deeply influences protein expression signatures in treated tissue with resultant increased synthesis of collagen and elastin with extracellular matrix remodeling (Beigvand et al., 2020). Conversely, non-ablative lasers primarily stimulate dermal activity without disrupting the epidermis, leading to a more gradual enhancement in skin quality through ongoing cellular activity, including fibroblast activation. This distinct difference in molecular response is critical for practitioners to consider when devising treatment planning strategies aimed at achieving optimal rejuvenation outcomes tailored to patient expectations. Understanding these variations can considerably impact therapeutic choices in the treatment centers for skin rejuvenation, thereby improving the overall efficacy of laser treatments.

Test Your Knowledge

1. What is the mechanism of action of a non-ablative fractional laser?
2. What is fractional skin treatment?

8.2. Types of Non-Ablative Lasers

Learning Outcome

1. Describe Nd:YAG lasers
2. Understand diode lasers for non-ablative skin rejuvenation
3. Describe erbium glass lasers

These are types of non-ablative lasers that play a very crucial role in rejuvenating the skin, especially when it comes to issues such as fine lines, wrinkles, and uneven skin texture, without the prolonged recovery associated with ablative procedures. Non-ablative lasers work by targeting deeper parts of the skin without damaging the epidermis to encourage the production of collagen and general improvement of skin texture. Among the common forms, there are the NIR lasers and PDL, based on two different mechanisms of action. NIR lasers use infrared light to reach deeper skin layers, to be then heated and subsequently remodeled by remodeling collagen. PDL acts differently because it has sites of action on the molecules in the blood within the blood vessels, hence being more productive on vascular lesions and pigmented lesions. Both are highly effective in enhancing skin quality with a lesser risk of side effects than their ablative equivalents. Fractional non-ablative lasers are a notable step forward in skin rejuvenation technology, enabling focused treatment of targeted skin areas without leaving untouched tissue behind. Fractional treatment decreases downtime and minimizes side effects, thereby making the treatment more patient-friendly. The two main forms of fractional non-ablative lasers include the Nd:YAG and Erbium-glass lasers. Nd:YAG lasers are usually deeper penetrating and are useful in treating vascular abnormalities and stimulating collagen production. In contrast, Erbium-glass lasers target the shallow skin levels, ideal for those who need to enhance skin texture and moderate photodamage. The application of these fractional lasers is indicative of ongoing advancement in non-surgical skin treatments and is an advancement toward achieving optimal results with minimal disruption to daily life, ultimately to achieve maximum patient satisfaction. The selection of the particular type of non-ablative laser treatment should be guided by the patient needs and skin conditions. Factors such as skin type, age, and desired outcomes all play a fundamental role in determining the most appropriate laser modality. For example, individuals with darker skin may benefit more from the Nd:YAG laser, which is less likely to induce post-inflammatory hyperpigmentation (PIH), a common concern with many laser treatments. Moreover, the flexibility of the fractional approach enables tailored treatment plans that address specific skin issues, maximizing effect and minimizing side effects. With ongoing research and emerging technology, lasers remain a dynamic therapy in the constantly evolving field of non-invasive aesthetic treatments. Continued interest in successful, low-risk rejuvenation methods underscores the relevance of these sophisticated laser-based treatments to contemporary dermatology (Barikbin et al., 2011; Baldin et al., 2023).

8.2.1. Nd:YAG Lasers

The neodymium-doped yttrium aluminum garnet (Nd:YAG) laser has become an important technology in nonablative rejuvenation, primarily due to its unique wavelength and interaction properties with tissue. It usually operates at 1064 nm, so it has the power to reach deeper layers of the skin without causing much disruption to the surface. This is, therefore, an important factor for patients who see real value in effective treatment with minimal downtime. This makes it possible to both thermally stimulate the production of collagen and treat a range of skin disorders, including those resulting from photoaging and skin texture abnormalities. The ability of the Nd:YAG laser to be tailored for use in fractional modes, wherein the beam is divided up into multiple microbeams targeting specific areas of the skin with minimal damage to the surrounding tissue provides for the most efficient healing and rejuvenation. The effectiveness of Nd:YAG laser is highlighted in comparative studies comparing its action with other technologies, including fractional CO_2 lasers. In one study, the treatment of atrophic acne scars was noted where Nd:YAG lasers showed pronounced safety and efficacy but less severe adverse effects than their ablative equivalents. In this study, both the picosecond Nd:YAG laser with holographic optics and the fractional CO_2 laser were administered in a controlled manner, showing no significant difference in physician-evaluated improvement despite the fractional CO_2 laser achieving better clinical outcomes in some aspects. Such results suggest that, although Nd:YAG might be inferior to all other laser types regarding aesthetics, its benefits in terms of safety and patient priority make it a precious tool for most applications in skin rejuvenation (Yuan et al., 2024). Additionally, the innovative application areas of Nd:YAG lasers also include the domain of combination therapies that prove to increase their efficacy in composite use with other treatment modalities. For instance, combining the Nd:YAG lasers with surface agents or alternative laser wavelengths, synergistic effects enhance outcomes, even in those who undergo correction of multiple skin concerns. Treatment protocols that respond effectively and can be obtained through the use of Nd:YAG lasers make them an integral component in comprehensive skin rejuvenation paradigms. These developments are supported by an increasing volume of research aimed at reducing risks, such as hyperpigmentation in diverse skin types that may be of especially great importance to darker skin tones. As further studies continue to develop the uses of the Nd:YAG laser in dermatology, its application in non-ablative rejuvenation of the skin will surely increase, providing patients with more individualized and effective treatments (Haykal et al., 2024) (Figure 8.5).

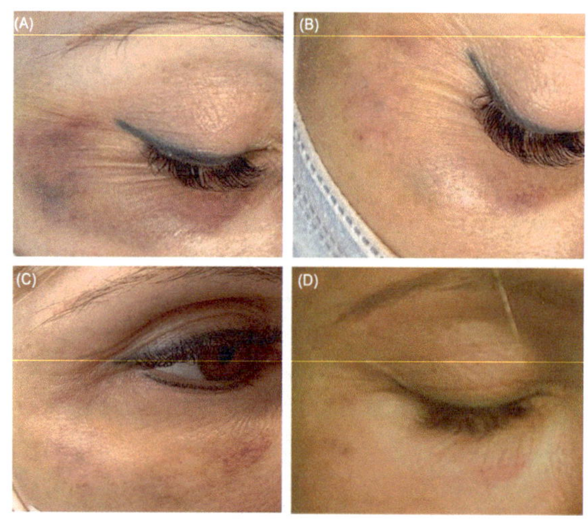

Figure 8.5. Gradual resolution of a bruise during seven days of Nd:YAG laser treatment. The bruise occurred after a dermal filler procedure. (A) Before the first laser session; (B) Two days after first laser session; (C) Two days after the second laser session; and (D) Two days after the third laser session.

Source: https://www.researchgate.net/publication/359282608/figure/fig1/AS:11431281172693931@1688639126052/Gradual-resolution-of-a-bruise-during-seven-days-of-NdYAG-laser-treatment-The-bruise.png.

8.2.2. Diode Lasers

This area of non-ablative skin rejuvenation has been to a great extent revolutionized by the diode lasers. These are promising and alternative means for classic ablative laser treatments. Different from their ablative peers, which remove the outermost layers of skin, diode lasers work through selective photothermolysis targeting specific chromophores in the skin without significant thermal damage to the surrounding tissue. This new mechanism not only allows for improved safety and reduced recovery periods but also minimizes the risk of adverse side effects such as dyspigmentation and scarring, which are common with more invasive techniques. The efficacy of diode lasers in skin rejuvenation stems from their ability to stimulate collagen synthesis, promoting a natural regenerative process that enhances skin texture and tone over time, thus making them a favored choice for many practitioners in cosmetic dermatology (Barikbin et al., 2011). The versatility of diode lasers extends beyond mere skin rejuvenation to encompass various dermatological applications, including the treatment of acne scars. For example, a dual-wavelength diode laser system provides simultaneous emission of different wavelengths, thereby targeting certain skin imperfections. Studies show that such systems can effectively manage atrophic acne scars by combining deep tissue penetration with superficial remodeling of the skin. Those treated with diode lasers have reported satisfactory improvements in skin texture and scar appearance. Patients who have been given treatments using the diode laser have testified to the technology's utility and capability. Evidence shows that downtime with these non-ablative procedures is significantly minimal, and in most cases, it goes a long way to reduce patient interference with daily activities as well as raise general satisfaction with aesthetic treatments (Amoruso et al., 2023). Apart from their effectiveness and low side effects, diode lasers have been known for their specific property of being easily incorporated into different fractional laser modalities. Fractional laser treatments, which subdivide laser energy into microbeams, enable precise targeting of skin tissues while preserving surrounding areas, thus promoting faster healing and allowing for a more tolerable overall experience. This fractional approach, combined with the advantages of diode laser technology, creates an innovative synergy that amplifies treatment outcomes in skin rejuvenation. Finally, the continued development of diode laser applications, combined with their coupling with fractional methods, underscores their critical position in modern cosmetic procedures aimed at promoting aesthetic enhancement with minimal downtime and maximum patient safety (Barikbin et al., 2011) (Figure 8.6).

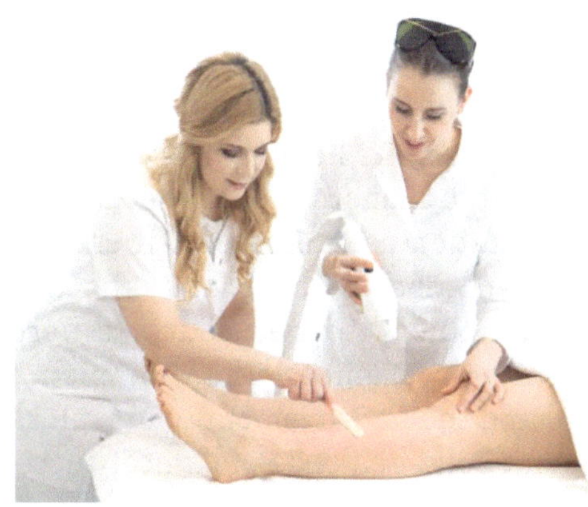

Figure 8.6. Diode laser treatment.

Source: https://www.konmison.com/wp-content/uploads/2024/01/diode-laser-treatment.webp.

8.2.3. Erbium Glass Lasers

A novel application for Erbium glass lasers is applied in non-ablative skin rejuvenation. These lasers work based on the principle of targeting water content in skin with minimal damage to the surrounding tissues. By using the fractionally treated approach, the intact remaining tissues can be preserved, making it less agonizing for the users, while giving the patients a beneficial outcome from the treatment process. Such a procedure ensures faster healing with necessary stimulation to produce collagen, which is a principal element in the successful rejuvenation of young skin. Clinical studies have indicated that the patients have less downtime as compared to the traditional ablative lasers, making Erbium glass lasers popular for effectively rejuvenated skin without increased dangers of complications due to postoperative morbidity, hence increasing wider acceptance in aesthetic dermatology (Allemann & Kaufman, 2018). Moreover, the special wavelength of Erbium glass lasers enables targeting deeper into skin imperfections, including fine lines, wrinkles, and textural irregularities, with much finer accuracy than its counterparts. With the Er:YAG laser, its controlled thermal effect vaporizes only the superficial layers of the skin, giving it much better precision control, which reduces the damage caused to the skin; the primary reason its healing process is more favorable and the chances of side effects such as hyperpigmentation are decreased. It enhances the growing number of clinicians who adopt this new technology to be used in different applications, for example, the treatment of acne scars and the improvement of overall skin texture. With solid evidence of clinical success, the effectiveness of the laser to resurface non-ablatively establishes its invaluable position in modern dermatology practices, corresponding to the increased call for non-invasive cosmetic procedures (Beigvand et al., 2020). In addition to their aesthetic applications, Erbium glass lasers have been shown to induce both histological and molecular changes that promote long-term skin rejuvenation. Studies indicate that these lasers stimulate the proliferation of fibroblasts and keratinocytes, leading to increased production of collagen and elastin within the dermal matrix. These changes are crucial in combating signs of aging and restoring skin elasticity. Additionally, the decrease in MMPs observed following laser therapy further highlights the therapeutic value of Erbium glass lasers, as MMPs break down extracellular matrix components. As ongoing research continues to elucidate the biological effects of laser treatments, it becomes evident that Erbium glass lasers stand out as a safe and effective modality for achieving younger, healthier skin, underscoring their relevance in the evolving landscape of non-ablative skin rejuvenation (Beigvand et al., 2020) (Figure 8.7).

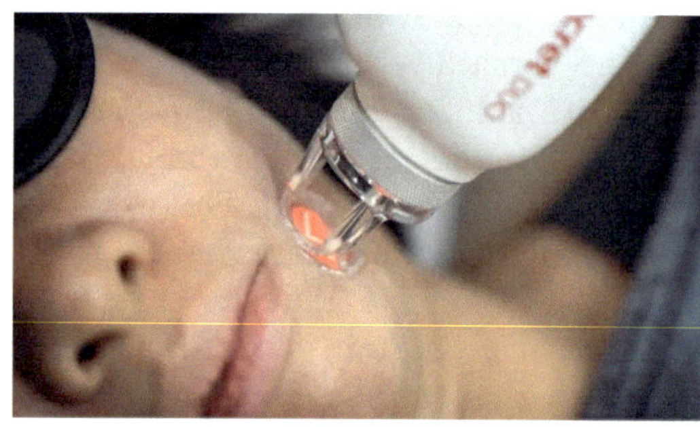

Figure 8.7. Erbium laser treatment.

Source: https://www.clearskin.in/wp-content/uploads/2024/07/Erbium-Glass-Laser-1.webp.

Test Your Knowledge

1. What does the Nd:YAG laser do for skin?
2. Is erbium laser ablative or non-ablative? Explain.

8.3. Indications for Treatment

Learning Outcome

1. Explain the role of skin tightening and lifting
2. Discuss the use in the treatment of acne scars
3. Understand how non-ablative fractional lasers reduce pigmentation and sun damage

The contraindications for non-ablative fractional laser treatment are extensive and include most skin issues that bother patients who would like cosmetic rejuvenation. Generally, the treatments are ideal for patients who show signs of aging, including fine lines, wrinkles, and loss of skin elasticity. In addition, patients who have photodamage in the form of uneven skin texture or tone benefit greatly from non-ablative laser treatments. The ability of these lasers to target deeper skin layers while minimizing damage to the outer skin makes them particularly attractive for those who wish to improve their skin quality without the downtime associated with invasive procedures. As the demand for minimally invasive cosmetic options increases, understanding the specific indications for these treatments becomes imperative for practitioners to tailor therapies to meet patient expectations effectively. Aside from aesthetic renewal, non-ablative fractioned lasers are also indicated for the treatment of some dermatological concerns. These include acne scars, large pores, and rosacea, which all lower one's self-esteem and quality of life. The lasers act by stimulating collagen growth, resulting in better texture and appearance of the skin over time. Research has confirmed that patients experience fewer universal side effects of the traditional ablative lasers, hence rendering non-ablative treatments more popular. As confirmed in literature, non-ablative fractional resurfacing reduces side effects without being less effective compared to other skin dermatological interventions, ultimately rendering higher patient satisfaction and adherence to treatment regimes in the long term (Barikbin et al., 2011). In addition, the flexibility of non-ablative fractional lasers enables practitioners to design customized treatment regimens according to the needs of individual patients. The settings on the laser can be adjusted according to the patient's skin type, treatment objective, and degree of dermatological condition to be treated. This flexibility is vital for delivering the best outcome, as well as for treating patients who are apprehensive about more intensive treatment. Evidence indicates that non-ablative treatments have increased in popularity because of their reduced rate of side effects and shorter recovery periods, and as such, they are a first-line option for most people (Stoian et al., 2019). With the evolution of non-surgical aesthetics, it is essential to learn about the numerous indications for therapy with these new technologies.

8.3.1. Skin Tightening and Lifting

The search for successful skin tightening and lifting has thereby led to great strides in non-invasive therapies, particularly through the development of fractional laser treatment. Unlike ablative treatments that remove skin layers, primarily leaving behind extensive recovery, non-ablative methods provoke collagen remodeling without destroying the outer layer of the skin. This less invasive approach sidesteps problems like dyspigmentation, residual erythema, and scarring, complications that have long dogged patients scheduled to receive conventional treatments. With each study that continues to validate the efficacy of non-ablative fractional lasers, practitioners now have a powerful tool for addressing lax skin and facial signs of aging that are mild to moderate in severity in the most patient-friendly and time-effective manner available (Barikbin et al., 2011). A pivotal aspect of skin tightening and lifting through non-ablative methods lies in the ability to stimulate the skin's natural regenerative processes. The fractional nature of the laser creates microscopic treatment zones within the dermis, inducing controlled thermal injury that triggers an immune response. This leads to the production of new collagen and elastin over time, thereby enhancing skin firmness and elasticity. As a result, patients often experience gradual and natural improvements in skin texture and tightness. The ability to tailor treatment settings based on individual skin types and conditions further amplifies the effectiveness of these procedures, making them a versatile option in aesthetic dermatology (Penev, 2022). Moreover, the integration of non-ablative skin tightening with other modalities enhances the overall rejuvenation experience. The use of fractional laser treatment together with RF or ultrasound technologies can produce a synergistic effect, yielding better lifting results for addressing deeper aspects of the skin. This multi-pronged therapy does not just stimulate collagen production but also enhances tissue cohesion and surface contours. Patients thus enjoy the benefits of immediate tightening as well as longer-term rejuvenation. Continual exploration of these combined techniques is necessary to refine protocols and optimize outcomes, ensuring that skin tightening and lifting methodologies remain at the forefront of non-invasive cosmetic treatments (Barikbin et al., 2011) (Figure 8.8).

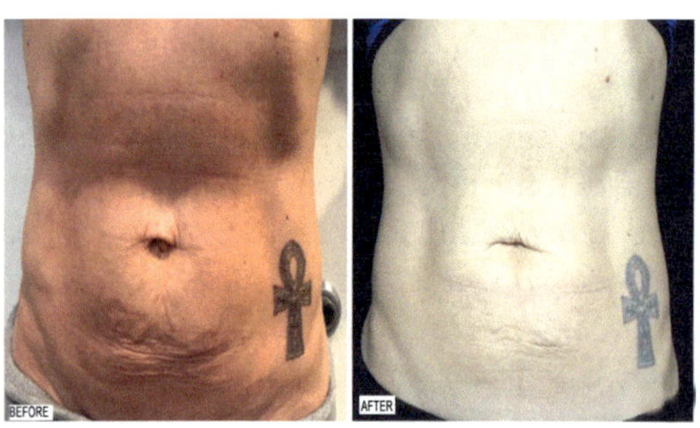

Figure 8.8. Before and after radiofrequency skin tightening.

Source: https://post.healthline.com/wp-content/uploads/2020/10/Before-and-after-radiofrequency-skin-tightening-1296X728-slide1.jpg.

8.3.2. Treatment of Acne Scars

The treatment of acne marks has gained much attention lately in dermatological practices due to the psychological and aesthetic burden imposed by such marks. Among the non-ablative methods of rejuvenating skin, fractional lasers stand out as a promising alternative for those seeking effective scar management. These lasers provide energy delivery to the dermis with minimal epidermal destruction, thus stimulating collagen generation and skin remodeling. Among these methods, the 1064-nm picosecond laser with holographic optics has demonstrated significant efficacy in addressing atrophic acne scars. A comparative study highlighted that this non-ablative nature results in fewer adverse effects compared to traditional ablative lasers, offering a safer alternative for many patients seeking improvement in their skin texture and appearance (Yuan et al., 2024). The 1565 nm non-ablative fractional laser is the other latest approach in acne scar treatment, besides the picosecond laser. This laser causes micro-injuries in the skin, hence stimulating collagen regrowth and improving the texture of the skin over a period. Dermatology has seen the increased use of this laser because of its efficacy in facial rejuvenation treatments and reduction of patient downtime. While certain individuals experience side effects like erythema and edema after treatment, they are generally transient and controllable. The addition of newer methods, for example, combining the 1565 nm non-ablative fractional laser with 30% super molecular salicylic acid, has been found to help mitigate side effects, thus enhancing patient satisfaction and global outcomes of the treatment (Zeng et al., 2024). Finally, the decision on which laser treatment of acne scars should be based on individual patient requirements, the unique nature of the scars, and side effects. Although both the picosecond and 1565 nm non-ablative fractional lasers have distinct advantages in the treatment of acne scars, continuous research and clinical experience are needed to refine protocols and increase efficacy. The integration of personalized treatment plans that may combine these technologies can lead to improved aesthetic results and minimize recovery times. As techniques continue to evolve within non-ablative skin rejuvenation, the future of acne scar treatment holds potential for safer, more effective therapies that can profoundly impact patients' self-esteem and quality of life (Figure 8.9).

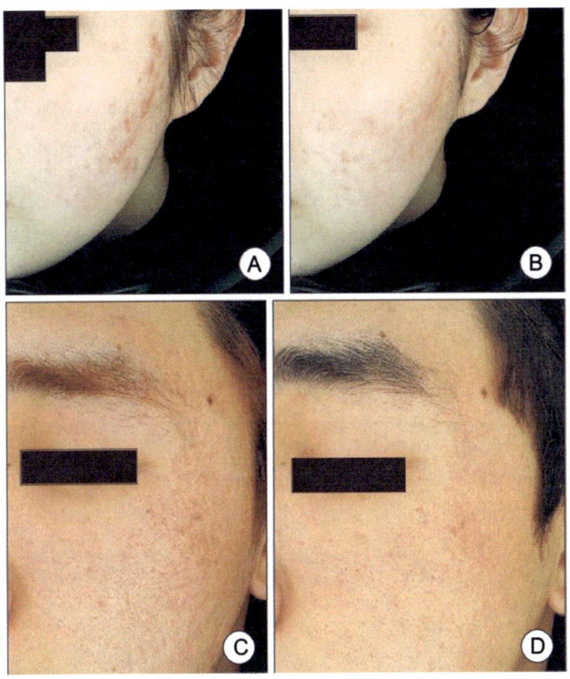

Figure 8.9. Acne scar cases treated with nonablative fractional dual laser. (A) Preclinical photograph; (B) Clinical photograph after treatment. Acute acne can be resolved after treatment; (C) Preclinical photograph; and (D) Clinical photograph after treatment. Improvement of the chronic acne scars can be seen.

Source: https://www.researchgate.net/publication/348085478/figure/fig3/AS:976076851404800@1609726264439/Acne-scar-cases-treated-with-nonablative-fractional-dual-laser-A-Preclinical.png.

8.3.3. Reduction of Pigmentation and Sun Damage

The increasing prevalence of sun damage and hyperpigmentation among individuals has prompted a significant interest in effective dermatological interventions. Non-ablative skin rejuvenation techniques, particularly fractional laser therapy, have emerged as notable solutions to address these issues. These procedures work by delivering targeted laser energy to the deeper layers of the skin, stimulating collagen production without the need for invasive methods. This results in a decrease in pigmentation, whereby the laser selectively removes melanin deposits but stimulates skin renewal. The benefit of non-ablative methods is their capacity to reduce downtime and thus are a desirable choice for patients who want aesthetic enhancement without prolonged recovery (Beigvand et al., 2020). As healthcare professionals learn more and more about these technologies, the incorporation of non-ablative procedures into general practice continues to grow, opening a multifaceted avenue for skin rejuvenation. In addition to working on pigment reduction, fractional lasers have proven to reverse the morphological and biochemical markers of sun damage. Studies show that the impact the lasers have had on the surface pigmentation induces positive histological changes in the skin. Activation of fibroblasts by non-ablative lasers enhances the formation of new elastin and collagen fibers in the dermis. This is essential to achieve the normal state concerning skin elasticity, firmness, and quality, usually compromised by the effects of sun exposure (Beigvand et al., 2020). There was also an induction of MMPs reduction, which might provide a restorative effect capable of countering the extracellular matrix deterioration otherwise triggered by UV radiation. These results highlight the rejuvenating power of fractional laser technology not only in treating current skin conditions but also in making the skin more resistant to future sun damage. As the science of aesthetic dermatology continues to advance, clinicians must also be aware of the nuances of pre- and post-treatment care that come with non-ablative procedures. Proper patient expectations, along with comprehensive knowledge of the advantages and disadvantages of procedures, is the root of achieving good results in skin rejuvenation. Clinicians must be well aware to educate patients regarding the expected improvements in pigmentation and texture while also making them aware of proper protective measures against exposure to the sun following treatment. A holistic approach also requires routine maintenance procedures to prolong the benefits gained from the initial treatments. The combined application of fractional lasers with adjunctive therapies such as chemical peels or topical therapy can also further increase efficacy and satisfaction, solidifying the position of these minimally invasive treatments in today's dermatologic practice (Figure 8.10).

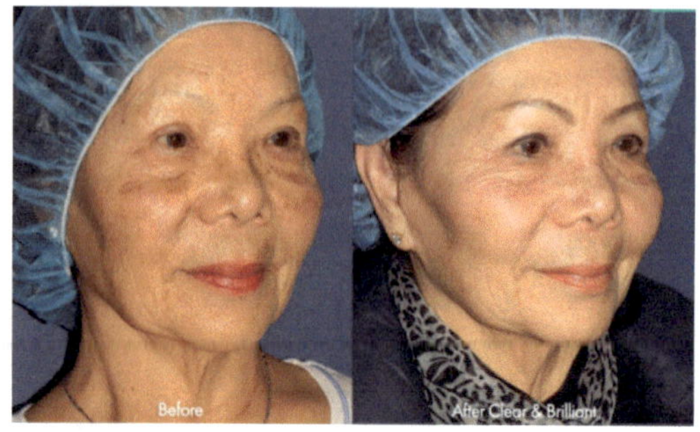

Figure 8.10. Before and after sun damage treatment.

Source: https://clderm.com/wp-content/uploads/2023/03/Clear_and_Brilliant_to_treat_sun_damage_Boen_CLDerm_San_Diego_ABCDE_653079_3-600x400.jpg.

Test Your Knowledge

1. What skin conditions are commonly treated with non-ablative fractional lasers, and how do these lasers benefit patients with these conditions?
2. How effective is non-ablative fractional laser treatment in improving skin texture and tone for individuals with post-acne scars or other forms of scarring?

8.4. Benefits of Non-Ablative Treatments

Learning Outcome

1. Explain how non-ablative treatments take minimal downtime compared to ablative methods
2. Discuss how non-ablative treatments are less risky
3. Understand the versatility in treating various skin types

Non-ablative treatments have gained increasing popularity in the realm of skin rejuvenation, primarily due to their multifaceted benefits. One of the most significant advantages is the minimized downtime associated with these procedures. Unlike ablative treatments, which remove layers of skin and often necessitate extensive recovery periods, non-ablative technologies enable patients to resume their daily activities almost immediately. This is especially attractive for people with active lifestyles who demand efficient solutions without the encumbrance of long healing periods. Further, the diminished risk of adverse effects, e.g., scarring or delayed redness, is reflective of a significant rise in patient satisfaction. Therefore, non-ablative treatments are not just more practical but also resonate with increasing societal needs for beauty with minimal disruption to daily life (Stoian et al., 2019). Another strong argument in favor of non-ablative treatments is their capacity to induce collagen remodeling without invasive techniques. By using technologies like fractional laser systems, they have been shown to induce deep dermal heating, prompting the body's natural healing processes to improve the elasticity and firmness of the skin. In their effectiveness, the sequential treatment protocols incorporating both ablative and non-ablative lasers point to such synergy in boosting skin rejuvenation outcomes. Specifically, research indicates that utilizing such complementary modalities can provide better outcomes while still enjoying the shallow healing pattern typical of non-ablative treatments (Viviano et al., 2022).

This seems to be the best of both worlds, wherein practitioners can provide better outcomes in skin texture and tone. Further, the versatility offered by non-ablative treatments is applicable to a broad array of cosmetic issues and is thus compatible with varied patient requirements. These treatments are able to take on concerns from fine lines and wrinkles to irregular pigmentation and skin texture. For those patients who want the benefits of facial rejuvenation without surgery, non-ablative treatments offer a strong option for creating dramatic changes. With understanding of these treatments continuing to grow, practitioners are better able to customize protocols that yield the most dramatic individual effects while carrying lower risks. Such personalization not only improves patient results but also creates an even greater sense of trust between practitioners and patients, which can result in long-term treatment compliance and overall satisfaction with the aesthetic experience (Stoian et al., 2019). The aggregate advantages of non-ablative treatments place them as a revolutionary force in modern skincare practices.

8.4.1. Minimal Downtime Compared to Ablative Methods

The development of non-ablative rejuvenation methods of the skin has thus touched on this major point of downtime caused by conventional ablative procedures. Though highly effective at managing an array of skin issues, ablative treatments typically go hand-in-glove with durations of long recovery surrounded by erythema, edema, and complications that can extend to scarring or hyperpigmentation. Side effects produce surgery downtime that can range from a few weeks to days, which is quite an inconvenience to patients who need cosmetic enhancement. Non-ablative lasers, however, can provide effective rejuvenation with much less downtime, and individuals can return immediately to their normal lives with minimal interference with their lifestyle. This aspect is crucial for many patients who prioritize convenience and accessibility in their skincare routines while still seeking effective treatment outcomes (Barikbin et al., 2011). The efficacy of non-ablative technologies, such as fractional lasers, complements their minimal downtime advantage, creating a compelling option for those wary of the prolonged recovery associated with ablative treatments. Fractional non-ablative lasers entail treating only a percentage of the skin, thus leaving the surrounding tissues intact and shortening healing time. Mild erythema and swelling are usually experienced by the patients. But according to many studies, this condition has been found to resolve in just days, unlike weeks wasted with ablative treatments. Low side effects also confirm that the low-risk aspect of the non-ablative procedures increases patients' satisfaction and acceptance. The dual-wavelength system described in the recently published article demonstrates how combined wavelengths can enhance results while preserving this minimal downtime benefit, driving the popularity of non-ablative techniques even more (Amoruso et al., 2023). The minimal downtime nature of skin rejuvenation through nonablative technology marks a significant advancement in dermatologic practice and represents how patients are addressing skin augmentation procedures. As social standards increasingly promote treatments that won't interrupt professional or personal schedules, non-ablative lasers provide a realistic solution without compromising efficacy. The toned-down recovery time is especially attractive to those with active lives or social obligations that bar prolonged downtime. This tactical realignment of emphasis away from invasively ablative methods toward non-ablative ones reflects an overarching trend toward patient-centered care in dermatology, wherein the pursuit of aesthetic enhancement is balanced against the necessity for convenience and minimal disruption to one's daily routine (Barikbin et al., 2011).

8.4.2. Lower Risk of Complications

The advent of non-ablative skin rejuvenation methods is a major improvement in cosmetic dermatology, especially because they carry less risk for complications than the conventional ablative treatments. Conventional ablative resurfacing treatments, though effective, are often associated with an array of side effects, including dyspigmentation, lasting erythema, and scarring, which can place a heavy burden on recovery for patients. The pursuit of higher cosmetic results with decreased adverse effects has driven the creation of non-ablative treatments, which are more manageable. With newer technologies in place, these interventions accomplish rejuvenation of the skin without the prolonged recovery time that goes along with their ablative counterparts and therefore increase the pool of patients interested in finding such low-risk, powerful therapeutic methods to make perfect and minimize skin imperfections and signs of aging (Barikbin et al., 2011). Non-ablative fractional lasers represent the critical breakthrough here, mainly due to their focused nature that diminishes the risk of complications. Such devices treat only a portion of the skin's surface and preserve adjacent untreated tissue, thus helping maintain the integrity of the skin as well as increasing the pace of healing. This novel modality not only decreases inflammation and the rate of adverse events but also enhances natural healing processes through enhancing tissue repair and remodeling of collagen. Disruption to the epidermal barrier was reduced, and the rate of complications such as infection or protracted erythema was reduced to a markedly lower rate than that reported for full-field ablative resurfacing treatments. As a result, patients can expect not only improved aesthetic results but also a more comfortable and safer recovery experience without the extensive downtime typically associated with more invasive laser treatments (Allemann & Kaufman, 2018). Moreover, the FDA's approval of non-ablative fractional lasers for a variety of dermatological conditions underscores their safety profile and clinical effectiveness. Such therapies are utilized not only for cosmetic enhancements but also for corrective treatments of conditions like acne scars and melasma, evidencing their versatility and lower complication rates. Research consistently indicates that patients experience fewer side effects, allowing for a broader demographic to safely engage in these procedures without the fear of severe postoperative complications. As clinical guidelines advance, practitioners prefer more non-ablative modalities, indicating an increasing amount of evidence and a growing consensus about their effectiveness and safety. This may further encourage compliance and patient satisfaction in achieving skin rejuvenation results with minimized risks of complications (Barikbin et al., 2011).

8.4.3. Versatility in Treating Various Skin Types

The fractional laser versatility and non-ablative skin rejuvenation is a significant factor that allows it to be used on all skin types. Unlike ablative procedures that target the superficial skin, non-ablative lasers penetrate further into the skin without disrupting the surface layer. Using this technique, the treatments can then target various problems like wrinkles, abnormal pigmentation, and texture imperfections in various skin types, from fair skin to darker complexions. As a result, patients may experience considerable improvement with minimal down time; today, in the era of aesthetic medicine, recovery time significantly impacts patient satisfaction and return on investment for practitioners. Moreover, the versatility of these technologies further enhances their acceptability and effectiveness and makes them the gold standard in modern dermatology (Stoian et al., 2019). Education and experience are critical to optimizing the adaptability of non-ablative therapies across different skin types. Practitioners familiar with diverse dermal properties, i.e., melanin density and epidermal thickness, can customize treatments to match specific requirements, maximizing outcomes while minimizing complications. For example, the use of fractional lasers can be modified to provide varying levels of energy and patterns of coverage, which improves their effectiveness on patients with distinctive skin textures and conditions. Therefore, customized treatment protocols not only consider the wide range of skin types but also enable practitioners to devise creative improvements and developments in techniques, resulting in effective outcomes and building patient confidence in non-ablative treatments. This bespoke approach is underscored by the evolutionary character of the field, where research and innovation are continually at the fore (Viviano et al., 2022). Further, the all-encompassing synergy of non-ablative rejuvenation technologies in the management of conditions like Striae distensae (SD) also underscores their versatility. Studies point to how patients from various backgrounds, including those with extensive stretch marks, have effectively gained from non-ablative fractional technologies like the Nd:YAP laser. In a recent study, treatment was significantly effective, with 88% of the patients showing excellent enhancements in the look of their SD after several sessions. The fact that such varied cases could be treated safely and effectively without significant side effects is testimony to the potential of non-ablative lasers as an important tool for aesthetic dermatology. This innovation gives more confident and trusting patients to opt for non-invasive solutions, thereby expanding the therapeutic space for a wider variety of skin issues (Viviano et al., 2022) (Figure 8.11).

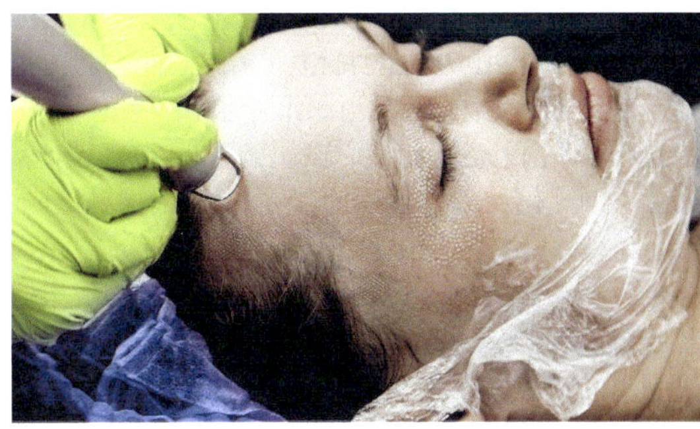

Figure 8.11. A patient undergoing fractional CO_2 laser resurfacing, a dermatological procedure that uses targeted laser energy to treat wrinkles, scars, and skin texture by promoting collagen remodeling and skin renewal.

Source: https://post.medicalnewstoday.com/wp-content/uploads/sites/3/2022/04/cosmetologist-face-co2-laser-header-1024x575.jpg.

Test Your Knowledge

1. What are the primary advantages of non-ablative treatments over ablative treatments?
2. How do non-ablative treatments reduce the risk of complications compared to more invasive, ablative procedures?

8.5. Potential Risks and Side Effects

Learning Outcome

1. Describe common side effects
2. Explain rare complications
3. Discuss the importance of patient selection and consultation

A new set of non-ablative skin rejuvenation techniques has taken the world by storm as they help rejuvenate the skin with minimal down time. However, no procedure is risk-free and side effect-free, especially fractional laser, and may depend quite essentially on the individual types and conditions of the skin. Commonly reported adverse effects include erythema, swelling, and discomfort following the treatment, which, although typically transient, can cause anxiety for patients who are unprepared for these reactions. Furthermore, individual responses to the treatment can differ, leading some patients to experience prolonged or more severe symptoms. For example, individuals with darker skin tones may be at a higher risk of PIH, presenting a considerable challenge for clinicians when assessing potential risks associated with fractional laser treatments (Penev, 2022). All potential risks must be meticulously communicated to patients before the procedure, emphasizing the importance of informed consent. Knowledge of the complete extent of side effects, including scarring or textural alterations, enables patients to make informed choices about their care. As set forth in today's clinical practice guidelines, professionals should initiate a multifaceted pre- and post-procedure care plan to address these potential problems. This involves advising patients to abstain from specific drugs or topical preparations that might increase the risk of adverse effects. Clinicians are encouraged to create a robust educational framework to ensure that patients are aware of the implications of choosing minimally invasive cosmetic procedures within the context of their skincare goals (Madnani et al., 2022). The emotional and psychological implications of experiencing side effects can also add layers of complexity to the treatment process. Patients may experience considerable distress following non-ablative skin rejuvenation if they develop unforeseen or extreme complications. The treatment of these psychological impacts is a critical aspect of postoperative care. Healthcare professionals must provide sufficient support and reassurance and utilize measures for managing and calming patients' anxieties and fears optimally. Moreover, scientific investigation of long-term results must take precedence in fractional laser effectiveness studies, as knowledge of the chronicity of adverse effects is indispensable to advancing patient care and satisfaction. Through the resolution of these possible risks as a whole, aesthetic dermatology can work to develop better treatment modalities while reducing the incidence of negative outcomes among patients.

8.5.1. Common Side Effects (E.g., Redness, Swelling)

Common side effects from this type of non-ablative skin rejuvenation and fractional lasers include redness and swelling, which are more commonly accepted as typical reactions after such procedures. These symptoms emanate from the skin's under-layer stimulation and also from the inflammatory response created by the lasers' energy. Redness is usually seen as erythema, which lasts anywhere from a few hours to several days post-treatment, depending on individual healing processes and treatment intensity. While redness often provides an appearance of concern for patients, it can be a sign that the procedure successfully encouraged collagen remodeling and cellular repair or was a part of the skin rejuvenation process. In most cases, these effects are transient, so minimal concern should arise, especially if watched for appropriately. This knowledge helps set realistic expectations among patients receiving these procedures and also enables informed discussion about possible outcomes. Swelling, another common side effect, often accompanies redness after non-ablative laser treatments. The degree of swelling can vary based on the treatment area and an individual's skin type. This localized edema results from increased blood flow and the influx of inflammatory mediators aimed at repairing the treated skin. While swelling generally resolves within days, it may prompt discomfort or sensitivity in some patients. Clinicians recommend post-procedure care, including cool compresses and proper hydration, to alleviate these symptoms and expedite recovery. By educating patients regarding these common contraindications, healthcare providers can minimize anxiety and promote compliance with aftercare protocols. Furthermore, awareness of these side effects can enhance the overall patient experience, allowing them to appreciate the restorative effects of the treatments upon the resolution of temporary discomforts. But within the overall context of aesthetic treatments, knowledge about general side effects such as redness and swelling is key in the teaching and aftercare of the patients. Adequate management pre- and post-procedure concerning such potential effects would make non-ablative treatments both more effective and safer. With increased understanding about how to avoid complications, clinicians can achieve greater consistency and enhance patient satisfaction. Many practitioners advocate for individualized treatment plans, taking into account patient sensitivity and tolerance, to further mitigate adverse effects. By balancing the benefits of skin rejuvenation with the potential for temporary discomfort, clinicians can create a supportive environment for their patients, fostering trust and open communication. Ultimately, understanding these common side effects reinforces the clinician-patient relationship, paving the way for improved aesthetic results and overall satisfaction (Madnani et al., 2022; Penev, 2022) (Figure 8.12).

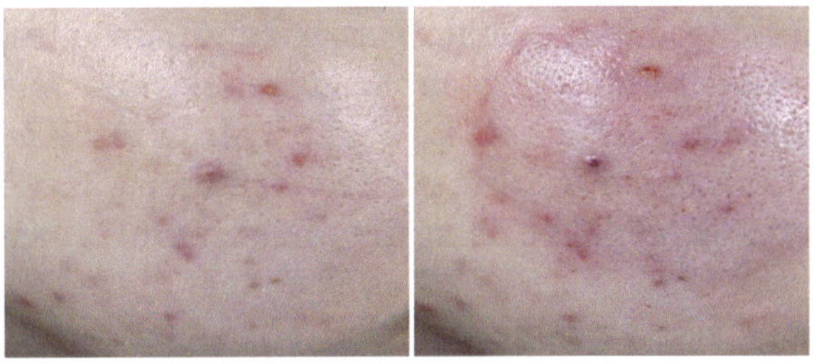

Figure 8.12. Before and after treatment with the 1565-nm nonablative fractional laser.

https://www.researchgate.net/publication/378639034/figure/fig2/AS:11431281245039087@1716049096579/Before-and-after-treatment-with-the-1565-nm-nonablative-fractional-laser.png.

8.5.2. Rare Complications (e.g., Hyperpigmentation)

Keeping in mind the developments in non-ablative facial rejuvenation, it is imperative to discuss the potential for infrequent complications arising from treatments, e.g., hyperpigmentation. Hyperpigmentation, by way of enhanced production of melanin in particular areas of the skin, can detract from the desired results of laser treatments. Especially in skin types with an inherent tendency towards pigmentation disturbances, the risk of such complications calls for judicious patient selection and tailored treatment protocols. Non-ablative fractional lasers, addressing only a fraction of the epidermis, are created to be as non-threatening as possible while still encouraging healing; yet they are not without some potential for adverse effects (Allemann & Kaufman, 2018). Knowledge of the mechanisms of pigmentation changes enables practitioners to anticipate, prevent, and control these events to the extent that patients are educated and ready for the realities of the rejuvenation processes. Practically speaking, the risk of hyperpigmentation as a complication of non-ablative lasers serves to emphasize the importance of adequate pre- and post-treatment care. Pre-op and post-op instructions must be dispensed to the patient about conditions most likely to result in complications, such as skin type, past history of pigmentation disorders, and solar exposure. Correct implementation of skin care regimens, including the application of broad-spectrum sunscreens, can significantly reduce the incidence of PIH and related complications. Secondly, adhering to a provided protocol of anti-inflammatory and soothing substances after treatment in place can help towards gaining an optimal healing process (Madnani et al., 2022).

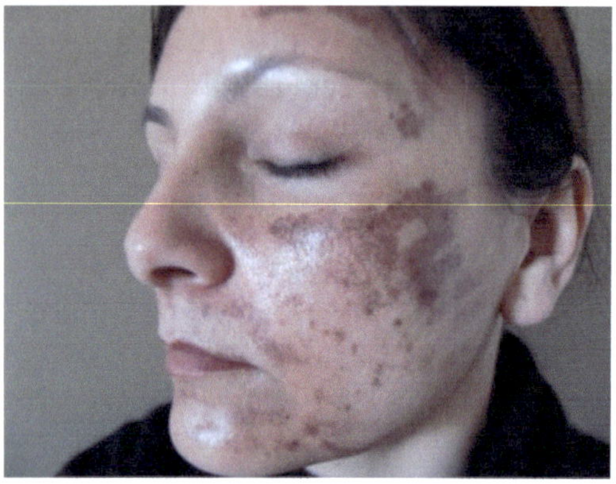

Figure 8.13. Hyperpigmentation after non-ablative laser treatment.

Source: https://goodskindays.co.uk/wp-content/uploads/2014/04/laser-burn.jpg.

By the use of an anticipatory approach that centers on awareness and preparation, medical professionals are better positioned to safeguard their patients against laser therapy's potential drawbacks. Clinicians and researchers must give attention to reporting and investigating the uncommon complications of non-ablative lasers, such as hyperpigmentation. Through greater knowledge of these events, treatment protocols can be enhanced, and overall patient satisfaction can be increased. With growing popularity in non-surgical dermatologic procedures, a strong evidence base that emphasizes the prevalence and management of complications will be crucial. Ongoing discussion in clinical practice and teaching sessions will help to refine methods, minimize rates of occurrence, and propagate the specialty of aesthetic dermatology. Ultimately, by giving high priority to research on this issue, the profession can help to ensure that non-ablative facial rejuvenation continues to be a safe and effective choice for patients with a desire for improved skin health and beauty (Figure 8.13).

8.5.3. Importance of Patient Selection and Consultation

The most important principle of effective nonablative skin rejuvenation and fractional laser therapy is the selection of patients. Each subject yields a distinctive set of skin types, conditions, and aesthetic goals, and proper evaluation must be conducted before any intervention on the part of the practitioner. This evaluation will not only provide an adequate match with specific laser modalities but also bestow an improved safety profile on the intervention. Knowledge of factors like skin phototype, past history of interventions and underlying dermatological illnesses can make a big difference in results. As Madnani et al. (2022) state, the clinicians' lack of information on benefits and risks worsens the need for selection of informed patients that ensures better preparedness of patients for physiological as well as psychological effects of intervention. Lastly, focusing on patient evaluation makes individualized strategies to therapy that optimize results while reducing complications. Consultation represents a vital part of the preselection process for patients, providing an avenue for education and mutual understanding between practitioner and patient. Indeed, during these consultations, practitioners can outline realistic expectations and clear potential outcomes associated with nonablative skin rejuvenation. This becomes such an important talk given the increased interest in less invasive cosmetic treatments as discussed by Bowler (2009). Patients often possess varying levels of knowledge regarding available treatments, making it imperative for dermatologic professionals to convey precise information. Comprehensive consultations empower patients to make informed choices, while simultaneously allowing practitioners to gauge the appropriateness of certain treatments. This pre-treatment dialogue not only establishes trust but also aligns the patient's desires with clinically achievable results. Attention should also be given in the post-procedural phase in terms of patient selection and consultation, considering that following aftercare practices is critical in the outcome of non-ablative treatments. For this reason, sometimes patients need carefully oriented support on skincare and what they should do post-procedure to heal best and effectively. An informed patient is much more likely to adhere to recommended aftercare practices, thereby reducing adverse effects such as hyperpigmentation or infection. Additionally, a robust follow-up strategy allows medical professionals to monitor progress and intervene promptly if complications arise. As underscored in the literature, including (Madnani et al., 2022), understanding pre- and post-procedural care is pivotal for both patient satisfaction and treatment success. Hence, thorough patient consultations not only set the stage for an effective procedure but also pave the way for ongoing support and management (Figure 8.14).

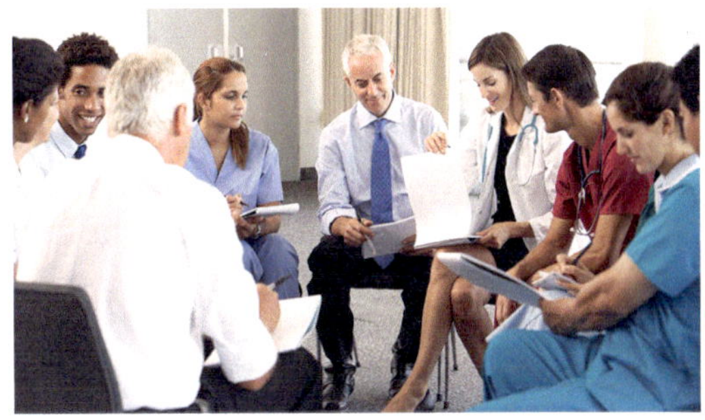

Figure 8.14. Performing tasks for client selection.

Source: https://www.patientsafety.com/hubfs/Campagnes/Pati%C3%ABntenparticipatie/blog%204%20selectie%20juiste%20persoon.jpg.

Test Your Knowledge

1. What are the common short-term side effects associated with non-ablative skin rejuvenation treatments?
2. How does non-ablative skin rejuvenation increase the risk of hyperpigmentation, and what factors contribute to its development?

8.6. Post-Treatment Care

Learning Outcome

1. Explain the importance of skincare routines
2. Discuss the importance of sun protection
3. Focus on follow-up appointments and monitoring

Post-treatment care is a valuable part of realizing maximum benefits from non-ablative facial rejuvenation and fractional laser therapies. Patients may develop redness of the skin, swelling, or heightened sensitivity following these treatments. Hence, adhering to certain aftercare guidelines is crucial to keep these effects at bay and promote skin healing. Clinicians often recommend avoiding sun exposure and applying broad-spectrum sunscreen to protect the treated areas, emphasizing that proper sun protection can prevent complications such as hyperpigmentation. Moreover, patients should avoid harsh skincare products, including those with retinoids or exfoliants, in the days immediately following treatment. This careful approach aids in the recovery process and enhances the efficacy of the treatment, laying the foundation for the expected rejuvenation results. Hydration plays a pivotal role in post-treatment skin care, as it helps facilitate the healing process after non-ablative treatments. Post-procedure, the skin's barrier may be compromised, necessitating the use of moisturizers and hydrating serums to restore moisture levels. Dermatologists often recommend the application of gentle, hydrating products free from irritants to encourage regeneration. Drinking plenty of water is equally important for topical hydration, as systemic hydration has a significant impact on skin health. This dual approach not only alleviates discomfort but supports skin resilience during the recovery phase; and by maintaining adequate hydration, patients can thereby maximize the aesthetic benefits obtained from laser treatments by supporting restoration of a healthy skin barrier. Finally, the success of non-ablative skin rejuvenation relies significantly on post-treatment care strategies. Clinicians and patients need to be aware of potential side effects and complications that can occur during healing. Proper awareness of pre- and post-procedure care can aid in maximizing the outcome of treatment and reducing risks involved with procedures. The practitioners should inform the patients of follow-up visits, in which such sessions enable them to evaluate the healing of the skin and even administer modifying care if required. The relationship promotes a collaborative practice and allows practitioners to win the trust of their patients and make the recovery process more convenient. Thorough post-treatment follow-up is not just an add-on to a cosmetic treatment; it is a critical element that affects global satisfaction and long-term outcomes (Madnani et al., 2022; Baldin et al., 2023).

8.6.1. Recommended Skincare Routines

Incorporating a recommended skincare routine is crucial for individuals seeking to enhance the effects of non-ablative skin rejuvenation and fractional laser treatments. A well-structured regimen can optimize skin health, improve treatment outcomes, and ensure long-lasting effects. Essential components typically include a gentle cleanser, an effective sunscreen, and targeted serums or creams. Cleansing preps the skin for treatment, while sunscreen protects against damage from the sun's UV, which is essential for maintaining the benefits of rejuvenation treatments. Additionally, introducing products that have active ingredients like hyaluronic acid and peptides can further assist in hydration and elasticity of the skin, promoting recovery as well as overall appearance of the skin. Emphasizing these elements within a skincare routine not only helps maintain results but also encourages patients to adopt behaviors that promote skin wellness long after their treatments have concluded. Complementing the primary skincare regimen, the timing and application of products play an essential role in maximizing the benefits of non-ablative treatments. After undergoing fractional laser therapy, the skin may be more sensitive and require a tailored approach to product application. For instance, patients are often advised to wait 48 to 72 hours post-treatment before reintroducing active ingredients, particularly those with exfoliating properties.

This consideration is crucial in preventing irritation and promoting healing. Gradually incorporating these products can provide ongoing support for skin renewal and texture improvement while mitigating potential adverse reactions. Additionally, maintaining open communication with skincare professionals regarding product usage ensures that the routine aligns with the treatment plan, allowing for a personalized approach that addresses individual skin concerns effectively. Lastly, patients require periodic review and adaptation of their skin care regimens in terms of changing skin needs and response to non-ablative therapy. Education on the signs of hydration, irritation, and overall well-being of the skin allows one to make informed choices with products. Periodic consultation appointments with dermatologists can offer individualized adjustments that serve as reminders of the specific skin type and response to therapy. From extraneous literature sources on the management of scars and wounds, including current guidelines on lasers and silicone, informed interaction with medical opinion maximizes knowledge in the sphere of skin wellness and may optimize the chance of success of non-ablative treatments. This helps patients extend the length of time rejuvenation results are maintained and improves their skin's texture and appearance for a considerable period (Téot et al., 2021) (Figure 8.15).

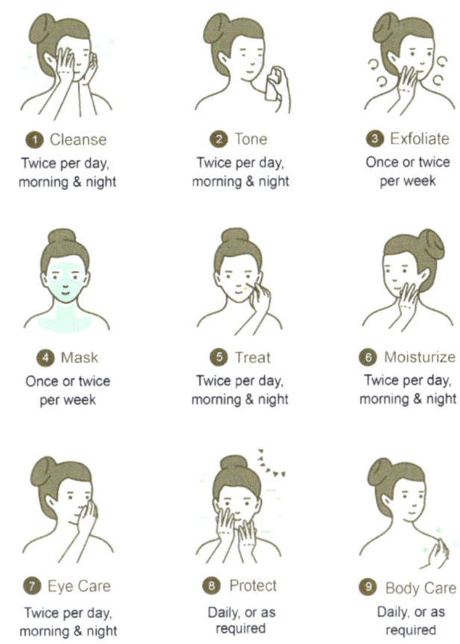
1 Cleanse
Twice per day, morning & night
2 Tone
Twice per day, morning & night
3 Exfoliate
Once or twice per week
4 Mask
Once or twice per week
5 Treat
Twice per day, morning & night
6 Moisturize
Twice per day, morning & night
7 Eye Care
Twice per day, morning & night
8 Protect
Daily, or as required
9 Body Care
Daily, or as required

Figure 8.15. How to build your best skin care routine?

Source: https://info.eminenceorganics.com/hs-fs/hubfs/eminence-organics-skin-care-steps-final.jpg?width=600&name=eminence-organics-skin-care-steps-final.jpg.

8.6.2. Importance of Sun Protection

Good sun protection not only maintains general skin health but is also a prerequisite for any type of skin rejuvenation therapy, such as non-ablative and fractional lasers. Sun ultraviolet (UV) radiation is one of the leading causes of skin injury, resulting in premature aging of the skin as well as a heightened risk of skin cancers. The harmful action of UV is further explained by the creation of dyspigmentation along with aggravation of any scar, like an acne scar, severely affecting the skin's overall appearance. Thus, those patients who undergo Q-Switched Nd:YAG laser therapy have to be educated regarding sun protection before and after the treatment, given the fact that this modality has been proven to be effective in scar improvement, especially for Fitzpatrick skin types III–IV (Viviano et al., 2022). The significance of protecting the skin from UV exposure extends beyond aesthetics; it plays a crucial role in the efficacy of non-ablative skin rejuvenation techniques. Research indicates that patients who utilize sun protection demonstrate better outcomes in laser treatments, as the skin's baseline health notably influences the healing process and overall results. Non-ablative lasers work by delivering focused energy that targets skin imperfections without damaging the surface layer. Therefore, ensuring that the skin is shielded from the harmful effects of sun exposure can facilitate a smoother, more effective treatment process. As laser systems have evolved, safety measures, such as educating patients about sun safety, have become integral to treatment protocols (Žužul, 2014).

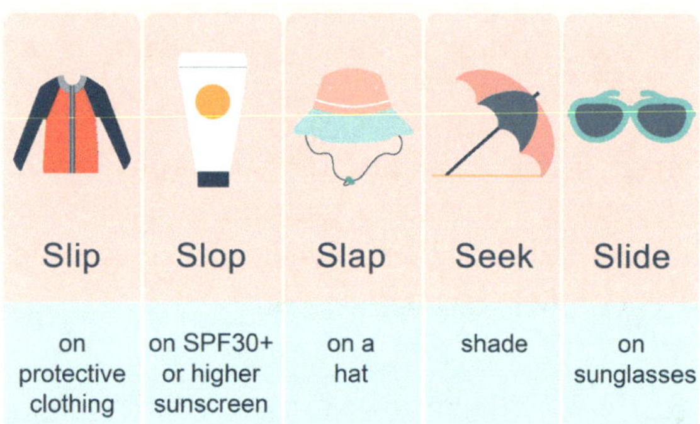
Slip
on protective clothing
Slop
on SPF30+ or higher sunscreen
Slap
on a hat
Seek
shade
Slide
on sunglasses

Figure 8.16. Sun protection.

Source: https://media.healthdirect.org.au/images/inline/original/hd_sun-protection_infrographic_v2024-93e0fb.png

Furthermore, the long-term benefits of sun protection include minimizing the recurrence of skin blemishes and preserving the results achieved through advanced laser therapies. Following non-ablative treatments, the skin is temporarily more vulnerable, thus requiring diligent care and protection against UV radiation. This protective measure not only aids in maintaining the rejuvenated skin's appearance but is also vital for preventing potential complications, such as hyperpigmentation or scarring, that may arise from exposure to the sun after treatment. In this respect, the implementation of sun protection measures is aligned with fractional laser treatments, and such an approach to skincare also seeks to further enhance recovery while strengthening the integrity of cosmetic results (Viviano et al., 2022). In conjunction with diligent sun protection, the patient is better assured of the sustainability and efficacy of rejuvenation efforts for their skin (Figure 8.16).

8.6.3. Follow-Up Appointments and Monitoring

Follow-up appointments are an important aspect of fractional laser and non-ablative rejuvenation treatments. The practitioner utilizes these appointments not just to assess the immediate status of post-procedure skin but also to monitor long-term outcomes. The practitioner's capacity to analyze skin responses to treatment can help fine-tune ongoing care programs to further optimize the rejuvenation process. Follow-ups can detect any unpleasant effects, such as hyperpigmentation or irregular scarring, so that quick intervention can be made. Patient feedback from these visits is also precious in aiding the modification of treatment protocols and ensuring patient satisfaction. Consistent follow-up appointments play an important role in maximizing the effects of nonablative treatments with minimal complications. Monitoring the progress of skin rejuvenation post-treatment presents numerous benefits for both the patient and practitioner. This can be used in the assessment of treatment efficacy, besides the identification of subsequent skin issues. This is crucial since non-ablative rejuvenation typically needs multiple sessions to be optimally maximized and effective. By close observation, clinicians can also see whether the skin has progressively improved in texture, tone, and elasticity over time. These findings inform decisions for future treatment or adjunct therapies that can further enhance results. Ultimately, effective monitoring keeps patients involved and creates a team approach to treatment in which the practitioner can adjust their approach to an individual's skin concern and goals. Advanced diagnostic techniques, such as dermatoscopy, can really enhance the follow-up process in non-ablative rejuvenation of the skin. Dermatoscopy allows practitioners to visualize skin structures not easily seen with the naked eye, thus facilitating the early detection of potential complications or changes in skin lesions that may require attention. This technique proves especially beneficial in monitoring any ongoing skin conditions or neoplasms, as outlined in the literature. The insights provided through dermatoscopic evaluation can inform treatment adjustments and contribute to a more personalized care plan. By utilizing such advanced methods in follow-up appointments, clinicians can offer a higher standard of care and ensure comprehensive monitoring of their patients' skin health, ultimately leading to more successful treatment outcomes in non-ablative rejuvenation protocols (Téot et al., 2021) (Figure 8.17).

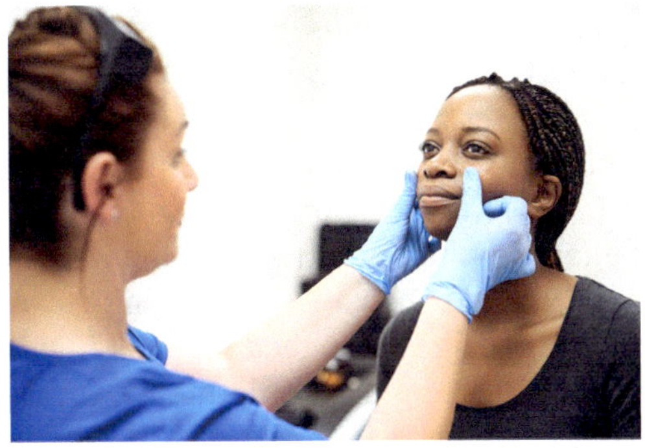

Figure 8.17. Dermatologist assessing a patient's skin to guide personalized treatment for diverse skin types.

Source: https://www.verywellhealth.com/thmb/iGUhYMvdx0TK40tUCTF2rpU8Xl4=/1500x0/filters:no_upscale():max_bytes(150000):strip_icc()/GettyImages-1154030721-974bcd6d70ff4489ba961317f1f3640f.jpg.

Test Your Knowledge

1. What are the essential steps in post-treatment care following non-ablative skin rejuvenation to ensure optimal results and minimize complications?
2. How long should a patient wait before resuming regular skincare routines?

SUMMARY

Non-ablative skin rejuvenation utilizing fractional lasers represents a significant advancement in aesthetic dermatology, offering effective treatment options with minimal downtime. These procedures effectively target various skin concerns, promoting collagen production and enhancing overall skin quality without causing extensive damage to the surrounding tissues. The evidence presented within the literature illustrates the efficacy of non-ablative technologies in addressing issues such as pigmentation, fine lines, and skin texture, indicating their role in modern cosmetic practices. Additionally, the incorporation of adjunctive therapies, such as exosomes and PRP, further amplifies the benefits of non-ablative treatments, enhancing both safety and patient satisfaction. Therefore, therapists need to consider combining these modalities in treatment protocols to maximize outcomes and address a growing need for less invasive treatments. The meta-analysis of existing literature about non-ablative skin treatments indicates a continued need for more research in order to determine standardized treatment protocols and parameters. Although promising results have been illustrated in recently published findings, as mentioned in studies determining the combination of ablative and non-ablative methods, variability in techniques, equipment, and patient responses call for a more unified approach. For instance, fractional lasers used in combination with other adjuvant treatments have reported better results in different forms of skin diseases, thus urging for good clinical trials to be conducted. Comprehensive studies using uniform methodologies, large sample sizes and longer follow-up information will not only elucidate further the treatment efficacy but also increase the credibility of non-ablative skin rejuvenation practice on a clinical basis. Future directions in non-ablative skin rejuvenation rely upon the exploration of newer techniques and technologies. As the field evolves, practitioners must stay abreast of innovative developments that could transform skin rejuvenation protocols. Research aimed at understanding the long-term effects and potential complications of these technologies is essential, considering the limited consensus on optimal practices noted in current literature. Furthermore, there is a rising interest in expanding the use of non-invasive treatments beyond traditional dermatological applications, such as non-invasive vulvovaginal rejuvenation, highlighting the versatility and potential of these therapies. Continued exploration and discourse among dermatologists and researchers will ultimately shape the landscape of aesthetic treatments, ensuring that patient safety and satisfaction remain paramount (Liedtke et al., 2023; Dhillon et al., 2024).

Advances in non-ablative rejuvenation of the skin, more so with the inclusion of fractional lasers, have been noteworthy and light up advances within aesthetic medicine. This procedure is characterized by the ability to produce collagen remodeling and elasticity that promotes no downtime, similar to the traditional ablative approach. The fractional laser helps target specific areas of the skin, causing controlled micro-injuries, which trigger the body's natural healing response. This method will not have harmful effects on the surrounding tissue of the area and, therefore, enhances faster recovery and fewer complications. With non-invasive methods becoming the first choice of practitioners, the success of fractional laser therapy has been well-established in various reports, thereby adding to a comprehensive understanding of its applications in the practice of skin rejuvenation. Addition of APCs enhances the efficacy of non-ablative rejuvenation. APCs, which are derived from the patient's own blood, contain a rich array of growth factors that facilitate tissue repair and skin rejuvenation, making them a promising adjunct therapy to fractional laser treatments. Clinical studies indicate that using preparations like PRP can significantly improve outcomes in facial rejuvenation applications, including treating acne scarring and enhancing skin texture. While studies have indicated that platelet-rich fibrin (PRF) produces better outcomes compared to PRP, limitations like limited sample sizes and different evaluation criteria highlight the need for more solid, well-designed randomized controlled trials for confirmation of these results (Davies & Miron, 2025). In addition, the safety profile of non-ablative treatments with the use of non-ionizing radiation (NIR) highlights the requirement for complete understanding and regulation. These aesthetic devices have become popular for their wide range of uses-from wrinkle improvement to scar reduction. However, the research has been largely concentrated on efficacy rather than side effects. Documented side effects included transient pain and erythema, to severe complications including burns and alteration of pigmentation. Pre-existing conditions such as darker skin tones and prior sun exposure may increase the risk of adverse outcomes. To protect patient safety, there is a pressing need for well-regulated practice in NIR cosmetic treatments and extensive studies that analyze both efficacy and safety to allow practitioners to make informed care decisions in the constantly changing field of aesthetic medicine (International Commission on Non-Ionizing Radiation Protection, 2020).

KEY TERMS FROM THIS CHAPTER

- Aesthetic dermatology
- Aesthetic medicine
- Biological responses
- Broad-spectrum sunscreens
- Chromophores
- Collagen synthesis
- Fractional laser technology
- Harmful effects
- Holographic optics
- Hydrating products
- Keratinocytes
- Liposuction
- Matrix metalloproteinases (MMPs)
- Proliferation
- Reduced recovery periods
- Skin texture abnormalities
- Striae distensae (SD)
- Ultraviolet (UV)

CRITICAL THINKING QUESTIONS

1. **Which of the following best describes non-ablative skin rejuvenation?**
   a. Removes the outer layers of the skin
   b. Heats the dermis without damaging the epidermis
   c. Causes complete epidermal ablation
   d. Requires extended downtime for healing
2. **What is the primary benefit of fractional laser technology over traditional laser resurfacing?**
   a. More aggressive treatment with deeper ablation
   b. Reduced collagen stimulation
   c. Higher risk of post-inflammatory hyperpigmentation
   d. Faster healing time due to microscopic treatment zones
3. **Which of the following wavelengths is commonly used in non-ablative fractional lasers?**
   a. 1064 nm (Nd:YAG)
   b. 2940 nm (Er:YAG)
   c. 1550 nm (Er:Glass)
   d. 10,600 nm (CO_2 laser)
4. **What is a key indication for using non-ablative fractional lasers?**
   a. Deep surgical scars
   b. Superficial wrinkles and photodamage
   c. Skin tag removal
   d. Tattoo removal
5. **Which of the following is a common side effect of non-ablative fractional laser treatment?**
   a. Temporary erythema and edema
   b. Severe bleeding
   c. Long-term skin thinning
   d. Full-thickness skin necrosis

Short Answer Questions

1. What is the primary mechanism of action for non-ablative skin rejuvenation treatments?
2. List two common types of non-ablative lasers used for skin rejuvenation.
3. What are the main indications for non-ablative skin rejuvenation therapy?
4. What are the advantages of non-ablative treatments compared to ablative procedures?
5. What is the difference between ablative and non-ablative fractional lasers?
6. What are the typical post-treatment side effects of fractional laser therapy?
7. Name at least two clinical conditions that can be effectively treated with fractional lasers.

Answer to Critical Thinking Questions

1. (b); 2. (d); 3. (c); 4. (b); 5. (a)

REFERENCES

1. Bogdan Allemann, I., & Kaufman, J. (2010). Fractional photothermolysis--an update. *Lasers in medical science*, *25*(1), 137–144. https://doi.org/10.1007/s10103-009-0734-8 (accessed on 11th June 2025).
2. Amato, S., Ciardo, S., Guida, S., Longo, C., Manfredini, M., Mercuri, S. R., Nistico, S. P., et al. (2023). Laser treatment monitoring with reflectance confocal microscopy. https://core.ac.uk/download/592024422.pdf (accessed on 11th June 2025).
3. Amoruso, G. F., Belletti, S., Bennardo, L., Fusco, I., Madeddu, F., Nistico, S. P., & Provenzano, E. (2023). An innovative dual-wavelength laser technique for atrophic acne scar management: A pilot study. https://core.ac.uk/download/614035653.pdf (accessed on 11th June 2025).
4. Stoian, Anca Pantea; Hainarosie, Razvan; Pietrosanu, Catalina; Rusescu, Andreea; Andronache, Liliana F.; Paunica, Stana; Balalau, Cristian; and Pituru, Teodora S. (2019) "Modern concepts in non-surgical esthetics; a review," Journal of Mind and Medical Sciences: Vol. 6: Iss. 2, Article 3. DOI: https://doi.org/10.22543/7674.62.P190195 Available at: https://scholar.valpo.edu/jmms/vol6/iss2/3 (accessed on 11th June 2025).
5. Baldin, G. C., & Liedtke, F. S. (2023). Use of ablative fractional CO_2 laser in facial rejuvenation: A prospective observational cohort study. https://core.ac.uk/download/622811929.pdf (accessed on 11th June 2025).
6. Barikbin, B., Ghavam, S. A., Karimi, S., Moravvej, et al. (2011). Nonablative fractional laser resurfacing. https://core.ac.uk/download/483636065.pdf (accessed on 11th June 2025).
7. Barnes, C., Chuang, J., & Wong, B. (2016). Overview of facial plastic surgery and current developments. https://core.ac.uk/download/617032104.pdf (accessed on 11th June 2025).
8. Viviano, M. T., Provini, A., Mazzanti, C., Nisticò, S. P., Patruno, C., Cannarozzo, G., Bennardo, S., Fusco, I., & Bennardo, L. (2022). Clinical Evaluation on the Performance and Safety of a Non-Ablative Fractional 1340 nm Laser for the Treatment of Stretch Marks in Adolescents and Young Adults: A Case Series. *Bioengineering (Basel, Switzerland)*, *9*(4), 139. https://doi.org/10.3390/bioengineering9040139https://core.ac.uk/download/592027176.pdf (accessed on 11th June 2025).
9. Bowler, P. J. (2009). Impact on facial rejuvenation with dermatological preparations. https://core.ac.uk/download/pdf/8289062.pdf (accessed on 11th June 2025).
10. Davies, C., & Miron, R. J. (2025). Autolougous platelet concentrates in esthetic medicine. *Periodontology 2000*, *97*(1), 363–419. https://doi.org/10.1111/prd.12582(accessed on 11th June 2025).
11. Madnani, N., Vedmurthy, M., Parthasarthi, A., Dhawan, S., Kandhari, R., Pillai, R., & Nischal, K. C. (2022). Expert opinion on pre and post procedure care in aesthetic dermatology. *International Journal of Research in Medical Sciences*, *10*(4), 991–1000. https://doi.org/10.18203/2320-6012.ijrms20220999(accessed on 11th June 2025).
12. Dhillon, J., & Jusuf, N. K. (2024). Non–invasive vulvovaginal rejuvenation: A review. https://core.ac.uk/download/639389933.pdf (accessed on 11th June 2025).
13. Duncan, D. I. (2022). Enhanced liposuction. https://core.ac.uk/download/534904133.pdf (accessed on 11th June 2025).

14. El-Kholy, B. M., Kandil, A. H., & Nawwar, E. M. A. (2022). New insight in the treatment of wide facial pores: Review article. https://core.ac.uk/download/524771765.pdf (accessed on 11th June 2025).

15. Téot L, Mustoe TA, Middelkoop E, et al., editors. Textbook on Scar Management: State of the Art Management and Emerging Technologies [Internet]. Cham (CH): Springer; 2020. Available from: https://www.ncbi.nlm.nih.gov/books/NBK586066/ doi: 10.1007/978-3-030-44766-3 (accessed on 11th June 2025).

16. Haykal, D., Cartier, H., Goldberg, D. J., & Gold, M. (2024). Advancements in laser technologies for skin rejuvenation: A comprehensive review of efficacy and safety. *Journal of Cosmetic Dermatology.* https://www.semanticscholar.org/paper/24ec0937d5b03213880a8a8bb056721844109481 (accessed on 11th June 2025).

17. Heidari Beigvand, H., Heidari, M. H., Mansouri, V., et al. (2020). Assessment of laser effects on skin rejuvenation. https://core.ac.uk/download/483636521.pdf (accessed on 11th June 2025).

18. International Commission on Non-Ionizing Radiation Protection. (2020). Intended human exposure to non-ionizing radiation for cosmetic purposes. https://core.ac.uk/download/552405446.pdf (accessed on 11th June 2025).

19. Liedtke, F. S., & Rajapaksa, S. W. (2023). Major clinical evidence of the optimization of the use of CO_2 fractional ablative laser with cells and molecules: A systematic review. https://core.ac.uk/download/622811954.pdf (accessed on 11th June 2025).

20. Penev, Y. (2022). Laser resources for facial rejuvenation and aestheticization // Възможности за лазерно подмладяване и естетизиране на кожата на лицето. https://core.ac.uk/download/578416857.pdf (accessed on 11th June 2025).

21. Pietkiewicz, P. (2022). Dermatoscopy. https://core.ac.uk/download/534901977.pdf (accessed on 11th June 2025).

22. Sjerobabski Masnec, I., & Šitum, M. (2014). Photorejuvenation–Topical photodynamic therapy as therapeutic opportunity for skin rejuvenation. https://core.ac.uk/download/33287089.pdf (accessed on 11th June 2025).

23. Yuan, Y., He, Y., Fang, J., Zhang, M., & Wu, Q. (2024). Comparison of the fractionated Nd:YAG 1064-nm picosecond laser with holographic optics and the fractional CO_2 laser in atrophic acne scar treatment: A prospective, randomized, split-face study. *International Journal of Dermatology.* https://www.semanticscholar.org/paper/1a040d07b94292209a6a02845840130403dba80c (accessed on 11th June 2025).

24. Zeng, Q., Wu, Q., Deng, L., Hong, L., Li, R., & Chen, A. (2024). Enhancement of facial rejuvenation through a combination of 1565 nm non-ablative fractional laser with 30% supramolecular salicylic acid. *Journal of Visualized Experiments: JoVE, 211.* https://www.semanticscholar.org/paper/65d86c4fd20f8441bfd393b9cf1f2b2137990b46 (accessed on 11th June 2025).

25. Žužul, K. (2014). The use of lasers in dermatology. https://core.ac.uk/download/197824559.pdf (accessed on 11th June 2025).

MESOTHERAPY

9

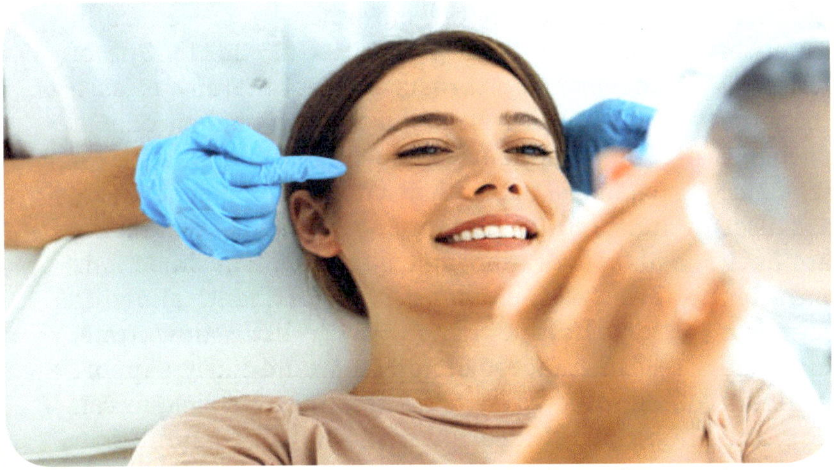

LEARNING OBJECTIVES

After studying this chapter, you will be able to:

1. Understand the mechanism of action of mesotherapy
2. Discuss about indications for mesotherapy
3. Explain the benefits of mesotherapy
4. Describe risks and side effects
5. Compare mesotherapy with other cosmetic procedures
6. Focus on current trends and innovations

Introduction

Cosmetic dermatology has seen an exponential rise in non-surgical methods used to improve aesthetic results for patients. Among these new practices, mesotherapy has seen much notice taken due to its capacity to rejuvenate and treat several skin-related issues. Mesotherapy is a method that requires the injection of small amounts of formulated solutions, such as vitamins, enzymes, and hyaluronic acid, into the mesoderm, the fat and tissue layer just below the skin. The rising popularity of mesotherapy lies in the fact that it is non-invasive and has less recovery time in comparison to conventional surgical intervention. With more people opting for effective yet less invasive alternatives, mesotherapy offers a powerful solution to cater to the needs of contemporary cosmetic treatment alongside being patient-friendly in choosing less invasive interventions (Stoian et al., 2019). Over the past few years, mesotherapy has been used not only for facial rejuvenation but also for body contouring and hair restoration. These uses have made mesotherapy a versatile cosmetic dermatology treatment that can be used to address a range of aesthetic issues. Due to the rising rates of conditions such as hair loss, practitioners are increasingly looking into mesotherapy as a potential solution over more aggressive forms of treatment. The method allows for targeted delivery of growth factors and nutrients capable of stimulating hair follicles, providing a non-surgical treatment for baldness (Cyran et al., 2024). Such applications mirror the active development of mesotherapy, with practitioners always seeking better effectiveness and safety of this therapeutic method in various dermatological disorders. In spite of the numerous benefits of mesotherapy, there is a need to thoroughly assess its effectiveness and safety on a sequence of applications. Emerging evidence still focuses on the impact of mesotherapy treatments, particularly with regards to the concentration of infused products and how many treatments are necessary to produce optimal results. The determination of these parameters in detail is essential to high patient satisfaction and minimizing side effects. Besides, with the continuously evolving non-surgical setting, it is imperative that practitioners continuously stay abreast of the newer trends in mesotherapy treatments and products to ensure that they meet the growing needs of their clients. Under strict surveillance and clinical fine-tuning, the field of mesotherapy can continue to solidify its position as a pillar of contemporary cosmetic dermatology, offering state-of-the-art treatments according to particular patient needs (Stoian et al., 2019).

Definition of Mesotherapy

Mesotherapy has been described as a treatment that essentially consists of intradermal injection of various agents. It opens the possibility of topically administered therapy where the drugs administered are much less than would otherwise have been administered through the customary systemic means, thus lessening side effects. The method is utilized in various fields such as pain and dermatology. Mesotherapy in dermatologic cosmetics serves to rejuvenate the skin, make it more beautiful, and even correct certain conditions like wrinkles, sagging, and localized fat deposition. Though this practice has been in popularity over time, despite the seriousness of the present lack of standard protocols, there is a tremendous voice calling for more systematic, extensive research and rigid safety testing for proper and responsible application of the mesotherapy procedure in clinical settings (Bifarini et al., 2021). One of the primary thrusts of mesotherapy is as a non-surgical means of cosmetic enhancement. The treatment can involve a combination of vitamins, enzymes, hormones, and plant extracts tailored to the patient's needs, enhancing skin hydration and elasticity. The injections are typically done for treatment, allowing for additive benefit with little downtime. Cosmetic dermatologists would likely support mesotherapy since a treatment technique can be put to use for a variety of different skin conditions, from the diminishment of cellulite to the treatment of anti-aging effects. However, although there is excellent patient satisfaction and anecdotal evidence, the results are badly documented in scientific literature. Various studies have shown the efficacy of mesotherapy in the improvement of skin appearance, but extensive clinical trials are required to confirm these results and study the treatment efficacy and safety in detail (Boshoff et al., 2016). The current discourse regarding mesotherapy points toward the necessity for a unified approach to develop its applications in cosmetic dermatology. Examples include differences in the injection technique, drug combinations and the course of treatment. Moreover, mesotherapy as a less-invasive intervention compared to surgery requires critical education to patients regarding potential benefits and risks in their elements. While professionals determine the viability of mesotherapy as an intervention in cosmetic procedures, there is a need for guidelines through robust research in the clinical area. These standards must encompass ideal formulations and techniques but also set criteria for choosing the patient; thus, mesotherapy might well be a safe aesthetic medicine tool (Bifarini et al., 2021) (Figure 9.1).

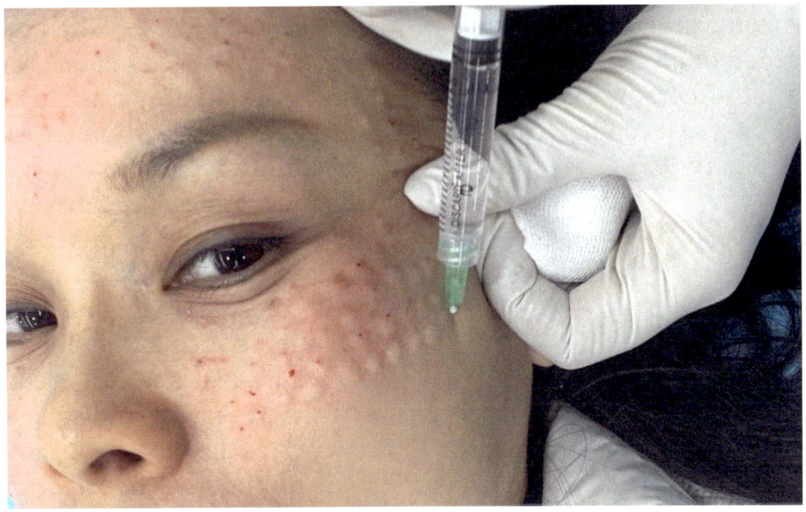

Figure 9.1. Mesotherapy treatment showing typical post-injection skin reactions.

Source: https://cdn.shopify.com/s/files/1/0871/7713/4375/files/lumps_after_mesotherapy_2.jpg?v=1727676611.

Historical Background

The development of mesotherapy started early in the 20th century with the French doctor Michel Pistor originally laying out the technique in 1952 as a therapy for a broad spectrum of medical conditions. Pistor's technique included the injection of drugs intradermally into the middle skin layer or mesoderm and therefore the treatment of localized conditions such as pain and inflammation. Over time, treatment became popular among cosmetic and aesthetic therapy physicians in Europe. Its gradual advancement was the manner mesotherapies evolved from curative treatment to emerge as one of the leading interventions in cosmetics focused on superficial aging, fat accumulation, and skin regeneration, therefore influencing its cosmetic use in dermatology. With the growing popularity of the method, more and more formulas began to develop in France and Belgium, thereby imparting a boost to the probable uses of mesotherapy. Medical experts delivered a variety of active ingredients like vitamins and amino acids, homeopathy, in attempting to achieve maximum results in all dermatological diseases. This diversification corresponded to increasing public fascination with non-surgical cosmetic treatments that made mesotherapy accessible to doctors' and patients' imaginations. The treatments had minimal downtime and localized treatment modality regained its popularity with the birth of an emerging trend towards esthetic treatments based on patient comfort and natural outcomes, and thus mesotherapy was a useful tool in cosmetic dermatology practice. However, despite its popularity, mesotherapy has been questioned in terms of its lack of solid scientific backing. Early trials provided anecdotal data but often were carried out without the rigorous methods demanded for medical licensure. In particular, the demand for controlled trials determining the effectiveness of several substances in mesotherapy was a pressing concern. For example, Herreros et al. (2018) is one such study that may have shown a potential advantage in the form of certain substances like silanol enhancing architecture in dermis, but were rarely broad in scope and replicable. With the increasing adaptation of mesotherapy in the department of cosmetic dermatology, proper research will be needed to fill these knowledge gaps, thus making mesotherapy a sound and effective treatment in the evolving trend of aesthetic medicine (Figure 9.2).

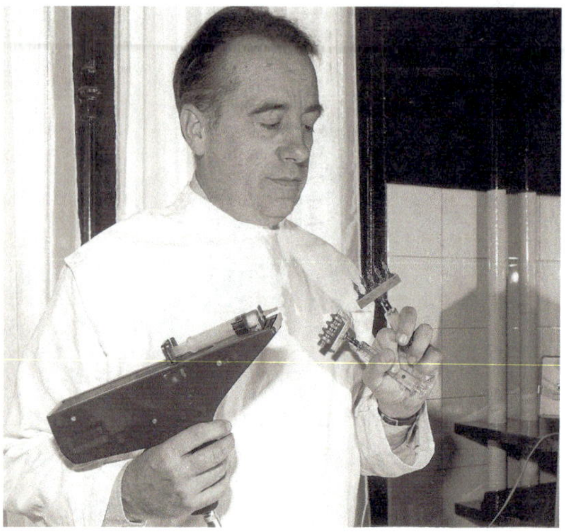

Figure 9.2. Michel Pistor performed clinical research and founded the field of mesotherapy.

Source: https://mi-medicalinnovation.com/img/cms/Pages%20CMS%20(Nx%20Sites)/M%20Pistor%201.jpg.

Importance in Cosmetic Dermatology

One of the most significant innovations within cosmetic dermatology is that treatments cannot be ignored when patient expectations are changing with advanced technology. The relatively new procedure of alternative non-surgical procedures has garnered much attention in recent years, hence fundamentally transforming the face of dermatology care. The therapy that has prominently featured in the list of most skin problems is mesotherapy; a convergent therapy to iron out wrinkles, remove cellulites, and rejuvenate the skin. According to research, therapies such as injectology have performed marvelously well with agents such as hyaluronic acid and botulinum toxin (BT), but mesotherapy excels in providing patient-specific solutions based on what a patient needs (Stoian et al., 2019). Rising interest in non-invasive treatment modalities emphasizes the role of mesotherapy in cosmetic dermatology, and there is a need for a proper and efficient technique that combines safety with efficacy, which eventually leads to patient satisfaction. Moreover, emphasis on beautification and well-being of the skin has witnessed the increasing use of mesotherapy as a component of multi-modality treatment modalities. By contrast, the traditional surgical treatments with their extensive recovery and side effects do not offer so much as the pleasing beauty of mesotherapy. This minimally invasive method not only eliminates the risk associated with surgery but also enjoys the modern patient's preference for not disturbing them unnecessarily. Notably, in regard to pre-and post-operative care, it is beneficial even in the scarring after surgery, as point out the studies about the effects of mesotherapy on postoperative treatment of scars (Boshoff et al., 2016). Such flexibility underlines the significance of mesotherapy within the context of cosmetic dermatology, where it functions both as a main treatment procedure and in support. Besides this, the fast development of technological innovations in cosmetic dermatology further underlines the opportunity for mesotherapy to change with the times and serve growing trends as well as patient needs. With a shift in aesthetic values and ever-increasing demand for tailored options, mesotherapy can employ diverse active ingredients to treat more specific skin issues and, therefore, enhance its therapeutic potential. Actually, the key principles of mesotherapy show that micro-injections of vitamins, enzymes, and other anti-aging agents into the skin are able to stimulate the production of collagen, hydration, and other sources of energy of the skin. Therefore, there are many practitioners who realize the benefit of mesotherapy in practice, not only for the short-term cosmetic effects, but also for the long-lasting impact on the health of the skin. For this reason, mesotherapy has become a fundamental component in the repertoire of cosmetic dermatology, making valuable contributions towards more holistic treatment strategies that focus on patient-centered principles.

9.1. Mechanism of Action

Learning Outcome

1. Explain injection techniques
2. Describe types of solutions used
3. Understand target areas for treatment

Mesotherapy, an innovative cosmetic dermatology procedure, is based on the idea of injecting an active mixture of ingredients into the mesoderm, the middle layer of the skin. This type of injection maximizes absorption and bioavailability so that healing factors selected , be they vitamins, minerals, or hyaluronic acid, are having their healing effect at the very points where they are required. Mesotherapy includes the subdermal injection of drug compounds at a precise depth, improving in general the texture, hydration, and nutrient supply of the skin. An added advantage is that mesotherapy can be beneficial in the treatment of hair loss and skin aging. Direct local effects should increase the microcirculation and metabolic activity in the treated area, which will eventually be translated to long-term improvement in the quality and health of the skin. Mesotherapy's mode of action also overlaps with other recent hair restoration therapies, particularly in patients with various types of alopecia.

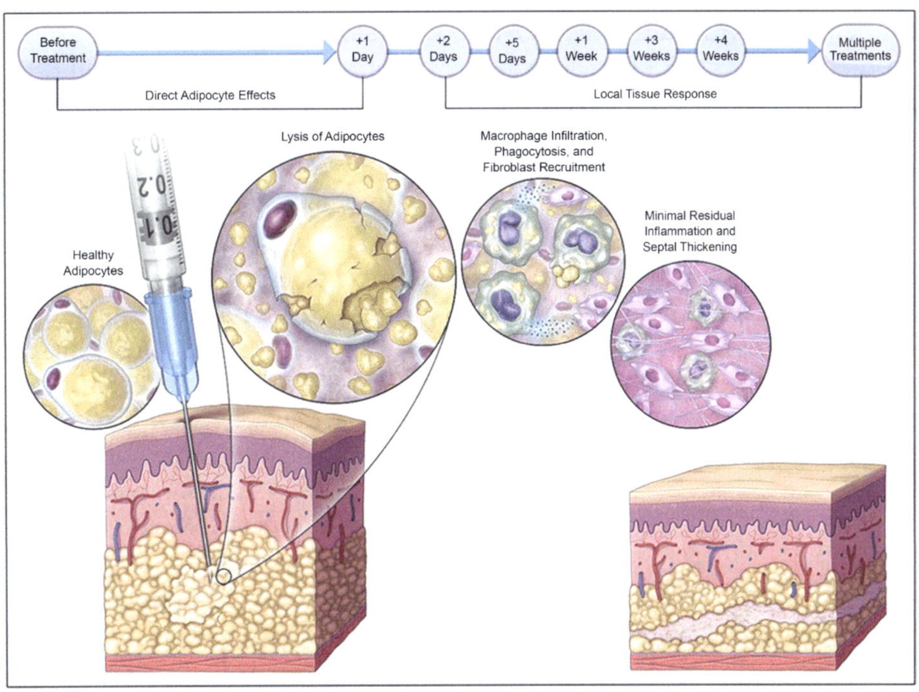

Figure 9.3. The mechanism of fat cell death in mesotherapy lipodissolve.

Source: https://www.researchgate.net/publication/327265146/figure/fig1/AS:664577020805120@1535458917075/Mechanism-of-action-of-deoxycholic-acid-Image-adopted-from-Ref-5.png.

Other scientists have examined the efficacy of mesotherapy with treatment modalities like PRP therapy, which involves using growth factors from the patient's own blood to excite hair follicles and ultimately trigger hair growth. Because mesotherapy enables these growth-enhancing factors to be targeted directly into the scalp, it provides maximum effectiveness of PRP with a synergistic modality that most optimally produces patient outcomes. The combined application of these treatments addresses both the cosmetic and physiological aspects of baldness and provides a multidimensional strategy that is fundamental in cosmetic dermatology, where hair loss can significantly impact quality of life (Altunel et al., 2017). Further knowledge about the mesotherapy as an agent of skin rejuvenation and hair loss treatment attests to its increasing role in modern dermatology. The personalized character of mesotherapy permits customized treatment protocols perfectly suited to the needs of the patient, thus increasing satisfaction and efficacy of treatment. The procedure has been combined with other therapy modalities, such as microneedling and low-level light therapy; these treatments have also had inconsistent success rates against hair loss. Combining multiple methods allows dermatologists to provide a multifaceted protocol that does more than just address short-term issues but actually encourages long-term outcomes. As research continues to evolve, further investigation into the precise mechanisms involved in these treatments will likely yield improved protocols and outcomes in the sphere of cosmetic dermatology (Cyran et al., 2024) (Figure 9.3).

9.1.1. Injection Techniques

This is, therefore, the secret to mesotherapy success in dermatological esthetics: good injection technique. Small quantities of the blend are injected into the skin by extremely thin needles into the mesoderm, i.e., the middle layer of the skin; it provides the vehicle for the administration of cocktails composed of vitamins, enzymes, hormones, and amino acids directly into the target tissue with local metabolic activity and tissue well-being. By choosing the injection method and location with precision, dermatologists are able to tailor treatments to patients' conditions and needs, whether tackling skin laxity, hyperpigmentation, or localized fat. Such injections depend not only on the agents delivered but also on the accuracy of the delivery method, which underscores the necessity of competent practitioners to reduce complications and maximize outcomes (Chirch et al., 2015). This trend of minimally invasive treatments, such as mesotherapy, necessitates additional insight into the injection techniques being used. Adequate technique can mitigate complications of cutaneous aesthetic treatment, e.g., bruising, swelling, infection, and a concern is the risk of nontuberculous mycobacteria (NTM) infections related to injection practices in cosmetic dermatology. Research has documented that such infections, among others, causing skin and soft tissue conditions, are contributed to by improper injection techniques (Chirch et al., 2015). Therefore, education and further training in the proper mesotherapy protocols should be implemented. By adherence to such proven best practices in injection techniques, dermatologists may improve the safety and efficacy of mesotherapy while also improving patient care. Beyond the generally popular uses of mesotherapy, new injection therapies are ongoing under the cosmetic dermatologic uses, particularly in alopecia. It is a challenge to treat various forms of hair loss; however, mesotherapy can be used as an adjunctive treatment for it. Microinjection techniques utilizing revitalizing agents, like PRP and growth factors, are mechanisms that try to induce regeneration of hair follicles and scalp well-being. These methods also represent a greater integration of mesotherapy in multi-modality treatment strategies in conditions over hair. Summarizing all, evidence hints that combination with mesotherapy will, in particular, achieve enhanced outcomes than either modality alone, especially in noncicatricial alopecias, such as androgenetic alopecia and alopecia areata. Techniques of injection continue to evolve, and mesotherapy is well-poised to add to the establishment of cosmetic dermatology practices (Figure 9.4).

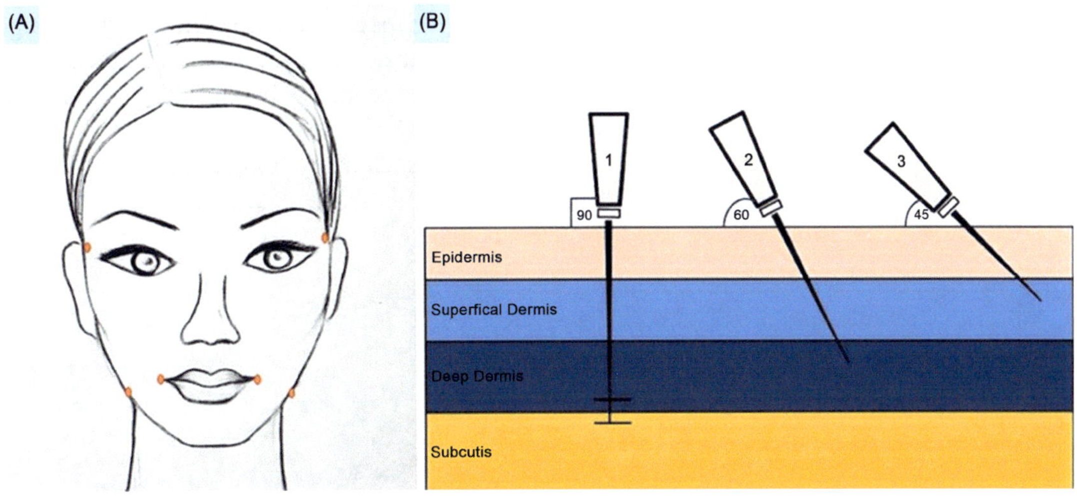

Figure 9.4. (A) Tensile column technique of mesotherapy; and (B) Angle and depth of injection.

Source: https://www.researchgate.net/publication/343810845/figure/fig2/AS:11431281173844637@1689056554209/A-Tensile-column-technique-of-mesotherapy-and-B-Angle-and-depth-of-injection.png.

9.1.2. Types of Solutions Used

Amongst the mesotherapeutic solutions, many solutions have emerged to prominence through their multi-faceted applications in cosmetic dermatology. They typically comprise hyaluronic acid, vitamins, minerals, and amino acids, each being intended to address a specific skin concern. Hyaluronic acid, due to its high water-holding ability, is engaged in maximizing the hydration and elasticity of the skin. At the same time, vitamins such as vitamin C are included for their antioxidant properties, which combat oxidative stress and promote skin renewal. This combination of active ingredients can prove to be highly effective in addressing conditions ranging from dry skin to the look of aging, thus making mesotherapy a multi-purpose procedure in dermatology. Furthermore, the ability to tailor these solutions enhances practitioners' ability to address specific patient requirements, further emphasizing the flexibility inherent in mesotherapy to improve skin well-being. More research is indicating that mesotherapy solutions are used to treat alopecia of different types, further highlighting their use in hair re-growth. For instance, in the context of androgenetic alopecia and other noncicatricial types of hair loss, specific formulations, including growth factors and botanical extracts, have shown promise in stimulating the hair follicles. Studies indicate that mesotherapy, utilized alongside other interventions like microneedling and PRP therapy, has the potential to yield variable results in promoting hair regrowth. The focus on such emerging techniques is shaped by the need for effective treatments in view of the partial ineffectiveness of traditional treatments. As mentioned above, various treatments applied for different types of alopecia, including mesotherapy, suggest growing awareness of this treatment as a potential panacea for hair loss amelioration in aesthetic dermatology (Altunel et al., 2017). Well, in addition to skin renewal and hair regrowth, the benefits of mesotherapy have been promoted as something new for post-surgery scarring. Because many women are on the lookout for how to avoid scarring from surgery, mesotherapy provides a non-surgical alternative toward helping such scar healing. This will be because the active ingredients applied may cause some inflammatory changes and trigger collagen remodeling and result in better scar appearance. In mammary reduction surgery, in the case of Mesotherapy Eporex treatments, effectiveness was to be determined; however, as the practice is given, a promising way towards diminishing the visibility of scars, it might very well be on the rise (Boshoff et al., 2016). This is why mesotherapy solutions may well have the capability of addressing a multi-aspect list of cosmetic issues, firmly reasserting its position in the arena of dermatology as an extensive tool (Figure 9.5).

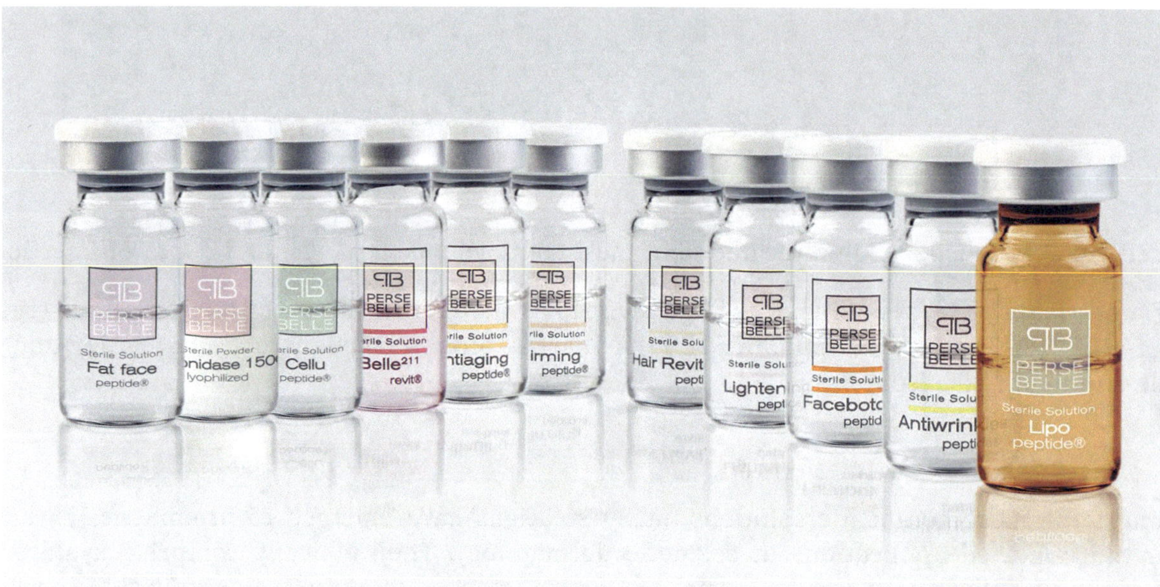

Figure 9.5. Solutions used for mesotherapy.

Source: https://www.cosmeditech.com/wp-content/uploads/2024/01/Top-Image-PBelle.jpg.

9.1.3. Target Areas for Treatment

In cosmetic dermatology, mesotherapy is a viable technique that is used to treat very specific areas that need to be treated. With the use of microinjections of drugs, vitamins, and other active ingredients, mesotherapy successfully treats issues like localized fat deposits, aging signs, and lax skin. Specifically, these areas are the abdominal and thigh areas and facial area, which most of the patients have the greatest aesthetic problems found in these areas. Tipping mesotherapy to localized treatment makes it more subject to customized care, and therefore enhances its efficacy and patient satisfaction. Although mesotherapy is promising in these regions, further studies are necessary to determine standardized procedures for maximizing its efficacy among various body sites and conditions so that practitioners can make effective decisions during practice (Bifarini et al., 2021). Mesotherapy is also becoming popular owing to possible advantages in the prevention of post-operative scarring. Because women are seeking alternatives to more aggressive interventions like mammary reduction surgery, efficient scar management is required. The Mesotherapy Eporex treatments that comprise an active substance blend promise a non-invasive alternative to surgically enhance the appearance of scars after a procedure. The stimulation of healing through injections of active material directly into scar tissue makes mesotherapy useful for healing and stimulating a better outcome. Yet, the absence of strong scientific evidence in specific support for the effectiveness of mesotherapy for this use requires further research. Specifically, rigorous clinical trials are needed to confirm the method and establish consistent results for patients looking to minimize post-operative scars (Boshoff et al., 2016).

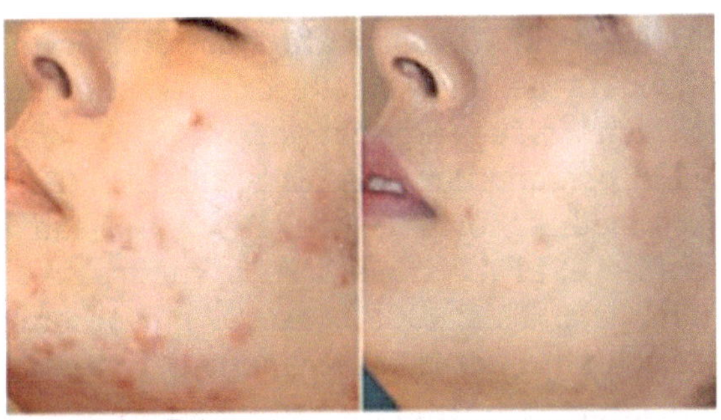

Figure 9.6. Mesotherapy for acne before and after treatment.

Source: https://www.researchgate.net/profile/Haqeeq-Ahmad/publication/344739896/figure/fig1/AS:948257303834625@1603093567476/Mesotherapy-for-Acne-before-and-after-Treatment.jpg.

Aside from alleviating aesthetic issues, mesotherapy can also be used for therapeutic intervention, especially in treating chronic diseases. This double potential contributes to its beauty as a treatment modality in multidimensional cosmetic dermatology. For instance, mesotherapy has also been used for the relief of pain in chronic states and for associating pharmacological agents with a desire to reduce inflammation and improve tissue health within targeted areas. At the convergence of health and beauty in mesotherapy, it opens up pathways for utilization in conditions of altering skin integrity, such as chronic venous disease and musculoskeletal disorders. By broadening the scope of target areas, mesotherapy not only addresses cosmetic improvements but also aids in the rehabilitation of underlying medical issues. Nevertheless, consensus among practitioners on appropriate indications and treatment protocols remains a critical hurdle that the field must overcome to maximize the therapeutic potential of mesotherapy (Bifarini et al., 2021) (Figure 9.6).

Test Your Knowledge

1. What are the main injection techniques used in mesotherapy, and how do they influence the treatment outcome?
2. What types of solutions are commonly used in mesotherapy, and what are their respective purposes?

9.2. Indications for Mesotherapy

Learning Outcome

1. Focus on fat reduction by mesotherapy
2. Define skin rejuvenation
3. Describe cellulite treatment

Mesotherapy has been a popular procedure in cosmetic dermatology, utilized particularly for aesthetic enhancement and treatment. Skin rejuvenation is one of the key indications for mesotherapy, and it is effective in addressing aging signs such as wrinkles and fine lines. The technique involves injecting a combination of vitamins, enzymes, and other bioactive substances directly into the mesoderm, the intermediate layer of the skin in which cellular processes are most vibrant. This intensive administration fortifies skin elasticity and texture and promotes hydration and a more youthful appearance. Because mesotherapy is a minimally invasive procedure, it is more and more favored by those patients who resort to non-surgical techniques of beauty treatment, following the trends of modern non-surgical esthetics discussed in recent medical literature (Stoian et al., 2019). Therefore, it is a major step forward in skin care techniques, providing several advantages that are attractive to a wide range of patient populations. The treatment of localized fat deposits and cellulite is another well-known use of mesotherapy. Such conditions tend to be major sources of dissatisfaction for patients and result in patients seeking out many different types of treatments. Mesotherapy is going to reduce fat and body contouring, as it could administer lipolytic agents that initiate the destruction of the fatty cells. This procedure has a high potential for patients who will struggle with resistant fat pockets that do not yield to standard weight loss mechanisms. As discussed in the overall review of non-surgical body contouring techniques, mesotherapy offers a unique approach with the benefit of minimal recovery time (Stoian et al., 2019). The practitioner will nonetheless be required to check individual patient records for assessment of appropriateness and ensure customized treatment targeting body objectives and particular physiological feedback. Mesotherapy is also used in treating hair loss, especially alopecia, of diverse presentations. Mesotherapy can be excellent for cases of androgenetic alopecia, alopecia areata, and even telogen effluvium, which is a process in which patients undergo excellent non-surgical treatment during which hair thickness and follicle condition improve. It can be described as the infusion of a mixture of growth factors, vitamins, and minerals that is administered into the scalp to reactivate hair follicles that help in further growth. Recent investigations and reviews suggest that mesotherapy, when used in conjunction with other treatments like microneedling or PRP therapy, may lead to variable yet promising results in the treatment of alopecia. This double use of mesotherapy adds to its versatility in cosmetic dermatology, confirming its position as an important choice for those who want to enhance their physical as well as psychological health.

9.2.1. Fat Reduction

The search for efficient fat reduction methods continues to be a major concern in cosmetic dermatology. Mesotherapy, an invasive procedure that entails the injection of diverse substances into the mesoderm, has also increased in popularity as an alternative for localized fat accumulation. This method is unique because it can act on localized regions, thus providing a specific treatment solution for body contouring without the need for surgery. Though conventional techniques like liposuction are likely to leave scarring and longer recovery periods, mesotherapy is a less invasive option. It is attractive due to the potential for fewer side effects and relatively faster results, consonant with modern aspirations for cosmetic procedures that best preserve everyday life. The efficacy and safety of mesotherapy for reducing fat, albeit popular, require thorough analysis. Scientific evidence on the results of mesotherapy is still limited for fat loss.

There is some research supporting mesotherapy treatment to obtain localized fat reduction, but no one knows how it works. Cosmetic dermatologists and patients are inconvenienced in determining if it has any benefits or not since there is a lack of strong clinical data. Current research raises issues about variability in findings, since patient responses can vary depending on practitioner ability and active ingredients employed. Hence, further research into how effective mesotherapy is and the best protocols for its use is necessary to validate its application in fat reduction. Additionally, the incorporation of mesotherapy into comprehensive fat reduction treatments is illustrative of a trend toward treating cosmetics by multifaceted methods. This paradigm would imply that mesotherapy can never be a lone solution but is better when used in conjunction with other procedures, including lifestyle changes or adjuvant therapies. For example, patients are likely to experience better results when undergoing a synergistic treatment plan comprising diet and exercise coupled with mesotherapy treatments. This holistic approach is commensurate with the prevailing trends in dermatology that focus on integrated patient management. Furthermore, understanding how mesotherapy interacts with other aesthetic modalities could lead to improved protocols and enhanced results for individuals seeking effective fat reduction methods, ultimately promoting greater patient satisfaction and treatment longevity (Figure 9.7).

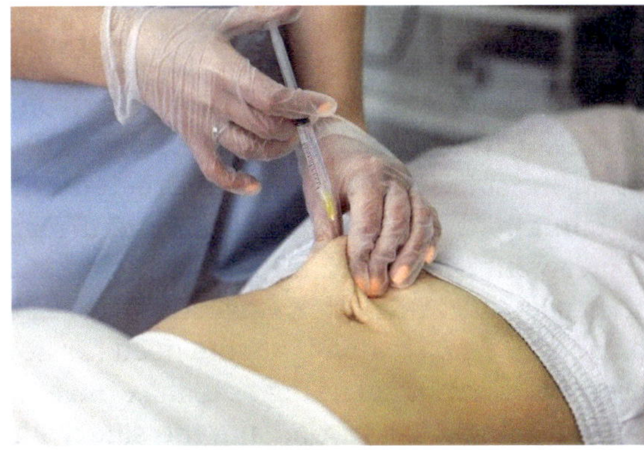

Figure 9.7. Mesotherapy for fat reduction.

Source: https://www.researchgate.net/profile/Seung- https://cdn.prod.website-files.com/66b127d3d0211e8547303fc6/6725c8e2c331b4affecd64f6_mesotherapy-fat-reduction.webp.

9.2.2. Skin Rejuvenation

The search for rejuvenation of the skin in cosmetic dermatology has been heavily researched, with the increase in individuals looking for non-surgical techniques to improve their appearance. Various technologies, including injectology, lasers, and mesotherapy, are examined for their safety and efficacy. Mesotherapy, in particular, has been developed as a rather versatile method that entails the injection of active substances and micronutrients within the mesodermal layer of the skin to address conditions like wrinkles, fine lines, and general skin health. As per the latest reviews, this novel combination of injectables, like hyaluronic acid and Botox, tends to create positive outcomes with regard to addressing clients' growing demands for non-surgical treatments. In addition, non-surgical lifting treatments are gaining popularity with great outcomes and minimal recovery periods, which indicates a preference for cosmetic enhancements without major surgical interventions (Stoian et al., 2019). The cumulative effects of the combination of several treatment modalities have contributed to the increasing demand for rejuvenation of the skin. An excellent study demonstrated significantly improved facial rejuvenation results with the concurrent application of autologous platelet-rich plasma (a-PRP) and hyaluronic acid (HA) than with either intervention applied in isolation. The patients treated with this combined therapy did have significant improvement in appearance and skin elasticity of the face and also better subjective scores of satisfaction. Thus, it highlights the need for new concepts of treatment strategies to maximize the outcome without compromising the safety and comfort of the patients. As patients continue to seek comprehensive solutions to skin aging, the integration of different modalities such as mesotherapy, a-PRP, and HA signifies a pivotal advancement in achieving optimal rejuvenation outcomes (Aboud et al., 2021).

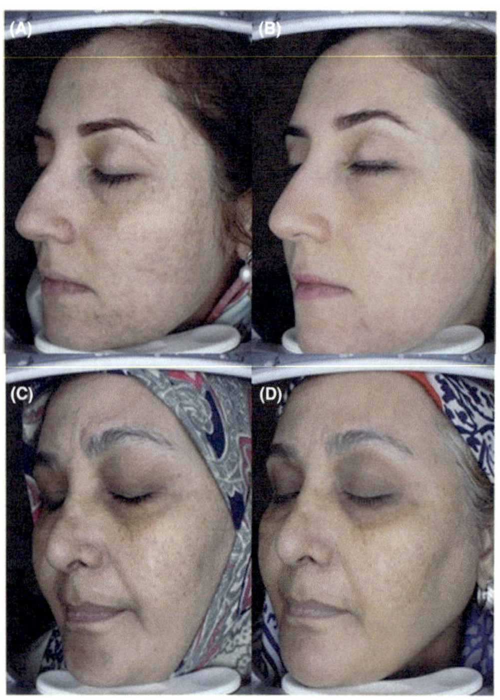

Figure 9.8. Photo of patients before (A, C) and after (B, D) mesotherapy.

Source: https://www.researchgate.net/publication/369596886/figure/fig1/AS:11431281158862542@1684248585659/Photo-of-patients-before-A-C-and-after-B-D-mesotherapy.png.

This relates mesotherapy, in itself, to an improvement in the landscape concerning skin rejuvenation, and it encourages the holistic approach to facial aesthetics. Injectable cocktails can be formulated to address the particular issues of the skin and all the different problems at the same time can be tackled. Putting all of these nutrients, vitamins, and regenerative agents together renders mesotherapy an active tool for boosting the production of collagen and rehydrating the skin. The flexibility of the technique matches current trends toward customized aesthetic therapy able to meet multifaceted patient demands. Finally, the higher level of evidence for mesotherapy as an adjunctive therapeutic regimen demonstrates its applicability for the continued development of cosmetic dermatology that would promote safer, more rewarding, and more effective results for rejuvenation-seeking patients (Stoian et al., 2019) (Figure 9.8).

9.2.3. Cellulite Treatment

The excessive prevalence of cellulite in women is a proven condition, with an approximate rate of 98% among females. It is an outcome of complex interactions between genetic, hormonal, and environmental determinants, leading to an architectural disorganization of connective tissue. Because of its prevalence, there has been an increasing demand for effective treatments of cellulite, hence creating some therapies. Of these, mesotherapy has drawn interest because of its non-surgical approach through the direct injection of bioactive substances into the targeted areas. Yet, the effectiveness of most treatments, such as mesotherapy, remains questionable since significant evidence of their efficacy is not yet determined, and there is still space for critical appraisal in the area of cosmetic dermatology (Couto et al., 2013). Cosmetic dermatology encompasses the treatment of cellulite with approaches that range from surgical to non-invasive methods. But since there is a growing interest in non-surgical cellulite removal, the risks of these procedures should also be taken into account. For example, though mesotherapy is seen as a relatively safe treatment, cases involving skin infections from cosmetic treatments tend to alert one to the possible complications. NTM have also appeared as major pathogens in this respect, implicating treatments such as mesotherapy in infections that can complicate the outcome of treatments. This issue underlines the importance of enhanced awareness and preventive measures in the use of cosmetic dermatological procedures (Chirch et al., 2015).

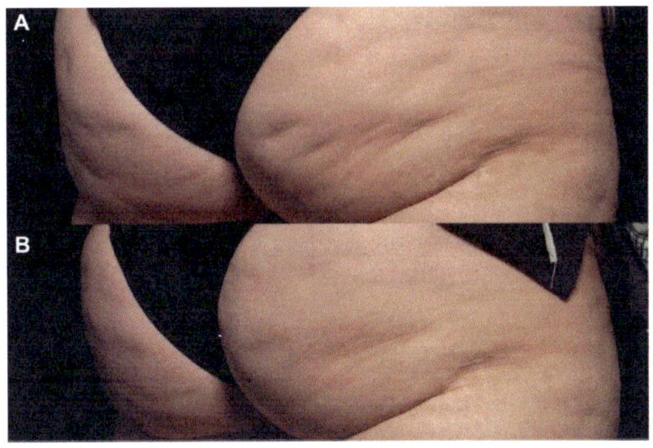

Figure 9.9. Significant improvement in cellulite of the buttocks 3 months following a single session of vacuum-assisted subcision (B) compared with baseline (A).

Source: https://www.researchgate.net/publication/312261231/figure/fig3/AS:11431281256215436@1719511190741/Significant-improvement-in-cellulite-of-the-buttocks-3-months-following-a-single-session.jpg.

In spite of the mounting interest in mesotherapy as a treatment for cellulite, the current controversy surrounding its overall efficacy continues. Although positive outcomes have been discovered in certain studies, the majority are undermined by the lack of large-scale controlled studies. The variable presentations of cellulite among persons also contribute to it becoming difficult to present a clear conclusion regarding the efficacy of the treatment. That is, while the safety of mesotherapy is indeed a valuable consideration for scientific research, choosing patient profiles that can benefit from the mesotherapy should also be extremely cautious. Only through aggressive scientific research can we determine what its real merits and limitations are, so it can be ensured that patients desiring cellulite treatments will have the correct expectation and realistic option, thereby creating a healthier cosmetic dermatology practice (Couto et al., 2013) (Figure 9.9).

Test Your Knowledge

1. Explain the mechanism by which mesotherapy helps reduce the appearance of cellulite.
2. What skin conditions can benefit from mesotherapy for rejuvenation, and what results are typically expected?

9.3. Benefits of Mesotherapy

Learning Outcome

1. Explain how minimally invasive procedures revolutionized patient care
2. Discuss the importance of quick recovery time in cosmetic procedures
3. Understand the notion of customizable treatments in mesotherapy

Mesotherapy's method in cosmetic dermatology has been in the spotlight for its multiple benefits since it is a widely sought-after practice for both aesthetic and cosmetic dermatology. It is a non-invasive, minimal procedure that uses a combination of vitamins, enzymes, and other bioactive substances injected directly into the mesoderm, which is the intermediate layer of the skin. One of its most important benefits is its versatility; mesotherapy can treat conditions as varied as a localized reduction of fat to rejuvenation of the skin, the fight against signs of aging, and many more. Targeted injections are what make it possible, through mesotherapy, for the local delivery of therapeutic agents that can offer more effective and enduring results than systemic therapy. Second, the ability to tailor it to individual patient needs makes it more appealing in cosmetic dermatology so that practitioners can devise custom regimens that achieve maximum patient response (Stoian et al., 2019). In addition to flexibility, mesotherapy has a lower recovery time, which makes it more appealing when compared to more invasive surgery methods. In most cases, patients can experience minimal downtime, thereby perfect with contemporary life demands because of their love of low disruption to daily routines. The fact that the procedures are non-surgical implies that individuals can generally go back to their routine shortly after treatment, a particular boon in a society increasingly enamored with fast, effective beauty fixes. Also, mesotherapy is generally less prone to have side effects than traditional surgical operations, and this factor enhances its attractiveness among patients who are not willing to undergo more invasive procedures. This factor makes it very popular among clients for cosmetic surgery without having to make the huge investment needed for surgery (Bifarini et al., 2021). It also leads to very customized treatment plans in mesotherapy, which may be used to target a variety of aesthetic concerns. Being an individualized method, a doctor can adjust the injectables preparation to focus on the particular client, which would depend on skin type, elasticity, or specific areas needing correction concerning its effectiveness. This personalization is vital in addressing various conditions, from cellulite to hyperpigmentation, thus fostering better satisfaction rates among patients. Moreover, as ongoing research continues to validate the effectiveness and safety, including evidence from randomized controlled trials, the procedure is expected to gain further acceptance among practitioners and patients alike. These attributes collectively underscore the profound impact mesotherapy can have within the field of cosmetic dermatology, promising enhanced outcomes and patient satisfaction (Stoian et al., 2019) (Figure 9.10).

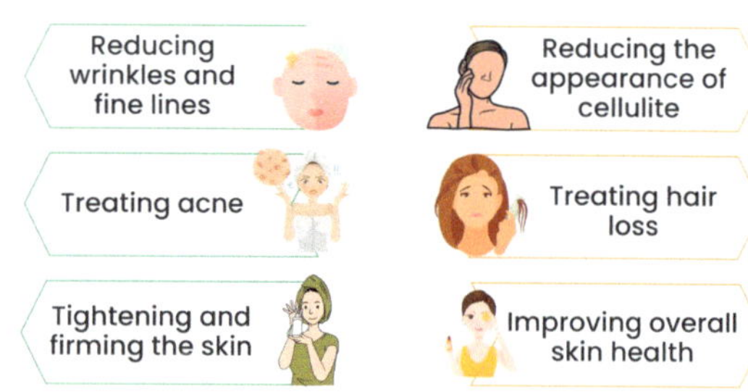

Figure 9.10. Benefits of mesotherapy.

Source: https://soulskinclinic.com/wp-content/uploads/2022/11/Soulskin-Clinic-1-1024x671.webp.

9.3.1. Minimally Invasive Procedure

In the realm of cosmetic dermatology, minimally invasive procedures have revolutionized patient care, particularly in how practitioners approach aesthetic enhancements. Mesotherapy exemplifies this innovation by providing a technique that delivers therapeutic agents directly to targeted areas of the skin, mitigating the need for extensive surgical interventions. This approach not only enhances the effectiveness of treatment but also reduces recovery time, leading to a lower burden on patients. Through the application of microinjections to deposit substances like hyaluronic acid and vitamins, mesotherapy addresses a multitude of cosmetic issues, ranging from fat dissolution to skin renewal. The increased popularity of such treatments highlights the changing face of cosmetic enhancements, where patients increasingly opt for less invasive procedures that are guaranteed to yield adequate results without the excessive downtime characteristic of conventional surgery. The more mesotherapy is accepted, the more vast would be its applications will be in the future in the treatment of various conditions. As an example, recently there came out the results of a study where a noncrosslinked hyaluronic acid filler was made to become effective by promoting the viability of human dermal papilla cells (DPC) and increasing VEGF release to combat oxidative stress problems faced by skin cells. In fact, these results further validate the use of mesotherapy as a cosmetic procedure and therapy, thereby justifying its position as one of the least invasive LITs. With the application of the regenerative properties of some agents, significant effects can be made in rejuvenating facial tissue, thereby justifying its place in line with the interests of patients for the enhanced aesthetic with reduced recovery barriers. With continued advances in research, mesotherapy's use could also move beyond aesthetic markings to more general dermatological therapies. The appeal of minimally invasive treatments such as mesotherapy is also heightened among the younger adult population, who are ever more attracted to aesthetic medicine as a way of realizing their ideal looks while meeting specific issues linked to their age group. It looks for remedies to skin defects and asymmetry in an endeavor to improve their natural beauty without radical procedures. The fact that one is able to fix asymmetries and outline facial contours using non-surgical treatments makes mesotherapy particularly appealing. Ethical concerns enter the scene since aesthetic medicine blurs the lines between therapeutic treatment and beauty standards in culture. The consequences that come with enhancing preventive aesthetics are significant enough to examine them in depth, particularly because young adults are undergoing such treatments as part and parcel of their grooming. Finally, mesotherapy and other micro-invasive methods not only indulge aesthetic needs but are indicative of the trend towards more affordable, sophisticated cosmetic dermatology solutions (Wollina & Goldman, , 2011) (Figure 9.11).

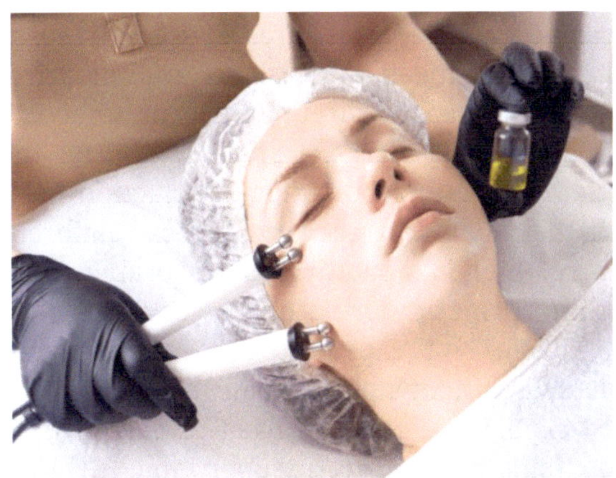

Figure 9.11. Mesotherapy facial with microcurrent for enhanced skin rejuvenation.

Source: https://www.inurskn.in/wp-content/uploads/2023/12/meso-cover-1.png.

9.3.2. Quick Recovery Time

There is a fast-growing allure to quick recovery time in cosmetic procedures that encourages both practitioners and patients toward mesotherapy. This is a relatively new approach where microinjections of vitamins, hormones, and other compounds are applied into the mesodermal layer of the skin. It is a procedure that is less likely to require much post-procedure downtime than the traditional counterpart. As patients seek less invasive solutions to their cosmetic problems, the rapid recovery from mesotherapy is a huge advantage in that it allows individuals to be back to their normal lives very shortly after the procedure. The benefit of a quick return to normalcy makes mesotherapy particularly attractive in the cosmetic medical tourism market, where convenience is as important as effectiveness in cosmetic treatments (Simpattanawong, 2016). Furthermore, the quick recovery time associated with mesotherapy is not only a matter of convenience but also contributes to its growing acceptance in the field of cosmetic dermatology. Many patients appreciate being able to avoid prolonged hospital stays or extensive recovery periods, which can often accompany more invasive surgical procedures. The non-invasive nature minimizes the risk of complications typically linked to surgery, such as infections and significant scarring. Studies indicate that patients tend to report high satisfaction levels with the results and recovery process, reinforcing the treatment's reputation as a favorable option within cosmetic dermatology (Castelanich et al., 2024). This expedited recovery may also bolster a patient's psychological well-being, as they experience enhanced self-esteem without the stigma of extensive recuperation. Including rapid recovery in the scope of mesotherapy within the greater perspective underscores its position as a revolutionary method in cosmetic dermatology. It reduces the procedures to the physical demands for recovery, thus being appealing to those who have hectic lifestyles. Mesotherapy is not only a flash in the pan because of the limited side effects and rapid healing, but it is also more than a quick fix; it offers long-term benefits that appeal to all kinds of consumers. This treatment's increased popularity is not only evidence of its effectiveness but also an indication of a cultural shift towards discovering beauty solutions that align with modern lifestyles. Mastering how to attain and regulate fast recovery time in mesotherapy allows practitioners to better address patient needs, fitting treatments into the realities of their patient's hectic lifestyle and demands (Simpattanawong, 2016).

9.3.3. Customizable Treatments

The concept of tailor-made treatments in mesotherapy is a milestone in cosmetic dermatology. Personalization is needed because it addresses the individual physiological characteristics of each patient and their beauty goals. Mesotherapy allows practitioners to create specially designed products and treatment methods for patients based on their main areas of concern, including localized fat elimination, skin revitalization, and cellulite elimination. Mesotherapy specialists have the option of tailoring treatment plans to include an integrated mixture of various active ingredients such as hyaluronic acid, vitamins, and amino acids. This personalization is especially crucial in the wake of increasing demand for non-invasive visible treatments free from extended recovery periods. Moreover, advancements in technology and clear clinical guidelines have improved the efficacy of customized treatments in mesotherapy. Recent literature outlines how innovative therapies and delivery mechanisms greatly enhance the efficacy of customized treatment approaches. The approach of using techniques such as ultrasound and electrical stimulation adjunctively during mesotherapy will allow for better absorption of active ingredients, thereby maximizing their therapeutic effects. Consensus on treatment protocols in foundational literature related to cosmetic dermatology supports evidence-based practices as being more likely to result in good patient outcomes. This evidence sustains personalization of treatments such that practitioners are provided with the best possible tools to manage the patient's requirements in the right way (Téot et al., 2021). Lastly, in addition to enhanced patient outcomes, customizable treatments in mesotherapy create an efficient collaborative practitioner-patient relationship. This could be accomplished as patients by giving them a chance to contribute to the development of their treatment plans, thus increasing engagement and adherence to proposed protocols. The collaborative decision-making experience promotes patient expression of expectations and wishes, as a result of which desired outcomes are better understood. As noted in instructional materials, patient engagement in treatment planning conveys congruence with contemporary trends in healthcare focusing on personalized care (Téot et al., 2021). Consequently, the incorporation of customizable treatments in mesotherapy not only improves aesthetic results but also empowers patients, creating a nurturing environment conducive to achieving their cosmetic goals.

Test Your Knowledge

1. Why is mesotherapy classified as a minimally invasive procedure, and how does this benefit patients?
2. What factors contribute to the quick recovery time associated with mesotherapy?

9.4. Risks and Side Effects

Learning Outcome

1. Describe common adverse reactions
2. Explain the long-term effects associated with mesotherapy
3. Understand contraindications essential for ensuring patient safety and treatment efficacy

The application of mesotherapy in cosmetic dermatology, while promising in terms of aesthetic outcomes, is not without its inherent risks and side effects. Patients often face both physiological and psychological risks, which can manifest in various forms. Physiologically, common side effects include bruising, swelling, and pain at the injection site, collectively contributing to discomfort and potential dissatisfaction with the procedure. More severe complications may include allergic reactions or infections because of introducing substances into the skin. The psychological factors that may hinder people from undergoing more procedures or having low self-esteem are anxiety regarding the results or dissatisfaction with the treatment. In conclusion, these risks inform practitioners and patients about preventing mesotherapy treatments by turning down these procedures and achieving realistic expectations from mesotherapy treatments (Simpattanawong, 2016). Risk perception plays a key role in the expansion and acceptance of mesotherapy as a treatment modality in cosmetic dermatology. The landscape of non-invasive aesthetic medical tourism, especially in locales like Bangkok, indicates that stakeholders such as patients and providers are often hesitant due to fears about efficacy and safety. Patients may fear physical risks, including complications from injection techniques or adverse reactions to the cocktails of mesotherapy. Economic risks are also involved, since patients may not get the results they were hoping for and may have to pay more for corrective treatments. As well as that, social pressure and psychological impacts due to perceived failures can exacerbate these concerns, possibly serving as barriers to obtaining mesotherapy treatments. Therefore, an understanding of these factors in context can inform the creation of effective risk reduction strategies, maximizing patient satisfaction and industry development (Simpattanawong, 2016). Interestingly, research into specific compounds used in mesotherapy, such as dimethylaminoethanol (DMAE) and amino acids, reveals their potential to mitigate aging-related skin issues. Studies have demonstrated that these substances can significantly improve skin structure when properly administered, which raises important discussions about risk-benefit ratios in mesotherapy. But even with these positives, such as heightened collagen level and skin thickness in some circumstances, the risks of improper use or application remain attached to these chemicals. Any therapeutic practice by definition is a matter of balancing likely benefits against possible unwanted side effects, so strict procedures must be laid down. Careful patient evaluations and appropriate treatment plans can help mitigate risks while optimizing the aesthetic benefits of mesotherapy, thereby sustaining its viability in the cosmetic dermatology arena.

9.4.1. Common Adverse Reactions

The technique of mesotherapy, as popular as it is becoming due to its minimally invasive nature in the field of cosmetic dermatology, has its own complement of common side effects. Patients quite often develop localized side effects in the form of swelling, redness, and tenderness at the site of injection. These are usually mild and tend to resolve spontaneously, but they can quite seriously inconvenience the patient. Also, bruising and hematoma are frequent side effects of mesotherapy. These side effects may discourage the patient from receiving repeated injections, and this is a drawback in terms of potential future treatment and patient satisfaction. Hence, the practitioner has to negate the issue of hyper-pronounced patient expectations by giving a meticulous explanation of such possible side effects before starting the treatment, so that they are adequately explained. Apart from local side effects, mesotherapy may cause more serious complications, although they are comparatively rare. Descriptions have mentioned instances of soft tissue and skin infections, some of which are caused by non-tuberculous mycobacteria like *M. chelonae* and *M. fortuitum*, especially in cosmetic treatments that break through the skin (Chirch et al., 2015). Infections can occur as a result of unsuitable injection methods or contaminated materials, highlighting the need for strict hygiene measures in the course of treatment. Infections, upon occurrence, can lead to delayed healing and may necessitate medical treatment, hence greatly affecting patient outcomes. These side effects can serve as cautionary tales both for the patients and practitioners, bringing the point home that patients have to select qualified experts who follow set health standards in the field of cosmetic dermatology. Moreover, the psychological impact of side effects cannot be over-looked in mesotherapy. Anxiety or dissatisfaction with the unintended side effects may lead to a biased perception of the effectiveness of treatments among patients.

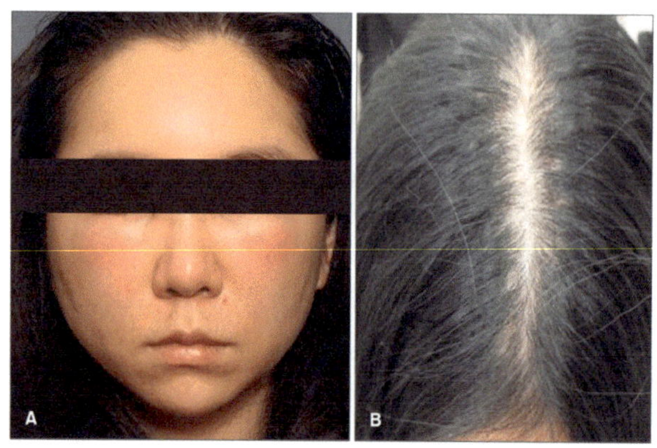

Figure 9.12. Initial photographs of a hypersensitivity reaction. Swelling on (A) face; and (B) scalp developed after intralesional injection of the mesotherapy mixture.

Source: https://www.researchgate.net/publication/331606044/figure/fig1/AS:734296222466048@1552081270142/nitial-photographs-of-hypersensitivity-reaction-Swelling-on-A-face-and-B-scalp.png.

Some allow their experiences to influence their willingness to undergo other cosmetic procedures, possibly hindering their quest for aesthetic ideals. Furthermore, as the body of literature grows regarding various treatments like PRP therapy for hair restoration, insights into the safety and efficacy of such alternatives become increasingly valuable (Cyran et al., 2024). This knowledge empowers patients to make well-informed decisions tailored to their specific needs and issues, highlighting the importance of comprehensive patient education in mitigating the psychological burdens associated with treatment-related adverse reactions (Figure 9.13).

9.4.2. Long-term Effects

The literature on long-term results of the use of mesotherapy in aesthetic dermatology is marked by bipolarity of potential benefit and severe danger. Mesotherapy is increasingly used because it can correct a number of dermatological conditions, such as alopecia, through local administration of active principles. Long-term efficacy is underway. Research has shown that mesotherapy has potential to increase the density of hair and regenerate hair follicles, particularly in non-cicatricial alopecia, such as androgenetic alopecia. Careful consideration must be given to the maintenance of these effects and side effects. While there are studies that support the potential of long-term improvement in looks, others confirm repeated intervention to maintain progress achieved, which may not be easy for patients seeking long-term solutions to dermatological concerns (Altunel et al., 2017). Biochemical mechanisms that underlie long-term effects of mesotherapy are primarily due to DPCs and their maintenance of hair follicle health and vitality. DPCs are the sites of maintenance and induction of hair growth, and therefore, they have a crucial role to play in providing sources of nutrients and growth factors to keratinocytes. The studies published in the recent years highlighted that certain mesotherapy preparations with hyaluronic acid and amino acids can confer protective actions against oxidative stress on DPCs. These therapies have been promising in maximizing cell viability and inducing vascular endothelial growth factor (VEGF) release, the most important of which is in maintaining hair follicles during their life cycle. While the scientific community uncovers these intricate interactions, the future of mesotherapy as a long-term treatment in cosmetic dermatology will be more apparent, especially for those with difficult conditions such as alopecia (Capillo et al., 2021). In the evaluation of the long-term consequences of mesotherapy, not only patient satisfaction but also the psychological dimensions of treatment outcomes should be taken into consideration.

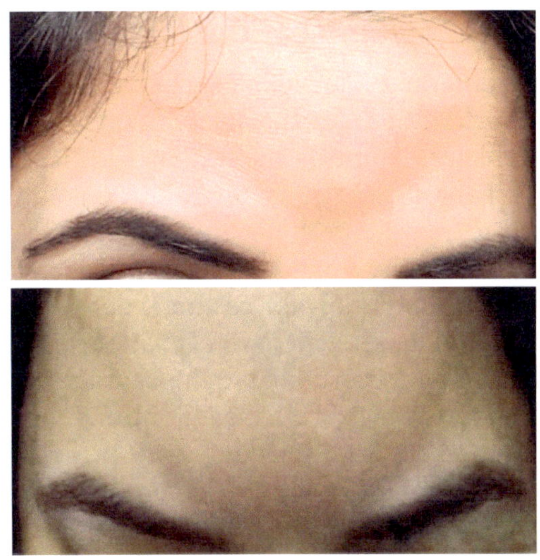

Figure 9.13. Patients presenting with an inverted triangle-shaped frontal edema after mesotherapy for androgenetic alopecia.

Source: https://www.researchgate.net/profile/Raquel-Carvalho-20/publication/356871238/figure/fig1/AS:11431281173720333@1689028730558/Patients-presenting-with-an-inverted-triangle-shaped-frontal-edema-after-mesotherapy-for.png.

The psychological impact of baldness can be very powerful and, in a great many instances, leads to decreased self-esteem and quality of life. Studies indicate that successful treatments like mesotherapy can enhance positive self-concept and the quality of life. However, such psychological benefits may rely on the persistence of the therapeutic effects. If the patient's outcomes vary or if they are subjected to multiple procedures to achieve and retain those results, his general satisfaction could wane and overall restoration effects that were based on mesotherapy would be negated. Thus, to truly evaluate this approach as an alternative mainstay for cosmetic dermatology, a thorough understanding of both the physiological and psychological implications of chronic mesotherapy is necessary (Figure 9.13).

9.4.3. Contraindications

In mesotherapy, knowledge of contraindications is important both for the safety of patients and for the success of treatment. Contraindications are a set of situations or conditions under which a treatment should not be carried out because there is a danger to a patient's health. In using mesotherapy for cosmetic dermatology purposes of fat reduction, rejuvenation, and hair loss treatment, certain patient characteristics disqualify them for this treatment. Individuals diagnosed with active skin infections, autoimmune disorders, or hypersensitivity to any of the ingredients in mesotherapy preparations are more likely to develop complications. Also, pregnant and breastfeeding women are usually warned against such treatments, as the long-term effects on fetal or neonatal health are not yet known. Identification of such contraindications is very important in minimizing complications and ensuring that mesotherapy is effective in the desired application. A broader definition of contraindications also encompasses the assessment of some dermatological conditions that may jeopardize the effectiveness of mesotherapies. For example, patients with cicatricial alopecia do not react in the same manner to mesotherapy compared with patients with noncicatricial types. Differential diagnosis is necessary because treatments offered for androgenetic alopecia or telogen effluvium won't provide a similar result when faced with the scarring or inflammatory cases. Therefore, practitioners are tasked with thorough assessments of predisposing conditions before commencing treatment.

Differential outcomes entail the possibility of differential results and, therefore, result in the paramount importance of contraindications for the selection of patients eligible for mesotherapy treatment of hair restoration, and other aesthetic treatments, thereby making it critical for an informed clinical decision. Last but not least, the ethical implications of ignoring contraindications in mesotherapy carry essential importance. Cosmetic enhancements are always in huge demand; however, the tendency to overlook or downplay risk factors may often lead to harmful effects on patients.

Therefore, a practitioner's responsibility is to initiate the welfare of a patient through the establishment of meticulous screening protocols that will effectively identify contraindicated conditions. Education about such implications is a must in the establishment of informed consent so that patients are fully aware of the potential benefits and risks involved with mesotherapy. Through compliance with established guidelines and contraindications, medical practitioners can improve the overall safety profile of mesotherapy in cosmetic dermatology, in addition to sustaining the tenets of medical ethics and a prioritization of patient safety. This strict methodology ultimately leads to an improved and responsible application of mesotherapy procedures to clinical practice.

Test Your Knowledge

1. What are the most common short-term side effects associated with mesotherapy?
2. Which factors can increase the risk of adverse reactions during or after mesotherapy?

9.5. Comparison with Other Cosmetic Procedures

Learning Outcome

1. Differentiate between mesotherapy and liposuction
2. Distinguish between mesotherapy and Botox
3. Explain mesotherapy and dermal fillers

The landscape of the cosmetic and aesthetic field is constantly changing, with one of the newer trends being mesotherapy as one of its more significant players for rejuvenation and treatment of alopecia among numerous other conditions. Mesotherapy is a relatively non-invasive treatment when it comes to skin rejuvenation and therapy of diseases like alopecia, in comparison to surgical procedures like hair transplants or facelifts. This treatment is especially attractive to those who want to have incremental improvements with the added advantage of not having lengthy recovery periods like in more invasive methods. Additionally, mesotherapy is flexible enough to address specific needs by modifying the formula according to individual skin issues, a luxury for many that traditional treatments cannot offer. This adaptability of mesotherapy thus makes it an attractive option over conventional cosmetic treatments, whose results may often be less personalized. In contrast to other non-surgical modalities, mesotherapy stands out because of its novel mechanism of action and variety of conditions it can treat. For example, other therapies like microneedling or PRP therapy have become popular for such uses in facial rejuvenation and hair growth. While it causes micro-injuries that stimulate the body's healing functions, mesotherapy is a direct injection technique utilizing rejuvenating substances that may contain vitamins, enzymes, and hyaluronic acid. Moreover, PRP therapy also aims at leveraging the body's natural growth factors; nonetheless, research has shown that the mixture of therapies, for example, the combination of hyaluronic acid with PRP, can lead to dramatically enhanced results for facial rejuvenation compared to each treatment executed in turn (Aboud et al., 2021). This comparison underscores the ongoing evolution of cosmetic dermatology, where synergistic effects among treatments signal a move toward comprehensive and multifaceted approaches. Moreover, mesotherapy's applicability in the treatment of hair loss further delineates its role within the domain of cosmetic procedures. The condition of alopecia, particularly the noncicatricial types such as androgenetic alopecia, has seen a growing repertoire of treatment options, including mesotherapy, low-level light therapy, and stem-cell therapy. Each technique has variable results; however, mesotherapy is reported to be superior and has been remarked as successful in enhancing the beauty, but also the quality of life for patients dealing with hair loss difficulties (Altunel et al., 2017). In contrast, other therapies may require more complex protocols or surgical procedures; the pragmatism and ease of mesotherapy might make it easier to achieve improved adherence among patients. The balance of efficacy, safety, and patient-centered care places mesotherapy in the vanguard of the ever-extending array of cosmetic dermatology, with potential for effective results while having fewer access limitations.

9.5.1. Mesotherapy vs. Liposuction

Liposuction versus mesotherapy has been the center of argument over which is one of the best treatments concerning excess fat and body sculpting. Mesotherapy includes the injection of a mixture of vitamins, enzymes, hormones, and herbal extracts into the mesoderm or middle layer of skin directly to attack localized fat. Advocates argue that this is a less risky and faster recovery treatment compared to the former surgery-based methods, such as liposuction. Liposuction, which is an invasive procedure, physically removes the fat from some parts of the body and the results are instantaneous and more visible. The issue with liposuction is that it has been in existence much longer and how efficient it is has been known in advance, but its invasive method of practice could result in complications that patients and practitioners of aesthetic medicine must carefully consider. The effectiveness of mesotherapy compared to liposuction is an area with marked disparities in their effects and impacts on patients. Research findings indicate that mesotherapy is associated with meager fat loss, typically requiring follow-up treatments for noticeable improvements. This method easily attracts those not eager to go under the knife but want something different-from-surgery. There are cases of full-scale changes for body contour through liposuction, in most massive corpulence conditions. An. Professionals within the field have articulated these distinctions, underlining that patient expectations must align with the chosen procedure. The need for comprehensive consultation and individualized treatment plans becomes paramount, allowing for a tailored approach that considers the nuances of each method's efficacy and potential side effects, as outlined in key texts on the topic (Simpattanawong, 2016). Ultimately, the choice between mesotherapy and liposuction may also reflect broader societal attitudes towards beauty and wellness, particularly in specific contexts such as Greece. As explored in recent anthropological studies, the consumption of cosmetic treatments goes beyond the physical results, embodying cultural meanings and personal narratives around beauty. These therapies, particularly cosmeceuticals, often carry significant emotional weight for users, who attribute personal and social value to them. This psychological aspect may be a consideration in selecting, as some patients will select mesotherapy only due to perception of safety and realization of philosophy of gradual perfection, whereas other patients will be attracted more towards liposuction due to its sensational and rapid results. With advancements in cosmetic dermatology over the years, it is significant to comprehend these nuances for making a judgment that may lead the patient toward a suitable decision compatible with his or her aesthetic pleasure and philosophy (Liakounakou et al., 2020) (Figure 9.14).

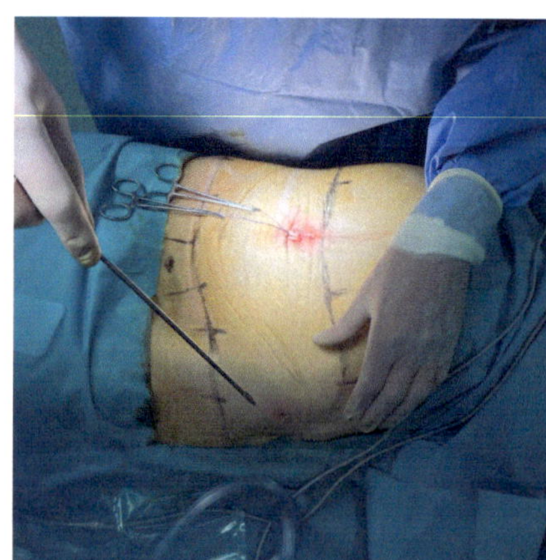

Figure 9.14. Liposuction. Visible dissected navel.

Source: https://www.researchgate.net/publication/383522140/figure/fig1/AS:11431281274380393@1724950783683/Liposuction-Visible-dissected-navel-own-work.png.

9.5.2. Mesotherapy vs. Botox

In the changing face of cosmetic dermatology, mesotherapy and Botox are two of the most well-known non-surgical cosmetic treatments. Mesotherapy, a procedure that entails intramuscular injection of a mixture of vitamins, minerals, and other therapeutic agents into the mesoderm, promises to rejuvenate the skin and treat localized fat deposits. Mesotherapy is much praised for its all-around nature, being able to treat various ailments, from cellulite to wrinkles on the face. This makes mesotherapy an adjustable treatment procedure, and therefore it can be devised to be specifically for the patient who wishes for a particular reaction. However, Botox's mechanism is different because this is a neuromodulator that temporarily paralyzes certain types of facial muscles to inhibit wrinkles; hence the role of each treatment towards facial beauty is through a different physiological pathway. Therefore, the choice depends on the assessment of the needs of the patient. The choice between mesotherapy and Botox often hinges on patient-specific goals and concerns. Mesotherapy is frequently favored by individuals desiring a holistic enhancement, as it focuses on improving skin texture and hydration. Recent research indicates that the ingredients of mesotherapy injections are significant determinants of success, with practitioners frequently altering the contents on the basis of patient type and status. In contrast, Botox is largely regarded as especially effective in the elimination of dynamic wrinkles, particularly those originating from facial movement. Botox's action is likely to be realized more quickly and to persist for several months, providing patients with a simple solution to the visible signs of aging. However, the calming effects on the muscles might not be harmonious with the specified aesthetic intentions of individuals who want to have more natural facial dynamics, thus emphasizing the relative subjectivity of aesthetic treatments in this regard. New evidence also clarifies the nuances of these cosmetic treatments, unveiling patient experiences and perceptions. For instance, a survey conducted in 2022 by The International Society of Aesthetic Plastic Surgery showed a prevalent use of injectables such as Botox in non-surgical procedures. Surprisingly, results showed varied perception of pain during such procedures, with some variation depending on age and phases of the menstrual cycle, with studies pointing to the possibility of patient satisfaction and outcome effects of these physiological factors (AlGhamdi et al., 2025). Since mesotherapy treatments highly depend on patients' reactions to various ingredients, knowledge of these variables can aid practitioners effectiveness in achieving expected outcomes. Furthermore, as the process of aging continues, substitute treatments like nutritional supplements such as Pure Gold Collagen are becoming more significant. The supplements aim to enhance skin quality through boosting collagen levels, proving how the industry constantly evolves to address varied aesthetic needs (Borumand et al., 2014) (Figure 9.15).

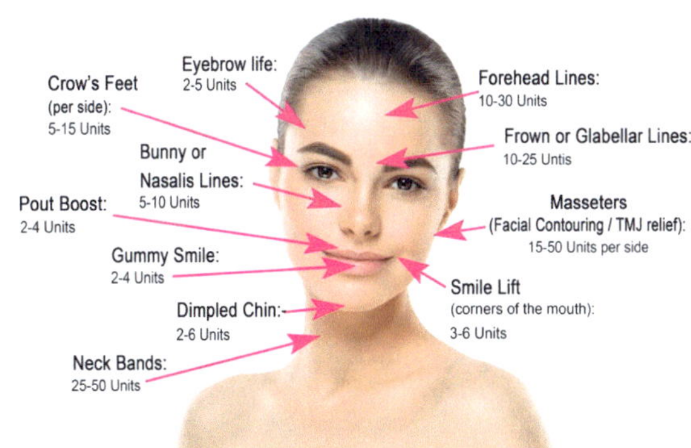

Figure 9.15. Site for Botox injections.

Source: https://www.researchgate.net/publication/352483617/figure/fig3/AS:1035679026913281@1623936530728/Site-for-botox-injections.ppm.

9.5.3. Mesotherapy vs. Dermal Fillers

The skin map has been revolutionized by the emergence of a plethora of minimally invasive procedures, and the most popular among them are mesotherapy and dermal fillers. Mesotherapy is the injection of an individualized blend of vitamins, enzymes, and hyaluronic acid directly into the mesoderm or the intermediate skin layer to stimulate and hydrate it. This treatment is aimed at the overall health and quality of the skin, targeting conditions like fine lines, irregular tone, and regional fat pads. Dermal fillers, on the other hand, have a specific function: to replace volume and fill out the skin by filling wrinkles and lines. Every treatment has distinct advantages, mesotherapy targets general skin rejuvenation, whereas dermal fillers deliver localized volumization, which assist prospective patients in making logical choices based on their skin requirements and expectations. Important distinctions in the modes of action for mesotherapy and dermal fillers again emphasize their diverse applications in cosmetic dermatology. Mesotherapy focuses on the introduction of nutrients into the skin, enhancing its hydration and flexibility and, in the long run, collagen synthesis. This treatment, therefore, not only beautifies but also provides healthier skin in a more holistic approach. On the other hand, dermal fillers are largely hyaluronic acid or collagen products that are volumizers and have instantaneous effects upon the procedure. Whereas fillers will bring instant gratification by reshaping the face, they will have to be topped up every couple of months to be able to persist in their effects. Therefore, understanding the individual character of each treatment becomes important for patients seeking tailored solutions for cosmetic flaws. Additionally, the ideal candidates for mesotherapy and dermal fillers can also differ by age and specific skin needs, making individualized treatment regimens important. As mentioned, age can significantly influence what aesthetic desires individuals have; young adults can look for procedures that treat asymmetries and add sculpting to the face, and older adults can look for treatments of wrinkles and sagging (Wollina & Goldman, , 2011). Furthermore, the evidence suggests that the effectiveness of mesotherapy in improving overall skin quality is notable, and clinical trials have demonstrated a statistically significant improvement in skin vitality after treatment, such as measured by hydration and texture parameters (Amuso et al., 2025). Therefore, both mesotherapy and dermal fillers have their own role to play in an integrated aesthetic treatment protocol so that practitioners can maximize results depending on the individual aims of their clients.

Test Your Knowledge

1. How does mesotherapy differ from liposuction in terms of mechanism, invasiveness, and recovery?
2. Compare the effects of mesotherapy and Botox in facial aesthetic treatments.
3. In what ways do mesotherapy and dermal fillers differ in their aesthetic outcomes?

9.6. Current Trends and Innovations

Learning Outcome

1. Focus on advances in injection techniques
2. Deal with new formulations and ingredients
3. Discuss integration with other treatments

With advancements in the science of mesotherapy remaining under the umbrella of cosmetic dermatology, the existing trends continue to shift toward less invasive approaches to ensure patient comfort and therapeutic outcome efficacy. Of these, the application of sophisticated pharmacological agents within the mesotherapy cocktail has been given priority, primarily to direct the therapeutic cocktail toward specific issues such as pigmentation, wrinkling, and balding. These preparations not only enhance the delivery of treatments but also cater to the rising demand for customized treatments in the field of aesthetics. Besides, the development of non-invasive aesthetic medical tourism also signals an emerging market where individuals seek quality mesotherapy treatments that balance efficacy and cost, and this makes it a competitive market for clinics and practitioners too. The investigation of such trends highlights the need to keep adapting to patient needs and market forces, especially as cross-border aesthetic service mobility grows, as emphasized by the new frameworks of risk perception for aesthetic medical tourism (Simpattanawong, 2016). The incorporation of technology into mesotherapy treatments has played a major role in the cosmetic dermatology landscape of innovations. Advances that have recently been made in the injection methods that have primarily centered on this use of microneedling and automated injections have made it possible to revolutionize the agents for mesotherapy. It had increased precision during delivery, which made it improve on absorption and distribution. Since patients demand more non-invasive treatments for their condition, fears of safety and effectiveness were addressed through embracing these new techniques. Moreover, the applications of digital platforms and telemedicine create a platform whereby the practitioner interacts with the patient and facilitates an informed consultation which creates a basis for individualized treatment plans. Therefore, through technology in mesotherapy, not only are patients' experiences improved, but also the standards of professionals in cosmetic dermatology (Micheal, 2014). The transforming face of mesotherapy is also targeted with educational efforts towards its changing scene. Professional training and development with a focus on best practices and innovative techniques are increasingly essential as complexity and sophistication characterize the development of practices. Organizations are gradually realizing the promise of curriculum development that shapes education to cover distinct challenges and skills relevant to aesthetic medicine. Curricula that detail comprehensive methods of mesotherapy treatments and include hands-on experience will ensure practitioners are competent in delivering contemporary industry benchmarks and patient satisfaction. By integrating industry expert feedback and scholarly studies, such education can provide future beauticians and dermatologists with the professionalism needed to manage the complexities of mesotherapy pragmatically while meeting the challenges of both domestic and global markets (Micheal, 2014; Simpattanawong, 2016).

9.6.1. Advances in Injection Techniques

Mesotherapy injection methods have evolved to be a major development in cosmetic dermatology, with the intention of treating a multitude of aesthetic issues, such as aging and skin-related problems. The traditional mesotherapy usually involved syringe-based manual procedures for the direct delivery of therapeutic agents into the mesoderm, which is the middle layer of the skin. The advent of mechanical devices, however, has revolutionized this procedure with enhanced precision and consistency. Recent research has shown that microneedling devices, for instance, offer a minimally invasive approach, reducing downtime while improving patient comfort and satisfaction, thus increasing the popularity of mesotherapy treatment among diverse populations (Sivaranjani, 2019). The technology in such injectables not only enhances clinical outcomes but also promotes new approaches to cure disorders like atrophic acne scars, dry skin, and other dermatological conditions. Furthermore, breakthroughs in the product injected through mesotherapy have transformed treatment efficacy. This advanced technology injectable carries hyaluronic acid and bio-identical hormones individually formatted to meet the skin's needs to revitalize and moisturize it on a cellular level. They have become clinically valuable in providing volume replacement and texture alteration (Elena et al., 2021). In addition, through nanotechnology, the introduction of nanoparticles with encapsulated active ingredients brings about targeted delivery along with sustained releases of therapeutic agents, thus further maximizing absorption and minimizing potential side effects. This innovative approach is further an improved treatment, not merely addressing signs of aging but also improving the overall healthiness of skin, making it an important milestone in cosmetic dermatology. Beyond improved results, the results of these advancements impact injection techniques: they ensure patient safety and satisfaction-essentials in clinical practice. Better training for practitioners in using automated devices and sophisticated injection techniques paves the way toward a higher standard of care while at the same time diminishing the associated risks with improper administration. The development of standardized protocols and the use of innovative technology, such as imaging techniques to guide injections, have significantly contributed to these safety measures (Sivaranjani, 2019). Furthermore, patient education regarding expectations, potential side effects, and post-treatment care has been prioritized, leading to higher satisfaction rates among patients seeking cosmetic procedures. Collectively, these advances not only elevate the practice of mesotherapy within cosmetic dermatology but also reinforce the commitment to providing effective and safe treatments tailored to individual patient needs (Figure 9.16).

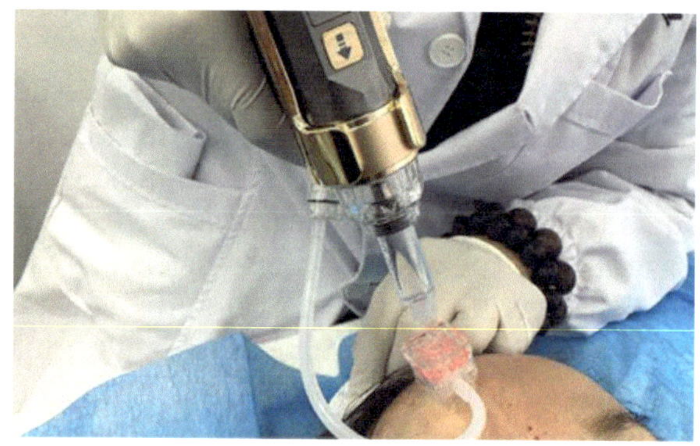

Figure 9.16. Mesogun technique for speed and consistency.

Source: https://cdn.shopify.com/s/files/1/0871/7713/4375/files/mesotherapy_injection_techniques3.jpg?v=1734679959.

9.6.2. New Formulations and Ingredients

The advent of mesotherapy in cosmetic dermatology has sparked innovative developments in formulations and ingredients aimed at enhancing treatment efficacy. One notable trend is the incorporation of multifunctional compounds into mesotherapeutic solutions. These formulations often include vitamins, minerals, and amino acids, which can synergistically address various skin concerns such as hydration, pigmentation, and aging. Through the utilization of these chemicals' biological profiles, practitioners are able to adjust treatment to meet the needs of a single patient. For example, the management of diseases such as melasma is a multi-factorial process in accordance with the complex etiology involving UV and hormones. The integration of compounds that inhibit melanin synthesis, such as kojic acid and ascorbic acid, will be particularly useful in conjunction with a standard mesotherapy protocol, leading to better patient outcomes and satisfaction (Para et al., 2024). Innovations in hyaluronic acid formulations constitute the backbone for innovation in mesotherapy. With HA traditionally revered for its hydrating properties, recent developments into HA-based injectables have significantly enhanced their functionality. For example, a variety of crosslinking methods have been reported in order to influence the rheological properties of HA gels, yielding products that would be more elastic and stable. New products now combine linear HA with other agents like antioxidants and vitamins forming a polycomponent system with anti-aging and rejuvenating action on the skin. These advanced HA formulations ensure that injectables not only fill and volumize but also nourish and protect the skin, addressing multiple age-related concerns simultaneously (Cassuto et al., 2021). This evolution demonstrates how mesotherapy can adapt and incorporate novel ingredients, ultimately enriching the therapeutic landscape in cosmetic dermatology. The exploration of tailored mesotherapy solutions reflects the ongoing demand for personalized dermatological care. Through the incorporation of innovative formulations that balance pharmacological and biological principles, clinicians are better able to address the individual needs of their patients. With the variety of ingredients available, customization is possible based on individual skin types and problems, making successful treatment protocols more achievable. In the case of patients suffering from difficult conditions such as melasma, there is a definite need for treatments that benefit not only cosmetically in the short term but also address the long-term health of the skin. The creation of products designed specifically for multifactorial cause conditions indicates the expansion of the specialty, which clearly demonstrates a demand for new formulations in advancing mesotherapy procedures in cosmetic dermatology (Para et al., 2024).

9.6.3. Integration with Other Treatments

The confluence of mesotherapy with other cosmetic treatments proves superior as it covers aesthetic needs under a multifaceted approach. For example, concurring skin problems related to pigmentation, texture, and hydration may be treated simultaneously by concurring mesotherapy with chemical peels or laser therapy. In this regard, mesotherapeutic agents will serve to optimize the benefits of a laser treatment by providing necessary nutrients to deeper layers after the treatment. This synergistic action allows for holistic care by treating surface and more in-depth dermatologic conditions together, thus ensuring more satisfied patients and better treatment outcomes. Strengthening these integrated treatments affirms that mesotherapy cannot be used alone but rather as part of a comprehensive aesthetic treatment plan aimed at catering to the heterogeneous needs of the patient in cosmetic dermatology. Additionally, new research on EVs and their use in mesotherapies indicates promising potential for incorporating regenerative methods into cosmetic treatment. Recent research has identified the regenerative capacity of EVs and their implications on reversing signs of aging and rejuvenating skin (Micheal, 2014). By combining mesotherapy with EV-based therapy, cosmetic dermatologists may be able to maximize tissue repair and rejuvenation, thereby providing patients with state-of-the-art solutions to fight skin aging and damage. This combination has the promise of utilizing the non-invasive benefits of mesotherapy while adding potent regenerative factors that may transform the discipline, eventually resulting in better aesthetic medicine outcomes. However, the inclusion of personality and psychological aspects in treatment protocols might also make mesotherapy and other aesthetic treatments more effective. Awareness of how personality influences a patient's acceptance of aesthetic treatments can inform the tailoring of treatment protocols (Stolić, 2020). For example, more conscientious individuals are likely to be more open to combining mesotherapy with other treatments, which can encourage a more active attitude towards their skincare routine. Taking patients through these psychological bases not only encourages improved compliance with combined therapy but also enhances their general aesthetic experience. Thus, the combination of mesotherapy and psychological consideration with physical treatment signifies a more holistic approach to cosmetic dermatology itself, providing further assurance that patient outcomes are optimized via a holistic care strategy.

Test Your Knowledge

1. What are some recent advances in injection techniques that have improved the precision and comfort of mesotherapy treatments?
2. What are some of the novel ingredients being incorporated into modern mesotherapy formulations?
3. How is mesotherapy being combined with other aesthetic treatments to improve outcomes?

SUMMARY

Mesotherapy emerges as a multifaceted approach in cosmetic dermatology, offering innovative solutions for various aesthetic concerns, ranging from skin rejuvenation to hair restoration. The versatility, characterized by the injection of active substances into the mesodermal layer of the skin, underscores its efficacy in addressing issues such as wrinkles, cellulite, and post-operative scarring. Research indicates that mesotherapy, particularly when combined with other treatments, can enhance overall results and patient satisfaction. The findings from recent studies reinforce its potential benefits, encouraging dermatologists to consider mesotherapy as a viable option in their practice. Furthermore, as the demand for non-invasive aesthetic interventions continues to grow, mesotherapy has the opportunity to evolve, aligning with patient expectations for minimal downtime and effective outcomes. This constantly expanding body of evidence propels forward the dialogue about the safety and effectiveness of mesotherapy. However, there is still a challenge in standardizing best practice due to variability in practitioner techniques and different formulation types. Therefore, proper training of practitioners in mesotherapy techniques and ensuring that every patient receives consistent information on treatment protocols remains critical. This notion resonates particularly in the context of emerging practices, such as PRP therapy and the investigation of mesotherapy for conditions like post-operative scarring following breast reduction, as observed in discussions around its impact on patient wellness and aesthetic improvement (Boshoff et al., 2016). Further research is needed to solidify its standing within cosmetic treatments, particularly in evaluating long-term outcomes and optimal protocol adherence. As the field of cosmetic dermatology grows, the use of mesotherapy with patients is both an opportunity and a challenge. Comprehensive research is essential to truly define its long-term safety and efficacy profiles. The potential in mesotherapy is stimulated by enhanced cooperation between cosmetic surgeons, dermatologists, and researchers toward better patient results and aesthetic outcomes. The focus on continued enhancement and improvement of injection techniques and formulations may help overcome some of the current deficits, therefore providing greater efficiency for mesotherapy in general. As knowledge continues to grow, as well as academic investigation into the subject, mesotherapy is ready to take its place within the future landscape of cosmetic dermatology as emerging studies in related fields of hair restoration often do (Cyran et al., 2024).

In recent years, the application of mesotherapy in cosmetic dermatology has garnered significant attention due to its minimally invasive nature and versatile uses. This technique involves the injection of various active ingredients into the mesoderm, the middle layer of the skin, thereby promoting localized treatment. Key points of interest in mesotherapy include its effectiveness in addressing conditions such as aging skin, cellulite, and localized fat deposits. Significantly, mesotherapy provides alternatives to surgery, especially for those who prefer non-invasive remedies that reduce recovery time and risks involved. With the changing aesthetic needs, clients are now more opting for mesotherapy as a good approach to obtain rejuvenated skin and a better look, which is easily fitting in with modern cosmetic needs. Additionally, mesotherapy is unique because it specifically targets all issues of the skin, such as post-surgical scarring. One major issue with women, particularly those who have undergone mammary reduction surgery, is the visibility of scars. Complications of the old ways of surgery are scarring and prolonged recovery. Mesotherapy, with procedures like Mesotherapy Eporex, has been proposed to be one solution to reduce such scars and improve skin texture after surgery. The implications of this application extend beyond superficial benefits, addressing deep-seated emotional and psychological factors related to body image. This approach invites further exploration into its efficacy against scarring as well as its broader role in enhancing recovery after surgical interventions, thus positioning mesotherapy as a promising alternative for improving patients' quality of life (Boshoff, 2016). Furthermore, the aging process manifests in various dermatological changes that necessitate thoughtful, targeted interventions to maintain skin health and vitality. As indicated in the literature, intrinsic factors such as hormonal fluctuations significantly alter the skin's structural integrity, particularly in adult women. Mesotherapy can effectively address these age-related changes by revitalizing the skin at a cellular level, promoting hydration, elasticity, and overall resilience. The treatment's focus on enhancing the skin's density and thickness aligns well with the need for ongoing and comprehensive skin care, especially in menopausal women who experience heightened challenges related to aging. By integrating mesotherapy into a holistic skin care regimen, practitioners can foster an environment conducive to sustained skin health and improved self-esteem, underscoring the importance of addressing both aesthetic and physiological aspects of skin aging (Herman et al., 2013).

KEY TERMS FROM THIS CHAPTER

Aesthetic therapy physicians	Architectural disorganization
Beauty goals	Botox's mechanism
Botulinum toxin (BT)	Harmful effects
Hyaluronic acid (HA)	Mesotherapy
Nontuberculous mycobacteria (NTM)	Vascular endothelial growth factor (VEGF)
Fat reduction	Cellulite treatment
Hair restoration	Nutrient cocktails
Anti-aging therapy	Localized fat loss
Vitamin infusion	Dermal hydration
Wrinkle reduction	Pigmentation control
Scalp therapy	Skin tightening
Injection technique	Tissue regeneration

CRITICAL THINKING QUESTIONS

1. **What is the primary purpose of Mesotherapy in aesthetic medicine?**
   a. To treat internal organ infections
   b. To replace surgical procedures entirely
   c. To deliver small amounts of medication directly into the skin
   d. To stimulate deep muscle contractions
2. **Which of the following is most commonly injected during mesotherapy?**
   a. Botox
   b. Hyaluronic acid
   c. Platelet-rich plasma (PRP)
   d. Vitamin C and other nutrients
3. **Who developed the technique of Mesotherapy?**
   a. Dr. Jean-Claude Aubert
   b. Dr. Michel Pistor
   c. Dr. Pierre Fournier
   d. Dr. Paul Langevin
4. **What is a common side effect of Mesotherapy?**
   a. Permanent scarring
   b. Severe allergic reaction
   c. Mild swelling and bruising
   d. Hair loss
5. **Which of the following conditions can mesotherapy potentially treat?**
   a. Hair loss
   b. Cellulite
   c. Wrinkles and fine lines
   d. All of the above

Short Answer Questions

1. What is mesotherapy, and what are its primary uses in medical aesthetics?
2. How does the technique of mesotherapy work in terms of injecting substances into the skin?
3. What are the common substances or ingredients injected during mesotherapy treatments?
4. What conditions or concerns can mesotherapy effectively treat?
5. Are there any potential side effects or risks associated with mesotherapy?
6. How does mesotherapy compare to other cosmetic procedures, such as liposuction or Botox, in terms of effectiveness and recovery time?
7. Who are the ideal candidates for mesotherapy, and are there any contraindications?
8. What is the typical recovery time after a mesotherapy procedure, and how many sessions are usually required for optimal results?

Answer to Critical Thinking Questions

1. (c); 2. (d); 3. (b); 4. (c); 5. (d)

REFERENCES

1. Aboud, C., Hersant, B., La Padula, S., et al. (2021). Synergistic effects of autologous platelet-rich plasma and hyaluronic acid injections on facial skin rejuvenation. https://core.ac.uk/download/541662302.pdf (accessed on 11th June 2025).
2. AlGhamdi, N. J., AlHemli, H. A., AlHuraish, D. S., Amir, B. A., Bin Rubaian, N. F., & Bukhari, A. E. (2025). Assessment of pain perception of aesthetic procedures during menstrual period in comparison to non-menstrual period days. https://core.ac.uk/download/651843299.pdf (accessed on 11th June 2025).
3. Altunel, C., Gencler, B., & Kartal, S. P. (2017). Cosmetic procedures in the treatment of alopecia. https://core.ac.uk/download/322430037.pdf (accessed on 11th June 2025).
4. Amuso, D., Desiderio, V., Qorri, E., et al. (2025). Mesotherapy with HA and choline against facial skin aging: An open-label uncontrolled, monocentric study. https://core.ac.uk/download/651715068.pdf (accessed on 11th June 2025).
5. Stoian, Anca Pantea; Hainarosie, Razvan; Pietrosanu, Catalina; Rusescu, Andreea; Andronache, Liliana F.; Paunica, Stana; Balalau, Cristian; and Pituru, Teodora S. (2019) "Modern concepts in non-surgical esthetics; a review," Journal of Mind and Medical Sciences: Vol. 6: Iss. 2, Article 3. DOI: https://doi.org/10.22543/7674.62.P190195 Available at: https://scholar.valpo.edu/jmms/vol6/iss2/3(accessed on 11th June 2025).
6. Bifarini, B., Brauneis, S., Collina, M. C., Di Campli, C., Di Marzo, R., Ferrara, P. E., Gori, F., et al. (2021). A call to action by the Italian Mesotherapy Society on scientific research. https://core.ac.uk/download/541504768.pdf (accessed on 11th June 2025).
7. Borumand, M., & Sibilla, S. (2014). Daily consumption of the collagen supplement Pure Gold Collagen® reduces visible signs of aging. https://core.ac.uk/download/186931355.pdf (accessed on 11th June 2025).
8. Boshoff, T. M. (2016). Mesotherapy EPOREX treatments on post-operative mammary reduction scarring. https://core.ac.uk/download/222967500.pdf (accessed on 11th June 2025).
9. Cai, X., Chen, Z., Liu, D., et al. (2014). Effects of dimethylaminoethanol and compound amino acid on D-galactose induced skin aging model of rat. https://core.ac.uk/download/28951119.pdf (accessed on 11th June 2025).
10. Capillo, M. C., D'Este, E., Di Francesco, S., et al. (2021). In vitro hair growth promoting effect of a noncrosslinked hyaluronic acid in human dermal papilla cells. https://core.ac.uk/download/491496546.pdf (accessed on 11th June 2025).
11. Cassuto, D., Bellia, G., & Schiraldi, C. (2021). An overview of soft tissue fillers for cosmetic dermatology: From filling to regenerative medicine. Clinical Cosmetic and Investigational Dermatology, 14, 1857–1866. https://doi.org/10.2147/ccid.s276676 (accessed on 11th June 2025).
12. Castelanich, D. G., Chacín, M., & Parra Hernández, L. A. (2024). Successfully nonsurgical epidermoid cyst management with recombinant hydrolytic enzymes: A case report. https://core.ac.uk/download/624336261.pdf (accessed on 11th June 2025).
13. Chandi, Garg, Shweta, Manchanda, S., & Garg. (2018). The wonder tool platelet-rich plasma in cosmetic dermatology, trichology and hair transplant. https://core.ac.uk/download/322432560.pdf (accessed on 11th June 2025).

14. Chirch, L. M., Grant-Kels, J. M., & Hypolite, T. (2015). Nontuberculous mycobacterial infections: A potential complication of cosmetic procedures. https://core.ac.uk/download/pdf/81164964.pdf (accessed on 11th June 2025).

15. Couto, M., Nobre, J., Noites, A., et al. (2013). Evaluation of ultrasound, ultra sonophoresis and homeopathic mesotherapy on cellulite treatment. https://core.ac.uk/download/232113110.pdf (accessed on 11th June 2025).

16. Cyran, P., Jaroszyńska, A., Jaroszyński, F., et al. (2024). Platelet-rich plasma (PRP) in hair restoration treatments: A comprehensive review of existing literature. https://core.ac.uk/download/620863922.pdf (accessed on 11th June 2025).

17. Domaszewska-Szostek, A., Krzyżanowska, M., Polak, A., & Puzianowska-Kuźnicka, M. (2025). Effectiveness of extracellular vesicle application in skin aging treatment and regeneration: Do we have enough evidence from clinical trials? International Journal of Molecular Sciences, 26, 2354. https://core.ac.uk/download/650323067.pdf (accessed on 11th June 2025).

18. Téot L, Mustoe TA, Middelkoop E, et al., editors. Textbook on Scar Management: State of the Art Management and Emerging Technologies [Internet]. Cham (CH): Springer; 2020. Available from: https://www.ncbi.nlm.nih.gov/books/NBK586066/ doi: 10.1007/978-3-030-44766-3f (accessed on 11th June 2025).

19. Giannouli, E. (2021). Anti-aging: Nanodrugs, monoclonal antibodies and biological therapies. https://core.ac.uk/download/553473048.pdf (accessed on 11th June 2025).

20. Goldman, A., & Wollina, U. (2025). Minimally invasive aesthetic procedures in young adults. https://core.ac.uk/download/pdf/8574728.pdf (accessed on 11th June 2025).

21. Herman, J., Rost-Roszkowska, M., & Skotnicka-Graca, U. (2013). Skin care during the menopause period: Noninvasive procedures of beauty studies. https://core.ac.uk/download/197740630.pdf (accessed on 11th June 2025).

22. Herreros, F. O. C. (2018). Remodeling of the human dermis after application of salicylate silanol. https://core.ac.uk/download/296846850.pdf (accessed on 11th June 2025).

23. Kalaskar, D. M., Butler, P. E., & Ghali, S. (2016). Textbook of Plastic and Reconstructive Surgery. https://core.ac.uk/download/79526588.pdf (accessed on 11th June 2025).

24. Liakounakou, A. (2020). The many faces of Botox: Beauty, crisis, and cosmeceuticals in Greece. https://core.ac.uk/download/323201712.pdf (accessed on 11th June 2025).

25. Micheal, S. 2014. The teaching methods in aesthetics in relation to the labour market needs in Cyprus. Masters thesis Middlesex University(accessed on 11th June 2025).

26. Parać, E., & Bukvić Mokoš, Z. (2024). Unmasking melasma: Confronting the treatment challenges. Cosmetics, 11, 143–143. https://doi.org/10.3390/cosmetics11040143 (accessed on 11th June 2025).

27. Simpattanawong, D. (2016). Non-Invasive Aesthetic Medical Tourism in Bangkok: A Qualitative Analysis of Stakeholder Risk. https://core.ac.uk/download/341769488.pdf (accessed on 11th June 2025).

28. Sivaranjani, J. Percutaneous Collagen Induction in the Treatment of Atrophic Acne Scars using an Automated Microneedling Device: A Novel Approach. Diss. Stanley Medical College, Chennai, 2019.(accessed on 11th June 2025).

29. Stolić, D. (2020). Attitudes Towards Aesthetic Interventions: Relations with Personality Dimensions and Tendencies Towards Personality Disorders. https://core.ac.uk/download/296595676.pdf (accessed on 11th June 2025).

30. Yussif, N. M. A. (2021). Periodontal Disease. https://core.ac.uk/download/478140632.pdf (accessed on 11th June 2025).

CRYOLIPOLYSIS AND BODY CONTOURING TECHNOLOGIES

10

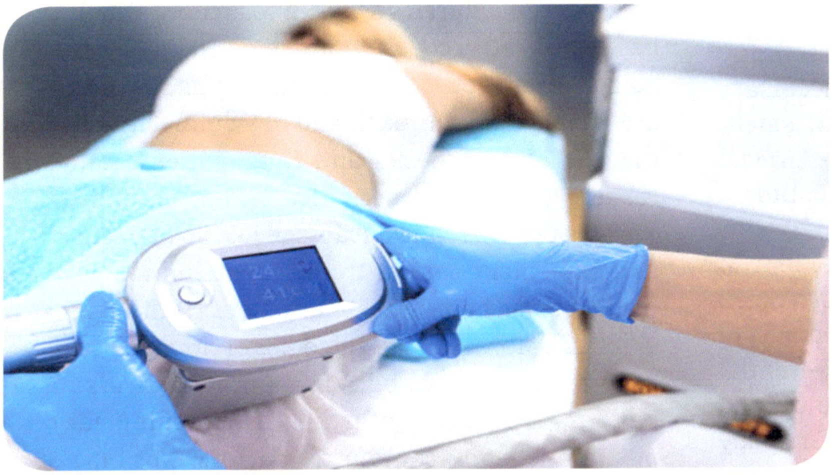

LEARNING OBJECTIVES

After studying this chapter, you will be able to:

1. Understand the history of body contouring technologies
2. Explain the mechanism of action underlying cryolipolysis
3. Discuss the benefits of cryolipolysis
4. Describe risks and side effects
5. Define the evolution of technology in cryolipolysis and body contouring technologies
6. Evaluate patient considerations for cryolipolysis and other body contouring technologies

Introduction

The quest for the ideal body shape has propelled innovation in aesthetic medicine, most notably in noninvasive body sculpting technologies. Traditional methods like liposuction, which became widely used because of their efficiency in eliminating localized fat and have been criticized for the invasiveness and downtime associated with surgery. With the shift in attitude in society to be less invasive, technologies like cryolipolysis have been offered as viable alternatives for sculpting, but without surgical alteration. These technologies offer treatment with a guarantee of quick outcomes and the least amount of downtime, ensuring the growing concern of body dissatisfaction due to more subcutaneous body fat and anomalies in the skin (Duncan et al., 2022). Cryolipolysis has come to be considered a current mode of non-invasive body contouring that relies on an endogenous process of selective cooling at the targeted sites to eliminate the fat cells. This has been proven to hold potential not only in the diminishment of localized fat deposits but also in skin quality. The inclusion of energy-based systems provides the practitioner with a three-dimensional method for body contouring. Additionally, maximizing the mode of treatment, i.e., the integration of high-intensity focused electromagnetic (HIFEM) therapy with radiofrequency (RF), has proved to have added value through treating fat and muscle laxity at the same time (Duncan et al., 2022). With an understanding of these non-surgical options, patients are able to make informed choices that satisfy their cosmetic goals. With advancing science of body contouring, ongoing research becomes necessary in order to establish the efficacy and safety of these emerging technologies. Non-surgical modalities are increasingly not only substitutes for liposuction but also the treatment of choice for most patients who desire improvement of their body silhouettes. Case series suggest mixed results, which supports the personalized nature of body contouring treatments. The potential for dramatic improvement in skin color and texture through modality pairing more forcefully argues in favor of individualizing the treatment with a view to a patient's specific requirements (Duncan et al., 2022). This obviously suggests that the field of body contouring is progressing towards better, patient-oriented practices with minimal invasiveness combined with optimized results.

Definition of Cryolipolysis

CoolSculpting, also known as cryolipolysis, is a non-invasive body contouring treatment used to remove localized fat deposits. It functions on the principle that fat cells are more susceptible to temperatures than other tissues. More specifically, the application of targeted cooling causes adipocytes to crystallize and subsequently undergo apoptosis, which is programmed cell death. The cells that have died break down naturally in the body over time and provide the treated skin with a slimmer appearance. Cryolipolysis requires less downtime, is much less harmful than more traditional approaches to liposuction and hence emerges as a respite for those seeking cosmetic transformation without surgery. The popularity of cryolipolysis rises with its simplicity and effectiveness in body sculpting. As body pressures get stronger, noninvasive treatments such as cryolipolysis counteract the demand for safe yet strong treatment.

The treatment is a comparison to more invasive procedures such as liposuction, which has prolonged recovery times and can be rather painful. On the other hand, cryolipolysis sessions are usually an hour each and are done without the use of anesthesia, and thus, patients can resume their usual activities within seconds. This procedure's side advantage just so happens to complement patient trends for less-invasive, pain-free body sculpting alternatives (Duncan et al., 2022). Moreover, the outcomes of cryolipolysis have been proven to be consistent with diverse patient populations, further establishing its position in body contouring devices. Not only is the treatment effective in removing fat, but also, it also has proven to enhance the quality of skin, and this is a critical factor in cosmetic treatments.

Through the treatment of stubborn areas of fat that are normally resistant to diet and exercise, cryolipolysis has the potential to drive worldwide body confidence in treated patients. As aesthetic technology continues to advance, it is worth considering cryolipolysis in combination with adjunctive noninvasive procedures, such as high definition LipoSculpture, which utilizes a combination of modalities for the best body contouring results (Soto et al., 2016). Combining these techniques highlights a groundbreaking shift in body contouring treatments, offering patients multiple channels for achieving their own set of desired results (Figure 10.1).

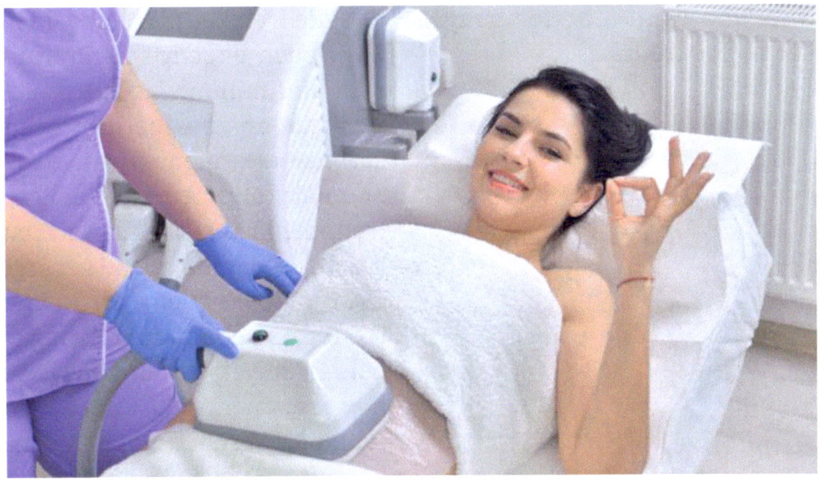

Figure 10.1. Cryolipolysis treatment for non-invasive fat reduction.

Source: https://www.kolorshealthcare.com/blog/wp-content/uploads/2023/09/Cryolipolysis.jpg.

Overview of Body Contouring Technologies

The body contouring technology environment has developed significantly from the earlier isolated surgery technique to many of the non-invasive options that are present today. Liposuction for centuries was the traditional way of fat removal from localized collections, but varied levels of recovery times, pains, and risks of complications demanded a shift towards less invasive techniques. As body image concern increases within society, non-surgical treatments have become popular among patients for successful, risk-free body reshaping without the inherent risks of conventional surgery (Duncan et al., 2022). The various advancements of new technology, such as HIFEM fields, radiofrequency (RF) energy, and combined treatment, have also expanded the range of options for consumers and working professionals alike. Non-surgical body contouring technologies mainly belong to two groups: energy-based modalities and cryolipolysis. HIFEM and RF therapies work together by enhancing muscle tone and fat reduction in targeted areas, while cryolipolysis freezes adipose tissue selectively to allow it to be removed naturally. A new freezing action selectively targets only fat cells without harming adjacent tissues, which has made it quite intriguing compared to conventional approaches (Duncan et al., 2022). By utilizing the body's own metabolic processes, patients can see changes in body shape that can be measured without significant downtime or discomfort. As the devices continue to evolve, the safety and efficacy of the technique still remain a priority for the practitioner to provide full-body contouring results. Adding to a variety of non-invasive body contouring modalities provides the practitioner with an alternative to aesthetic improvement. For example, synergy of HIFEM with RF: Not only does it tone up the muscle, but also provides a glabrous surface of the skin, uniting both into an integral method of the issues of body contouring (Duncan et al., 2022). Optimization of outcomes can also be enhanced by incorporating concomitant treatments such as targeted pressure energy (TPE) for improvement in skin laxity and overall quality. Through clinical investigation and patient assessment, such combination procedures demonstrate widespread body aesthetic improvement with fewer opportunities for potential risk and side effects than invasive procedures (Duncan et al., 2022). Accordingly, the body contouring industry is becoming a future where non-surgical technology offers efficient, patient-centered procedures for those who want a better body shape and self-esteem (Figure 10.2).

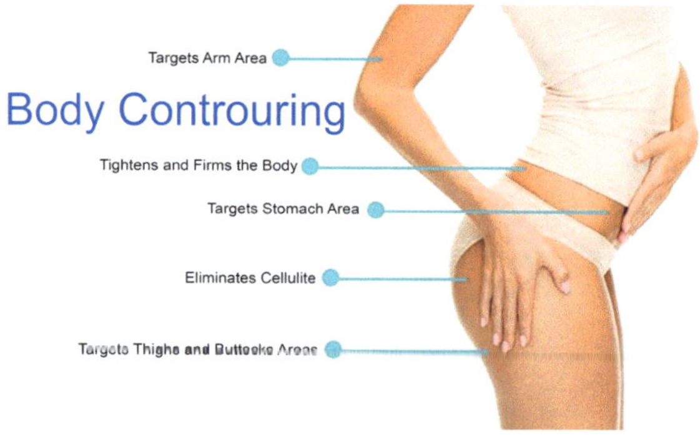

Figure 10.2. Body contouring.

Source: https://plasticsurgery.in/storage/files/body-contouring.png.

Importance of Non-Invasive Aesthetic Procedures

The increasing demand for non-invasive aesthetic procedures reflects a broader societal shift towards minimally invasive alternatives for body contouring. Traditional surgical methods, such as liposuction, while effective, are often accompanied by significant discomfort, recovery time, and potential complications. As individuals become more aware of their body image and seek solutions without the burdens associated with surgery, non-invasive techniques gain popularity. Treatments such as cryolipolysis and HIFEM ensure strong body contouring with significantly reduced risks and negligible downtime. Such developments not only address an interest in looking better but also fit into people's lifestyles, enabling them to incorporate treatments into their daily life without prolonged interruptions (Duncan et al., 2022). Apart from fitting well in modern lifestyles, non-invasive body contouring technologies seem to add a more holistic approach to health and beauty. While society is trying to deal with the challenges of body dissatisfaction owing to fat buildup and skin irregularities, the need for non-invasive procedures emerges. Advancements in aesthetic medicine, like the use of synchronized RF alongside other modalities, have been effective in improving the quality of skin and minimizing the buildup of fat without surgical or anesthetic procedures. With non-surgical treatments, patients undergo a gradual and natural process of change, sharply differing from the instantaneous and sometimes dramatic results frequently found in surgery (Duncan et al., 2022). This is such a trend that not only altered the forms of body contouring but also the values held in society about beauty and its acceptance. New treatments like CBL-514 injectables serve as examples of significant non-surgical interventions in modern cosmetic treatments. From available studies, it is found that CBL-514 significantly reduces abdominal subcutaneous fat without the disadvantages of surgical procedures, including increased recovery time and trauma. The added benefit of this non-invasive treatment is that a noticeable reduction of fats through targeted injections makes such procedures an attractive method for those searching for safe, effective, and efficient remedies against localized fat deposits. With continued research confirming these methods, non-invasive aesthetic procedures are no longer alternatives; they are forming the future of body contouring. With their proven safety and efficacy, these technologies provide patients with confidence in managing their body image while minimizing the risks traditionally tied to surgical options.

10.1. Historical Background

Learning Outcome

1. Understand the development of cryolipolysis
2. Focus on the evolution of body contouring techniques
3. Describe milestones in aesthetic medicine

Evolution in body contouring technologies traces back to the emergence of liposuction, which began in the late 20th century. From its initial introduction as simply a direct technique for localized fat reduction, liposuction has evolved to become a complex procedure involving multiple techniques and applications. Advancements in this area have resulted in a range of minimally invasive and non-invasive alternatives, enabling practitioners to respond to the intricacies of body contouring with enhanced accuracy. Medical professionals have written thorough manuals that map the evolution of these methods, describing their practical uses and limitations. As a means of being the first to pioneer body sculpting, liposuction opened the doors for even more developments that focused on attempting to find the demand for less invasive options and safety in cosmetic treatments. This established precedent allowed for further treatments to be pushed towards innovation, with cryolipolysis being an evolutionary treatment based on the premise of an innovative and non-surgical means of body contouring. The emergence of cryolipolysis therefore, is rooted in scientific observation of the effect of cold exposure upon the adipose tissue. The early research indicated that targeted cooling had the potential to kill fat cells through apoptosis without damaging surrounding tissues, thereby laying the ground for this revolutionary therapy. This finding led the way to the creation of cryolipolysis as a safe, non-surgical fat reduction procedure, which became commercially available to the public in the mid-2000s. Specifically, the technology exploits the inherent metabolic function of the body so that patients can experience perceivable enhancements with corresponding minimal risks of surgery. As with current research, including the promising results regarding CBL-514 injections, body contouring technology improvements indicate an increased focus on treatments that reduce the procedure's risk but enhance efficiency (Goodman et al., 2022). This shift is not only addressing patient concerns over safety but also emphasizing the potential of innovation in aesthetic medicine. The background to the technologies of body contouring shows that there was a profound change in popular attitudes towards cosmetic treatments. The consumer of today is better educated and requires procedures to meet high levels of safety, effectiveness, and convenience. As body contouring techniques advance, the use of new technologies and techniques remains the top priority. Therapists are nowadays enabled with the employment of various minimally invasive techniques that can be formulated according to the specific patient, thus improving satisfaction and outcomes. Moreover, a comparative analysis of studies on the reporting of new treatment effectiveness and safety through incorporation of CBL-514 enhances the understanding of the mechanistic drivers resulting in the reduction of fats (Duncan et al., 2022). Such an evidence-based practice facilitates the ability of practitioners to provide modern solutions for individuals seeking body recontouring procedures, as a reflection of historical progression that has culminated in the present status of cosmetic procedures.

10.1.1. Development of Cryolipolysis

Cryolipolysis constitutes one of the important advances in non-surgical body sculpting innovations. It was a spin-off from the invention that localized reduction of fat deposition was attainable through regulated cooling, where the adipocytes were targeted and not the surrounding tissue. Researchers have since been contemplating this technology for its effectiveness in targeting much greater health dangers of deposits, e.g., abdominal regions, which lead to long-term maladies like diabetes and cardiovascular diseases. Research has brought cryolipolysis into the spotlight as a workable solution for those who find it hard to shed stubborn body fat via conventional ways of diet and exercise. That it is non-invasive has made it especially appealing to such individuals in search of cosmetic enhancement without the risks bundled with surgical procedures, thus noting its place in today's aesthetic practice (Assis et al., 2022). Current literature has reviewed the efficacy of cryolipolysis in comparison to other body contouring methods, acknowledging its pros and cons. For example, the treatment alone was capable of producing a marked decrease in subcutaneous fat, with research studies being able to report a thinning of the fat layer by about 20–30% following a solitary treatment session. This has inspired the incorporation of cryolipolysis into multimodal treatment plans to improve cosmetic results. The consolidation of cryolipolysis with other technologies, including ultrasound therapy and RF, has proven promising in optimizing the reduction of fat and improving skin laxity, especially when aesthetic demands are at play. Combined therapies have demonstrated greater potential for circumferential reductions than cryolipolysis alone, underscoring the need for holistic treatment strategies within cosmetic practices (Cunha et al., 2019).

While the advancement of cryolipolysis marks a pivotal step in non-invasive fat reduction, ongoing research remains essential for optimizing its application in clinical settings. Exploring different protocols and combination treatments will also aid in the development of standardized treatment practices that take into account patient-specific needs and optimize efficacy. Furthermore, knowing the mechanisms of tissue response to cryolipolysis, including reperfusion and cell apoptosis, will increase the understanding of fat metabolism during treatment. With increasing evidence regarding the safety and efficacy of cryolipolysis, subsequent studies will be conducted to legitimize such claims and take the techniques applied clinically to a more advanced level. This research will eventually develop well-established, evidence-based answers to the clients seeking body sculpting services that would solidify the position of cryolipolysiss in the burgeoning aesthetic medicine industry (Cunha et al., 2019) (Figure 10.3).

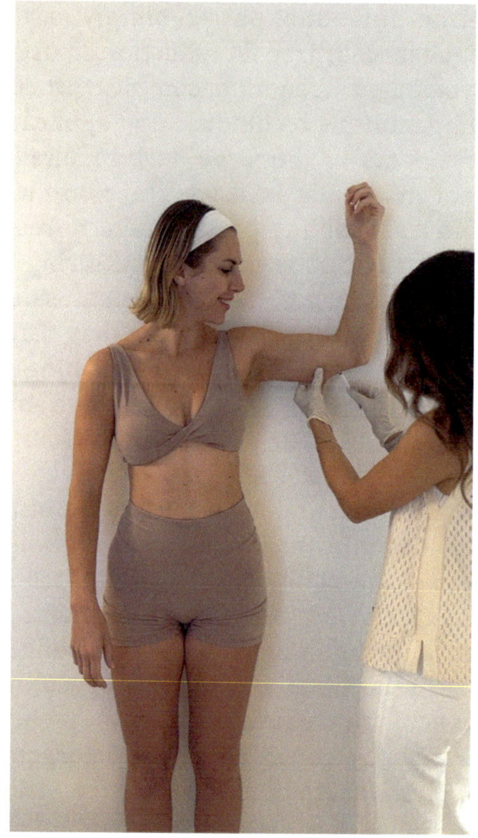

Figure 10.3. Fat freezing (cryolipolysis).

Source: https://images.squarespace-cdn.com/content/v1/61e76e4169daa00f3b3a2d92/74e7b6c5-e718-420f-847d-78f7c99daad1/IMG_8409.jpg.

10.1.2. Evolution of Body Contouring Techniques

The evolution of body contouring techniques reflects the intersection of aesthetic desires and advancements in medical technology. Initially, procedures such as liposuction emerged as minimally invasive methods aimed at reducing localized fat deposits. Over time, the field has witnessed significant innovations, with various energy-based devices gaining prominence in body contouring. These advancements not only offer improved precision and safety but also cater to a broader spectrum of treatment options. This has, therefore, led to the evolution of lipolytic techniques, including the use of lasers and ultrasound to melt and reduce fats with results that are less painful with reduced downtime. Therefore, one can say that practitioners now rely on a complete toolkit comprising all forms of minimally invasive and non-invasive procedures to ensure a customized answer to the needs of their patients, according to recent literature on modern methodology in the practice of body contouring (Duncan et al., 2022). Cryolipolysis came to herald a great deal in body contouring with the best demonstration of non-invasive fat reduction through controlled cooling. Since cryolipolysis implies apoptosis caused in adipose tissues while maintaining the integrity of the structure surrounding such tissues, it is effective in recontouring body aesthetics without hindering the quick recovery needed post-surgery. It is becoming popular since one would see and feel the benefits without being threatened by surgical risks. Additionally, modern technologies further advance this as the base method and investigate extensions like combination treatments where cryolipolysis is used in combination with other methods to achieve increased effects. The evolution of such techniques above shows an increasing trend of patient-centeredness in aesthetic medicine. Thus, a treatment can be made even more customized based on individual body composition and aesthetic intent (Ockell et al., 2023). In such a changing landscape, integration of patient feedback and clinical outcomes dictates the path of further advancement in the field. Research on post-bariatric patients' experiences has identified the risk of complications related to excess skin following dramatic weight loss and illustrated that contouring techniques need to not only affect these outcomes but also, somehow, address the problems of excess skin as well. Innovations on modified abdominoplasty techniques are being developed to cater to these patients, signaling a commitment towards patient satisfaction improvements. The development of models for predicting post-operative discomfort helps practitioners predict complications, therefore improving patient outcomes. Therefore, the development of body contouring methods not only focuses on technological improvements but also serves in compliance with the core human aspects of individuals undergoing aesthetic enhancements, connecting clinical know-how with patient welfare (Ockell et al., 2023) (Figure 10.4).

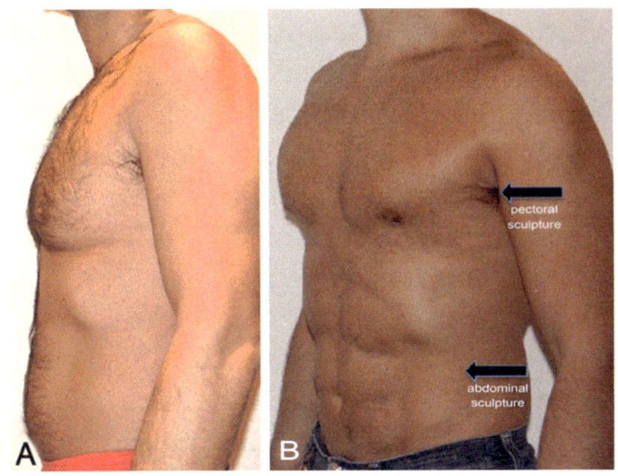

Figure 10.4. New male body contouring (muscular sculpture, MS) in normal-weight patient.

Source: https://www.researchgate.net/profile/Cristiano-Monarca/publication/271596747/figure/fig1/AS:392151142813728@1470507527007/New-male-body-contouring-muscular-sculpture-MS-in-normal-weight-patient.png.

10.1.3. Milestones in Aesthetic Medicine

The development of aesthetic medicine has been punctuated by some milestones that have transformed the landscape of body contouring technology. Cryolipolysis is one such trailblazing non-surgical treatment that can reduce localized fat. Ever since it made its entry during the late 2000s, this groundbreaking treatment employs controlled cold temperatures to kill fat cells by crystallizing them, and these subsequently get expelled out of the body naturally. Clinical trials have shown the effectiveness of cryolipolysis, indicating its ability to decrease subcutaneous fat without damaging adjacent tissue. The success of the technology represented a considerable change in aesthetic treatments, reflecting increasing consumer demand for effective treatments with minimal recovery time. The safety profile of cryolipolysis has also promoted its use, making it a leading option for aesthetic practices worldwide. While the aesthetic medicine market grew, there came innovations in body sculpting technologies that accompanied cryolipolysis. RF and ultrasound technologies have progressed, each with its own series of benefits to offer in the field of fat reduction and skin tightening. Together, these technologies give a solution to body contouring from many directions, which can be utilized to tailor treatment based on the needs of specific patients. For instance, RF promotes collagen production, enhancing skin elasticity while reducing fat layers, thus addressing dual concerns of fat reduction and skin rejuvenation. Moreover, the synergy of these modalities enables practitioners to create comprehensive treatment plans, optimizing results and patient satisfaction (Swanson, 2018). Thus, the evolution of body contouring techniques reflects both technological advancements and an increasing understanding of aesthetic medicine. The impact of milestones in aesthetic medicine, particularly in cryolipolysis and body contouring technologies, extends beyond individual treatments; it fosters a broader cultural shift towards body positivity and self-acceptance. As procedures have become more accessible and regarded as routine transformations rather than extreme interventions, society's perception of aesthetic treatments has evolved. Non-invasive treatments such as cryolipolysis give a person control over one's body without the shame once experienced in seeking cosmetic alteration (Swanson, 2018). Second, technological advancements have been instrumental in leading the revolution in personalized medicine, enabling a customized approach to body contour following individualistic characteristics and objectives (Swanson, 2018). This points out the need to understand that aesthetic medicine is not simply about changing how one appears, but also about improving one's body image.

Test Your Knowledge

1. What were the key scientific observations and breakthroughs that led to the development of cryolipolysis as a non-invasive fat reduction technique?
2. How have body contouring techniques evolved from invasive surgical methods like liposuction to modern non-invasive procedures?
3. What are the major milestones in the history of aesthetic medicine that have significantly shaped current practices?

10.2. Mechanism of Action

Learning Outcome

1. Describe how cryolipolysis works?
2. Compare with other body contouring methods
3. Understand physiological effects on fat cells

The mechanism of action underlying cryolipolysis, a non-invasive body contouring technology, is based on the targeted application of cold temperatures to adipose tissue. During the procedure, controlled cooling is used to induce apoptosis, or programmed cell death, in fat cells while sparing surrounding structures such as skin and muscles. This process occurs because adipocytes are more susceptible to cold than other types of cells. Once the temperature is low enough, the fat cells are crystallized, and within several weeks, it slowly gets metabolized and removed from the body by the lymph system. This treatment has now proved to be a great advancement in body contouring procedures, which allows patients the facility of having a slimmer figure without surgery, thus eliminating concerns over the invasiveness and recovery time required for conventional liposuction procedures (Duncan et al., 2022). The effectiveness of cryolipolysis is further enhanced by understanding the physiological responses of the body to fat cell reduction. Following the procedure, patients often experience localized inflammation as part of the natural healing process, which paradoxically promotes cellular repair and regeneration. This inflammatory response contributes to the gradual and sustained reduction of adipose tissue in the treated areas. Studies indicate that cryolipolysis may result in various levels of fat reduction, typically within the range of 20% to 25% in treated areas after one session, but could vary with individual situations and the nature of the tissue (Badran et al., 2023). Not only does this technology redefine the body shape, but it could also give confidence to those who prefer non-invasive treatments to overcome body dissatisfaction as a result of localized fat buildup. Apart from its direct cosmetic effects, cryolipolysis has potential metabolic effects that can be investigated. While the primary goal remains aesthetic enhancement, some studies have suggested that the reduction in local fat deposits could influence systemic metabolic factors, potentially improving metabolic health over time. For instance, the process may result in alterations in fat distribution and a decrease in metabolic markers associated with obesity-related conditions (Badran et al., 2023). These findings are preliminary and require further research in order to establish some kind of clarity on cryolipolysis-associated metabolic effects, especially concerning diverse populations. Ideally, the full mechanism of action and secondary effects associated with cryolipolysis will push forward further work into similar non-invasive technologies to offer comprehensive solutions in body contouring and management of body composition within the modern aesthetic landscape.

10.2.1. How Cryolipolysis Works

The underlying mechanism of cryolipolysis is based on the principle of selective cryo-lipolysis, wherein subcutaneous fat cells are targeted without causing harm to surrounding tissues. This process involves cooling the adipose tissue to a temperature that induces apoptosis, or cell death, solely in fat cells. When exposed to cold, the lipid-rich membranes of these cells undergo crystallization, which disrupts their structural integrity and eventually leads to cell death. This approach allows for the emulsification and gradual elimination of fat through the body's lymphatic system over a period of weeks. Consequently, cryolipolysis provides a non-invasive alternative to traditional liposuction, appealing to individuals seeking body contouring without the associated downtime or risk of surgical procedures, a significant factor noted in recent studies discussing the efficacy and safety of non-invasive techniques in aesthetic practice (Duncan et al., 2022). Moreover, several technical and physiological factors influence the effectiveness of cryolipolysis, such as cooling parameters and individual body composition. Optimal results depend on variables like treatment area, fat thickness, and individual patient characteristics. Several devices have been developed with different applicators and cooling mechanisms, designed to increase fat reduction while preserving the integrity of the skin. As evidenced in clinical results, uniform pressure and uniform cooling are important in order to guarantee effective cryolysis of fat cells while avoiding discomfort. In addition, although research indicates that cryolipolysis can cause a significant reduction of localized fat deposits, elucidation of the metabolic adjustments after treatment, such as temporary changes in the metabolic markers, indicates a field with much to be studied (Badran et al., 2023). Finally, the integration of cryolipolysis in body contouring regimens reflects a broader trend in aesthetic medicine toward minimally invasive treatments that align with patient preferences for safety and efficiency. By offering a method that combines safety, minimal downtime, and visible results, cryolipolysis has gained considerable popularity among those reluctant to undergo traditional surgical procedures. Patient satisfaction is commonly driven by the patient having realistic expectations of the results, along with the understanding that these results are not overnight but instead develop over several months. Of note, the development of combination therapies, using such technologies as HIFEM fields or synchronized RF in conjunction with cryolipolysis, may further improve outcomes, allowing for a comprehensive body-contouring treatment for a number of aesthetic concerns (Duncan et al., 2022). This relates to the changing scenario of non-invasive fat reduction practices, which is a kind of surging demand for new treatments in aesthetic medicine (Figure 10.5).

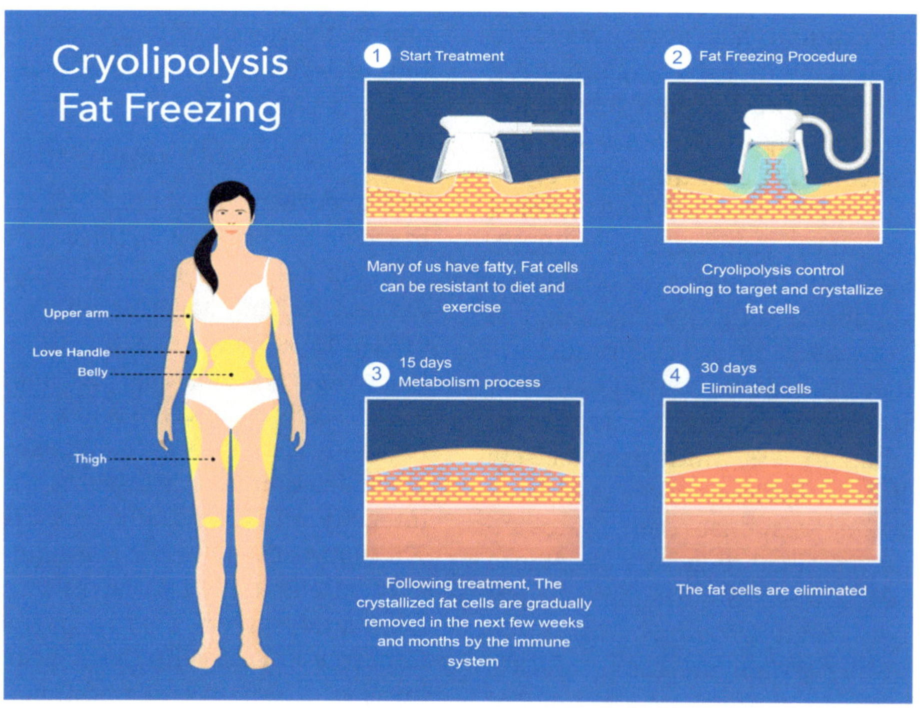

Figure 10.5. Cryolipolysis fat freezing mechanism.

Source: https://www.shumailas.com/wp-content/uploads/2022/07/Cryolipolysis-fat-freezing-procedure-.jpg.

10.2.2. Comparison with Other Body Contouring Methods

In the realm of body contouring technologies, cryolipolysis stands out as a non-invasive alternative to traditional methods such as liposuction. Liposuction, while effective at producing immediate physical improvements, often involves discomfort, significant downtime, and potential complications due to its invasive nature. In contrast, cryolipolysis employs a targeted cooling process to selectively eliminate adipose tissue without damaging surrounding structures. Such a technique has become increasingly popular among patients requiring effective body contouring with minimal recovery time. Furthermore, advancements in other non-invasive platforms, such as high-intensity focused electromagnetic field (HIFEM) treatments, have synergistic effects when combined with cryolipolysis, expanding further the variety of techniques available for body sculpting in the medical aesthetic industry (Duncan et al., 2022). In addition, a developing literature emphasizes the metabolic impact of different body contouring techniques, with emphasis on terrain complexity. Scientific studies have established that nonsurgical techniques for subcutaneous fat excision, like cryolipolysis, may possess differing metabolic profiles from classic invasive techniques like liposuction. For example, while both methods can induce changes in body composition, NSSFR maintains its effect on body composition for an extended duration, albeit with initial negative impacts on lipid profiles (Badran et al., 2023). Such differentiations are crucial for practitioners and patients alike, as they navigate their options based on desired outcomes and potential side effects. The combining of two or more technologies, e.g., the fusion of cryolipolysis with RF therapy, is essential in furthering the overall treatment effectiveness. Studies reveal that the concurrent application of technologies, like HIFEM or synchronized RF, can meet numerous body contouring demands at the same time, correcting for muscle laxity while also targeting adipose tissue (Duncan et al., 2022). Accordingly, the demand for a more integrated approach to body contouring procedures is rising, and professionals need to remain up to date with changing practices. Because demand for non-invasive techniques is growing further, continued research is needed to guide best practices and provide the best results for patients in search of optimal and safe body sculpting methods (Figure 10.6).

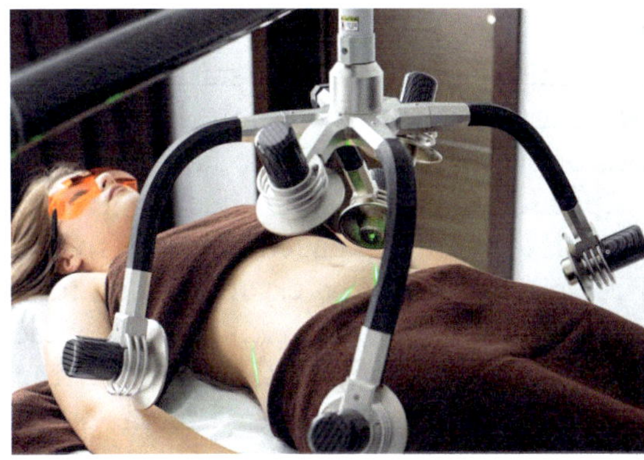

Figure 10.6. Nonsurgical subcutaneous fat removal (NSSFR).

https://dryusra.com/wp-content/uploads/Most-Popular-Non-Invasive-Fat-Loss-Procedures-1.jpg.

10.2.3. Physiological Effects on Fat Cells

The physiological effects on fat cells are critical to understanding the efficacy of noninvasive body contouring technologies like cryolipolysis. This method strategically targets subcutaneous fat by inducing controlled cooling, promoting apoptosis in adipocytes without damaging surrounding tissues. As adipocytes succumb to this cooling process, they gradually release their contents, which are then metabolized and eliminated by the body's lymphatic system. Notably, the treatment is more than a decrease in volume of fat; it also impacts the metabolic profile of the treated region, with effects on variables like insulin sensitivity and inflammation markers. Thus, in addition to producing the desired aesthetic changes, cryolipolysis can also trigger favorable metabolic alterations in line with enhanced health results, making it a convergence of cosmetic enhancement and physiological advantage. Interest in body contouring technology mirrors increasing societal anxiety over body image and the psychoemotional effects of perceived flaws in fat distribution. The fat cells, especially in problem areas that are hard to lose through diet or exercise, have a major effect on an individual's self-esteem and general mental state. Noninvasive treatments such as cryolipolysis provide a workaround for conventional surgical choices like liposuction, which are effective, involves potential drawbacks based on invasiveness and recovery. Contrarily, cryolipolysis induces fat loss over time, making it more acceptable for those desiring body enhancement without resorting to surgery. As such treatments become more popular, it's important to appreciate their physiological effects on fat cells, both to predict the outcomes of treatment and discover any permanent metabolic advantages of adipose tissue reduction (Duncan et al., 2022). Current studies indicate that the transitory and significant metabolic effects of reducing subcutaneous fat, regardless of the method used, are achieved through surgery or nonsurgical interventions. Of importance, improvements in fat mass after interventions such as cryolipolysis have been documented, indicating potential benefits to body composition and metabolic health. Although nonsurgical fat removal can yield short-term benefits, including increased insulin sensitivity and changes in blood lipid profiles, the duration of these benefits has been controversial. Emerging evidence suggested that some metabolic benefits were short-term, but these insights provided a more profound understanding of the effect of fat reduction on hormonal regulation and metabolic pathways. In addition, this diversity of response might offer a useful explanation of the interaction between the fat cell physiology and the prior weight loss history and acute adipocyte behavior (Badran et al., 2023) (Figure 10.7).

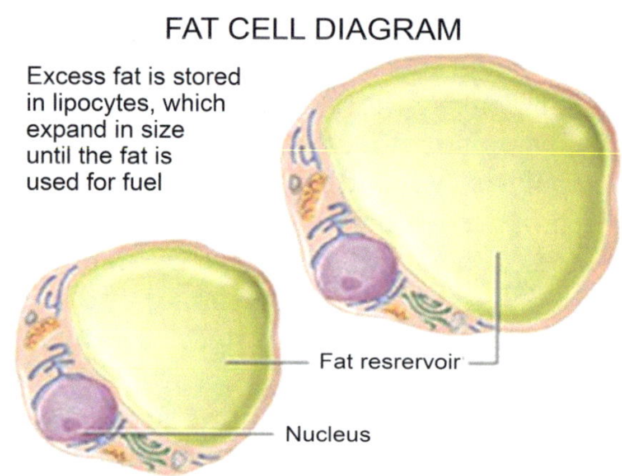

Figure 10.7. The incredible shrinking of fat cell.

Source: https://media.springernature.com/lw685/springer-static/image/art%3A10.1186%2Fs42269-019-0238-z/MediaObjects/42269_2019_238_Fig3_HTML.png?as=webp.

Test Your Knowledge

1. How long does it take for cryolipolysis to work?
2. How does cryolipolysis selectively target fat cells without damaging surrounding tissues?

10.3. Benefits of Cryolipolysis

Learning Outcome

1. Describe the non-invasive nature of cryolipolysis
2. Explain that minimal recovery time is crucial in the context of cryolipolysis
3. Deal with long-lasting results in body contouring technologies

Cryolipolysis is one of the growing non-invasive body contouring procedures, especially because of its focused approach that reduces localized fat stores. Differing from traditional surgical practices, cryolipolysis procedure utilizes controlled cooling for the targeted selective destruction of fat cells with non-affected tissues around them. It has been known to effectively cause apoptosis within the adipocytes, which would then lead to slow fat volume reductions without cuts and extensive recovery periods. The ease of the procedure has contributed to its widespread acceptance among individuals seeking aesthetic improvements without the risks associated with surgical interventions. As studies suggest, the method not only promotes significant fat loss but also aligns with contemporary demands for minimally invasive aesthetic solutions in the cosmetic field, enhancing its appeal to both patients and practitioners engaged in body contouring technologies.

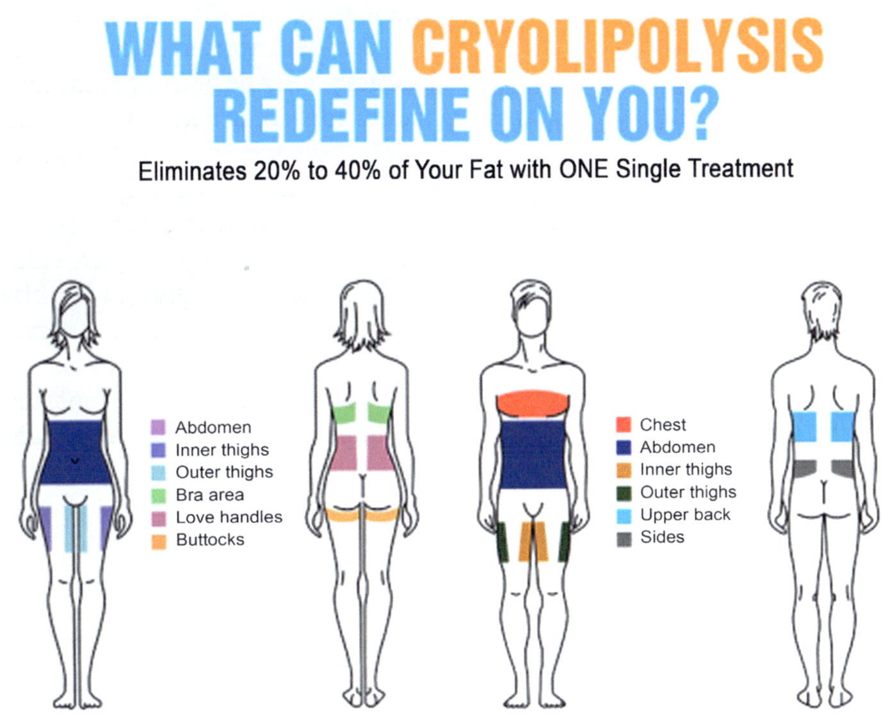

Figure 10.8. Benefits of cryolipolysis.

Source: https://dimyth.com/wp-content/uploads/2021/06/cryolipolysis-3-480x363.png.

In support of cryolipolysis efficacy are also recent clinical studies that underline its potential in fat reduction. In particular, some results reported imply an ability to yield considerable fat loss over time using cryolipolysis at optimal dosages. For example, significant reductions in volume and thickness of abdominal fat have been recorded post-treatment in patients who have been treated for body contouring applications. As presented in many of the studies, the procedure is safe and very tolerable to patients, thus avoiding the usual side effects common with other minimally invasive fat reduction procedures. The ability to deliver a reduction in fat stores in a safe manner places cryolipolysis firmly into the market of body contouring technologies, offering patients a surefire approach to defeating unreachable fat repositories that diet and exercise tend to fail. Furthermore, the advantages of cryolipolysis go beyond simple fat loss; it is a move towards patient-focused aesthetic treatments. The non-invasive nature of the procedures enables patients to return to their normal activities nearly immediately after the treatment, minimizing the psychological and practical burdens typically created by surgical means. Further, the minimal downtime makes it desirable for busy individuals seeking to achieve desired outcomes without large time investments. These are the factors that will help in improving the satisfaction and adherence of patients, for a patient will be more likely to seek treatments that easily fit into their lives. Mainly, the incorporation of cryolipolysis into body sculpting treatments portrays how technological advancements may result in safer, more accessible beauty services with multiple benefits to the patients (Goodman et al., 2022Soto et al., 2016; Chang et a;., 2022) (Figure 10.8).

10.3.1. Non-Invasive Nature

The non-surgical aspect of cryolipolysis is one of its most attractive features in the field of body contouring devices. This technology utilizes controlled cooling to address and destroy subcutaneous fat cells without compromising the integrity of adjacent tissues. In contrast to the more invasive surgical alternatives, such as liposuction, cryolipolysis avoids the use of anesthesia, incisions, and prolonged recovery times, developing a more convenient path for those who seek body composition enhancement. The ability to perform cryolipolysis in an outpatient setting enhances its appeal, providing a convenient alternative that aligns with the contemporary consumer's lifestyle. The reduced downtime associated with non-invasive procedures aligns favorably with patients' preferences for less disruptive treatment options, ultimately contributing to the growing popularity within the aesthetics market (Duncan et al., 2022). Additionally, the non-invasive feature of cryolipolysis favors patient diversity in treatment. The technology is especially beneficial for those who may not be comfortable with conventional treatments that they deem insufficient or too cumbersome due to considerations such as risks associated with surgery, long periods of recovery, or permanent conditions that rule out surgeries. Substantial evidence supports that non-invasive treatment for abdominal adiposity, which is a universal issue for most people, is possible using methods such as cryolipolysis, particularly since this form of fat carries greater health consequences (Assis et al., 2022). Since increasing numbers of people are looking for safe, efficient, and less invasive means to contour their bodies, cryolipolysis has become a viable option that meets these demands while encouraging general health. The implications of the non-invasive framework extend beyond mere aesthetics; they encapsulate broader societal shifts toward health and well-being. Given the increasing prevalence of body dissatisfaction and the desire for improved self-image, non-invasive procedures like cryolipolysis offer individuals a means to enhance their physical appearance while maintaining their commitment to health. As the procedure necessitates no significant downtime, patients can integrate treatments into their regular routines with minimal disruption. This is a part of a growing high-lighted whole-wellness emphasis, demanding not just physical transformation but also emotional well-being. The integration of cryolipolysis into the mainstream body sculpting signifies a dramatic change in demand for less invasive, less costly alternatives to the traditional methods, further solidifying its position among the current body aesthetic treatments (Duncan et al., 2022) (Figure 10.9).

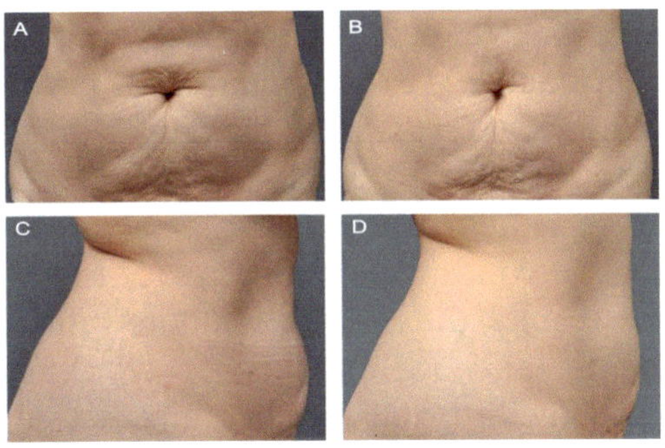

Figure 10.9. (A, C) This 51-year-old woman presented for fat reduction and abdominal contouring. The patient's pretreatment weight was 56.4 kg, her body mass index (BMI) was 22.8, and her body fat was 36.4%. (B, D) Six months after cryolipolysis treatment of her entire lower abdomen with a large applicator in a single session, the patient showed a clinical reduction of fat (weight, 56.7 kg; BMI, 23.0; body fat, 35.7%).

Source: https://www.researchgate.net/publication/260562146_Noninvasive_Selective_Cryolipolysis_and_Reperfusion_Recovery_for_Localized_Natural_Fat_Reduction_and_Contouring/fulltext/55f1755008aedecb69000003/Noninvasive-Selective-Cryolipolysis-and-Reperfusion-Recovery-for-Localized-Natural- Fat-Reduction-and-Contouring.pdf?origin=publication_detail&_tp=eyJjb250ZXh0Ijp7ImZpcnN0 UGFnZSI6Il9kaXJlY3QiLCJwYWdlIjoicHVib GljYXRpb25Eb3dubG9hZ CIsInBy ZXZpb3VzUGFnZSI6InB1YmxpY2F0aW9uIn19&__cf_chl_tk=VNxIz gEwNmc.Xh.n tyvl8JIMkxFRjoT QQs.ClX6ZnEI-1747546771-1.0.1.1-wyneNx3D5 JYjRJd3PjJucJlPSi1 bsAErT GUNnR52a3o.

10.3.2. Minimal Recovery Time

The topic of minimal recovery time is crucial in the context of cryolipolysis and body contouring technologies, particularly as these procedures gain traction among individuals seeking effective yet non-invasive solutions for fat reduction. Unlike traditional liposuction, which often necessitates significant recovery periods due to surgical invasiveness, cryolipolysis allows patients to resume their daily activities almost immediately following treatment. This factor significantly lowers the psychological and logistically cumbersome impediments that patients can encounter in the process of deciding on body contouring treatments. The low downtime aspect of cryolipolysis is a welcome relief, particularly to people who lead fairly hectic lifestyles or responsibilities that would not permit them to take weeks off work for recuperation, hence its popularity among larger numbers of people. In terms of clinical effectiveness, the minimal treatment recovery required by cryolipolysis does not sacrifice results. While the controlled cooling used in this procedure certainly aims to target and eliminate fat cells, its non-invasive nature leaves other tissues relatively undamaged, avoiding bruising and swelling associated with more invasive treatments. So, patients mostly complain only mildly of discomfort, and most side effects, such as temporary redness or numbness, resolve within days to hours. This elevates patient satisfaction with the treatment and contributes to the overall positive experience, that cryolipolysis can indeed help people achieve the desired body contouring results while providing a much easier recovery process compared to the conventionally used treatment modes such as liposuction, which inherently involve risks of complications from the post-operative period and a longer recovery period (Duncan et al., 2022). Additionally, the trend of minimal recovery time procedures complements societal changes to find more non-invasive aesthetic treatment options.

Body dissatisfaction, heightened by extreme societal pressures regarding personal and physical appearance, has been the cause for many different body contouring solutions. While conventional invasive procedures such as liposuction have long been thought to be the gold standard of body contouring, their negative aspects, including the recovery time and the associated problems of these procedures, are mostly responsible for the growing popularity of alternatives such as cryolipolysis. As evidenced by the successful use of HIFEM and RF technologies, non-invasive options not only afford minimal downtime but also exhibit remarkable efficacy in addressing issues such as muscle laxity and skin texture improvement (Duncan et al., 2022). This shift highlights a broader trend in aesthetic medicine, where the demand for efficiency, safety, and aesthetic satisfaction underscores the evolving landscape of body contouring technologies.

10.3.3. Long-Lasting Results

The search for long-lasting results in body contouring technologies is a critical element in the evaluation of their efficiency. As the noninvasive trend gains momentum, patients now seek alternatives to liposuction, a surgical intervention that is effective but extremely painful and involving lengthy recovery times. Among the techniques, cryolipolysis is considered one of the preferred because it selectively applies cold temperatures to targeted fat areas and removes them, leaving the rest of the tissues intact. It is based on controlled cooling to cause apoptosis in the adipocytes, thus encouraging decreased subcutaneous layers of fat. The reason that it is non-invasive means not only are the risks associated with surgical treatments minimized, but also provides a desirable option for individuals looking to attain gradual and permanent solutions to body contouring, meeting the culture's demand for safe beauty enhancement as per recent literature (Duncan et al., 2022). Additionally contributing to the popularity of cryolipolysis is the fact that it works effectively in delivering enduring results. The technology not only allows for instant aesthetic improvement but also provides patients with confidence about the permanence of their outcomes, especially when paired with lifestyle changes such as diet and exercise. In fact, clinical research has determined that the decreases in a patient's fat layer persist well beyond the time of treatment because the body naturally processes and eliminates crystallized fat cells. There is no other body sculpting technology that compares. There are some technologies that need repeated sessions or continuous maintenance to achieve similar results. Such advancements reflect the expanding acknowledgment of cryolipolysis as a satisfactory non-invasive alternative and highlight the possibility of longer-lasting results when used within a balanced regimen of body aesthetics (Duncan et al., 2022).

In addition, breakthroughs with combination treatments further maximize the durability and efficacy of cryolipolysis results. Combining cryolipolysis with other technologies, such as HIFEM therapy or synchronized RF, can enhance fat reduction while also enhancing skin quality at the same time. An example is the combination of HIFEM and RF, which not only aims at fat but also muscle laxity and skin defects, hence providing a better solution for body contouring. Results from multiple clinical cases indicate that such synergistic approaches produce substantial improvements, fostering a more appealing and maintained body shape for patients. As non-invasive technologies evolve, their capacity to yield long-lasting results will likely solidify their position as preferred options for effective body contouring, demonstrating their significant role in modern aesthetic practices (Duncan et al., 2022) (Figure 10.10).

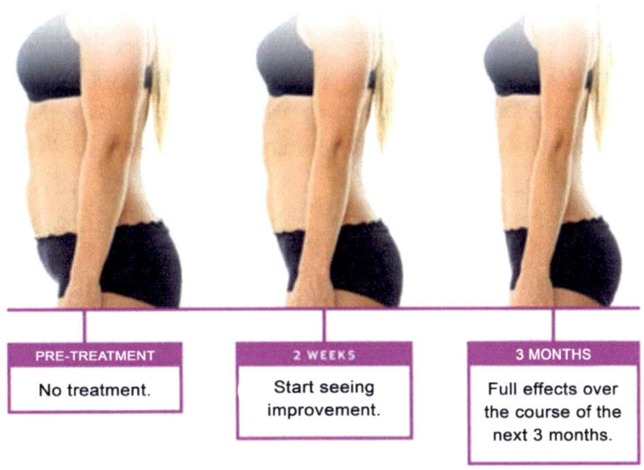

Figure 10.10. After 3 months of results from body contouring treatment.

Source: https://aestheticsmedspa.com/wp-content/uploads/2021/05/ultrashape-power.jpg.

Test Your Knowledge

1. How does the non-invasive nature of cryolipolysis compare to traditional fat-reduction procedures like liposuction?
2. What are the typical recovery times associated with cryolipolysis, and how do they impact a patient's daily routine?

10.4. Risks and Side Effects

Learning Outcome

1. Describe common side effects
2. Explain rare complications
3. Focus on contraindications for treatment

Cryolipolysis is not an invasive body contouring technology and carries a host of risks and side effects. Even though usually not harmful, temporary adverse effects that the patient may feel because of it are redness, swelling, bruising, or tingling at the treatment site. These side effects usually resolve within a few days to weeks, but differ from one individual to another based on the sensitivity of the skin and the intensity of the treatment. Moreover, some patients may report discomfort during the procedure, although it is usually mild compared to invasive techniques. Such experience underscores the need for thorough patient consultation to assess their suitability for cryolipolysis, ensuring that they are well-informed about these temporary inconveniences and the overall realistic expectations regarding results. In addition to mild side effects, cryolipolysis carries a risk of more serious complications, albeit rare. A case of paradoxical adipose hyperplasia (PAH), in which treated fat cells expand instead of diminishing, has been reported in a minority of patients. This effect can cause a detectable thickening of the fat, which runs counter to the desired outcome of the treatment. Awareness of this risk is critical since it can result in the need for additional procedures to correct the unwanted result. Because of such potential, consultation with proper experts who have better expertise should be done in the case of new patients. Education for these comparatively distant risks needs to be done as part of a complete strategy of decision-making, where aesthetic objectives are balanced suitably against complications. Besides this, consideration of alternative technology, such as CBL-514, provides a comparative perspective of risks and side effects associated with non-invasive procedures for fat reduction. Research on CBL-514 highlights it as a novel injectable treatment promoting fat reduction while boasting a favorable safety profile. Clinical studies demonstrate that while CBL-514 induces adipocyte apoptosis to reduce subcutaneous fat, the side effects associated with its usage remain manageable and generally mild. Patients opting for such alternatives may find a balance of efficacy and reduced risk of complications compared to cryolipolysis. A proper understanding of the full spectrum of risks related to these contouring technologies-beyond cryolipolysis, and now including its alternatives like CBL-514-can lead to informed decisions in line with health and aesthetic goals and would ultimately result in safer and more satisfactory outcomes in body contouring endeavors.

10.4.1. Common Side Effects

Cryolipolysis is one of the non-invasive body contouring technologies that has gained acceptance in aesthetic medicine based on the selective activation of cell death in fat cells through controlled cooling. However, the patients must be informed about the commonly known side effects accompanying the procedure. Generally, the patients often experience numbness, tingling, or pain in the treated areas after the treatment, resulting from the mechanisms of cooling used in the procedure. These sensations generally resolve within a few hours to several days, but understanding their occurrence helps manage patient expectations and enhances the overall satisfaction with the treatment experience. Besides transient feelings, another frequent side effect of cryolipolysis is erythema or the formation of redness at the treatment sites. This reaction is mostly benign and tends to subside within a week. Less commonly, patients might also notice swelling or firmness in the areas that are treated, which typically denotes the healing process of the body due to its metabolism of the crystallized fat cells. Recognition of these responses enables practitioners to assure patients, thus alleviating anxiety regarding the treatment's immediate consequences and affirming the non-invasive procedure. As the art of body contouring evolves, it is still necessary to understand the nuances in side effects with cryolipolysis.

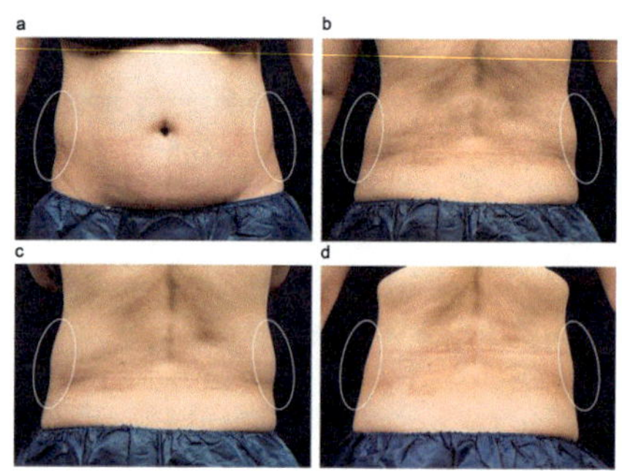

Figure 10.11. This 42-year-old female received two sequential cryolipolysis cycles to each flank. Clinical photographs show flank fat reduction between baseline (a, c) and 12 weeks post-treatment (b, d). This subject lost only 0.9 lbs. from her baseline visit to her final photographic evaluation, 12 weeks later.

Source: https://www.researchgate.net/profile/Eric-Bernstein-2/publication/268235431/figure/fig2/AS:282615706865666@1444392243242/This-42-year-old-female-received-two-sequential-cryolipolysis-cycles-to-each-flank.png.

Significant adverse effects are rare, but the potential for complications such as PAH (growth of fat cells in the treated area) underscores the importance of careful patient selection and thorough pre-procedure counseling. Investigating other nonsurgical approaches, as reported in recent literature, is needed to expand practitioner awareness and promote patient results. By taking into account diverse treatment options along with knowledge of their impact, practitioners can more effectively customize interventions to address specific patient needs and preferences while maximizing benefits from cryolipolysis and other body reshaping devices (Goodman et al., 2022; Duncan et al., 2022) (Figure 10.11).

10.4.2. Rare Complications

Advanced body contouring technology, especially cryolipolysis, revolutionized the world of cosmetics in the realm of fat reduction without the need for surgery. But on the very same years that these technologies have revolutionized the cosmetic market, unwarranted side effects of such procedures can no longer be ignored. Cryolipolysis is considered generally safe, but PAH has been identified as a very rarely occurring complication, in which treated areas experience an unexpected increase in fat volume. This complication not only presents aesthetic difficulties but may also decrease patient satisfaction remarkably. Incidence of PAH is low, but the consequences are great enough that clinicians must take care to carefully select patients and provide extensive pre-treatment consultation for discussing possible risks and consequences of treatments. Since there are various ways of reducing fat, developments like CBL-514 also suggest that the complications might vary across technologies, emphasizing the need for ongoing research in this evolving sector (Goodman et al., 2022). Additionally, the complications from body contouring procedures, including those related to cryolipolysis, remain an essential area of investigation. A clear knowledge of the possible side effects, from mild to severe, is necessary for specialists in this area. An example is that although cryolipolysis has lower rates of complications than invasive treatments, on rare occasions, there have been skin necrosis and neuropraxia reported. These can result from inadequate technique or inherent patient conditions, making it important to have personal treatment plans. Such complications have been encountered with the traditional liposuction technique when hematoma and seroma formations are noted. If such complicated procedures are learned and known, best practice among practitioners would be enhanced with procedure results and patient safety, encouraging such an attitude of knowledge and readiness within clinical practice (Robb & Gold, 2022). The requirement of ongoing training and education for the healthcare professionals who run cryolipolysis and similar body contouring treatments is essential.

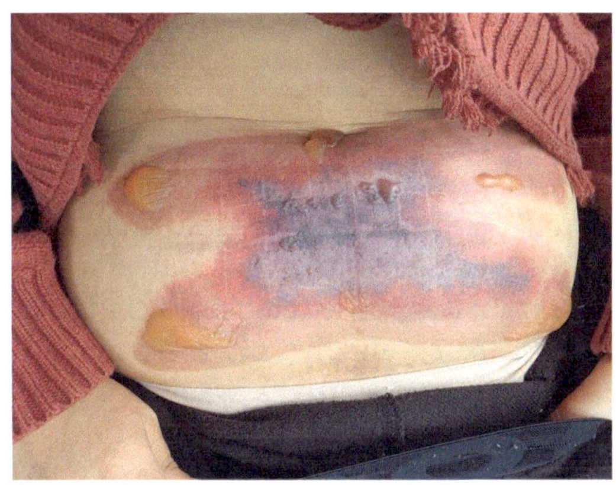

Figure 10.12. Severe abdominal fat necrosis following complications of cryolipolysis.

Source: https://s3.amazonaws.com/production.scholastica/public/attachments/5165ee5e-3c60-48d3-b120-f73bf812c1c2/large/fig_1._day_two_following_the_procedure__prior_to_presentation_at_local_emergency_department.jpg.

They should be properly trained to recognize the early warning signs of rare complications so that appropriate intervention can be facilitated. Technical proficiency is not enough; acquiring good communication skills with patients is necessary to provide realistic expectations. With innovative and newer techniques for fat reduction, like the upcoming technology CBL-514, practitioners are required to remain aware of the distinctive risks related to each modality. This could be done through group practice by the practitioners, exchange of experiences and information about complications that will bring in a learning community for ongoing improvement. Finally, resolution of unusual complications will not only improve the safety of treatment but also improve patient confidence in the fast-changing era of body contouring devices (Goodman et al., 2022) (Figure 10.12).

10.4.3. Contraindications for Treatment

Cryolipolysis, being a technology applied in body contouring, has several contraindications; hence, there are specific medical conditions relating to the skin that render its application inappropriate. Cryoglobulinemia or cold agglutinin disease patients fall into this category, as such diseases tend to provoke adverse effects when exposed to cold temperatures inherent in the use of cryolipolysis. Contraindications also involve those patients who have disease conditions such as liver or kidney damage. Fat could not be metabolized and eliminated by the body. This information about contraindications is quite necessary for practitioners as it enables them to safeguard their patients and prevent complications that could arise due to improper candidates receiving such treatment. Beyond certain specific health conditions, there are lifestyle factors that may make prospective patients inappropriate for cryolipolysis. Such as individuals who are severely overweight or who anticipate intense results without taking on accompanying lifestyle modifications may be left with less-than-optimal results. Cryolipolysis is not a replacement for conventional weight loss strategies; it is, rather, a method meant to sculpt the figure by removing localized fat deposits. Therefore, it is the responsibility of clinicians to assess the overall health, weight, and expectations through a comprehensive consultation process. This thorough evaluation ensures practitioners that the person is not only compatible physically but also psychologically with the expected outcome of the treatment. In addition, it has been noted that surgical interventions in the area to be treated may interfere with both the safety and efficacy of cryolipolysis. For instance, prior liposuction procedures may alter the skin's structure or elasticity, leading to unpredictable results from cryolipolysis. As noted in the broader context of body contouring techniques, emerging energy-based technologies require an understanding of individual patient histories to optimize results and minimize complications, particularly in cases of prior surgical interventions. Therefore, medical professionals must have a very elaborate conversation with a patient about their treatment history in order for it to be controlled properly to deliver the best results in the area of body contouring technologies (Khanna et al., 2021; Duncan et al., 2022).

Test Your Knowledge

1. What are the most common side effects experienced by patients after undergoing cryolipolysis treatment?
2. What rare but serious complications have been reported following cryolipolysis, such as paradoxical adipose hyperplasia?

10.5. Technological Advancements

Learning Outcome

1. Focus on innovations in cryolipolysis devices
2. Deal with integration of other technologies (e.g., RF, ultrasound)
3. Describe future trends in body contouring

The fast-changing advancements in technology in the aesthetic sector have brought along a series of innovations that highly improve body contouring treatments like cryolipolysis. Unlike the conventional invasive procedures, contemporary noninvasive treatments treat body dissatisfaction without causing much pain and discomfort, as well as reduced recovery periods. The change from traditional surgery alternatives like liposuction to noninvasive treatments is driven by growing consumer demand for less harmful procedures that provide good results without surgery. For example, technologically advanced modalities, such as HIFEM treatment or synchronized RF, can treat excess fat and muscle laxity at the same time in order to enhance both physical and cosmetic well-being. The combination of these technologies not only widens the range of treatment possibilities but also raises the standards of care for patients in noninvasive body contouring, making it an essential field of investigation in contemporary aesthetic medicine (Duncan et al., 2022). With the plastic surgery environment progressing over time, methods like High Definition LipoSculture are remarkable developments in the realm of body contouring technology. This new method of liposuction is an advancement over the conventional liposuction as it gives improved sculpting properties that produce lean, athletic physiques. With the help of technology, experts are now in a position to achieve cleaner contours and tailored results, which satisfy contemporary ideals of beauty for good body proportions. Research has found that such high-definition treatments can minimize possible complications as well as significantly enhance patient satisfaction rates, which is a major change in surgical trends. This shift toward less invasive and more secure procedures not only represents evolving patient needs but also highlights the need for continued innovation in plastic surgery. The development of these sophisticated methods is therefore a foundation of current body contouring methods, encouraging further research and refinement within aesthetic practices (Soto et al., 2016). Additionally, the science behind the technological push of cryolipolysis points to the essential convergence of science and patient autonomy in cosmetic procedures. Cryolipolysis uses controlled cooling to destroy fat cells, and it is a noninvasive method for body contouring that appeals well to patients looking for effective body weight management. Gradual fat loss with this technology can result in remarkable changes without the risks that come with surgery. It is not just the action of cryolipolysis that makes it so attractive, but also the fact that it provides a sustainable and controllable course toward aesthetic objectives-which makes the necessity of proper patient education and informed consent at the center of this process. Continued advances in aesthetic technologies continually direct focus to safe, patient-oriented methods; hence, cryolipolysis represents a paradigm shift in the healthcare environment and places it at the forefront of body contouring techniques in modern times.

10.5.1. Innovations in Cryolipolysis Devices

The cryolipolysis market also indicated impressive development recently as new technology that can enhance the efficiency and safety of fat loss therapy is being formed. One of the significant breakthroughs is the development of technology that is able to treat multiple areas at once in order to increase patient throughput as well as reduce the overall treatment time. Newer machines in the cryolipolysis family have more ergonomic features and adjustable suction settings, offering not only a pleasurable experience for the user but also allowing for tailored treatments dependent on patient anatomy. This is critical; as practitioners push to give the best possible results, the ability to tailor treatment parameters ensures that efficacy and safety are maximized. Moreover, enhanced cooling technologies have been integrated to optimize fat cell crystallization, resulting in more effective adipocyte destruction while preserving surrounding tissues. Further contributing to the evolution of cryolipolysis is the integration of complementary technologies that combine various energy modalities with cryolipolysis. These hybrid devices can offer a multifaceted approach to body contouring, addressing cellulite and skin laxity alongside targeted fat reduction. For example, treatments that combine RF or ultrasound with cooling technology optimize collagen remodeling and tightening following the treatment. Indeed, aside from optimizing aesthetic outcomes, integrative treatments optimize indications for cryolipolysis since patients demand holistic solutions to their issues. Such convergence of technologies is one part of a greater trend in non-surgical aesthetics, where combination treatments are increasingly among the leading new trends. Therefore, practitioners must be aware of these new technologies' distinct mechanisms and advantages in order to optimize patient satisfaction and treatment outcomes. Technical progress aside, the field of cryolipolysis is also influenced by dynamic training and education systems for practitioners. Since new technology devices are coming into the market, it is important to provide detailed education on how to use them properly and their potential complications. Education programs for practitioners to learn about advanced cryolipolysis procedures have been introduced in line with the demand for evidence-based practice for non-surgical aesthetics. There is a need for a curriculum with a formal framework consisting of hands-on practice, case studies, and assessment techniques such as objective structured practical exams to enhance the competence and confidence of the practitioners. Development of such learning frameworks, based on thorough literature reviews and global assessments, guarantees that the practitioners are well prepared to handle the issues introduced by cryolipolysis technology. Innovation and education in sync are important elements in keeping up excellence, perpetually to the advantage of patient and practitioner (Kumar, 2021; Duncan et al., 2022) (Figure 10.13).

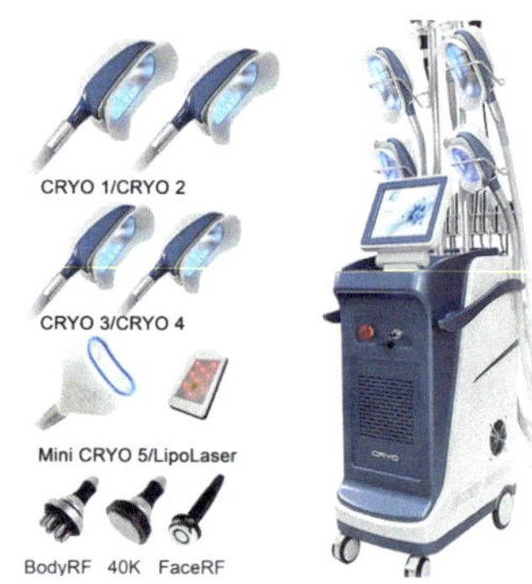

Figure 10.13. Cryolipolysis devices.

Source: https://sdcosmeticscare.com/cdn/shop/files/cadcfa-069c0f8c69e145628dd420f58dc9a2a2_mv2.jpg?v=1708845991&width=1445.

10.5.2. Integration of Other Technologies (e.g., RF, Ultrasound)

The combination of synergistic technologies like RF and ultrasound with cryolipolysis is an enormous leap in body contouring. These modalities have the potential to increase the efficacy of the fat removal treatment because they are able to consider and treat the varied tissue characteristics of the patient, which will ultimately enhance the outcome. RF technology achieves this by delivering thermal energy to the planes of subcutaneous fat. Therefore, cell metabolism is initiated and ultimately tissue tightening. The combination method might have contributed more advantages to body contouring clients when utilized in conjunction with cryolipolysis, which is a method of controlled cooling applied to trigger apoptosis of adipocytes. Additionally, it has previously been established through the literature that the combination of RF and cryolipolysis not only minimizes recovery times but also widens the spectrum of body types that may be treated, which is a more adaptive treatment possibility in clinical practice. Ultrasound technology also encompasses dynamic incorporation into non-invasive body contouring. Pulsation of sound waves into the fat tissues may help emulsify the fat tissue, and thus, when combined with cryolipolysis, it enhances its efficacy. The synergistic action of both techniques would allow for further fat cell disruption before freezing actually occurs, thus promoting more fat reduction in general. Moreover, ultrasound could potentially be incorporated with cryolipolysis for optimal aesthetic results in terms of skin texture and elasticity, which could be another appealing addition for those practitioners interested in body contouring approaches. Besides bringing the potential clinical benefit from the use of ultrasound in conjunction with cryolipolysis, it helps meet patients' expectations for safer, more effective, and less invasive aesthetic procedures (Duncan et al., 2022). It also highlights the importance of formal training and education for practitioners when combining other technologies such as cryolipolysis, especially for non-surgical aesthetic treatments. Providers are properly trained in delivering these more complex combination treatments with a well-defined curriculum dedicated to these combining techniques. There is a lack of real-world training and education in this area, according to a recent study (Kumar, 2021). Educational systems compatible with technological progress will remain in front of the curve with regard to the treatment that will change with time, thus encouraging patient care and outcomes. Further, evidence-based education would most likely stimulate the safe combination of several modalities, promoting both successful treatment outcomes as well as safety satisfaction for the patients who receive such body-contouring treatments (Figure 10.14).

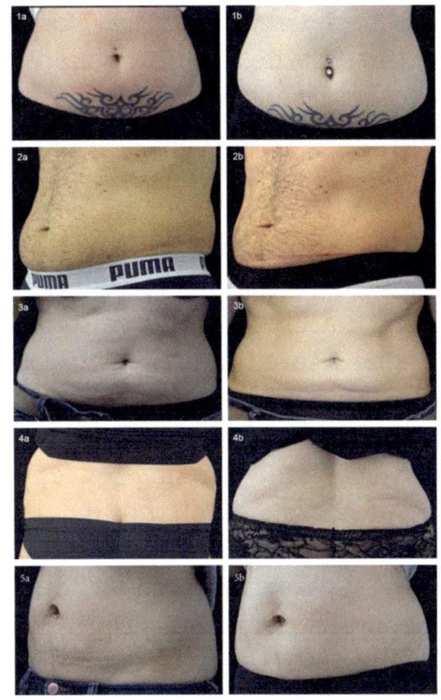

Figure 10.14. RF-assisted cryolipolysis accelerates the removal of fat excess. Either lower abdominal (1, 2, 3, and 5) or bilateral flanks (4); unwanted fat excess were treated by combining RF and cryolipolysis. Pictures were taken immediately before (a) as well as 6 weeks (b) after on single treatment session. A significant clinical difference could be observed as a consequence of RF-assisted cryolipolysis.

Source: https://www.researchgate.net/publication/339118508/figure/fig1/AS:1084231891591170@1635512435328/RF-assisted-cryolipolysis-accelerates-the-removal-of-fat-excess-Either-lower-abdominal.jpg.

10.5.3. Future Trends in Body Contouring

There are new trends in body sculpting that signal a move away from invasive procedures that are patient satisfaction and comfort-focused, with minimal recovery time. Procedures like HIFEM treatments are being used more for their muscle contraction effects and fat burning without the invasiveness of surgery. As increasingly more worry arises over invasive treatments like liposuction, demand has skyrocketed for alternatives that deliver equivalent results with less discomfort. Solutions that combine HIFEM and synchronized RF are being found to yield improved outcomes, specifically in addressing muscle laxity and overall skin quality. This multi-dimensional philosophy emphasizes an increasing recognition of the multi-planar nature of body contouring that not only seeks to eliminate fat but enhance the quality of muscle and skin, providing a more holistic aesthetic improvement (Duncan et al., 2022). With the evolving concept of body contouring, the sustainability of outcomes and metabolic considerations are becoming focal areas of interest. New research on both surgical subcutaneous fat reduction (SSFR) and non-surgical subcutaneous fat reduction (NSSFR) procedures has unearthed interesting metabolic outcomes. Whereas SSFR can have transient effects associated with body composition and insulin sensitivity, NSSFR has a sustained effect on body composition lasting up to two months, even though there are initial lipid profile disturbances (Badran et al., 2023). This differentiation in metabolic outcomes suggests that patient selection based on individual characteristics is critical. Consequently, future body contouring practices will likely integrate personalized approaches, tailoring procedures to optimize both aesthetic outcomes and metabolic health, thus improving patient satisfaction and safety over the long term. The incorporation of newer technologies within the realm of body contouring not only indicates the evolving patient population but also highlights the significance of safety and efficiency. With increasing evidence proving the efficacy of non-surgical approaches, practitioners are spurred to look for novel combinations of technologies like TPE with monopolar RF to deliver better outcomes. What complements these practices is that, therefore, healthcare professionals can provide better solutions to the highly complex problems of cellulite and skin laxity facing body contouring. The trend of advancement in body contouring procedures is observed, consistent with the industry that has always focused on total care. With improved clinical outcomes through technological advancements, ongoing research will be inevitable, eventually paving the way towards a future where patient-specific needs are addressed through tailored body contouring treatments (Duncan et al., 2022; Badran et al., 2023).

Test Your Knowledge

1. What recent technological advancements have improved the precision, comfort, or treatment time of cryolipolysis devices?
2. In what ways are next-generation cryolipolysis systems addressing limitations of earlier models, such as treatment area flexibility or uneven fat reduction?

10.6. Patient Considerations

Learning Outcome

1. Identify ideal candidates for cryolipolysis
2. Describe consultation and assessment process
3. Set realistic expectations

In considering patient factors for cryolipolysis and other body contouring devices, pre-treatment evaluation takes precedence. A comprehensive review of the patient's medical history, lifestyle, and expectations is essential to ensure that the selected procedure is in line with individual requirements. Clinicians should address areas of concern, likely outcomes, and procedural steps to ensure realistic expectations and maximum patient satisfaction. Since cryolipolysis is associated with different experiences and is characterized by minimal downtime and non-invasiveness, there is an immediate need for practitioners to correct any misconceptions that are mentioned regarding its efficacy against surgical interventions. This will help healthcare providers minimize dissatisfaction levels and further strengthen the suitability of such treatments in the realm of body contouring options. Considerations after the treatment are an indispensable feature for the patient as well. Monitoring for adverse effects, although rare, is essential to ensure that complications are addressed promptly. Patient education regarding postoperative care can significantly influence recovery and enhance the longevity of results. It is important for patients to understand the timeline for visible improvements, which may not be immediate. Other complications from other technologies in body contouring, liposuction being one of them, underline the need to select the appropriate patient. As these methods have their unique potential risks along with variable outcomes, cryolipolysis would work as a wise decision for patients who desire non-invasive treatments with less postoperative issues and safety concerns (Duncan et al., 2022). Another aspect of body contouring is the psychological arena. Patient motivations often vary, with some seeking cosmetic enhancements for self-esteem improvements rather than purely aesthetic goals. Knowledge of the psychological undertones involved in body image and weight can inform practitioners in providing individualized advice and guidance during the course of treatment. Evaluation of these motivations helps to align treatment options with patient expectations and can be used to determine which body contouring technology is best suited. As body contouring continues to advance, incorporating new solutions such as CBL-514 may bring compelling opportunities for patients requiring safe, efficient fat reduction without the risks of surgery. Early reports indicate that the effectiveness of these treatments implies that they could well be a welcome addition to the non-invasive armory, highlighting the necessity for ongoing debate around patient factors within this changing landscape (Goodman et al., 2022).

10.6.1. Ideal Candidates for Cryolipolysis

Suitable candidates for cryolipolysis, the non-invasive body contouring technology, typically possess certain physical characteristics and health profiles. Mostly, those patients with localized small pockets of fat that persist even with a healthy lifestyle, including diet and exercise, are prime candidates for this treatment. Cryolipolysis is designed to target and reduce these localized fat deposits, making it particularly attractive to those seeking improvement in body contour without resorting to more invasive techniques like liposuction. Additionally, as body dissatisfaction linked to subcutaneous fat becomes increasingly prevalent, non-surgical options like cryolipolysis emerge as appealing alternatives, particularly for individuals hesitant about surgical procedures. The suitability stems from its ability to produce tangible results with minimal downtime, allowing candidates to resume their daily activities quickly, thus enhancing its overall appeal in contemporary aesthetic practices (Duncan et al., 2022). Moreover, ideal candidates should possess realistic expectations regarding the outcomes of cryolipolysis. This treatment is not intended as a weight loss solution; instead, it serves to sculpt and enhance specific body areas. Patients seeking dramatic changes or those with extreme weight loss aspirations might find cryolipolysis to be lacking in their ability to address their needs. Candidates are usually advised to maintain a consistent weight, as extreme fluctuations will impact the efficacy of the treatment. Patients with pre-existing medical conditions, including cryoglobulinemia or cold agglutinin disease, can also be excluded based on the nature, which is selective cooling of fat cells. Accordingly, the successful candidates can comprehend the concept of cryolipolysis, preferably being used to complement a well-balanced lifestyle rather than a standalone solution for body reshaping and contouring (Duncan et al., 2022). The other significant factor will be the anatomical locations that can be targeted for cryolipolysis. Classical and ideal candidates who present with fat deposits in anatomical locations often targeted by the treatment procedure include the abdomen, flanks (love handles), and thighs. Skin elasticity and overall skin condition also play vital roles in determining candidacy; individuals with loose or sagging skin may not achieve the desirable tightening effect post-treatment. Furthermore, prospective patients should participate in thorough consultations with qualified healthcare providers to assess their suitability and discuss possible outcomes. By providing an understanding of the procedures mechanics and expected results, practitioners can better guide candidates toward achieving their desired aesthetic goals. This process has, through thorough assessment, ensured cryolipolysis meets the needs of those patients seeking effective and non-invasive body contouring solutions, according to Duncan et al. (2022) (Figure 10.15).

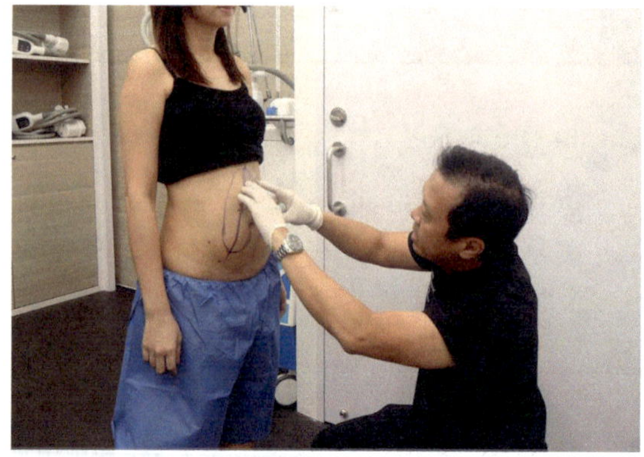

Figure 10.15. A patient receiving CoolSculpting, a popular fat-freezing procedure that uses controlled cooling to reduce stubborn fat deposits without surgery.

Source: https://halley.com.sg/wp-content/uploads/2022/09/CoolSculpting-in-Singapore-Is-CoolSculpting-the-Same-as-Fat-Freezing.jpeg.

10.6.2. Consultation and Assessment Process

The consultation and assessment procedure is a critical process in the use of cryolipolysis and body-shaping technology. During the initial consultations, practitioners receive thorough medical histories and assess patients' aesthetic wants to develop a personalized strategy. This consultation not only informs patients about the potential outcomes but serves to create clinician-patient rapport and trust as well. Key considerations during this assessment include understanding the patient's body shape, fat distribution, and skin quality, which directly influence the effectiveness of cryolipolysis. Additionally, the assessment process often involves discussing the patient's lifestyle, weight history, and any previous body contouring procedures, ensuring a holistic understanding of their needs and expectations. Following the initial evaluation, a detailed physical examination may be conducted, focusing on areas targeted for cryolipolysis. This step is essential, as successful body contouring is contingent upon accurate assessments of subcutaneous fat deposits and skin laxity. For instance, practitioners must evaluate the thickness and characteristics of the adipose tissue to determine the suitability of cryolipolysis as a non-invasive option for fat reduction. Furthermore, advancements in techniques, such as those highlighted in High Definition LipoSculture, emphasize the importance of precise assessment to achieve desired aesthetic results while minimizing complications (Soto et al., 2016). By establishing a thorough understanding of each patient's anatomical and physiological attributes, practitioners can better advise on realistic expectations and potential outcomes, ultimately enhancing patient satisfaction. Refinement of consultation strategies, combined with new technologies, has revolutionized the assessment process in body contouring clinics. As noted in the recent advancements, technologies based on energy can be added to the conventional liposuction, creating new lines for less invasive treatments (Khanna et al., 2021). The advancement requires practitioners to remain knowledgeable about recent developments to be able to advise patients fully on the available options. In this context, the assessment process becomes not just a preliminary step but a dynamic exchange of information that empowers patients to make informed choices. Thus, the consultation and assessment process is integral to ensuring safety and efficacy in body contouring procedures, highlighting the convergence of clinical expertise and patient-centered care in achieving optimal results.

10.6.3. Setting Realistic Expectations

A change of body contouring technologies requires changes in how patient expectations are managed so as to meet their desired expectations. Cryolipolysis, branded popularly as a less invasive option relative to the conventional liposuction technique, ensures dramatic fat reduction with minimal downtime. Reality dictates that outcomes vary generally depending on numerous determinants, anatomically speaking, on the area treated, and post-procedure compliance. Educating patients on these variables not only fosters a more accurate understanding of potential outcomes but also enhances their overall satisfaction with the procedure. As outlined in recent literature, the importance of clarifying the limitations and possible results of cryolipolysis cannot be overstated, as it directly impacts patients' psychological and physical responses to treatment. Moreover, it is essential to consider the long-term implications of cryolipolysis when formulating patient expectations. While many patients seek immediate results, the body's natural processes can take weeks to months to reveal the full effects of the treatment. This delayed gratification can lead to frustration if not anticipated adequately. Surgeons should communicate that the results, although permanent in terms of targeted fat cells, may vary due to ongoing lifestyle factors and metabolic changes. Integrating discussions surrounding the complementary nature of various body contouring technologies, including liposuction, allows for a comprehensive understanding that may empower patients in making informed decisions about their choices. Enhancing a patient's confidence in their physician benefits them in a multi-faceted way, as they can immerse themselves in the process and look at their expectations from a healthier perspective. Lastly, discussing the psychological aspects surrounding body image and aesthetic goals is crucial to setting appropriate expectations. Cryolipolysis is not a weight-reducing measure but only a way to fashion and refine the contours of the body. Having such differentiation in mind allows patients to properly place their goals so that they aim at improvement, not perfection. According to Robb & Gold (2022), having such subtleties in mind is essential for both surgeons and patients to appreciate the complexity of body contouring surgeries. Moreover, the multi-faceted nature of patient care necessitates an ongoing dialogue about concerns and dissatisfaction potentially arising from complications or unmet expectations. Engaging patients in conversations about what they can realistically achieve through cryolipolysis and related technologies ultimately leads to more fulfilling outcomes and contributes to a broader understanding of body image and personal satisfaction. As treatment methodologies continue to advance, maintaining transparency between practitioners and patients will be the bedrock for fostering enduring trust and achieving desired results.

Test Your Knowledge

1. What physical characteristics make someone a good candidate for cryolipolysis treatment?
2. Why is cryolipolysis not recommended as a weight-loss solution for obese individuals?
3. What questions should practitioners ask during the consultation to identify potential contraindications or risks for cryolipolysis treatment?

SUMMARY

Cryolipolysis is a body contouring technology, an upgraded form, which differentiates itself from conventional methods of liposuction by the lack of invasion. This process uses localized cooling that directly impacts and limits subcutaneous fat, hence free from the risk and recovery that is often inherent with surgeries. Ongoing technological and clinical evolution of cryolipolysis demonstrates that it is not only a surface treatment but with potential for cosmetic enhancement as well as metabolic impact. New literature expresses a need for more research into its long-term implications, particularly on metabolic alterations and overall patient satisfaction, an interesting field to study in ongoing research and clinical application (Duncan et al., 2022). Moreover, the integration of cryolipolysis with other body contouring technologies may enhance treatment outcomes and patient experiences. Combining different modalities can optimize fat reduction and improve skin laxity, creating a comprehensive approach to body contouring. Studies highlight that the effectiveness of such combinations could address broader patient needs, particularly those seeking non-invasive solutions for body shaping and weight management. The interplay between these technologies underscores the necessity of personalized treatment plans tailored to individual patient anatomy and metabolic health outcomes. Understanding the nuances of these combinations could pave the way for more sophisticated, efficient interventions that extend beyond surface-level improvements (Badran et al., 2023). As the understanding of body contouring continues to grow, so must the research findings from the application of cryolipolysis be considered for clinical practice and further research. Metabolic implications of fat reduction with non-invasive techniques, especially when done in conjunction with surgery, will provide valuable insights into how these treatments work in the long run. Improved insight into how cryolipolysis affects such variables as glucose homeostasis and insulin sensitivity will not only be beneficial in terms of individual treatment planning but also toward a greater understanding of obesity-associated health hazard. As we proceed forward, interdisciplinary collaboration among cosmetic surgeons, endocrinologists, and researchers will be highly crucial to advance the field of body contouring, thereby ensuring innovative and safe and beneficial inventions to diverse patient populations (Duncan et al., 2022).

The advent of cryolipolysis as a body shaping technology represents an important milestone in aesthetic medicine, defined by its non-surgical approach to reducing fat. As opposed to the conventional surgical interventions that typically demand considerable recovery time and possible side effects, cryolipolysis presents a comparatively painless solution for patients who require the physical improvement of their appearance without the risk of invasive interventions. As detailed in newer literature, this technology works on the basis of cooling targeted fat deposits, resulting in adipocyte apoptosis without damaging adjacent tissues. These developments offer a better alternative to surgical fat reduction methods and demonstrate increasing demand for minimally invasive body contouring. Understanding these methods and their implications is pivotal as the industry continues to evolve, necessitating further investigation into both aesthetic outcomes and metabolic effects of these technologies. In assessing the metabolic implications of subcutaneous fat removal procedures, current research presents a spectrum of findings that merit attention. Whereas SSFR has demonstrated short-term metabolic improvements, chiefly enhancements in insulin sensitivity, nonsurgical methods such as cryolipolysis have divergent long-term metabolic influences. Recent work emphasizes the paucity of definitive evidence for the long-term influence of NSSFR on metabolic status and proposes variability in outcomes as a function of patient history and physiological parameters. This intricate relationship between fat removal technologies and metabolic health emphasizes the need for ongoing research to uncover the complexities that underlie these interactions. Notably, the connection between body contouring methods and their metabolic repercussions requires further exploration to optimize treatment protocols and patient experiences effectively. The comprehensive evaluation of body contouring technologies, including cryolipolysis, underscores the necessity for continuous dialogue among medical practitioners and researchers in the field. As the landscape of aesthetic medicine shifts towards more innovative solutions, it remains crucial to understand the capabilities and limitations of these advancements, both from a clinical and a patient-centered perspective. The traditional reliance on surgical interventions has prompted a collaborative exploration of non-invasive techniques involving multiple practitioners, with a consistent emphasis on informed patient decision-making. Through the synthesis of knowledge from different specialties and ongoing awareness of developing technologies, practitioners can more effectively negotiate the intricacies involved with body contouring. As defined in recent scholarly literature, the importance of these developments goes beyond visual attraction, bringing with them wider metabolic implications that need further attention to guarantee safety and efficacy in the treatment of body contouring (Duncan et al., 2022; Badran et al., 2023).

KEY TERMS FROM THIS CHAPTER

- Adipocytes succumb
- Beauty enhancement
- Cosmetic enhancement
- Dissatisfaction
- Homeostasis
- Liposuction
- Lymph system
- Natural healing process
- RF technologies
- Adjacent tissues
- Conventional treatments
- Cryolipolysis
- Fat removal treatment
- LipoSculture
- Localized fat,
- Modern methodology
- Post-procedure compliance
- Subcutaneous fat

CRITICAL THINKING QUESTIONS

1. **What is the primary mechanism of Cryolipolysis for body contouring?**
   a. Heat application to break down fat cells
   b. Cold application to freeze and destroy fat cells
   c. Ultrasound waves to target fat cells
   d. Laser energy to break down fat cells
2. **Which of the following body areas can Cryolipolysis effectively treat?**
   a. Belly, thighs, and arms
   b. Wrinkles and fine lines
   c. Hair regrowth
   d. Muscle toning
3. **Which of the following is a key advantage of Cryolipolysis over traditional liposuction?**
   a. It requires a long recovery period
   b. It is a non-invasive procedure
   c. It is suitable for individuals with high body fat percentages
   d. It provides immediate, dramatic fat removal
4. **Which body contouring technology utilizes focused ultrasound to target and reduce fat?**
   a. Liposuction
   b. Cryolipolysis
   c. High-Intensity Focused Ultrasound (HIFU)
   d. Radiofrequency therapy
5. **What is the typical duration of a Cryolipolysis treatment session?**
   a. 30 minutes to 1 hour
   b. 2–3 hours
   c. 15–20 minutes
   d. 5–10 minutes

Short Answer Questions

1. What is Cryolipolysis, and how does it work to reduce body fat?
2. What are the main benefits of Cryolipolysis compared to traditional fat-reduction methods like liposuction?
3. What types of body areas are most commonly treated using Cryolipolysis technology?
4. Are there any potential side effects or risks associated with Cryolipolysis treatments?
5. How long does a typical Cryolipolysis session last, and how many sessions are typically required for optimal results?
6. What is the science behind Body Contouring Technologies, and how do they compare to Cryolipolysis?
7. How do non-invasive body contouring techniques like radiofrequency, ultrasound, and laser compare to Cryolipolysis in terms of effectiveness and recovery time?

Answer to Critical Thinking Questions

1. (b); 2. (a); 3. (b); 4. (c); 5.(a)

REFERENCES

1. Soto, J., Aguilar, H. A., & Barajas-Gamboa, J. S. (2016). High Definition Liposuction: A Challenge for a Perfect Body Contouring. InTech. doi: 10.5772/65811 (accessed on 11th June 2025).
2. Assis, T. D. de, & Ferreira, T. C. (2022). *Criolipólise: Eficácia No Tratamento Da Gordura Localizada / Cryolipolysis: Effectiveness in Treating Localized Fat.* https://core.ac.uk/download/597567687.pdf (accessed on 11th June 2025).
3. Badran, S., Habib, A. M., Aljassem, G., Musa, O. A. H., Clark, J., Hamdi, M., Abou-Samra, A. B., Glass, G. E., & Doi, S. A. (2023). Metabolic changes after surgical fat removal: A dose-response meta-analysis. *Journal of plastic, reconstructive & aesthetic surgery : JPRAS, 76*, 238–250. https://doi.org/10.1016/j.bjps.2022.10.055(accessed on 11th June 2025).
4. Goodman, G. J., Ho, W. W. S., Chang, K. J., Ling, Y. F., & Sheu, A. Y. (2022). Efficacy of a Novel Injection Lipolysis to Induce Targeted Adipocyte Apoptosis: A Randomized, Phase IIa Study of CBL-514 Injection on Abdominal Subcutaneous Fat Reduction. *Aesthetic surgery journal, 42*(11), NP662–NP674. https://doi.org/10.1093/asj/sjac162(accessed on 11th June 2025).
5. Irvine Duncan, D., Chilukuri, S., Kent, D., Hoffmann, K., & Tingsong, L. (2022). Non-invasive Alternatives for Liposuction. IntechOpen. doi: 10.5772/intechopen.101396(accessed on 11th June 2025).
6. Da Cunha, N. B., Nascente, F. M., Sobrinho, H. M. da R., et al. (2019). *Uso do Ultrassom Terapêutico E Criolipólise Aliados a Outras Terapias Estéticas Combinadas No Tratamento Da Lipodistrofia Localizada.* https://core.ac.uk/download/230349025.pdf (accessed on 11th June 2025).
7. Duncan, D. I. (2022). *Enhanced Liposuction.* https://core.ac.uk/download/534904133.pdf (accessed on 11th June 2025).
8. W. Robb, C., & H. Gold, M. (2022). Complications and Solutions for Post-Operative Liposuction Deformities. IntechOpen. doi: 10.5772/intechopen.101284(accessed on 11th June 2025).
9. Khanna, J., & Saheb-Al-Zamani, M. (2021). *Enhanced Lip Contouring of The Arms.* https://core.ac.uk/download/479934754.pdf (accessed on 11th June 2025).
10. Kumar, Narendra; (2021) Design, Development and Implementation Framework for a Postgraduate Non-Surgical Aesthetics Curriculum. Doctoral thesis (Ph.D), UCL (University College London). (accessed on 11th June 2025).
11. Ockell, J. (2023). *Breast Measurements and Excess Skin Before and After Bariatric Surgery and In the Normal Population.* https://core.ac.uk/download/620668213.pdf (accessed on 11th June 2025).
12. Swanson, E. (2018). *Evidence-Based Body Contouring Surgery and VTE Prevention.* Springer. https://play.google.com/store/books/details?id=1QdGDwAAQBAJ&source=gbs_api (accessed on 11th June 2025).

BOTULINUM TOXIN: TYPES, INDICATIONS, TECHNIQUES

11

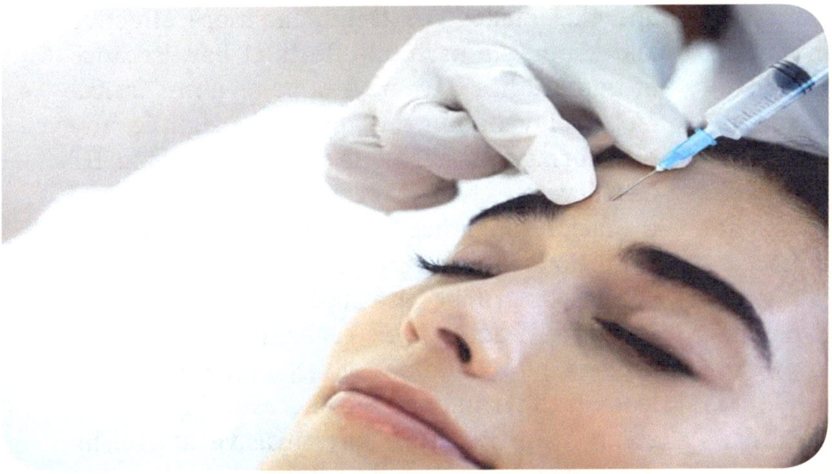

LEARNING OBJECTIVES

After studying this chapter, you will be able to:

1. Explain the types of botulinum toxin
2. Understand the mechanism of action of botulinum toxin
3. Discuss about indications for use
4. Describe injection techniques
5. Focus on safety and side effects
6. Deal with patient experience and satisfaction

Introduction

Botulinum toxin (BT) in cosmetic dermatology has been in the limelight recently, and it is the leading non-invasive therapeutic agent in facial rejuvenation. Corrective dermatology is progressing, and both patients and practitioners are attracted to appearing youthful with little time off and fewer complications. According to research, application of procedures such as BT injections has been on the rise due to their instantaneous visible effect and comparative safety compared to more invasive procedures. The trend has opened up to continuous innovations and evolution of application procedures, ultimately leading to patient satisfaction and acceptance of cosmetic dermatologic procedures (Lipozen et al., 2010). Thus, the addition of BT to a variety of treatment protocols speaks to its efficacy and diversity in correcting a wide variety of aesthetic concerns, paving the way for its greater acceptance among cosmetic procedures. The cosmetic application of BT extends beyond cosmetic ideals; it is also being investigated for therapeutic applications in a variety of dermatologic diseases. Recent studies indicate its use in treating extensive dermatological disorders such as acne vulgaris and acne scars, giving rise to new frontiers in clinical practice (Podraza et al., 2025). This possibility emphasizes the role of BT in cosmetic dermatology but also requires its use in less prevalent issues of dermatology. Its expansion of indication is quite a paradigm change in the therapeutic process, making it possible for practitioners to venture into multimodal treatment of patients. Furthermore, as an increasingly rich amount of evidence confirms its efficacy, the application of BT in the treatment of intricate skin diseases is assuming an increasingly pivotal role, thus opening up new horizons to the clinical practice of cosmetic dermatology. Hence, details about the products of the BT available in the market are significant to attain maximum care on the dermatologist's side. Every preparation having different strengths and modes of action can be made suitable according to individual aesthetic and medical requirements of clients. Second, application techniques themselves will determine outcomes; hence, practitioner expertise and experience are especially relevant in the delivery of safe and effective treatments. Continuous education and training in the agents and techniques used for BT application will keep dermatologists up to date with changing best practices. Growing interest in combining BT with other corrective procedures justifies learning these products and techniques. Cosmetology in dermatology, as well, keeps evolving, and this evolving relationship of BTs with use as an all-encompassing treatment option heralds a new era towards improved skin health and appearance.

Definition of Botulinum Toxin

A potent neurotoxin produced by the bacterium *Clostridium botulinum*, BT has found its vast uses in therapy and cosmetic applications. Because of its inhibitory effect on the neurotransmitter release of acetylcholine (Ach) at the neuromuscular junction, BT is utilized to induce potent and reversible paralysis. It is utilized in nearly every branch of medicine, and in cosmetic dermatology in particular, the reduction of appearances due to dynamic wrinkles and fine lines is treated by BT. Various preparations are present in the market, placed as the drug, i.e., Botox, Dysport, and Xeomin, differing in terms of potency and diffusion profiles. They make it simple to treat muscular groups in a few words, and this makes the treatment more effective and keeps the harmful effects at bay. Because of this, BT has become a popular non-surgical facial rejuvenation therapy. It has significantly transformed the aesthetic dermatology field. BT has more uses than just cosmetic rejuvenation of the facial skin; it has future use in other medical conditions like migraine, hyperhidrosis, and spasms. Its primary use in cosmetic dermatology is for anti-aging, i.e., reversal of the aging process, i.e., treatment of facial muscle spasms leading to wrinkling. The success of BT largely stems from its minimally invasive approach: with treatment usually offered in outpatient clinics, this provides quick recovery times. In fact, the patient begins noticing the results in just a few days, big turnoff for those who want a quick turnaround. Apart from that, additional research keeps pursuing additional indications for BT, expanding its uses even more and further solidifying its central place in aesthetic and medical dermatology. Legal control of the use of BT, while widespread and accepted, is intensely complicated even with extensive utilization. Advertising control and medical norms must therefore be followed since, in most nations, the drug is a prescription drug. Non-adherence is common; recent research has shown that the majority of the clinics have endorsed BT treatment without the use of pre-established standards (Davies et al., 2023). More than an ethics problem, it is also a possible hazard to the safety of the patients, so it is critical that there ought to be greater regulation and monitoring in the aesthetics clinic. With more demand for cosmetic surgeries, priority should be assigned to proper education and safety protocols to make sure that the patients are well taken care of when dealing with this growing sphere of cosmetic dermatology (Figure 11.1).

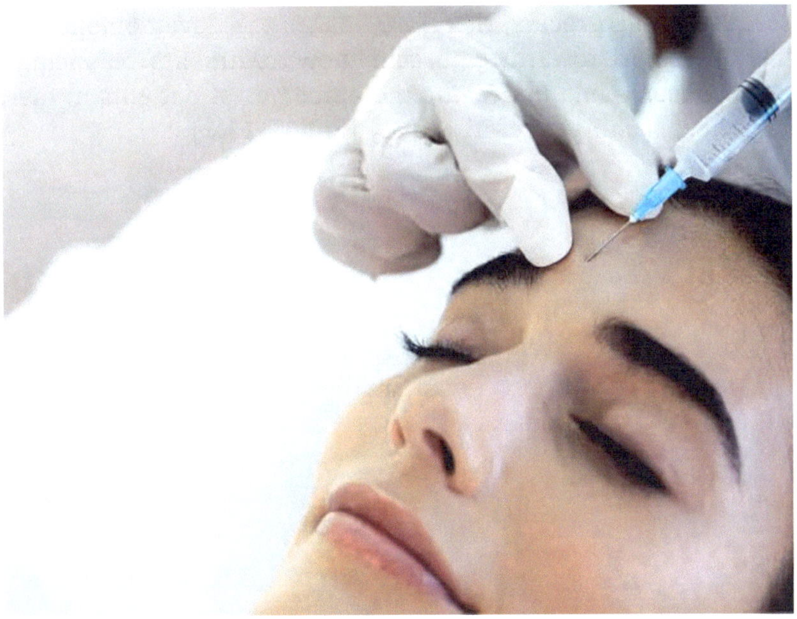

Figure 11.1. A medical professional administering botulinum toxin injection for cosmetic purposes, commonly used to reduce the appearance of facial wrinkles and fine lines.

Source: https://media.post.rvohealth.io/wp-content/uploads/2020/08/732x549_THUMBNAIL_The-Cosmetic-Use-of-Botulinum-Toxin.jpg.

Historical Context of Its Use in Dermatology

History within dermatology has also employed BTs, from being a lethal neurotoxin to a routine cosmetic treatment. *Clostridium botulinum* was initially recognized as the etiological agent of foodborne botulism in the late 19th century. Investigation work was primarily focused on observing its toxic nature, the paralyzing effect that the toxin induces. But the medical profession began to realize potential therapeutic uses as early as the 1970s, which were related to the state of disease in strabismus and blepharospasm. That model led to further studies on using BT cosmetically, specifically for the condition of wrinkles and fine lines, an innovation that improved its use in dermatology. Cosmetic use of BT became very popular by the early 2000s, making it necessary to have some training and education in non-surgical aesthetic procedures. Although extensively accepted, a lack of uniform training within the field meant that there was no proper way to send practitioners to obtain effective evidence-based techniques for injecting BT. Those knowledge deficiencies actually had come to the extent of still reacting to gigantic efforts to develop standardized curricula, bearing witness to strict training in non-surgical aesthetics being necessary. This professional education call was reflected by the onset of postgraduate programs in non-surgical aesthetics because the industry quickly evolved to a specialist branch of dermatology requiring specialist training and qualifications for safe and effective use (Kumar, 2021). Continued studies, though, in the safety and efficacy of BT further rooted it in dermatology. Plentiful research has guaranteed, not just its cosmetic usefulness, but also possible curative uses, like the eradication of chronic migraines and hyperhidrosis. This has resulted in the approval of different BT types for different indications, increasing their application in clinics and making rational its application in dermatological procedures. This process, therefore, makes the development of BT in dermatology an example of a wider movement towards embracing new treatments, balancing between scientific evidence and aesthetic concerns and improving the outcomes of patients in therapeutic as well as cosmetic practice together (Inchingolo et al., 2021) (Figure 11.2).

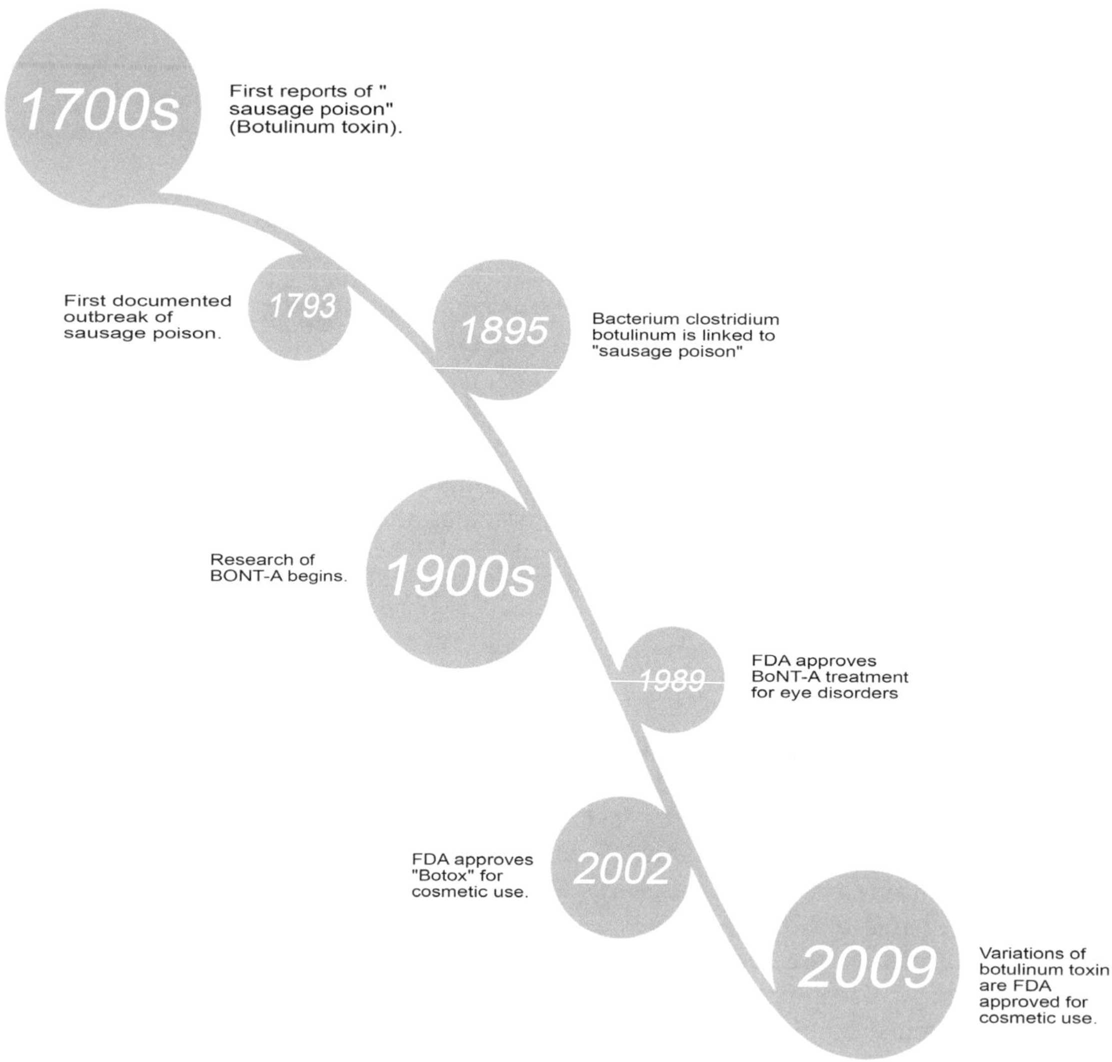

Figure 11.2. Timeline of the use of botulinum toxin.

Source: https://anue.co.nz/wp-content/uploads/botox-timeline2-1024x919.png.

11.1. Types of Botulinum Toxin

Learning Outcome

1. Understand different serotypes of botulinum toxin (BT)
2. Discuss commercially available formulations of BT
3. Deal with the comparison of efficacy and safety among types

The five various forms of botulinum toxin (BT), i.e., A, B, C, D, E, and F, have composed the landscape of cosmetic dermatology, primarily with type A used most widely in aesthetic applications. BT type A therapeutically, is found to have temporary paralyzing effects on muscles, which minimizes the appearance of lines and wrinkles, especially in the forehead and the periorbital areas. Such formulation is commercially available in a number of different formulations, some of which are onabotulinumtoxinA (Botox), abobotulinumtoxinA (Dysport), and incobotulinumtoxinA (Xeomin). Each of these formulations has distinct characteristics, including diffusion profile and potency, which may influence the overall clinical effects. Practitioners need to understand the differences between these formulations in order to avoid incorrect usage or interchangeability assumptions that may cause suboptimal outcomes or reactions in patients (De Boulle et al., 2010). BT type B, while less commonly used than type A, has become popular as a second-line therapy, especially in those who experience resistance to type A products. Type B works via the same mechanism of acetylcholine blockade but is otherwise typically preferred for certain clinical situations, i.e., when patients manifest undesirable side effects following use of type A products. Type B will also be useful for patients who need to be relieved from spasticity or muscle tension, as its pharmacological composition can be more ideally targeted towards their needs. The practitioner should consider the potential difference in dosing and effectiveness of the two types. With the advancement of cosmetic treatments, knowledge of these differences and choosing the correct type of BT can make a big difference in patient satisfaction and treatment success (Proietti et al., 2021). Additionally, emerging research explores the applicability of other BT types, such as C and D, particularly within dermatological contexts. These less commonly used forms are not yet as ubiquitous in cosmetic use, but research highlights their promise for use in treating diseases such as hyperhidrosis and dynamic facial wrinkles. The relative safety profiles of various BTs continue to be issues of debate among medical professionals, especially as regulatory models develop and additional research sheds light on their risks and benefits. With a focus on improving the quality of life of the patient, the inclusion of these alternatives may open doors to more individualized and efficient dermatologic treatments. An understanding of each can not only provide clinicians with the information required for optimal patient management but also develop an appreciation for how BT may be designed to meet individual aesthetic needs (De Boulle et al., 2010) (Figure 11.3).

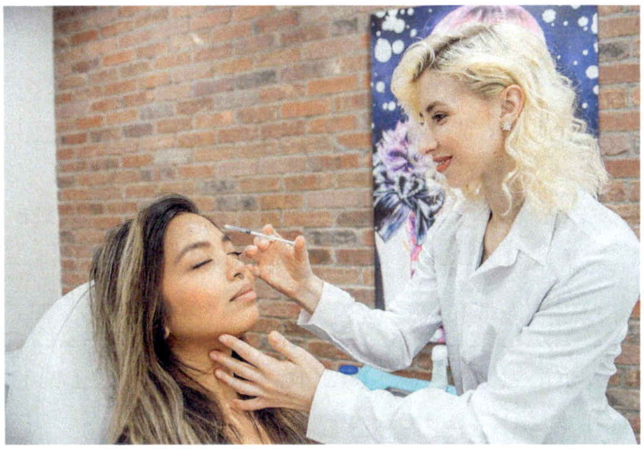

Figure 11.3. Doctor performing botulinum toxin injection.

Source: https://upload.wikimedia.org/wikipedia/commons/thumb/4/43/Doctor_performing_Botox_injection.jpg/1280px-Doctor_performing_Botox_injection.jpg.

11.1.1. Different Serotypes of Botulinum Toxin

The profile of BT in cosmetic dermatology is characterized mainly by its serotypes, which vary in characteristics and application. Of the seven types found, types A and B are utilized mainly in aesthetic dermatology. BT type A is widely used due to its efficacy and longer duration of action, and it has become a workhorse for several indications, particularly to avoid facial wrinkles such as glabellar frown lines. Clinical trials underscore the importance of respecting the nuances of each serotype since the preparations are not equally substitutable and dosing regimens dramatically differ. A new review reports that clinicians need to understand that dosing recommendations can't be done based on a standardized conversion ratio, mainly because different preparations have different pharmacologic profiles and this is going to impact the outcome in terms of both safety and efficacy (De Boulle et al., 2010). Although more frequently utilized within cosmetic therapies, the BT type B is less frequently utilized but is held in reserve for those developing immunity to the type A preparation. Type B is of shorter duration of action and necessitates more frequent injections in order to produce the desired aesthetic results. Although both serotypes decrease muscular hyperactivity successfully, the selection can be based on the patient's individual treatment history, tolerance, and certain characteristics of regions being treated. The awareness of these differences underlines the necessity of a personalized aesthetic analysis, ensuring the modality selected is appropriate for the individual patient's anatomical and aesthetic needs (Bouzouaya et al., 2018). This is important to effective patient satisfaction as well as positive outcomes, and it highlights that cosmetic dermatology cannot work under the one-size-fits-all model. The variability in serotypes goes beyond just the efficacy and duration of action; it also implies that there may be differences in mechanisms of action and safety. For example, the differential effects on neurotransmitter release as well as the different receptors targeted by the various serotypes require a more tailored approach to treatment planning. In addition, there is increasing evidence that this understanding enables practitioners to come up with co-operative treatment protocols integrating BOT with other cosmetic treatments, e.g., dermal fillers or thread lifting, for best outcomes. Not only is the global treatment aesthetically rewarding but also deals with longevity and reducing repetition of repeated treatments. Therefore, a multidisciplinary understanding of the different serotypes is critical for aesthetic practitioners that aim to harmonize treatment methods and optimize patient outcomes in cosmetic dermatology (Bouzouaya et al., 2018) (Figure 11.4).

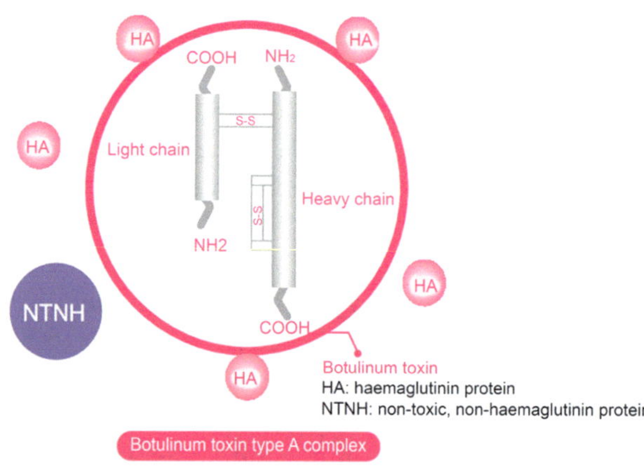

Figure 11.4. Schematic illustration demonstrating the structure of botulinum toxin type A complex.

Source: https://www.researchgate.net/profile/Nark-Kyoung-Rho/publication/287919414/figure/fig5/AS:668310307885064@1536349002499/Schematic-illustration-demonstrating-the-structure-of-botulinum-toxin-type-A-complex-In.png.

11.1.2. Commercially Available Formulations

In fact, commercially available formulations of BT have significantly altered and continue to evolve with advances in current cosmetic dermatology. There are, in fact, multiple formulations, each with diverse properties and uses in the clinic. One of the most well-known comprises onabotulinumtoxinA, abobotulinumtoxinA, and incobotulinumtoxinA, each being applied to particular aesthetic functions. While all of these preparations basically act by preventing acetylcholine release from neuromuscular junctions, their variation in molecular weight and biochemical features poses a need for prudence by clinicians in dosing and administration. As per recent textbooks, the variations should be observed, as the FDA-based revision of labeling requirements is to highlight the fact that dosing among formulations is not the same. This is in appreciation of the importance of individualized treatment plans that correspond to patients' aesthetic requirements and the unique characteristics of each product (De Boulle et al., 2010). The safety and efficacy profiles of these commercially sold formulations of BTs have been well documented, giving credence to their use in cosmetics. Therefore, e.g., therapeutic application has shown that onabotulinumtoxinA is extremely effective for glabellar frown lines relaxation, while abobotulinumtoxinA would be the first-line option for large areas due to its diffusion characteristics. Their versatility can be reversed for off-label use, and it is smoothing out numerous varieties of cosmetics-related problems like horizontal lines and crow's feet to make it even more desirable for clinicians and patients alike. Nevertheless, an in-depth understanding of anatomical nuances of facial musculature has to be obtained to derive maximum benefit with the least amount of risk. This level of comprehension, in addition to the insights derived from decades of clinical practice, reinforces that the treatment process with BT must be accompanied by an artistic sense as well as a sound foundation in anatomical science (Amer et al., 2021). Even more than this, the commodification of such product types has conditioned and determined the attitudes and expectations of patients towards noninvasive treatments for cosmetics. Knowledge of BT's potential to enhance physical looks and self-esteem has raised patient demand. Numerous licensed practitioners offering such product types are available, from dermatologists to plastic surgeons. However, patient satisfaction is also based on not just the suitable use of these preparations but also the practitioner's skill to conduct a suitable aesthetic evaluation. Proper determination of the correct formulation, dose, and injection technique specific to the patient is therefore required. Therefore, this tailored approach provides the foundation to initiate the most favorable cosmetic results and to ensure long-term patient satisfaction in BT treatments (De Boulle et al., 2010) (Figure 11.5).

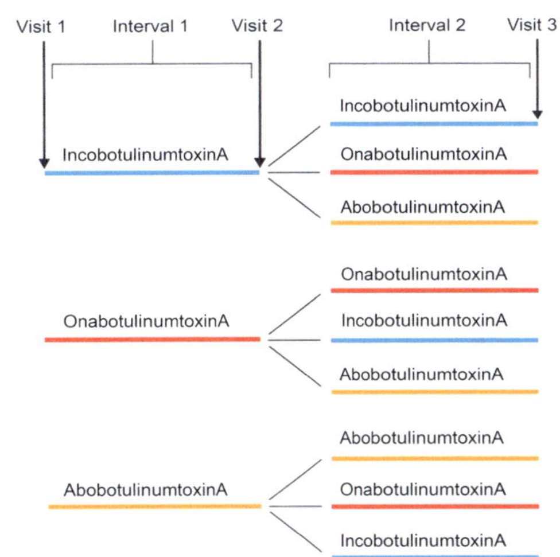

Figure 11.5. Diagram showing treatment flow.

Note: The three possible treatments and treatment intervals are shown, along with the nine possible treatment combinations.

Source: https://www.researchgate.net/profile/Welf-Prager/publication/229082997/figure/fig1/AS:202961742503966@1425401258756/Diagram-showing-treatment-flow-Note-The-three-possible-treatments-and-treatment.png.

11.1.3. Comparison of Efficacy and Safety Among Types

The effectiveness of BT types A in cosmetic dermatology is also greatly based on their proprietary formulation and FDA-approved uses. The effectiveness also differs not only among the types but also in different patient populations based on age and patient-specific skin type. For example, onabotulinumtoxinA and abobotulinumtoxinA contain different formulations, which result in different potency and onset of action. Research has indicated that these differences need to be taken into consideration seriously, as specialists cannot rely on dosing interchangeability or results between the products on the market. As demonstrated by recent research, patient satisfaction and treatment continuation possibilities have a direct correlation with the proper formulation selection with proper patient evaluations and the desired treatment objectives in mind, promoting the need for individualized practices in aesthetic treatments (De Boulle et al., 2010). In addition to effectiveness, safety is a major consideration when the different types of BTs are compared. Side effects may range from minor localized swelling to life-threatening complications. The course, of course, would largely be a function of the specific formulation used as well as the skill of the clinician. Reports indicate that while all types of BT possess an excellent safety profile, side effect frequency does differ by product. For example, onabotulinumtoxinA has an extensive safety database confirming its usage over several years, while newer products may have less longitudinal data. Patient education about these potential complications is thus the key to establishing realistic expectations and obtaining informed consent. Knowledge by the practitioner of each product's specific safety issues is crucial to optimizing patient benefit and minimizing harm (De Boulle et al., 2010). Furthermore, age factors also play a significant roles in both efficacy and safety in BT treatments in different age groups. Young adults, particularly those in their third decade of life, often seek minimally invasive treatments due to aesthetic ends that may involve correction as well as facial sculpting. Motivation and need for treatment in this age group are quite dissimilar from those in older patients who might be seeking to reduce wrinkles or be rejuvenated. Actually, almost the same issues that are at stake with aesthetics because of its literature are involved in the moral obligation of utilizing cosmetic procedures as a preventive measure. Concurrent management of elderly patients, a specific lifestyle, and aesthetics preferred by them optimizes outcomes and safety, yet another reason why age should be an important variable when the strategy for these BT treatments is determined.

Test Your Knowledge

1. What are the main serotypes of BT, and how do they differ in terms of potency and clinical applications?
2. Which BT serotypes are most commonly used in medical and cosmetic procedures, and why are they preferred?

11.2. Mechanism of Action

Learning Outcome

1. Define the neuromuscular junction and muscle contraction
2. Explain the role of acetylcholine in muscle activity
4. Discuss how BT inhibits muscle movement

Botulinum neurotoxins toxin (BoNT) works mostly by preventing the release of acetylcholine from the neuromuscular junction and inducing transient paralysis of muscles. This has major implications in cosmetic use, especially in diminishing the visibility of dynamic wrinkles created by muscle contractions of the facial region. By blocking acetylcholine, BoNT temporarily lowers muscle movements, which relaxes wrinkles like frown lines or crow's feet. The effectiveness of BT is attributed to its ability to selectively bind and enter presynaptic terminals of motor neurons. Since it interferes with neurotransmitter discharge, the decline in muscle contraction not only extends to aesthetic enhancement but also the disappearance of conspicuous manifestations of age, which further adds to the overall aesthetic results for non-surgical cosmetic clients. More recent studies broaden the wider implications of BoNT mechanism beyond aesthetics and suggest potential therapeutic uses. BoNT neurotoxicity has been of potential interest for the potential use in treating chronic pruritic disorders. Though there are still nascent data, evidence supports the likelihood that BT can modulate neuronal, glial, and immune-mediated mechanisms of itch as described in recent reports. The mechanism through which BoNT produces its antipruritic actions could form a solid foundation for the further study of its application in dermatologic conditions outside those for which it is used for purely aesthetic reasons. Emphasis is placed on the fact that clinical validation, through controlled, rigorous trials, will be crucial to ensuring wider acceptance of BoNT as a therapeutic agent in contexts beyond irritation and inflammation management (Gazerani, 2022). Additionally, the efficacy of BoNT in dermatological disorders like acne vulgaris and acne scars reflects its multi-modal mechanism of action. New research indicates the therapeutic potential of BoNT to inhibit inflammatory responses and sebum secretion that facilitate acne, allowing for better treatment outcomes of this prevalent disease (Podraza et al., 2025). Its inhibitory action on local muscle contraction can also serve to restrict scarring during healing. However, a compelling requirement for more thorough research is clear to securely place it in the treatment regimen of acne therapy. In progress, the growing knowledge of BoNTs complex mechanisms will create new grounds for cosmetic as well as therapeutic dermatology applications, securing its place as a valuable tool for improving skin health and appearance (Figure 11.6).

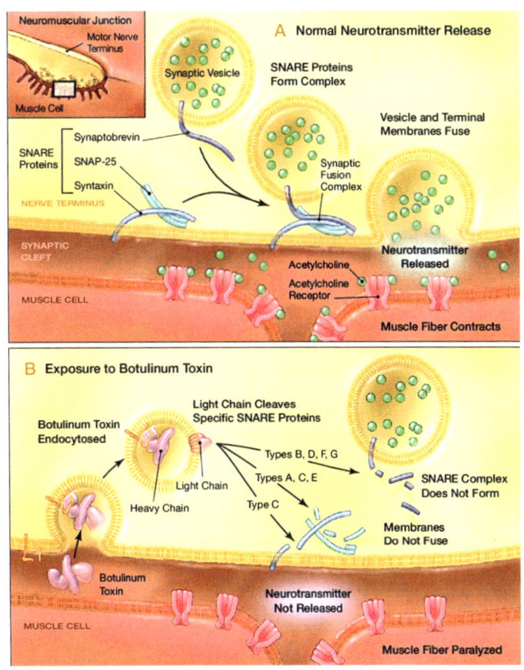

Figure 11.6. Mechanism of action of botulinum toxin.

Source: https://www.researchgate.net/profile/Trish-Perl/publication/236309435/figure/fig1/AS:645024287055880@1530797182653/Mechanism-of-Action-of-Botulinum-Toxin.png.

11.2.1. Neuromuscular Junction and Muscle Contraction

The neuromuscular junction, or NMJ, is a basic location of muscle contraction that is the motor neuron-skeletal muscle fiber interface. The motor neuron at the NMJ releases the neurotransmitter acetylcholine (ACh) onto the sarcolemma receptors of the muscle fiber, causing a wave of depolarization. It triggers a series of events in the muscle cells that ultimately lead to the generation of muscle contraction by the sliding filament mechanism. Successful communication during this phase is not just crucial for voluntary movement but also for the normal muscle tone and function itself. A knowledge of the dynamics at the NMJ is therefore key when it comes to intervening with something like BT that acts directly on the complex system of signaling. The implications of these events are significant in cosmetic dermatology, in which beauty is cultivated by modulating muscle contractions and wrinkle relief and fine line reduction. BT, derived from *Clostridium botulinum*, exploits the NMJ to produce its effects therapeutically by blocking the release of ACh. This process, ultimately, creates a flaccid muscle contraction or temporary paralysis that makes it useful cosmetically. As the release of ACh is inhibited, those muscle contractions involved in the creation of dynamic wrinkles are greatly reduced, and the skin becomes smooth. With its calculated position in the forehead and around the eyes, the toxin has become a very sought-after procedure for cosmetic enhancement. The mechanisms of action of BTs have been thoroughly studied to demonstrate how they halt the cycle of muscle contraction, thereby providing immediate and long-term relief for those desiring to treat the signs of aging. Those practitioners injecting BT cosmetically need to understand this mechanism since it will enable them to target appropriately and produce optimal results for their clients. Since the cosmetic application of BT is established, its safety profile after injecting the toxin at the NMJ must be scrutinized in detail. A portion of the side effects are infrequent but are potentially a result of interaction between the toxin and the neuromuscular transmission pathway. The complications, like weakness at the local site or accidental paralysis of the muscle, remind one of the need for accurate dosage and administration. Additionally, patients who have pre-existing neuromuscular disorders should proceed slowly with treatment since their starting neuromuscular condition is already compromised.

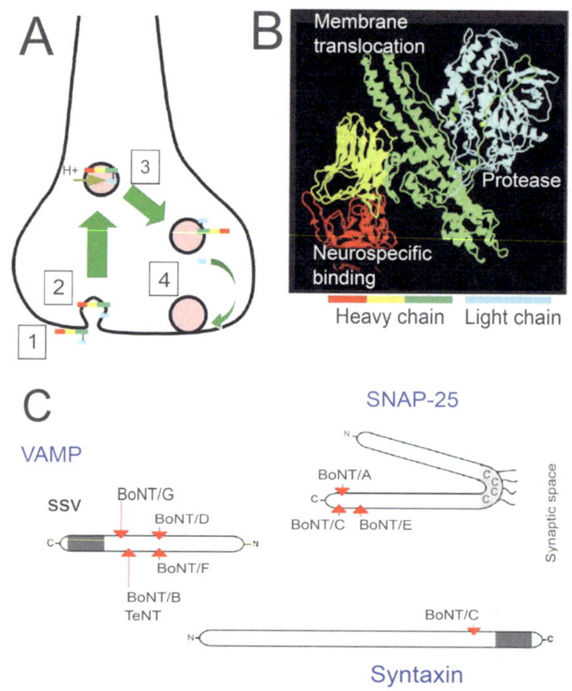

Figure 11.7. Mode of action of botulinum neurotoxins at the neuromuscular junction.

Source: https://www.researchgate.net/profile/Jordi-Molgo/publication/11601496/figure/fig1/AS:276992743231488@1443051624270/Mode-of-action-of-botulinum-neurotoxins-at-the-neuromuscular-junction-A-The-neurotoxin.png.

There are also ethical issues with the application of BT since, in the majority of cases, such treatments are motivated by societal pressure to comply and maintain beauty ideals.

Equilibrium of these ethical implications and physiological basis of NMJ dynamics enables clinicians to discuss the case with patients in an intelligent manner so that expectations are met with probable results and probable hazards of BT treatment (Fico et al., 2018; Akuma et al., 2024) (Figure 11.7).

11.2.2. Role of Acetylcholine in Muscle Activity

Acetylcholine plays a fundamental role in the intricate process of muscle contraction as a neurotransmitter at the neuromuscular junction. Upon arrival of an action potential at the terminal of a motor neuron, acetylcholine is released into the cleft of a synapse. The chemical messenger binds to nicotinic receptors on the muscle fiber membrane, opening for sodium ions. This ion flow depolarizes the muscle cell membrane and ultimately leads to muscle contraction. It is essential for voluntary movement and overall muscular coordination. Dysfunctional disruption of acetylcholine transmission can cause severe neuromuscular disorders, demonstrating its indispensable contribution to skeletal muscle function. BT, which is derived from the bacterium *Clostridium botulinum*, inhibits normal acetylcholine release and hence muscle contraction. Specifically, BT irreversibly binds cholinergic nerve endings, thereby preventing the exocytosis of acetylcholine from synaptic vesicles (Inchingolo et al., 2021). It is therefore able to cause a temporary paralysis of the targeted muscles, thus the compound proves to be highly useful in cosmetic dermatology. With its use to retard muscle activities, BT has aesthetic uses, e.g., reducing the apparent visibility of dynamic wrinkles. The modulation of acetylcholine release exemplifies how understanding its role in muscle activity has led to innovative treatment modalities in cosmetic applications. Clinical studies have elucidated the various therapeutic applications of BT beyond cosmetic enhancements, particularly regarding conditions linked to abnormal muscle activity. Research indicates that the toxin can effectively cure conditions in neurological patients such as chronic migraines and hyperhidrosis (abnormal sweating) (Podraza et al., 2025). Such findings indicate the multifaceted nature of BT as a treatment, as well as its extensive uses in the dermatology community and beyond. By inhibiting acetylcholine release, doctors are able to deliver targeted therapy that not only enhances bodily appearance but also the patient's quality of life in the presence of some medical conditions. Therefore, the intersection of BTs' pharmacological activity and the biochemical role of acetylcholine is a rich area for ongoing research.

11.2.3. How BT Inhibits Muscle Movement

The BT, a very potent neurotoxin of *Clostridium botulinum*, is popular for its capability of blocking muscle movement. This property has been found to be valuable in cosmetic dermatology. It does so by blocking the normal action of acetylcholine, which is the neurotransmitter needed for muscle contraction. Injection of BT into a muscle makes it migrate along the nerve terminals to block the release of acetylcholine from the neuromuscular junction. Hence, the injected muscle is relaxed and causes temporary flattening of the display of dynamic wrinkles, primarily in the forehead and eyes. It is a mechanism showing how BTs work to be beneficial in cosmetic applications in eliminating shiny features on the face due to numbing unnecessary lines caused by facial expressions. BTs grow more intricate as their effect cascades down to the neuronal and its supporting cellular framework. When it invades nerve endings, the toxin binds to particular receptors. It is this way that it is internalized and cleaves particular proteins, which enable docking and subsequent release of synaptic vesicles. This particular mechanism of action results in the possibility that even small doses of toxin can be effective. Such properties, in cosmetic dermatology, are widely utilized by practitioners in extrapolating treatment effects. Anatomical variability and variability of the structure of the muscle in individuals present a challenge. These differences should be considered, as they could impact the technique and volume of injection to achieve a desired cosmetic outcome, all once more underlining the injector's skills and anatomical knowledge to ensure safety and efficacy in these treatments (Bartosiński et al., 2025). In addition, clinically relevant effects of BT extend beyond cosmetic applications; due to its capacity to alter neuronal excitability, other areas of use have been evaluated. For instance, some studies showed the potential for botulinum neurotoxins in the management of chronic pruritus with the possibility of preventing the propagation of signals of itching (Gazerani, 2022). Further studies are required to establish robust clinical evidence for such applications; the mechanisms involved imply that BT could also serve to inhibit muscle contraction and neuronal transmission in a wide range of scenarios. This feature presents the prospect of a broadening of BTs application in dermatology and beyond, and one should keep looking into its broader functions in the treatment of both cosmetic and therapeutic disease.

Test Your Knowledge

1. What is the role of acetylcholine in muscle contraction, and how does it interact with the neuromuscular junction to initiate muscle activity?
2. Explain the process by which BT inhibits acetylcholine release at the neuromuscular junction and its impact on muscle contraction.

11.3. Indications for Use

Learning Outcome

1. Understand the treatment of dynamic wrinkles
2. Describe therapeutic applications beyond cosmetics
3. Explain patient selection criteria

BT application in cosmetic dermatology is increasingly popular, and its primary role is to treat dynamic wrinkles of the face. The wrinkles result from repeated muscle contractions with facial expression movement and typically appear in areas such as the forehead, glabellar region, and lateral canthal folds. By blocking the release of acetylcholine at the neuromuscular junction, BT functionally paralyzes muscles for a temporary period, resulting in a reduction in the appearance of such wrinkles. Patients often remark on enhanced self-esteem and mood upon completion of treatment, citing psychological benefits of these cosmetic treatments. The beneficial influence on patient satisfaction and treatment continuation highlights the importance of giving heed to specific indications for use in the range of clinical situations, as emphasized by recent studies (De Boulle et al., 2010). In addition to the wrinkles treatment, one of the additional ranges of application for BT is for other therapeutic uses in cosmetic dermatology. Hyperhidrosis, migraine headache, and temporomandibular joint disorders are great instances of its broader use. For hyperhidrosis, intradermal injection of BT in the affected areas can lead to a great decrease in sweating and thereby help the patient's quality of life for this incapacitating disease. Additionally, research shows that migraines have had patients report alleviation of symptoms after being administered BT injections, proving its application outside of simple cosmetic improvements. This multi-faceted treatment underscores the fact that professionals need to make detailed aesthetic assessments to tailor treatment to suit patient requirements and objectives, which are of prime importance for effective results in cosmetic medicine (De Boulle et al., 2010). Furthermore, it is important to realize that BT products are not interchangeable and necessitate a precise knowledge of their specific attributes and dosing regimens. Practitioners are urged to be well-informed about the distinct products available, such as onabotulinumtoxinA and abobotulinumtoxinA, because of differences in potency that may affect clinical effect as well as patient safety. Each formula contains unique attributes and dose recommendations, which must be closely adhered to in order to realize maximum effectiveness with minimal adverse effects. As the art evolves, ongoing research enhances our understanding of BT, determining a new paradigm for optimal practice and guaranteeing treatments uphold present safety and efficacy measures. Thus, professionals must keep an eye out to integrate advances into their practice in an attempt to sustain the optimum quality of care in cosmetic dermatology (De Boulle et al., 2010).

11.3.1. Treatment of Dynamic Wrinkles

The dynamic wrinkles are increasing because of BTX injections, wherein folds and lines are created when the muscles are contracted. Impressions are created over time due to temporary contractions of the muscles below the skin during facial expressions. The effect of BTX, and Botox more specifically, is a direct way to reverse these aging signs by inhibiting the release of acetylcholine from the nerve endings, thereby paralyzing the wrinkle-producing muscles. This effect is especially relevant in aesthetic dermatology as it directly addresses the muscle action responsible for dynamic wrinkles. By selective facial muscle relaxation, patients can achieve a smoother appearance without diminishing their ability to express emotion, thereby underlining the therapeutic potential of BT in enhancing both appearance and self-esteem in patients receiving treatment for signs of aging (Eckstein, 2009). Treatment is often a series of precisely controlled injections given by an experienced practitioner, who must have in-depth knowledge of facial anatomy to prevent injury and ensure maximal effect. Botox dosage and placement are also major determinants of treatment outcomes that require individualized treatment planning. Akin to this, however, is a balance between wrinkle diminution and maintenance of facial motion. Over-treatment can result in a frozen appearance, the reverse of what one wishes for. In addition, side effects, although usually minor and fleeting, can involve bruising and swelling, or, in the case of very occasional instances, weakness in surrounding muscles. Thus, effective patient-practitioner communication can consequently be critical to the formation of realistic expectations about outcomes and the risk of side effects that further support the general efficacy of Botox as an ideal treatment option for controlling dynamic wrinkles (Fernández-Varela-Gómez et al., 2024). Still more critical is the attainment of patient satisfaction through proper pre-treatment evaluation and monitoring. The clinicians would take into account each patient's unique skin quality, age, and lifestyle factors that would affect the result of Botox injections. It is crucial to appreciate the delicate play of aging as well as skin physiology; the dynamic wrinkles are contributory and due to sun damage and smoking, which need a full skincare regimen program along with injectables. Teaching practices aimed at the maintenance of skin health, i.e., application of sun protection and topical treatments such as retinoids, can be complementary to Botox interventions. With this diversified treatment, not only are the actual wrinkles corrected, but also wrinkles that may appear in the future, inducing long-term skin wellness while enhancing aesthetic outcomes in an ever-changing area with new devices and products (Eckstein , 2009; Fernández-Varela-Gómez et al., 2024) (Figure 11.8).

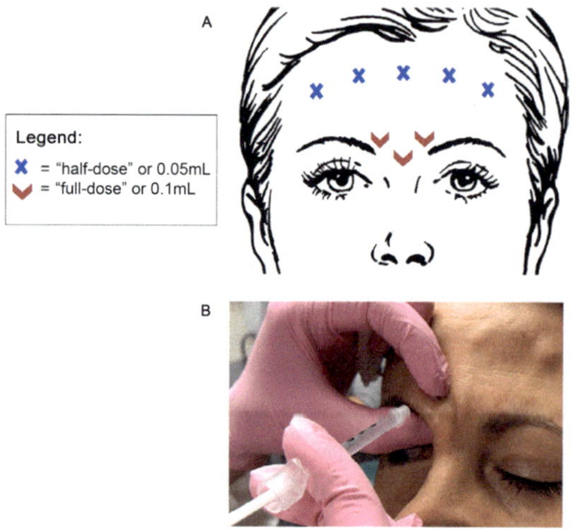

Figure 11.8. (A) Botulinum toxin injection for forehead wrinkles and frown lines. Glabellar injections may be performed without treatment of the frontalis, but frontalis injections must always be accompanied with glabellar treatment to avoid brow ptosis; and (B) demonstration of injection technique whereby pinching and elevating the tissue protects the underlying neurovascular bundle. While these figures offer a guide, dosing may vary between patients according to their musculature and anatomy.

Source: https://www.researchgate.net/publication/328465061/figure/fig1/AS:1159224885288967@1653392158486/A-Botulinum-toxin-injection-for-forehead-wrinkles-and-frown-lines-Glabellar-injections.jpg.

11.3.2. Therapeutic Applications Beyond Cosmetics

Aside from its significant use in cosmetic dermatology, BT is also becoming increasingly well-known for medical use in the therapy of numerous medical conditions. Originally marketed to shrink facial wrinkles, BT type A is increasingly being utilized as therapy for chronic migraines, debilitating headaches that may not be eased by standard drugs. Some clinical trials have demonstrated that BT injections lower the frequency and severity of migraine attacks to a great extent. The effect of this neurotoxin is obtained by avoiding the release of pain pathway neurotransmitters, a feature which has been proven to be effective not only in enhancing the quality of life of patients but also in lowering pain drug dependence. With ongoing research revealing the multi-functional nature of BT, its therapeutic use for pain control is one of the primary developments of its utility beyond esthetics (De Boulle et al., 2010). Another potential area of utilization of BT is the treatment of movement disorders such as focal dystonias and spasticity. These diseases usually arise due to neurological disorders leading to impairment of motor function with the consequent involuntary contraction of the muscles and extensive disability. BT has been shown to result in advantageous effects in the relief of these symptoms effectively by inducing paralytic blockade of the overactive muscles involved. The exact mechanism is the inhibition of the release of acetylcholine in the neuromuscular junction, thus preventing hypertonic contraction and relieving patients. Further, the functional and quality of life improvement facilitated by BT in such patients has promoted further interest in designing customized treatment regimens. Therefore, BT's use in movement disorders is a reflection of its multidimensionality, and this gives clinicians an important instrument in the therapy of multidimensional neurological disorders (De Boulle et al., 2010). Aside from its uses in the treatment of pain and movement disorders, BT has proven to be useful in the treatment of certain dermatological diseases, specifically chronic pruritus and hyperhidrosis. A number of clinical case reports cite its application with anti-pruritic effects, yet not for itch control. Once more, neurotoxins' effect appears to be relaxing the channels of itch perception, but is being applied off-label. Moreover, BT is also effective in controlling excessive sweating or hyperhidrosis, involving the armpits and palms. Such therapeutic usages have the potential to substantially decrease levels of perspiration by inhibiting the transmission of the sympathetic nervous system signal to sweat glands. Growing evidence for such usages also indicates an extensive spectrum of usage for BT and thus growing demand for further research and perhaps licensure for the likes of chronic itch control (Figure 11.9).

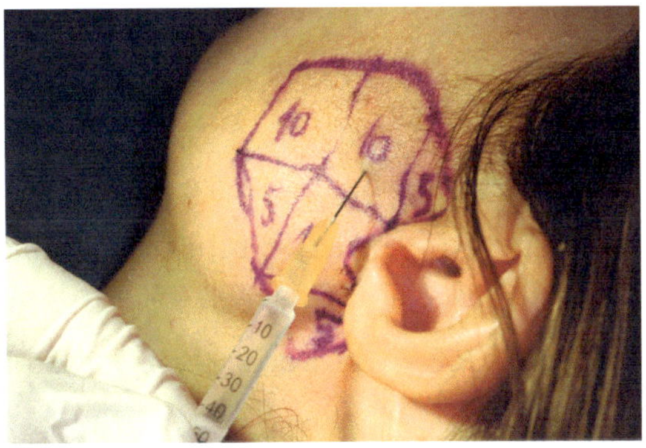

Figure 11.9. Intracutaneous application of Botulinum toxin-10 IU and 5 IU of Dysport® into skin areas of 4 cm 2 and 2 cm 2, respectively.

Source: https://www.researchgate.net/publication/277859777/figure/fig2/AS:669038023819267@1536522503155/ntracutaneous-application-of-Botulinum-toxin-10-IU-and-5-IU-of-DysportR-into-skin-areas.ppm.

11.3.3. Patient Selection Criteria

Any such inherent efficacy of BT in cosmetic dermatology relies upon proper selection criteria for a patient. The ideal patients typically possess dynamic wrinkles, which tend to be exacerbated with increasing age or even by persistent facial movements. Therefore, the psychological as well as physiological status of the patients must be evaluated properly by the practitioners to ensure optimal outcomes. Past history of psychological illness or unrealistic expectations can cause trouble, and an initial consultation beyond cosmetics is needed. Additionally, the candidates should have a clear idea about the procedure, risks associated, and potential results. This first approach to patient selection not only increases the percentages of patients' satisfaction but also decreases complications resulting from BT injections, thereby contributing to the long-term acceptance of the treatments in cosmetic clinics (Blugerman et al., 2016). The medical history of the patients must also be incorporated into the process. Some contraindications, such as neuromuscular disease, pregnancy, or use of certain medications, make it more probable that adverse effects will occur during or following the treatment. A good medical evaluation therefore, must be done in order to identify people who may be inappropriate for BT treatments. Doctors have to discuss openly any adverse reactions to other aesthetic treatments, drugs, or allergies; this enables them to make the treatment particularly appropriate to each client. The rising need for non-surgical treatments, as stressed by recent research, underlines the importance of following strict patient selection criteria to guarantee efficacy and safety within cosmetic dermatology (Pereira et al., 2022).

Finally, the changing face of cosmetic dermatology has highlighted the value of patient education during the process of selection. Also, educating patients regarding the nature of BT, mechanism of action, and what to expect in this regard, including side effects, would be beneficial for setting up the patient's expectations based on the clinical situation. In addition, patients should be instructed regarding some treatment alternatives and techniques such that patients become participants in decision-making. This combined practice has therefore enhanced patient satisfaction as well as improved better results of standards of postoperative care and reduced the possible complications. In conclusion, proper patient selection criteria, complemented by extensive education as well as realistic expectation management, therefore, constitute the pillars of successful BT treatments in cosmetic dermatology (Blugerman et al., 2016) (Figure 11.10).

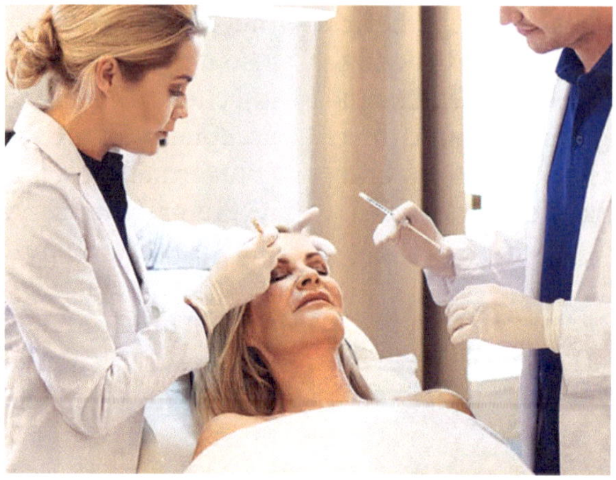

Figure 11.10. A healthcare professional performing a botulinum toxin (Botox) injection, a minimally invasive procedure widely used in aesthetic medicine to temporarily reduce dynamic facial wrinkles.

Source: https://media.post.rvohealth.io/wp-content/uploads/2020/08/5514-Doctor_Applying_Botox-732x549-thumbnail-732x549.jpg.

Test Your Knowledge

1. What are dynamic wrinkles, and how does BT help in their treatment?
2. Beyond cosmetic use, what are some therapeutic applications of BT, and what conditions can it help manage?
3. What factors should be considered when selecting a patient for BT treatment for cosmetic purposes?

11.4. Injection Techniques

Learning Outcome

1. Describe preparation and dosage considerations
2. Focus on injection sites and techniques
3. Explain the importance of precision and technique in outcomes

In cosmetic dermatology, the success of BT injections is largely dependent on accurate injection technique. Skill in these techniques is crucial for the best aesthetic outcomes with minimal side effects. Techniques are highly site-specific based on the particular anatomic location being treated, the desired final effect, and the patient's unique facial musculature. For instance, when treating glabellar lines, a grid pattern is often employed in order to evenly place the neurotoxin throughout, while for other areas linear or fan-shaped patterns can be employed in order to achieve maximum relaxation of the muscles in a safe manner. Utilizing proper technique not only achieves maximum therapeutic effect but also ensures minimum risk of unwanted effects such as bruising or asymmetry. Therefore, constant education and competence in injection skills are important for cosmetic procedure practitioners to give patients the safest and most effective treatments available. As the uses of BT expand into new indications beyond classic facial cosmetic treatment, injection skills must also develop to address new areas of interest that are emerging. The focus on current literature have been injections for many body rejuvenation therapies, with new techniques being introduced over recent years. The face, neck, chest, and even the hands are being treated with injectables and dermal fillers to replace volume and improve skin quality (Marie-Christen, 2022). The modalities of injection in these non-facial areas require a subtle knowledge of the underlying anatomy and laxity patterns of the skin to attain satisfactory results. Techniques like deep dermal injections are specifically designed for these regions, highlighting the importance of tailoring injection techniques to patient- and anatomy-based considerations. These advances highlight the dynamic characterization of injection techniques and place them at the forefront of responsible aesthetic practices. BT applications, although beneficial, also necessitate a cautious critique of patient evaluation protocols for determining the best approaches to injection. The detailed evaluation that includes wrinkle severity, quality of the skin, and patient expectations is required for treatment customization. Like in other medical treatments, the sophistication of the treatment necessitates a clear understanding of the patient's anatomy and aesthetic goal. Working toward this objective, practitioners are required to prioritize informed consent and educate patients regarding the risks and benefits of different injection methods. This patient-centered approach not only increases safety but also trust and satisfaction in the treatment process. In general terms, injecting BT is a mix of technical skill, aesthetic sensibility, and commitment to patient care, all of which are included in delivering cosmetic dermatology services effectively.

11.4.1. Preparation and Dosage Considerations

In organizing the preparation and dosage of BT in cosmetic procedures, one should have respect for the variations that follow due to patient anatomy and desired effect. Each protocol must be cautiously individualized according to age, facial musculature, and treated areas. For instance, the glabellar lines may need diverse dosing and methods of injection as compared to those that have been used in the forehead or around the eyes because their muscle power and skin elasticity are dissimilar. A clear-cut baseline test before the administration can render the dosing even more appropriate to achieve the final aesthetic effect without many complications (Kennedy et al., 2010). By actual dosage, the practitioners must follow established guidelines, but be prepared to adjust according to real-time feedback from the patient. Conservative doses are usually a standard beginning, particularly in areas that experience side effects. Overdosage in even moderate levels can lead to unexpected effects such as eyelid drooping or bracketing of facial expressions. Because dosage accuracy is so critical to both safety and efficacy, ongoing monitoring of patient response following treatment is a critical component of refining dosages and future protocol modification. This feedback loop is critical and can be further optimized through clinician experience and ongoing education about new practices and studies of BT therapy in cosmetic dermatology (Ratyna et al., 2024). Furthermore, informed consent and patient education are essential components of the whole preparation process. Communication regarding potential risks, benefits, and the approximate duration of action can significantly affect patient satisfaction and compliance with aftercare. As adverse effects of BT have been reported, having an understanding of the causes of the complications is important. Open lines of communication allow clinicians to have confidence that the patients not only know the esthetic objectives but are aware of what safety measures can be taken to prevent potential risks. These precautionary steps are particularly critical in the face of evidence that reveals a rate of severe adverse effects from BT treatment that may inadvertently discourage patient participation if unreported data are not addressed quickly (Kennedy et al., 2010; Ratyna et al., 2024) (Table 11.1).

Table 11.1. Total Recommended Treatment Dose

Treatment Area	Total Recommended Treatment Dose
Glabellar lines	20 Units in 0.5 mL
Lateral canthal lines	24 Units in 0.6 mL
Forehead lines and glabellar lines	40 Units in 1 mL
Platysma bands	One band on each side: 26 Units in 0.65 mL 1 band on one side, 2 bands on the other side: 31 Units in 0.78 mL Two bands on each side: 36 Units in 0.9 mL

Source: https://www.drugs.com/dosage/botox-cosmetic.html.

11.4.2. Injection Sites and Techniques

Selection of injection points for BT injections is important in obtaining the best cosmetic results with minimal chance of complications. Typical injection points are the glabella, forehead, and crows feet that relate to dynamic facial movements that cause wrinkles to form. Each of these points needs precision; for example, glabellar injection should safely avoid nearby muscles to avoid undesired brow ptosis. Further, the clinician must conduct an entire aesthetic analysis to ascertain individual patient needs because anatomical differences may influence site and dosage of injection. Though there are general technique and site guidelines, practitioners must consider each product of BT's individual characteristics because dosing guidelines vary significantly among products. This personalized approach optimizes patient satisfaction and guarantees outcome longevity, thereby contributing to the widespread popularity of these minimally invasive treatments (De Boulle et al., 2010). Injection techniques utilized during treatment with BT also play an important role in optimizing the effectiveness and safety of treatment. Tensor technique or fan technique are techniques utilized depending on the treatment zone and the patient's personal aesthetic goals. Utilization of a strategic multi-point approach also allows for more even toxin distribution, which may optimize its action with minimized side effects. Practitioners should also emphasize the importance of needle gauge and depth of injection to further optimize patient comfort and outcomes. Research has proven that employing a careful and methodical injection method not only guarantees the realization of the intended aesthetic results but also guarantees protection from unwanted side effects, such as bruising or swelling (Wollina & Goldman, , 2011). Attention to detail is paramount since the precision of injections can directly translate into an overall patient experience and the degree to which the patient feels satisfied. Individual demographics and anatomical features strongly dictate both potential sites and methods of BT injection. For younger individuals, cosmetic treatment may aim largely at prevention, such as smooth, subtle enhancers rather than true correction of established wrinkles. Injector techniques may thus differ to maintain a cosmetic, unaltered look while addressing potential asymmetry in the face and re-establishing symmetry to youthful contours. Conversely, older individuals typically seek procedures that reverse or reduce outward signs of aging, which calls for a different regimen in both location selection and injection style. Ethical issues also come into play, as practitioners have to walk the line between aesthetic medicine and the simple business of following cosmetic fashions. Finally, individualized evaluation and individualized treatment plans based on an integrated concept of these determinants are required to maximize BT treatment and provide patient satisfaction (De Boulle et al., 2010) (Figure 11.11).

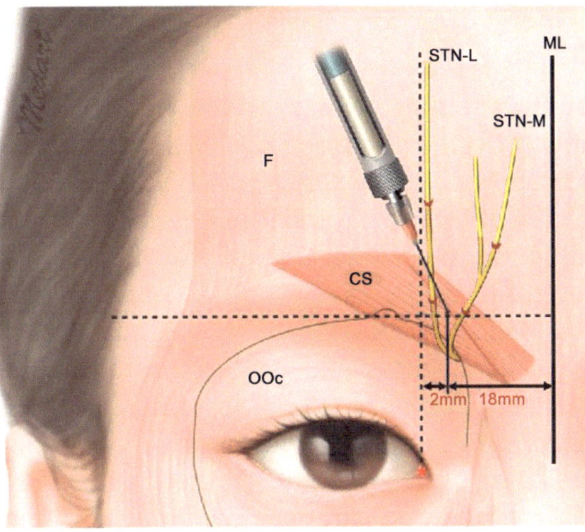

Figure 11.11. Guideline for the injection site of botulinum toxin for achieving successful anesthesia in patients.

Source: https://www.researchgate.net/profile/Shin-Hyo-Lee/publication/317614214/figure/fig3/AS:647102971518978@1531292779736/Guideline-for-the-injection-site-of-botulinum-toxin-for-achieving-successful-anesthesia.png.

11.4.3. Importance of Precision and Technique in Outcomes

Application of BT in cosmetic dermatology has transformed far more aesthetically pleasing treatment by providing the least invasive methods to address wrinkles as well as other cosmetic anomalies of the face. However, achievement is still largely technique- and injection-related. Knowledge of complex facial anatomy is crucial to practitioners; an erroneous injection might result in complications such as eyelid ptosis or asymmetry, thereby negatively affecting the intended aesthetic outcome. As explained in recent literature, the correlation between anatomical variation and injection techniques is paramount, once again highlighting the injector's necessity to be extremely familiar with facial musculature and patient-specific personal variation to produce the best results with a minimal number of unwanted side effects (Bartosiński et al., 2025). The technique used during the administration of BT influences not only immediate cosmetic outcomes but also the length for which a patient will be content. Any placement of administration points or dosing will require the methodologies to be precise. Techniques need to be standardized but flexible to apply to individual patients with differing anatomy or needs, potentially impacting the result. Clinicians should utilize evidence-based methods driven by peer consultation and resulting clinical experience accumulation. A literature review demonstrates the fact that although the chances for complications might be minimal as experienced practitioners perform procedures, such complications are transitory, thus impairing patient satisfaction and confidence immensely (Ratyna et al., 2024). Therefore, technical perfection is necessary in aesthetic medicine to maintain professional standards and patient confidence. For survival of good outcomes in cosmetic dermatology, education refreshers and attendance at the latest injection techniques are crucial for practitioners. With the ever-changing field at a faster pace through new findings and information, injectors must keep enthusiasm in honing their skills and acquiring new information surrounding BT therapy. This is not only meant to provide protection against complications and risk but also to improve the overall efficacy of treatments. Finally, the ability of the practitioner to make injections accurately not only enhances patient experiences but also ensures the reputation of BT treatments as a reliable and effective option in cosmetic dermatology. By cultivating a culture of technical excellence and accuracy, the cosmetic dermatology practice will sustain its success and make its role as an aesthetic leader even more secure.

Test Your Knowledge

1. What are the key considerations when preparing BT for injection, and how does the preparation process impact the effectiveness of treatment?
2. How is the appropriate dosage of BT determined for different patients or conditions, and what factors influence this decision?

11.5. Safety and Side Effects

Learning Outcome

1. Describe common side effects associated with treatment
2. Discuss serious complications by using BT
3. Understand the guidelines for minimizing risks

The use of BT in cosmetic dermatology is preceded by a detailed consideration of safety and possible side effects. It is indeed the case that, under the hands of skilled practitioners, the treatment is reasonably safe, but it can cause adverse reactions. Adverse reactions or side effects are usually reported as injection-site pain, swelling, bruising, and erythema. Apart from this, a few patients might experience temporary muscle asymmetry or weakness because of unintentional diffusion of the toxin to other muscles. These adverse effects are reversible and vanish after a few days; however, severe complications, though infrequent, may arise in the form of respiratory problems or allergy. Practitioners must therefore perform thorough checks of patient health and tailored treatment processes in order to prevent the danger of toxicity and provide optimal patient safety. The consequence of BT transcends the aesthetic issue since safety will be more crucial in patients with existing medical conditions. Current debate suggests that cancer survivors undergoing aesthetic procedures might utilize BT to improve quality of life and body image. Nevertheless, this patient group commonly presents with special medical complications that require multidisciplinary treatment, prioritizing safety over offering a cosmetic effect. Care providers need to exercise caution in managing the safety profile of BT for cancer patients, adjusting the treatment protocols based on potential complications of earlier therapies. The tailored treatment is an indication of the need to establish not just the advantages but also the risks of BT for the therapeutic intervention not to compromise a patient's wellbeing or health status (Proietti et al., 2021). With growing evidence for the therapeutic effectiveness of BT in diseases beyond cosmetic use, safety awareness and side effects remain most paramount. Research indicates promising results in BT utilization for acne vulgaris and acne scars, which leads to its expanding use in dermatology (Podraza et al., 2025). However, before such BT can be adopted as a standard of care therapy for such disorders, rigorous clinical studies need to be undertaken to evaluate its safety and side effects among different groups of patients. Caution should be exercised, particularly in weighing the adverse effects risk against possible therapeutic gain. Additional research into patient response and long-term results will contribute to the expanded safety profile of BTs, such that cosmetic dermatology can utilize these new treatments responsibly and effectively.

11.5.1. Common Side Effects Associated with Treatment

Cosmetic dermatology has thus witnessed a huge increase in the use of BT, with its efficacy in reducing facial wrinkles and rejuvenating the skin. However, as is the case with most medical procedures, it is equally important to be aware and realize what the common side effects are with this treatment. Patients experience some localized reactions at the site of injection, which can be redness, swelling, or even bruising in nature and are usually mild and temporary. Additionally, some individuals report transient headache and discomfort following the procedure. Understanding these effects is crucial as they can impact patient satisfaction and decision-making regarding future treatments. As the popularity of BT increases, awareness of these potential side effects allows for better patient education and preparation for what to expect following the procedure. This knowledge benefits both clinicians and patients alike, promoting an atmosphere of transparency and trust in cosmetic treatment outcomes (Goldust et al., 2022). Another prevalent side effect associated with BT treatment is the possibility of muscle weakness or asymmetry, particularly when injections are administered in areas requiring precise muscle control. For instance, injections aimed at the masseter muscle for cosmetic slimming or therapeutic benefits can lead to unintended alterations in facial asymmetry or difficulties in chewing if improperly administered. The intricacies involved in facial anatomy highlight the importance of skillful techniques to minimize these adverse effects. Recognizing that while these complications are often temporary, they can significantly impact patient confidence and satisfaction is vital for practitioners. Additionally, continuous efforts in learning mechanisms behind these complications will be required to improve techniques as well as patient outcomes in cosmetic dermatology (Ratyna et al., 2024). Aside from immediate side effects, some minor yet vital long-term effects may arise from BT injections. Although such serious complications are relatively infrequent, systemic spread of the toxin has been documented to cause complications, including respiratory distress or generalized muscle weakness in susceptible patients. Such findings are significant because they potentially undermine patient health and safety. Therefore, when providing any treatment, it is always prudent that health care professionals perform adequate preservice assessments for the procedure. They should also alert the patients about the possible risks involved in performing the specific treatment. By creating an informed understanding of the benefits and risks, practitioners will be able to steer patients toward well-informed choices consistent with their aesthetic desires while maintaining best possible safety for the administration of BT therapies (Goldust et al., 2022) (Figure 11.12).

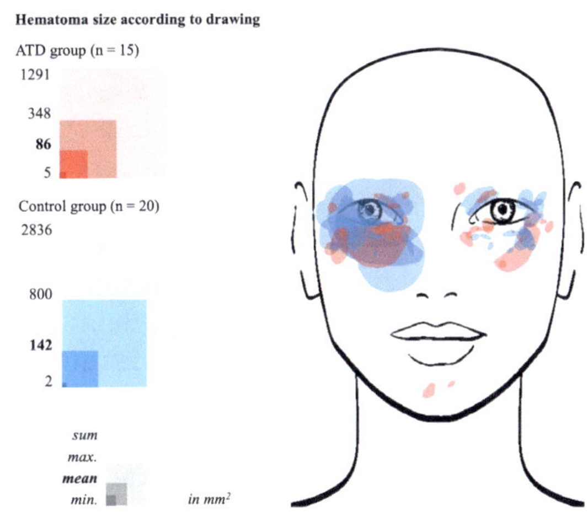

Figure 11.12. Depiction of hematomas drawn in a facial image after current BoNT/A injection according to their size and localization.

Source: Wenninger FC, Wabbels B. Frequency of Hemorrhagic Side Effects of Botulinum Neurotoxin Treatment in Patients with Blepharospasm and Hemifacial Spasm on Antithrombotic Medication. Toxins. 2022; 14(11):769. https://doi.org/10.3390/toxins14110769

11.5.2. Rare But Serious Complications

Although BT has become popular in aesthetic dermatology because of its efficacy in smoothing out fine lines and rejuvenating facial appearance, practitioners need to be cautious of the uncommon but serious complications that may result from its administration. Severe adverse effects, although uncommon, may result in considerable patient dissatisfaction and possible long-term consequences. For instance, complications such as dysphagia, respiratory distress, and even the onset of botulism-like symptoms have been reported in rare cases, particularly when the dosage exceeds the therapeutic threshold or when injected improperly. Understanding these risks is essential for practitioners, as the success of these aesthetic procedures hinges not only on the aesthetic outcome but also on the safety of the treatment approach, highlighting the necessity for proper training and patient selection before intervention (Goldust et al., 2022). Moreover, complications can vary based on the anatomical region targeted during BT injections. For example, while treating the masseter muscle for aesthetic lower facial contouring, patients may experience unintended weakness in adjacent muscles, leading to difficulties with chewing or facial asymmetry. This area is particularly sensitive, and despite the low incidence of adverse effects, the potential for complications necessitates thorough anatomical knowledge and precision during injection. Studies emphasize the importance of employing established guidelines when injecting this muscle to mitigate risks (Ratyna et al., 2024). Furthermore, obtaining informed consent regarding possible adverse effects can enhance patient understanding and satisfaction, ensuring they are aware of both the benefits and risks associated with the procedure. In conclusion, although BT injections are typically deemed safe and effective, clinicians must navigate the realm of rare but serious complications associated with their use. A comprehensive approach to patient assessment, injection technique, and post-operative monitoring is crucial in minimizing such risks. By adhering to established protocols and engaging in continuous education regarding emerging research on complications, practitioners can better safeguard both their clients and their own professional reputations in the competitive field of cosmetic dermatology. Ultimately, the goal remains not only to enhance aesthetic outcomes but also to ensure that patient safety is paramount in every aspect of treatment (Goldust et al., 2022).

11.5.3. Guidelines for Minimizing Risks

In the realm of cosmetic dermatology, particularly concerning BT use, the establishment of stringent guidelines for minimizing risks is essential to safeguard patient well-being. An effective approach begins with thorough patient assessment, which includes detailed medical histories and consideration of any existing conditions that could amplify the potential for adverse reactions. The elective nature of such procedures underscores the responsibility of practitioners to ensure that patients are well-informed about both the risks and benefits. As noted in Gomes et al. (2023), elective procedures can have unintended consequences, including effects on the ocular surface. Thus, practitioners must adopt a comprehensive consultation model that prioritizes informed consent, enabling patients to make educated decisions regarding their treatments and potential outcomes. Furthermore, adherence to standardized injection techniques significantly reduces the likelihood of complications associated with BT administration. This includes meticulous attention to anatomical landmarks and the selection of appropriate dosages tailored to individual patient needs. Proper knowledge of facial musculature is crucial, as variations in anatomy may lead to unintended results or side effects, such as asymmetrical facial expressions. The recovery process following injection is also vital, as described in Ratyna et al. (2024), outlining stages that can influence general recovery. By informing patients on post-care and potential complications, professionals can take a key role in facilitating the best recovery and risk reduction with botulinum injections. Lastly, ongoing education and professional development of professionals in cosmetic dermatology cannot be ignored in risk management. Continuing professional development may improve the practitioners in terms of skills and expertise and thus ensure they are current with new techniques and safety standards. Attendance at workshops, conferences, and peer-reviewed publications keeps practitioners abreast of new research and best practices. Additionally, building a peer review and experience-sharing network can add value to the collective expertise on risk reduction. The potential impact of interventions, as highlighted in Gomes et al. (2023), reinforces the importance of evaluating not only the immediate aesthetic outcomes but also the long-term implications on patient health and quality of life.

Test Your Knowledge

1. What are some of the most common side effects associated with BT treatment?
2. What are some rare but serious complications that may occur after BT injections, and how can they be recognized and treated?

11.6. Patient Experience and Satisfaction

Learning Outcome

1. Discuss pre-treatment consultation and expectations
2. Understand the process of post-treatment care and follow-up
3. Describe the factors influencing patient satisfaction

The evaluation of patient experience and satisfaction in cosmetic dermatology, particularly regarding BT treatments, is an essential component of effective clinical practice. Understanding the factors that contribute to a positive experience can significantly enhance patient outcomes, fostering trust and encouraging treatment adherence. In the context of BT, clinicians must recognize the psychological dimensions of facial aesthetics, which can influence a patient's self-perception and emotional well-being. Research indicates that procedures targeting specific areas, such as frown lines, have profound implications for how patients view themselves and how they are perceived by others, ultimately enhancing their overall satisfaction with the treatment (De Boulle et al., 2010). This awareness allows practitioners to tailor interventions more effectively, ensuring that they align with the individual expectations and goals of their patients. However, not to be taken lightly is the importance of patient-reported outcomes in satisfaction assessment. These provide very crucial insights into the efficacy and tolerability of different formulations of BT, guide both clinical decision-making and education of the patient for one's physician, and ensure that not all formulations are considered to be used interchangeably. Differences in dosing and administration can directly affect patient satisfaction and compliance with ongoing treatment. A thorough and individualized aesthetic evaluation is necessary to navigate these complexities, ensuring that the selected product meets the unique needs of the patient (De Boulle et al., 2010). By prioritizing these assessments, practitioners can address specific patient concerns, fostering a collaborative environment that enhances overall satisfaction and encourages positive treatment experiences. Additionally, taking into account the age-related considerations in aesthetic medicine is vital for optimizing patient experience. Young adults, particularly those in their third decade of life, exhibit distinct aesthetic needs and priorities that can differ significantly from older populations. Procedures aimed at correcting facial asymmetries or enhancing facial sculpting are particularly salient in this demographic, as they may align with societal perceptions of beauty and self-image. Thus, understanding the ethical implications surrounding these interventions is essential, as they often blur the lines between medical necessity and cosmetic desire. As practitioners navigate these challenges, it is paramount to engage in open dialogues with patients, ensuring they feel supported and informed about their choices, ultimately contributing to a more satisfactory and meaningful aesthetic journey.

11.6.1. Pre-Treatment Consultation and Expectations

The pre-treatment consultation serves as a foundational element in the administration of BT for cosmetic purposes. This phase allows practitioners to conduct a thorough assessment of the patient's medical history and specific aesthetic goals. By engaging in an open dialogue, practitioners can address concerns, clarify expectations, and evaluate any potential contraindications. A detailed interview not only assists in refining the treatment plan but also in aligning the procedure with the patient's desired outcomes. According to recent studies, such consultations are instrumental in tailoring procedures that optimize safety and efficacy, as they facilitate the selection of the most appropriate treatment methods for each individual. With this targeted approach, practitioners can enhance patient satisfaction and minimize post-treatment complications, thus ensuring a well-considered pathway towards achieving aesthetic harmony. Addressing patient expectations during pre-treatment consultations is paramount to the success of BT procedures. Patients often arrive with preconceived notions about the outcomes, influenced by social media and peer experiences. Practitioners need to spend time informing patients about realistic outcomes with BT and both its strengths and limitations. Creating a clear definition of what the treatment can and cannot do serves to minimize dissatisfaction and build trust in the clinician's expertise. Additionally, the consultation process enables practitioners to psychoprepare patients, reminding them of the need to follow post-treatment aftercare to maximize outcomes. By clarifying these expectations, practitioners not only enhance the overall patient experience but also cultivate a professional environment that prioritizes informed consent and ethical practice, ultimately reinforcing the therapeutic alliance between patient and provider. Furthermore, the significance of pre-treatment consultations extends to the consideration of various factors that influence the safety and efficacy of BT treatments. Various elements, such as the patient's age, skin quality, and health conditions, must be assessed to define the most suitable approach to treatment. For instance, individuals with underlying chronic conditions may require special consideration or alternative strategies to ensure successful outcomes. Additionally, understanding the patients' lifestyle, including their smoking status and medication use, can impact their recovery and results. Through careful evaluation during these consultations, practitioners can outline potential complications and realistic timelines for recovery, thereby establishing an informed path forward. This comprehensive approach integrates not only medical assessment but also patient education, ultimately fostering an environment that supports optimal aesthetic outcomes and minimizes adverse events (Kumar, 2021; Nieć et al., 2024) (Figure 11.13).

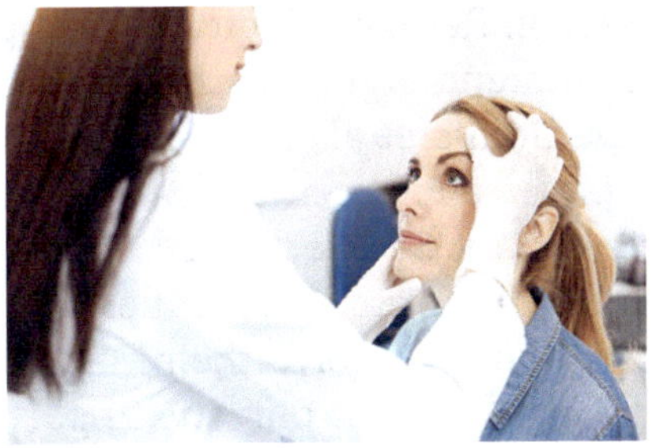

Figure 11.13. Pre-treatment consultation.

Source: https://media.istockphoto.com/id/684098354/photo/nice-pleasant-woman-looking-at-her-doctor.jpg?s=612x612&w=0&k=20&c=OPFbdkqSmejzP3vI13nYgLTcy3hbhMjqC2VEuepZRYQ=.

11.6.2. Post-Treatment Care and Follow-Up

Post-treatment care and follow-up are crucial components in ensuring the safety and efficacy of BT treatments in cosmetic dermatology. Once patients have undergone the procedure, they are advised to avoid strenuous activities and not to touch or massage the treated areas for at least 24 hours. Such care plan is crucial to reduce the risk of diffusion of the toxin into unwanted muscles, which may result in less-than-optimal results like facial asymmetry or other complications. As described in the literature, the fact that BT works and how it interacts with the muscular anatomy of the face guarantees a better-informed practice of post-treatment counseling. Steps taken during this phase can significantly enhance patient satisfaction and results, underpinning the importance of diligent follow-up protocols in clinical practice. Regular follow-up appointments play an integral role in managing patient expectations and monitoring outcomes after BT treatments. During these consultations, practitioners assess the effectiveness of the treatment, address any potential complications, and provide recommendations for future care. Detection of adverse effects, while rare, can contribute to significant patient concern; hence, the establishment of an open line of communication is paramount. Patients should be educated about the possibility of temporary reactions such as bruising or swelling, as highlighted by the findings that indicate these effects, though typically mild, can impact patient confidence (Ratyna et al., 2024). Therefore, establishing a timeline for follow-up not only reassures patients but also allows clinicians to implement necessary interventions if complications arise, reinforcing a culture of safety and efficacy in aesthetic procedures. Furthermore, a comprehensive post-treatment care plan should incorporate recommendations for skin care and lifestyle modifications that support the treatment effects. Educating patients about the appropriate skincare regimens, such as the use of gentle cleansers and sun protection, can enhance outcomes and prolong the effects of BT. Practitioners need to provide guidance tailored to individual skin types and conditions, acknowledging the diverse responses to treatments. Besides skincare recommendations, referencing the possible requirement for touch-up treatments every now and then can keep patient satisfaction levels (Bartosiński et al., 2025). Recognizing the complexities of post-treatment care ensures that the provider not only prevents risks but also initiates long-term aesthetic goals consistent with patients' expectations. Following the overall strategy in follow-up reflects dedication to quality care in cosmetic dermatology.

11.6.3. Factors Influencing Patient Satisfaction

Cosmetic dermatology patient satisfaction, particularly for BT treatment, is increasingly recognized as a key factor in the success of treatment. Quality communication between practitioners and patients, as well as the competency of the clinician, are some of the elements behind the satisfaction level. In addition, adequate communication of the interventions, results, and management of patient expectations by the clinician is at the heart of establishing levels of satisfaction. Research indicates that patient-reported outcomes, detailing individual experiences after treatment, significantly influence their overall satisfaction and likelihood of continuing treatment (De Boulle et al., 2010). When patients feel adequately informed and understood, their confidence in the treatment and the practitioner invariably rises, suggesting that the relational aspect of care cannot be overlooked. Another vital factor influencing patient satisfaction is the clinical effectiveness of BT procedures themselves. The visible results of cosmetic treatments directly impact how patients perceive their value. Studies evaluating the efficacy of BT in addressing aesthetic concerns highlight not only the importance of achieving desired outcomes but also the role of factors such as dosing and individual skin responses. For instance, promising results have been observed in the treatment of conditions like acne, where BT shows potential in reducing acne lesions and improving the appearance of scars, which could lead to higher satisfaction levels among patients seeking these specific outcomes (Podraza et al., 2025). Therefore, balancing effective treatment techniques with a thorough understanding of indications is crucial for enhancing overall patient satisfaction. Finally, patient demographics and inter-individual variability have a significant impact on levels of satisfaction in cosmetic dermatology. Age, gender, and psychological profile can influence the way patients experience and perceive their treatment. Younger patients may have more challenging aesthetic aspirations, whereas older patients may value subtlety and elegance. Moreover, dominant social and cultural beauty ideals also have the power to influence expectations, and practitioners need to navigate these sensitively. Understanding these nuances allows dermatologists to tailor treatments and foster an environment that prioritizes individual patient needs. Ultimately, addressing these varied influences is essential for practitioners aiming to improve patient satisfaction in BT procedures, thus ensuring that aesthetic goals are not only met but exceeded (Figure 11.14).

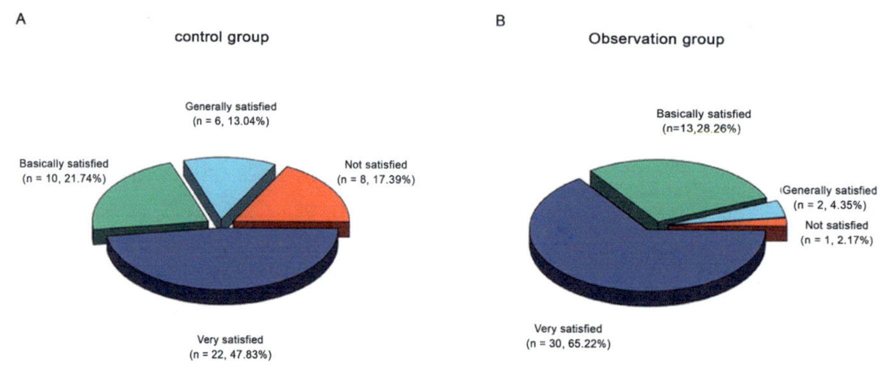

Figure 11.14. Patient satisfaction distribution chart (A) the distribution of patients' satisfaction in the control group; (B) Distribution of patients' satisfaction in the observation group.

Source: https://www.researchgate.net/publication/383827792/figure/fig4/AS:11431281279779726@1727194138308/Patient-satisfaction-distribution-chart-Fig-A-the-distribution-of-patients.jpg.

Test Your Knowledge

1. What factors influence patient satisfaction with BT treatments in cosmetic dermatology, and how can these be addressed by practitioners
2. How do patient expectations regarding the results of BT treatments impact their overall experience?

SUMMARY

Over the last two decades, development in various techniques and rising interest in cosmetic procedures have helped put BT in an increasingly cornered market. In short, BT has become the most transformative advancement within the field of cosmetic dermatology and has opened up vast options for aesthetic enhancement. As dermatological innovations progress, patients increasingly favor procedures that yield immediate results with minimal downtime and limited risks. This trend is particularly evident in light of the growing preference for nonablative techniques, which have largely overshadowed ablative resurfacing methods. The synergistic use of BT in conjunction with other corrective procedures significantly bolsters aesthetic outcomes, demonstrating its unparalleled efficacy in modern dermatological practice (Lipozen et al., 2010). The versatility of BT extends beyond mere aesthetic improvements, revealing promising avenues for therapeutic applications within dermatology. Its potential in treating conditions such as acne vulgaris, rosacea, and acne scars has garnered considerable attention in recent research. Findings indicate an impressive efficacy of BT treatment of acne and its related scars, which not only increases patient satisfaction but also expands the range of treatment options for dermatologists (Podraza et al., 2025). Nevertheless, it is essential to note that additional research is required to validate these findings and further develop application methods across a range of patient populations. Such inquiries will aid in establishing standardized protocols for dosage and treatment frequency, thereby optimizing therapeutic outcomes and expanding the clinical understanding of BT. Ultimately, the integration of BT into cosmetic dermatology reflects an evolution in aesthetic practices that prioritize safety, efficacy, and patient satisfaction. As practitioners continue to explore the boundaries of dermatological treatments, the need for comprehensive evaluations and ethical considerations becomes paramount. The potential benefits of combining BT with other procedural interventions must be carefully balanced against inherent risks. By fostering an environment of continued research and innovation, the field can enhance the quality of care provided to patients seeking cosmetic and therapeutic interventions. The future of BT in dermatology is not just about accomplishing desired cosmetic results but also about perfecting therapeutic procedures to treat a wider range of dermatological concerns, ultimately enhancing the field as a whole.

In summation, the exploration of BT in cosmetic dermatology highlights its prominent role as a foundational treatment within minimally invasive aesthetic procedures. The various formulations of BT type A, such as onabotulinumtoxinA and abobotulinumtoxinA, serve distinct purposes in enhancing facial aesthetics. Clinicians and patients increasingly recognize the significance of facial expressions, particularly regarding frown lines, in influencing self-perception and emotional well-being. Further, changes in the conventions on nonproprietary naming required by the United States FDA highlight the need for practitioners to distinguish between these preparations to provide accurate dosing and application methods. As detailed in recent literature, it is evident that thorough patient assessments during consultations are imperative, as individual treatment plans tailored to personal aesthetic goals optimize patient satisfaction and the likelihood of ongoing treatment engagement (De Boulle et al., 2010). Furthermore, ongoing advancements in the understanding of BTs mechanisms of action have revolutionized approaches to a variety of dermatological conditions. While traditional applications primarily focus on cosmetic enhancements, burgeoning research suggests potential therapeutic benefits beyond aesthetics. The anti-pruritic effects of botulinum neurotoxins, as observed in various chronic itch conditions, exemplify these emerging applications.

Although clinical evidence remains mostly anecdotal, with limited randomized controlled trials, the case studies presented offer insights into the potential utility of these toxins in managing itch-related ailments. Such findings indicate a broader scope for BT treatments, yet underscore the necessity for rigorous research to enhance the evidence base supporting these off-label applications (Gazerani, 2022). Lastly, the discussion surrounding BT in cosmetic dermatology emphasizes not only the current consensus on its applications but also the future directions necessary for its continued evolution. Achieving regulatory approval for additional indications, such as anti-itch therapies, necessitates well-designed studies that can establish robust primary and secondary outcomes. The mechanisms underlying the therapeutic benefits of BTs engage various biological processes, including neuronal and immune modulation, which warrant further investigation. As the field of cosmetic dermatology advances, integrating scientific research with clinical practice will be crucial for refining treatment protocols and expanding the therapeutic horizon of BT applications. By fostering collaboration between clinicians and researchers, the potential for innovative treatments in aesthetic and therapeutic contexts can be fully realized, ultimately enhancing patient care and satisfaction (Gazerani, 2022).

KEY TERMS FROM THIS CHAPTER

- Conspicuous manifestations
- Dissatisfaction
- Multi-point approach
- Neuromuscular junction
- Quality communication
- Botox
- Xeomin
- Myobloc
- Facial wrinkles
- Co-operative treatment
- Dysfunctional disruption
- Neurological disorders
- Poly-L-lactic acid (PLLA)
- Regulatory models
- Dysport
- Jeuveau
- Muscle relaxation
- Glabellar lines

CRITICAL THINKING QUESTIONS

1. **Which of the following is the most common cosmetic indication for botulinum toxin injections?**
   a. Hyperhidrosis
   b. Wrinkle reduction
   c. Acne treatment
   d. Hair loss
2. **Which of the following types of botulinum toxin is most commonly used in cosmetic dermatology?**
   a. Botulinum toxin A (Botox)
   b. Botulinum toxin B (Myobloc)
   c. Botulinum toxin C
   d. Botulinum toxin D
3. **What is the primary mechanism of action of botulinum toxin in the treatment of wrinkles?**
   a. Stimulating collagen production
   b. Increasing blood flow to the skin
   c. Blocking acetylcholine release at neuromuscular junctions
   d. Contracting the underlying muscles
4. **Which of the following is a common side effect associated with botulinum toxin injections in cosmetic procedures?**
   a. Hypertrophic scarring
   b. Bruising and swelling at the injection site
   c. Increased pigmentation
   d. Hyperpigmentation of the treated area
5. **Which technique is commonly used to minimize the spread of botulinum toxin beyond the target area?**
   a. Massaging the injection site
   b. Injecting large volumes at once
   c. Injecting into the superficial dermis
   d. Using a small-gauge needle and precise injection points

Short Answer Questions

1. What are the main types of Botulinum toxin used in medical and cosmetic treatments, and how do they differ?
2. List at least three common medical indications for the use of Botulinum toxin.
3. What are some common cosmetic indications for Botulinum toxin?
4. Describe the general technique for administering Botulinum toxin for aesthetic purposes.
5. What are the potential side effects of Botulinum toxin treatment, and how can they be minimized?
6. What are some contraindications or precautions to consider before administering Botulinum toxin?

Answer to Critical Thinking Questions

1. (b); 2. (a); 3. (c); 4. (b); 5. (d)

REFERENCES

1. Aghaei, S. (2022). *Recent Advances in Wound Healing*. https://core.ac.uk/download/534900218.pdf (accessed on 11th June 2025).
2. Akuma, O. M., Azi, C. I., Carsrud, N. D. V., et al. (2024). *BOTOX's Mechanism, Diversity Considerations, And Therapeutic Potential in Cosmetic, Medical, And Dental Practice*. https://core.ac.uk/download/621451720.pdf (accessed on 11th June 2025).
3. Gomes, J. A. P., Azar, D. T., Baudouin, C., Bitton, E., Chen, W., Hafezi, F., Hamrah, P., Hogg, R. E., Horwath-Winter, J., Kontadakis, G. A., Mehta, J. S., Messmer, E. M., Perez, V. L., Zadok, D., & Willcox, M. D. P. (2023). TFOS Lifestyle: Impact of elective medications and procedures on the ocular surface. *The ocular surface*, *29*, 331–385. https://doi.org/10.1016/j.jtos.2023.04.011(accessed on 11th June 2025).
4. Bartosiński, R., Dutkiewicz, J., Kaźmierczak, J. M., Kąpa, et al. (2025). *Complications and Anatomical Considerations in Botulinum Neurotoxin Type A Injections for Upper Face Rejuvenation: A Systematic Review*. https://core.ac.uk/download/646079970.pdf (accessed on 11th June 2025).
5. Blugerman, G., Martinez, L., Schavelzon, D., Wexler, et al. (2016). *Botulinum Toxin in the Nasal Area*. https://core.ac.uk/download/322425961.pdf (accessed on 11th June 2025).
6. Ratyna, K., Bochenek, O., Koper, M., Kałuża, J., Konaszczuk, A., Nowak, A., ... Skarbek, M. (2024). Adverse effects of treating bruxism and masseter muscle hypertrophy with botulinum toxin injection - a literature review. *Quality in Sport*, *21*, 54012. https://doi.org/10.12775/QS.2024.21.54012(accessed on 11th June 2025).
7. Bouzouaya, C., & Feiner, R. (2018). *Adjuvant Botulinum Toxin Harmonization in Minimally Invasive Facial Aesthetic Surgery*. https://core.ac.uk/download/322438270.pdf (accessed on 11th June 2025).
8. Podraza, A., Sacher, K., Maciaszek, O., Turemka, M., & Chmiel, M. (2025). Botulinum Toxin: An Innovative Approach to Treating Acne and Acne Scars: A systematic review. *Journal of Education, Health and Sport*, *79*, 57875. https://doi.org/10.12775/JEHS.2025.79.57875(accessed on 11th June 2025).
9. Christen, M. O. (2022). Collagen stimulators in body applications: A review focused on poly-L-lactic acid (PLLA). *Clinical Cosmetic and Investigational Dermatology, 15*, 997–1019. https://doi.org/10.2147/ccid.s359813.
10. Cosma, P., Fini, P., Gubitosa, J., et al. (2021). *Nutricosmetics in Skincare—The Fascinating World of Skin–Brain Connection: A Review to Explore Ingredients, Commercial Products for Skin Aging, And Cosmetic Regulation*. https://core.ac.uk/download/541255577.pdf (accessed on 11th June 2025).
11. Davies, J., Mosahebi, A., Sousi, S., et al. (2023). *Cosmetic Business Mechanics in London: A Cross-Sectional Analysis and Audit of ASA Compliance*. https://core.ac.uk/download/564422122.pdf (accessed on 11th June 2025).
12. De Boulle, K., Fagien, S., Sommer, B., & Glogau, R. (2010). Treating glabellar lines with botulinum toxin type A-hemagglutinin complex: a review of the science, the clinical data, and patient satisfaction. *Clinical interventions in aging*, *5*, 101–118. https://doi.org/10.2147/cia.s9338(accessed on 11th June 2025).

13. Nieć, M., Olejarz, Z., Nowak, K., Drygała, Z., Wyrwał, J., Zielińska, Z., ... Krasuska, M. (2024). Factors influencing the length of the recovery period after blepharoplasty: a review of the latest data. *Journal of Education, Health and Sport, 59*, 183–208. https://doi.org/10.12775/JEHS.2024.59.012(accessed on 11th June 2025).

14. Eckstein, R. (2009). *BOTOX and Its Effect on Wrinkles.* https://core.ac.uk/download/428373214.pdf (accessed on 11th June 2025).

15. Fernández-Varela-Gómez, F., Sandoval-García, A., & Valeria Cabrera-Rios, K. (2024). Signs of skin aging: a review. *International Journal of Research in Medical Sciences, 12*(7), 2674–2679. https://doi.org/10.18203/2320-6012.ijrms20241935(accessed on 11th June 2025).

16. Fico, G., Laneri, S., & Pero, R. (2018). *Botulinum Toxin Adverse Events.* https://core.ac.uk/download/322438576.pdf (accessed on 11th June 2025).

17. Gazerani, P. (2022). *How Does Botulinum Toxin Inhibit Itch?* https://core.ac.uk/download/541300994.pdf (accessed on 11th June 2025).

18. Goldman, A., & Wollina, U. (2025). *Minimally Invasive Aesthetic Procedures in Young Adults.* https://core.ac.uk/download/pdf/8574728.pdf (accessed on 11th June 2025).

19. Goldust, M., Gupta, M., Kassir, M., Kroumpouzos, E., et al. (2022). *Complications of Botulinum Toxin A: An Update Review.* https://core.ac.uk/download/621756021.pdf (accessed on 11th June 2025).

20. Gregoriou, S., Sidiropoulou, P., Kontochristopoulos, G., & Rigopoulos, D. (2019). Management strategies of palmar hyperhidrosis: Challenges and solutions. *Clinical Cosmetic and Investigational Dermatology, 12*, 733–744. https://doi.org/10.2147/ccid.s210973.

21. Inchingolo, A. D., Wegierska, A. E., Scarano, A., Lorusso, F., Inchingolo, F., Dipalma, G., Charitos, I. A., et al. (2021). *Botulinum Neurotoxins (BoNTs) and Their Biological, Pharmacological, And Toxicological Issues: A Scoping Review.* https://core.ac.uk/download/541257581.pdf (accessed on 11th June 2025).

22. Inchingolo, A. D., Wegierska, A. E., Scarano, A., Lorusso, F., Inchingolo, F., Dipalma, G., Amer, A., Amer, M., & Nofal, H. (2021). *Botulinum Toxin for The Face.* https://core.ac.uk/download/387219624.pdf (accessed on 11th June 2025).

23. Kennedy, N. R. (2010). *Taming the Perfect Poison: A Comparative Analysis of the EMEA's EPAR System and the FDA's Improved Warning Protocol.* https://core.ac.uk/download/71461728.pdf (accessed on 11th June 2025).

24. Kumar, N. (2021). *Design, Development and Implementation Framework for A Postgraduate Non-Surgical Aesthetics Curriculum.* Narendra Kumar A dissertation submitted in partial fulfilment of the requirements for the degree of Doctor of Philosophy of University College London Division of Biosciences, University College London(accessed on 11th June 2025).

25. Li, K., Meng, F., Li, Y. R., Tian, Y., Chen, H., Jia, Q., Cai, H., & Jiang, H. B. (2022). *Application of Nonsurgical Modalities in Improving Facial Aging.* https://core.ac.uk/download/571657020.pdf (accessed on 11th June 2025).

26. Lipozenčić, J., & Bukvić-Mokos, Z. (2010). *Korektivna Dermatologija Danas.* https://core.ac.uk/download/14451790.pdf (accessed on 11th June 2025).

27. Proietti, I., Skroza, N., Mambrin, A., Marraffa, F., Tolino, E., Bernardini, N., Marchesiello, A., Rossi, G., Volpe, S., & Potenza, C. (2021). Aesthetic Treatments in Cancer Patients. *Clinical,*

cosmetic and investigational dermatology, 14, 1831–1837. https://doi.org/10.2147/CCID.S342734(accessed on 11th June 2025).

28. Pereira, J. G. D., Manganaro, N. L., & da Silva, R. H. A. (2022). *Complications in Orofacial Harmonization Procedures: A Systematic Review*. https://core.ac.uk/download/548337240.pdf (accessed on 11th June 2025).
29. Popescu, M., Berteanu, M., Beiu, C., Popa, L. G., Mihai, M. M., Iliescu, M. G., Stănescu, A. M. A., et al. (2022). Complementary strategies to promote hair regrowth in post-COVID-19 telogen effluvium. *Clinical Cosmetic and Investigational Dermatology, 15*, 735–743. https://doi.org/10.2147/ccid.s359052.
30. Sivesind, T. E., Szeto, M. D., Kim, W., & Dellavalle, R. P. (2021). Google Trends in dermatology: Scoping review of the literature. *JMIR Dermatology, 4*, e27712. https://doi.org/10.2196/27712.

DERMAL FILLERS: TYPES, INDICATIONS, AND INJECTION TECHNIQUES

12

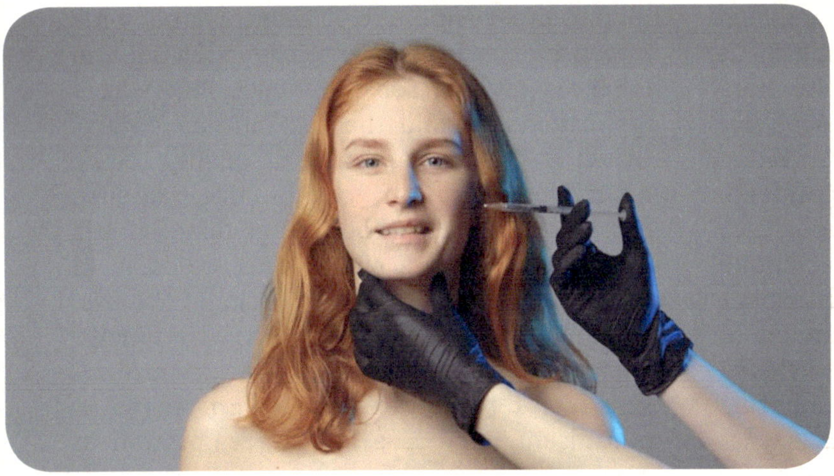

LEARNING OBJECTIVES

After studying this chapter, you will be able to:

1. Define the types of dermal fillers
2. Understand indications for the use of dermal fillers
3. Discuss the benefits of dermal fillers
4. Discuss risks and side effects
5. Define methods of injections
6. Highlight post-treatment care in guaranteeing the safety and durability of dermal filler treatments

Introduction

Aesthetic medicine has lately seen the popularity of dermal fillers rise as a minimally invasive facial rejuvenation procedure. This has been spurred by the heightened recognition of individualized aesthetic treatment for confronting the varied demographic needs that include varied ethnic groups and age concerns. As physicians have been seeking solutions to the many faces of facial aging, dermal fillers have stepped in as valuable tools in aesthetic medicine. The synergy of hyaluronic acid (HA) fillers, botulinum toxin (BT), and minimal-invasive treatments has shifted the emphasis to the depth of knowledge within patient-specific needs and anatomical variability (Moon et al., 2021). Such depth will ultimately enhance patient satisfaction and achieve the best aesthetic outcome. The development of multiple dermal filler varieties has further propelled the specialty, and operators are now able to customize treatment protocols according to unique facial anatomy and patients' cosmetic preferences. HA fillers are now the most widely used option because they are versatile and have a relatively low incidence of adverse effects. Their ability to restore lost volume, rebuild the face, and restore skin texture and hydration has made them extremely valuable in aesthetic medicine (Moon et al., 2021). The behavior of the different filler materials and their indications should thus be well known to practitioners for safety and effectiveness. The growing popularity of injectable treatments further highlights the importance of continuing education and training in aesthetic medicine practitioners, alongside a strong commitment to evidence-based practice. Since the field of aesthetics is dynamic, clearly procedural manipulations like injection maneuvers need to be balanced cautiously in combined treatments like dermal fillers alongside other modalities like BTs. Learning to master proper technique ensures not only the safety of the treatment but is a requirement for the achievement of harmonious outcomes. Anatomical knowledge of the face must be acquired, and it cannot be stressed enough that it will learn clinicians what complications can occur and how to avoid them. As treatment of such complexities becomes ever more the domain of clinicians, patients will increasingly demand better aesthetic outcome, and these in their turn will redefine the standards of beauty and of aging within populations. Strategic application and use of dermal fillers are thus at the center of modern aesthetic practice.

Definition of Dermal Fillers

Dermal fillers are injectable biocompatible substances that restore lost volume, soften the look of wrinkles, and rejuvenate the contours of the face. Composed primarily of hyaluronic acid, calcium hydroxylapatite (CaHA), and poly-L-lactic acid (PLLA), fillers vary in their physical and chemical makeups; hence, treatments are tailor-made according to what the client requires. The effect of the fillers is tissue volumization and the stimulation of collagen growth, which contributes to the youthful appearance. They are applied most commonly to the cheeks, lips, and nasolabial folds, with near-instant results and minimal downtime. Knowing the definition of dermal fillers is most important because it provides the foundation for learning their types, uses, and nuances of injection technique so that one can administer such beauty treatments to patients safely and effectively. The increasing popularity of dermal fillers points towards a wider cultural trend towards noninvasive cosmetic treatments. It not only reflects the need for facial rejuvenation but also enhances patients' self-confidence. Fillers have applications beyond the cosmetic advantage, including the enhancement of quality of life in survivors of cancer. It is possible that such patients can develop body image disturbances due to treatment side effects, thus providing an added therapeutic benefit to dermal filler use. Flexibility in filler injections, such as in the use of patients with a history of complicated medical illnesses, demonstrates their importance in multidisciplinary care for the restoration of appearance as well as emotional comfort. Hence, the implication of the term dermal fillers extends the cosmetic to encompass their therapeutic use in a broader paradigm of health (Proietti et al., 2021). Since patients need safety and efficacy from their cosmetic treatments, increased knowledge regarding dermal fillers assists in decision-making. Even the definition of dermal fillers may result in a more vigorous discussion on quality, longevity, and patient satisfaction among products. For instance, hyaluronic acid fillers benefit from having an immediate action with biocompatibility but are essentially different from other, longer-lasting options like polymethyl methacrylate fillers. Such a radical variation places greater importance on the choice of an adequate filler to satisfy a particular patient's needs and expectations. The practitioner must also possess skills in injection methods that provide the best aesthetic results with the best safety to the patient. With each new breakthrough in filler technology and its use, continuous education and ethical self-reflection regarding their use become essential so that dermal fillers are used wisely to achieve the desired outcome in patients (Figure 12.1).

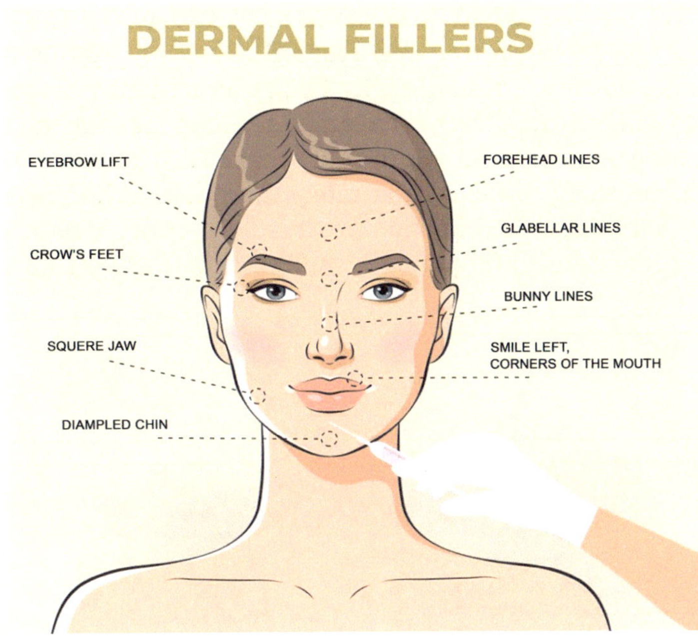

Figure 12.1. Dermal fillers.

Source: https://syraaesthetics.com/blog/wp-content/uploads/2023/11/Dermal-filler-Infographics-v2-1024x1024.jpg.

Historical Context and Evolution

The evolution of dermal fillers is observed to depict an intriguing trend based on advances in medical technology and rising societal concern about aesthetics. From initial attempts at facial enhancement as far back as the late 19th century, when paraffin wax was employed as an injected substance to address wrinkles and augment facial structures. Though these earlier treatments held more propensity for complications and unwanted side effects, their evolution set a goal for safer and more effective techniques. The tipping point came in the form of late 20th-century technology in hyaluronic acid fillers, which transformed the safety profile and outcome possible with dermal fillers. This shift represented a turning point in cosmetic dermatology history, opening the door for mass adoption and acceptance by both popular culture and the medical profession and enabling ongoing innovation and new applications. The ongoing evolution of dermal fillers has, at least in large part, been driven by the acceptance of minimally invasive techniques in dermatologic therapy, a reflection of overall changes in medicine toward minimizing risk to the patient and time off from activities. These minimally invasive dermatosurgical therapies, as discussed in recent critiques, have reshaped the treatment model of aesthetic medicine with recognition of patients' increasing demand for immediate gratification with minimal downtime. The evolution of various fillers, collagen fillers to biostimulants, is a testament to ongoing advancement in the practice, each to restore facial volume, improve skin texture, or to stimulate collagen. It is not a technological revolution per se; it is also a sign of changing cultural values embracing cosmetic alteration as the new norm and even desirable, broadening the scope of possibility in aesthetic medicine even further (Meghe et al., 2024). To this, the history and culture of dermal fillers is enhanced with clinical trials and studies that are continuously being done for the sake of enhancing the technique of injection and outcome. Conferences like the Italian Association of Plastic Aesthetic Surgery (AICPE) annual congress are part of the process of sharing new studies, reflecting product development progress and procedural technique advancements (Riggio, 2024). Practitioner-to-practitioner experience and knowledge sharing reinforce the direct correlation between maximizing technique and patient satisfaction, as well, putting distinct, customized solutions to each patient's needs foremost. Future developments will focus on safety, efficacy, and integrating new technologies such as biosensors and imaging technology that make the injection process even easier, demonstrating how the field is progressing for scientific interest and patient requirements (Figure 12.2).

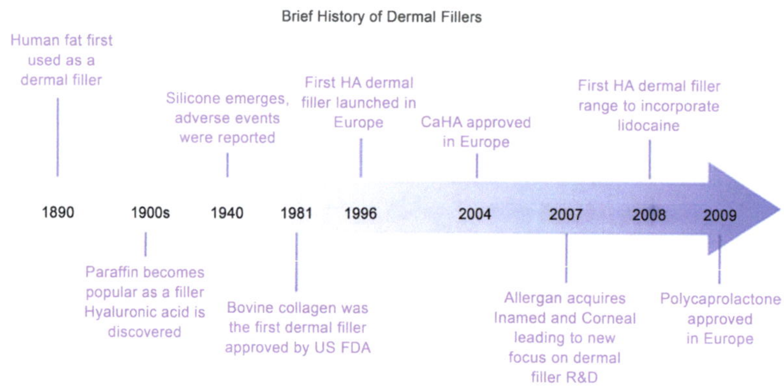

Figure 12.2. Brief history of dermal fillers.

Source: https://media.springernature.com/lw685/springer-static/image/chp%3A10.1007%2F978-3-662-55844-7_1/MediaObjects/272536_1_En_1_Figa_HTML.gif.

Importance of Understanding Dermal Fillers

It is necessary to know dermal fillers because they have become very popular in esthetic medicine, and therefore a similar need for safety as well as efficacy. With increasing market, the sophistication of the products and techniques also increases. Clinicians must be familiar with the various types of fillers, their indications, and also with the possible complications associated with their application. Most of the side effects are benign, although there are dangerous risks such as ischemic complications of accidental arterial injection, which are responsible for serious complications like skin necrosis or irreversible blindness (Ciesielska et al., 2025). Thus, sufficient knowledge of the various filler substances and the intricacies of their injection processes grants doctors the authority to handle these hazards appropriately. Technical and artistic skill in dermal filler injections necessitates anatomy and patient-specific information. Each patient possesses a unique anatomical space, and customized procedures are needed while developing treatment plans. For instance, the periorbital area is particularly challenging, necessitating acute caution and improved facial anatomy understanding to avoid complications (Ciesielska et al., 2025). Symmetry of the face, skin status, and patient expectation must be addressed by practitioners in order to create aesthetically pleasing results. Furthermore, specialized training in combination with the application of imaging modalities such as ultrasound can significantly reduce the risk of negative effects so that practitioners may control the complexity of the facial architecture and achieve maximum effect on each patient. The importance of dermal fillers extends beyond cosmetic purposes since the substances are required to enhance the quality of life in numerous cohorts of patients, including cancer patients. Alterations in body image experienced by patients during cancer therapy adversely affect their psychological well-being. The integration of aesthetic procedures such as dermal fillers with supportive therapy may be used to treat these conditions and thus result in improved quality of life and self-esteem. This necessitates an ethical responsibility to the practitioners to be cautious in the use of dermal fillers and employ them appropriately in a multidisciplinary regimen of patient management. With the explicit comprehension, practitioners are then capable of curing not only physical illnesses but also contributing a positive impact on the psychology of patients.

12.1. Types of Dermal Fillers

Learning Outcome

1. Define hyaluronic acid fillers
2. Explain the role of calcium hydroxylapatite fillers
3. Describe the biocompatibility and biodegradability of PLLA fillers

Of all the dermal fillers, HA fillers are likely to be the most popular and utilized. With their ability to replenish volume and hydration, HA fillers are perfectly suited to the body's tissues, and the skin looks at its best. Thanks to formulation advancements, such as the Vycross® range, their use has been further refined. Of particular note is the introduction of VYC-25L (Juvéderm Volux®), which has revolutionized facial contouring, and of special note to areas such as the chin and lower face third. Not only is the innovation paramount in aesthetic correction, but it would also converge treatment modalities, paving the way for practitioners to deliver maximum results (Segurado et al., 2021). These technologies make the selection of the most appropriate types of fillers based on the requirements of each patient necessary to achieve customized treatments that work. In addition to HA fillers, other fillers are available, such as calcium hydroxylapatite (CaHA) and poly-L-lactic acid (PLLA), each with specificity and clinical applications. CaHA has mineral-like substances that naturally exist in bones that restore volume immediately and induce collagen production in the long run. It is therefore extremely suitable for deeper folds of the face and cheek volumization. Further, PLLA is a biostimulatory filler that encourages the body to create collagen over time, with a very subtle and natural look that gets even better over months. These features allow clinicians to make treatment modifications based on various categories of patients, i.e., volumization or rejuvenation (Segurado et al., 2021). Understanding the differences between these mechanisms of action can play a very significant role in overall aesthetic outcomes and patient satisfaction. Safe administration of dermal fillers is also based on comprehensive knowledge of injection techniques. Incorrect administration leads to complications such as vascular occlusion or skin necrosis and hence demands practitioners who are experienced in advanced techniques. These include preinjection aspiration and imaging guidance that play a critical role in avoiding such side effects. Also, the periocular region, which is full of anatomical complexity, requires conservative technique and meticulous observation because complications here could lead to irreversible damage. The intersection of patient anatomy-specific, end-result-specific, and filler material-specific treatment strategies, therefore, serves to provide maximum safety and efficacy with dermal fillers. This integrative concept not only merges the effectiveness of the aesthetic procedures but also minimizes the risks of injection with fillers.

12.1.1. Hyaluronic Acid Fillers

Hyaluronic acid (HA) fillers form a popular tribe of dermal fillers and are well accepted due to their biocompatibility and cosmetic multifunctionality. HA is a naturally occurring polysaccharide component of connective tissues, which preserves water content and structure needed to maintain the look of young-looking skin. Since HA fillers can attract water molecules, they provide the skin with moisture and volume, and therefore, there is a noticeable reduction in wrinkles and fine lines. In clinical practice, injection technique is not standardized and practitioners use different techniques based on various facial areas, i.e., lips, cheeks, and nasolabial folds. This versatility range not only facilitates personalized treatments according to the patient's requirement but also guarantees the growing popularity of HA fillers as a surgical alternative. Hyaluronic acid fillers' applications are not limited to just cosmetic enhancements but are employed to treat various medical conditions as well. For example, HA fillers have been successfully employed in nonsurgical rhinoplasty as a fully acceptable alternative for patients ready to fix postoperative deformities or enhance the nasal appearance without the risk of revision surgery. There ought to be a thorough understanding of the surgical anatomy and probable deformities for physicians applying HA fillers in such sensitive areas, as highlighted in recent literature. Their non-invasive nature also adds to higher patient satisfaction and an acceptable level of complications, typically 7% in the event of post-rhinoplasty application (Valente et al., 2018). That is an aspect that is reflective of the significance of HA fillers as a highly sought procedure for aesthetic and functional applications in the majority of clinical settings. Injection techniques of hyaluronic acid fillers are critical to the success of aesthetic procedures and underscore the importance of practitioner skill. Various techniques, such as linear threading, serial puncture, and retrograde techniques, are employed based on the region of treatment and desired result. Choice of technique also has implications for long-term filler stability in tissue because proper positioning can enhance tissue integration and reduce potential complications. In addition, filler development, including cross-linking technology, improved the long-term and shelf-life effectiveness of HA fillers to render them more suitable for use in many indications. With new techniques and media, there is a need for regular training and education of practitioners to ensure efficacy and safety, thereby addressing the growing demand for non-surgical aesthetic treatments (Makvandi et al., 2021) (Figure 12.3).

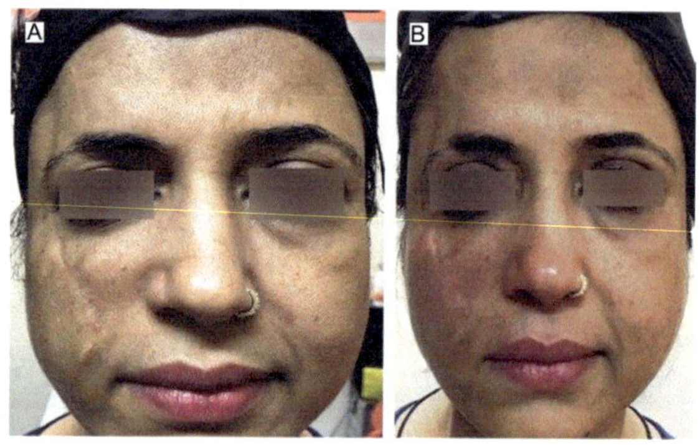

Figure 12.3. (A) Patient before scar correction with hyaluronic acid fillers; and (B) Patient after 2 mL of hyaluronic acid filler.

Source: https://www.researchgate.net/publication/318902798/figure/fig1/AS:11431281256167995@1719511170988/A-Patient-before-scar-correction-with-hyaluronic-acid-fillers-B-Patient-after-2-mL.jpg.

12.1.2. Calcium Hydroxylapatite Fillers

CaHA fillers are a paradigm shift in the use of dermal fillers, approved by the authorities for the treatment of medium to deep wrinkles and loss on the face. As CaHA fillers consist mostly of calcium and phosphate, they possess a biocompatible formula that not only supports replacement of lost volume but also induces natural collagen stimulation in the long run.

These two features render them of most value to those patients needing a permanent, aesthetically satisfying change without surgery. Clinically, CaHA has been noted to also improve laxity of the skin, with a more generalized application than just volume replacement. The ability to address shallower and deeper skin concerns in one session adds to the multi-faceted function of CaHA fillers in aesthetic dermatology, transforming the facial non-surgical rejuvenation paradigm (Goldie et al., 2018). The injection technique used with CaHA fillers is critical to obtaining maximum benefit and avoiding complications. Extremely skilled practitioners prefer the precise use as per the specific anatomical areas treated, which can continue to benefit the cosmetic result immensely. Injection of the mid-face with CaHA, for instance, can yield excellent cheek volume augmentation, whereas hyperdiluted CaHA methods have been determined to enhance skin texture and laxity on the neck and décolletage. Side effects, though comparatively rare, can be bruising, swelling, and induration, particularly in thinner, darker skin (Goldie et al., 2018). It is thus crucial that aesthetic practitioners abide by best practice guidelines to ensure safe and acceptable results for patients. Ongoing advancements in injection practice reflect the ambition to optimize the full potential of these fillers in clinical use. Also, the application of CaHA fillers in treatment is not merely for general use but involves special applications, like in nonsurgical rhinoplasty. Since the procedure is gaining popularity, CaHA has been utilized to correct deformity after rhinoplasty or augment nasal shape without the necessity for further surgical intervention. Retrospective results verify that application of CaHA fillers after surgery has yielded good outcomes, reducing the necessity of extensive revision and maintaining a natural appearance. This adaptability verifies that CaHA fillers offer not only a solution to facial volume loss in aging but also have an inherent place in surgical deformity correction. With the current advancements in aesthetic procedures, more studies of CaHAs properties will certainly be utilized in newer techniques to continue solidifying its position in numerous procedures, as a valuable tool within the cosmetic dermatologist's arsenal (Figure 12.4).

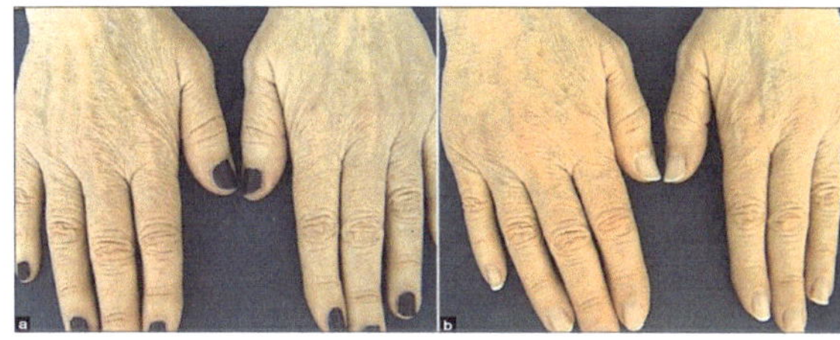

Figure 12.4. Injection with calcium hydroxylapatite (1.5 mL) and prilocaine (0.3 mL) in each hand: A 65-year-old female patient (a) before treatment; and (b) 6 months after treatment.

Source: https://www.researchgate.net/publication/232742253/figure/fig5/AS:203003865899031@1425411301769/Injection-with-calcium-hydroxylapatite-15-mL-and-prilocaine-03-mL-in-each-hand-A.png.

12.1.3. Poly-L-Lactic Acid Fillers

PLLA fillers are the newer generation of dermal fillers that are biocompatible and biodegradable. It is now a key part of cosmetic medicine. Although older hyaluronic acid fillers have been formulated to restore volume immediately, PLLA stimulates the body's natural collagen production over a period of time. This novel mechanism of action is optimally in line with the novel trend toward long-duration and natural results in aesthetic treatments. PLLA fillers are ideally suited to correct volume loss associated with aging, such as in the cheek and temple, for contour refashioning of the youthful shape at the cost of permanent fillers (Ciesielska et al., 2025). The temporary but lasting volumization is based on the education of the patient since patients will ask for subtle modifications in order to avoid the overfilled look of more conventional treatments. One of the better aspects of PLLA fillers is that their effects are long lasting, typically two years, through the natural process of collagen remodeling. Nonetheless, the mode of injection is essential to attain complete benefits, and practitioners need sufficient knowledge of facial anatomy and aesthetics to achieve it right.

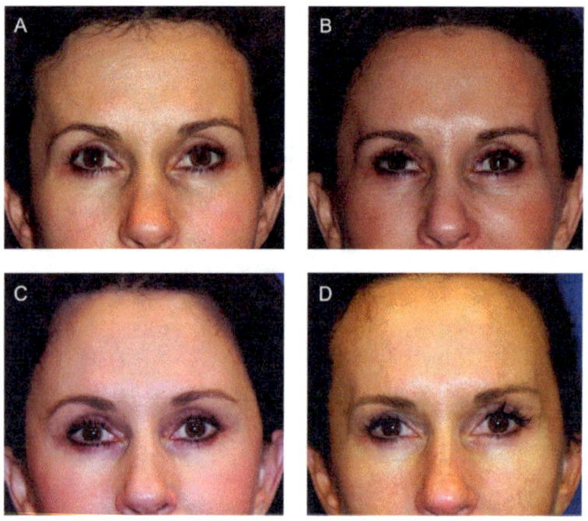

Figure 12.5. Poly-l-lactic acid (PLLA) can effectively restore temporal volume loss with stable improvement. (A) A 45-year-old female patient is shown preoperatively; (B) The patient is shown 2 years after high superficial musculoaponeurotic system (SMAS) facelift and fat injections with temporal hollowing; (C) The patient is shown 4 years after facelift with fat injections and 2 years after PLLA injections in 2 sessions with 1 vial/session concentrated on temporal hollowing; and (D) The patient is shown 7 years after facelift and fat injections and 5 years after PLLA injections.

Source: https://www.researchgate.net/publication/359016337/figure/fig4/AS:11431281097179667@1668488568255/Poly-l-lactic-acid-PLLA-can-effectively-restore-temporal-volume-loss-with-stable.png.

As PLLA takes several sessions of injections to add volume incrementally, customized treatment is necessary. Such treatments enable the specific facial anatomy and desired outcome by the patient, which poses the significance of customized treatment in aesthetic surgery (Burgess, 2006). Apart from that, the aggregate consequence of PLLA augmentation makes it feasible to change treatment options throughout one's life, thus optimizing satisfaction and ongoing confidence in the practitioner's skill. There are serious issues of concern, however, relating to side effects and complications despite the fact that numerous advantages accompany PLLA fillers.

Although most side effects are temporary and self-limiting, practitioners should exercise caution in the event of severe complications such as granuloma formation, which can be managed by surgery (Ciesielska et al., 2025). Therefore, knowledge of potential risks is critical for practitioners to prevent complications with meticulous injection technique as well as patient selection. Since the patient population that requires cosmetic treatment is dynamic, increased demand for products that have the function to beautify and extend supports ongoing usage of PLLA fillers in current aesthetic medicine. In combination with adequate injection technique and cautious patient selection, overall treatment success and patient satisfaction in the fast-evolving field of dermal fillers can be enhanced (Burgess, 2006) (Figure 12.5).

Test Your Knowledge

1. What are Hyaluronic Acid Fillers and how do they work in the skin?
2. What are the primary differences between hyaluronic acid fillers and CaHA fillers in terms of texture and use cases?
3. How long do hyaluronic acid fillers and CaHA fillers last, and what factors can influence their longevity?

12.2. Indications for Use

Learning Outcome

1. Discuss facial volume restoration
2. Understand wrinkle reduction by the use of dermal fillers
3. Focus on lip enhancement

Indications of dermal filler injection include several cosmetic and clinical applications that vary from facial aging to functional rehabilitation. The most important applications are the replacement of lost volume, relaxation of wrinkles, and the enhancement of facial contours, which all play a role towards younger-looking skin. Above all, fillers hold different materials that could be hyaluronic acid and calcium hydroxyapatite, polymethyl methacrylate, and each one of them treats very specific issues on the skin, like nasolabial folds, marionette lines, and cheek volume loss. Each of them has very unique properties to achieve a specific cosmetic outcome, so a suitable filler choice must be determined based on the individual patient's need and anatomy. This selection is important because it influences both the visual results and the possibility of side effects that can be sensed when using these products (Medeiros, 2013). Outside of aesthetic use, dermal fillers are also important in clinical and functional restorations. Diseases such as facial lipoatrophy, which are common in HIV patients, are significantly improved by fillers' ability to volumize, not just improving appearance but confidence as well. Fillers are used in reconstructive surgery, for example, the reconstruction of post-traumatic face or the correction of congenital deformities. The uses of fillers in these situations demonstrate their versatility of use beyond beauty; they give patients an improved quality of life by curing various physical conditions. Additionally, advancements in the technology of injection have allowed professionals to inject such products with greater precision and fewer complications so that the desired aim is achieved as per the expectation of the patient and safety (Medeiros, 2013). The efficiency and safety of dermal fillers depend mainly on the injection techniques used for treatment. The ideal injection achieves the desired effect with a minimum of unwanted effects, by placing the filler in the right plane of tissue. The provider should know the anatomy of the face and volume measurement for a natural outcome. In addition, knowledge of the potential complications and being prepared for such side effects also facilitates the proper use of fillers. This not only gives a better aesthetic outcome but also fosters patient confidence and satisfaction through the process of informed consent and management of realistic expectations. Advances in minimally invasive techniques contribute to the continued education and professional development of the practitioner to ensure safe use of dermal fillers to maintain patient satisfaction and safety (Medeiros, 2013).

12.2.1. Facial Volume Restoration

Aesthetic medicine now also includes restoration of facial volume, especially with the advent of improved dermal fillers. Age-induced diminution of HA and collagen leads to loss of facial volume and sagging of the skin, along with protrusion of wrinkles. A reversal of this change is brought about by the use of HA-based fillers, an appropriate method for filling volume and rejuvenating the face. For example, the release of VYC-25L (Juvéderm Volux®) has made it possible to have procedures that are uniquely applied for remodeling of the lower third of the face and chin (Segurado et al., 2021). In addition to volume replacement, this filler makes subtle contouring possible, which is essential in achieving aesthetically enhanced outcomes. Information on the properties of these fillers is crucial to ensure ideal patient benefit and compliance with best practices in clinical usage. The choice of the dermal filler and the technique of injection applied are very important to reach ideal natural results of facial volume replacement. Each of the fillers has unique characteristics based on its cross-linking technology, viscosity, and elasticity, which ultimately shape its performance and longevity in the tissue (Catalano et al., 2016). For example, fillers like Aliaxin® have certain formulations that can provide full restoration of facial features with differential lifting and hydration levels. Their biochemist characteristics, such as water adsorption and rheologic behavior, lend support to a customized treatment protocol, achieving optimized results in varied patient populations.

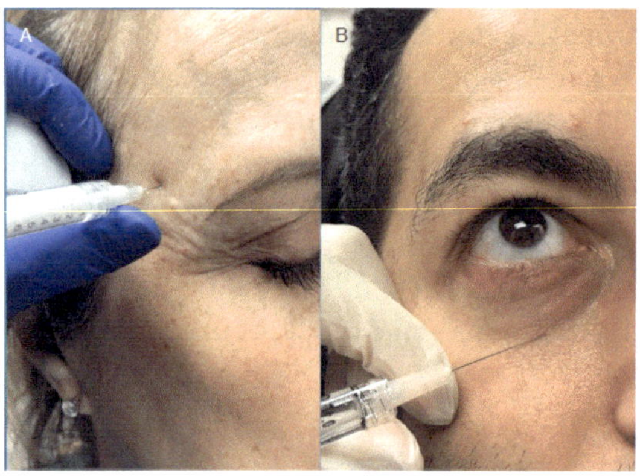

Figure 12.6. Volume restoration with dermal fillers. Common periocular treatment areas include the temple (A); and tear trough (B).

Source: https://www.researchgate.net/publication/328465061/figure/fig4/AS:1159224885293075@1653392158662/Volume-restoration-with-dermal-fillers-Common-periocular-treatment-areas-include-the.jpg.

Practitioners are urged to consider the patient's skin type, end result desired, and aesthetic goal when selecting the appropriate filler and modality. By considering these elements in a smart approach, practitioners can achieve maximum treatment efficacy, resulting in higher patient satisfaction and safety. In addition, the advent of minimally invasive methods has transformed the field of facial volume replacement. Putting patient comfort at the top, most practitioners have embraced comfort- and safety-based techniques. Improved injection methods, from old-school to newer ones such as microcannulas, have minimized downtime and dermal filler-related complications (Segurado et al., 2021). These technologies are not only enhancing outcomes for patients but also extending the shelf life of results. The more clinicians become familiar with these technologies, the more they will be able to shape treatment plans for the numerous disparate needs of their patients. Last but by no means least, proper filler choice, injection technique, and knowledge of facial anatomy come together to emphasize the role of facial volume repletion in the big picture of aesthetic treatments (Figure 12.6).

12.2.2. Wrinkle Reduction

Increased use of cosmetic procedures for the purposes of anti-wrinkling has encouraged tremendous progress in the field of dermal fillers. The substances that are injected to provide volume and smoothness to the skin surface have been used almost exclusively to treat areas of wrinkled skin on the forehead, nasolabial folds, and crow's feet. Various fillers, including hyaluronic acid and collagen stimulators, are applied to serve a particular function based on the ingredients and purpose they are designed to achieve. For example, hyaluronic acid fillers give immediate results with natural consequences, and thus are in great demand by patients who desire instant and minimally invasive procedures. Knowledge of the different fillers on the market is pivotal for physicians wishing to get the most effective result of wrinkle diminishment with patient satisfaction and safety. Furthermore, the mode of administration by injection when administering dermal fillers has a great impact on the outcomes of wrinkle reduction treatments. Precise usage is needed not only to deliver efficacy but also to limit complications. There are techniques ranging from bolus injection to more sophisticated methods such as the linear retrograde technique, which has more control in filling in the filler. Providers should be familiar with facial anatomical structures in order to avoid complications such as vascular occlusion or nodules. In addition, the application of novel techniques, such as the use of microcannulas that reduce cutaneous trauma, has enhanced the safety profile of the procedures. Continuing education about injection techniques is necessary to maintain optimal levels of clinical quality and aesthetic results. Of the newer generation of dermal fillers, polycaprolactone (PCL)-based materials are emerging as potential options for long-term correction of wrinkles.

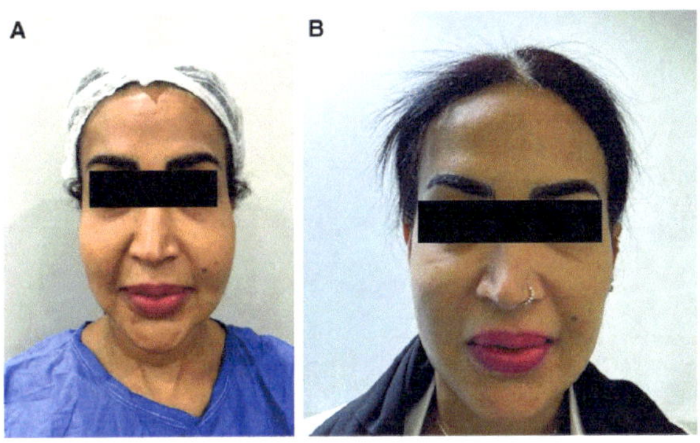

Figure 12.7. A 46-year-old female patient with permanent filler in the cheeks and malar area operated upon by face lift and permanent filler excision. (A) Preoperative view. Note the size of the cheeks preoperatively; and (B) Postoperative photograph with the size of the cheeks reduced after material removal.

Source: https://www.researchgate.net/publication/362199929/figure/fig3/AS:1180834119856143@1658544201461/a-46-year-old-female-patient-with-permanent-filler-in-the-checks-and-malar-area-operated.png.

PCL is a biocompatible, biodegradable polymer with superior mechanical characteristics that makes it a very good candidate to be employed in aesthetics. It is also a collagen stimulator, providing long-term volumization benefits when paired with immediate benefits, thereby providing instant gratification as well as maintenance of long-term skin health. With a new composition that stimulates collagen formation, fillers like these do not just superficially correct wrinkles but also tighten and improve skin texture in the long term. The evolution of the dermal filler context requires research and technique advancement to always provide safe and effective treatments for wrinkle reduction to clients (Marie-Christen et al., 2020; Makvandi et al., 2021) (Figure 12.7).

12.2.3. Lip Enhancement

The pursuit of fuller lips has evolved into a current high-growth trend that mirrors wider social trends in the pursuit of enhanced aesthetics. Lip augmentation-most commonly done by injection of dermal fillers-may help fulfill the desire to achieve a fuller-looking appearance of the lip and compensate for slight asymmetry or loss in volume due to the consequences of aging. Different materials are used in lip fillers, and among the most popular is HA because of its water-holding capacity and biocompatibility. As mentioned, there are many different therapeutic modalities available for cosmetic lip augmentation, ranging from temporary injectable fillers to surgery, such that there is some level of tailoring depending on patient desire and preference as well as outcome desired (Reddy et al., 2012). Thus, greater access to such choices is an indicator of a shift in the value accorded to facial appearances by individuals, and lip augmentation is both a standard of beauty and a form of self-expression. Injectable fillers, particularly hyaluronic acid-based fillers, have been discovered to be successful in providing naturally occurring outcomes with lip augmentation. These fillers achieve this by the deposition of volume and definition to the lips, thereby enhancing the shape and form of the lips as well as hydrating.

The flexibility of HA fillers also enables practitioners to customize the treatment based on the anatomical features of each patient, thereby optimizing aesthetic results. They are also appealing as their treatment is less invasive, and they do not usually have much downtime and immediate results. Findings of the study highlighted favorable effects of HA fillers in varied situations, such as treatments for aesthetic augmentation of the lip, showing high patient satisfaction (Cortese et al., 2021). The above finding reflects growing mainstream beauty treatments as dermal fillers, to restore lip volume and balance. Despite the benefits of lip enhancement with dermal fillers, side effects and complications must be taken into consideration. Complications occurring at a rate of inclusion include bruising and swelling at the injection site, which are typically transient in nature and resolve within a few days. Severe but rare complications have led to lifelong aesthetic morbidity in some patients, thereby requiring attention from an experienced injector and education of the patient to prevent such risks. With expertise in injection technique and patient choice, however, the safety record of such aesthetic procedures also increases. On top of this, as development remains to occur in filler technology and injection methods, the business is likely to see further enhancements in patient outcomes and satisfaction levels. The attraction of lip augmentation, therefore, is not only to get the desired physical outcomes but also safety and effectiveness in achieving such outcomes (Reddy et al., 2012) (Figure 12.8).

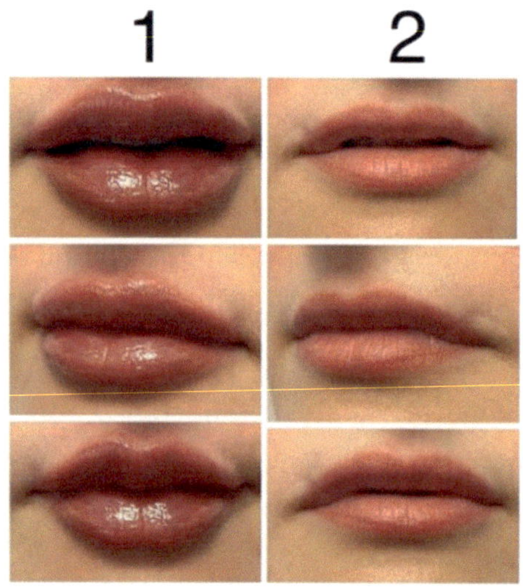

Figure 12.8. Dermal filler application to the lip: (1). Three months after the filler; and (2). Before the filler application, B filler application to the nasolabial fold.

Source: https://www.researchgate.net/publication/390920895/figure/fig2/AS:11431281385579088@1745027450614/Dermal-filler-A-Filler-application-to-the-Lip-1-Three-months-after-the-filler-2.jpg.

Test Your Knowledge

1. How do dermal fillers restore facial volume?
2. What is the mechanism by which dermal fillers reduce wrinkles?
3. What are the key factors to consider when using dermal fillers for lip enhancement, and what outcomes can patients expect?

12.3. Benefits of Dermal Fillers

Learning Outcome

1. Talk about the instantaneous outcome of dermal filler treatment
2. Discuss how dermal filler treatment is defined as a minimally invasive procedure
3. Understand the versatility in treatment areas

Dermal fillers provide a myriad of advantages that have rendered them a mainstay of aesthetic medicine. At the forefront of these benefits is their capacity for the restoration of volume loss related to aging, a process that compromises the structural integrity of the skin. Natural fat, collagen, and elastin within the skin decrease as people grow old, causing sagging and wrinkle formation. Dermal fillers like HA not only provide volume to the skin but also help improve hydration, resulting in a more youthful appearance. That fillers have the ability to correct facial areas, from the lip to nasolabial folds, makes practitioners able to accommodate patients' individualized needs. This versatility provides fillers with the opportunity to be incorporated into a total facial rejuvenation protocol, perhaps with other treatments such as BT, thereby achieving maximum aesthetic benefit and an enhanced harmonious facial appearance (Makvandi et al., 2021). In addition to their action of filling out, dermal fillers also contribute towards smoother skin texture and contour, further enhancing facial beauty. These products fill in bare areas and diffuse thin lines, making them look brighter and fresher. This can be seen in the use of fillers to make the lips look better or defining the jaw line, where it can drastically reshape through a mastery of precision and skill. Meanwhile, fillers stimulate collagen to grow over time and their effects lead to sustained improvement of skin elasticity and tightness. This natural response speaks to their effectiveness as not merely a temporary solution, but as an investment in skin treatment in the long term. Practitioners are now realizing that combined use of fillers and bioabsorbable suspension threads, particularly to correct not only volume but laxity of facial tissue as well, can be a breathtaking improvement in facial rejuvenation (Moon et al., 2021). Convenience and lack of invasiveness are important benefits that clearly resonate with the present patient's need for fast and effective cosmetic procedures. In contrast to the traditional surgery option, recovery time for dermal filler injections is minimal or zero and patients can get on with their regular activities in the twinkling of an eye. This will be most appealing for those who seek subtle but observable alterations with no commitment and downtime of such more invasive approaches. The fact that dermal fillers allow patients to achieve perceivable results with minimum treatment sessions stands as supportive for enhanced patient satisfaction rates and also repeat treatment inclination. Improved injection techniques, for example, micro-cannula technology, have seen improvement in safety profiles and reduced complications, hence being a reasonable choice for those who want to attain complete aesthetic results without much risk (Makvandi et al., 2021) (Figure 12.9).

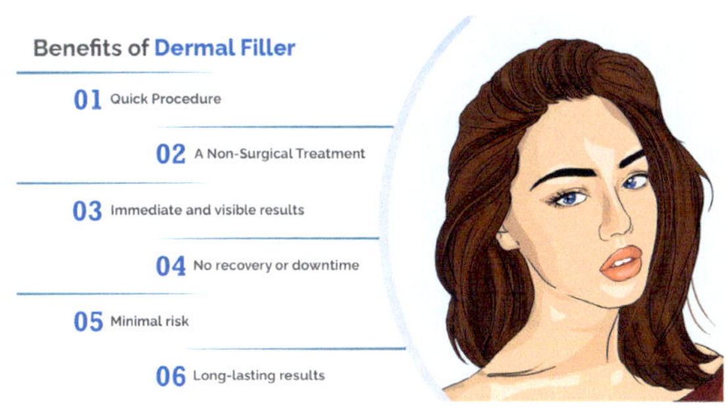

Figure 12.9. Benefits of dermal fillers.

Source: https://www.cosmedocs.com/wp-content/uploads/2021/07/benefits-of-fillers.jpg.

12.3.1. Immediate Results

The popularity of dermal fillers is basically attributed to their rapid effect, which enables patients to notice the difference within mere minutes after a procedure. Most commonly employed in the restoration of volume at places such as cheeks, lips, and nasolabial folds, fillers can completely alter the facial appearance as well as even out defects once injected. Rapid turnaround is the first choice of most patients, who see it as a readily available option compared to other more intrusive procedures requiring weeks or months of recuperation time. Use of hyaluronic acid fillers in particular, has become more popular due to the fact that they have immediate results combined with the ability to touch up as needed. As hinted in the recent studies, the real-time efficacy of the fillers provides them as a commonly acceptable solution for individuals needing instant cosmetic improvement for better confidence and satisfaction in a productive time period (Ciesielska et al., 2025). Clearly visible in lip filling, the activity is exceptionally prominent, as fillers can instantly change the lips' size and shape within a few minutes. With different ingredients present in varying combinations, treatments may be designed to suit individual taste, with a more voluminous set of lips representing the new definition of beauty. Results not only offer instant satisfaction to oneself but also act as a canvas for further aesthetic improvements. The reported success of such procedures underscores the need to use correct filler agents and methods that deliver maximal results upon administration. Most patients are interested in such cosmetic procedures because they want not just temporary results but also to undergo drastic changes without surgery downtime (Reddy et al., 2012). Additionally, advances in injection methods have played a pivotal role in providing instant and satisfactory outcomes with less risk of complications. For instance, the use of micro-cannulas instead of regular needles allows for precise filler placement with reduced bruising and swelling risks. The technologies enhance the patient experience through immediate cosmetic enhancement while offering reduced risk. To ensure outcomes integrity, practitioners are encouraged to adhere to the standards in place, for instance, proper product and injection methods. With safety of the patient and patient-specific treatment plans at the forefront, aesthetic practitioners can now deliver genuine exceptional results, meeting the promise of instant effects, thus solidifying the position of dermal fillers in contemporary cosmetic treatments (Ciesielska et al., 2025) (Figure 12.10).

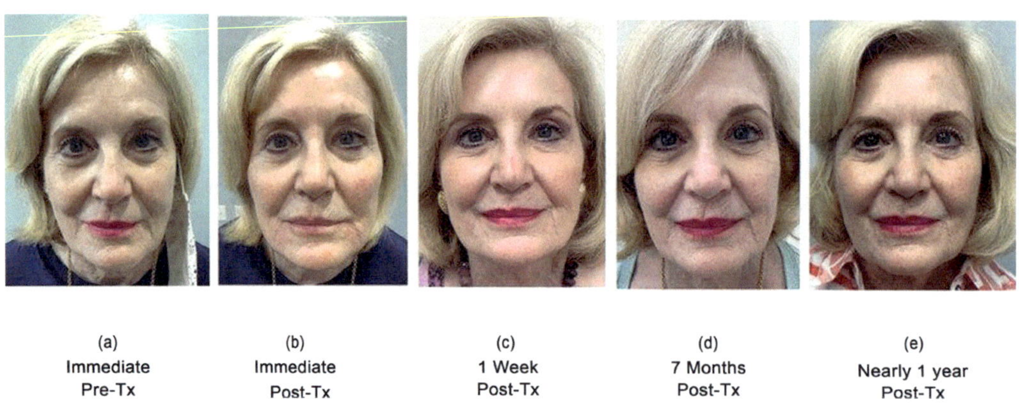

Figure 12.10. (A) Immediately before the procedure; (B) Immediately after the procedure; (C) One week after the procedure; (D) Seven months after the procedure; and (E) Nearly one year after the procedure.

Source: https://www.researchgate.net/publication/354884566/figure/fig1/AS:1112547763728404@1642263465887/A-Immediately-prior-to-the-procedure-B-Immediately-after-the-procedure-C-One-week.jpg.

12.3.2. Minimally Invasive Procedure

Over time, minimally invasive treatments of aesthetic medicine have completely revolutionized patient expectations from cosmetic procedures. Non-surgical dermal fillers revise imperfections such as loss of facial contour, defect of shape, and asymmetry. This is quite different from what conventional surgical procedures achieve because they tend to have long recoveries and enormous risks, while minimally invasive treatment and recovery are brief. Indeed, formulation innovations, i.e., the creation of hyaluronic acid fillers like VYC-25L, introduce safety and versatility to the practitioner in trying to optimize outcomes in patients. With increased familiarity with more sophisticated products, practitioners are now able to standardize injection methods and personalize treatments for unique patient profiles, thus achieving reproducible and fulfilling results in facial aesthetics (Segurado et al., 2021). In addition to this, age is also the critical benchmark for determining the appropriateness and effectiveness of minimally invasive treatments. For example, young adults in their early twenties will opt for facial shaping rather than fixing asymmetry when they are entering aesthetic medicine for the first time (Wollina & Goldman, , 2011). In such a situation, attention to inquired nuances of subtlety is the last worry over transformative makeovers, adopting a preventative approach to beauty. Awareness of the specific objectives of young patients not only influences the selection of filler material but also the technique of injection. The practitioners must be competent to modify their practice to accommodate varying anatomical frameworks and patient tolerance. Familiarity with age-related incentives can aid in informed decision-making to ensure treatment remains safe and efficacious. Other than age, the ethics of undergoing minimally invasive procedures bring into stark relief the subtleties of aesthetic medicine. While the procedures can go a long way to improve one's sense of self-esteem and satisfaction with how one looks, they do bear implications about the societal expectations and pressures to fit one into accepted models of beauty. With advancements in the specialty, practitioners need to ensure that they provide an environment conducive to well-informed decision-making and realistic anticipation of treatment outcomes of treatments such as dermal fillers. The integration of proper patient assessment, such as stress laid on the use of VYC-25L in the consensus guidelines, assists in the provision of safety as well as efficacy. Lastly, maintaining ethical practices with a transition towards higher demand for less invasive treatments is of the utmost importance to long-term reputation in aesthetic medicine (Segurado et al., 2021).

12.3.3. Versatility in Treatment Areas

The diversity of dermal fillers is inherently expressed through the numerous fields of treatment, and therefore, the fillers are inevitable components of aesthetic medicine. Comprised mostly of HA, the fillers not only serve volume replenishment but also facial contour enhancement and facial skin texture irregularity correction. The diversity of the fillers makes them applicable in numerous facial areas, including cheeks, lips, nasolabial folds, and under-eye areas. Because of the possibility of tailoring injectables to meet every patient's specific requirement, fillers can easily fill the gaps between on-the-rise aesthetic demands and unique anatomical variations. Such a level of customization in use demonstrates the utmost importance of practitioner skill and facial anatomical understanding in providing the best results. The ability of HA fillers to effectively volumize some areas makes them a mainstay in non-surgical aesthetic procedures, solidifying further their position within current aesthetic treatments. Their pairing with other modalities, such as BT and bioabsorbable threads, places into limelight their synergistic effect and enhances the scope for use. This multidisciplinary strategy is imperative in the treatment of complex facial aging patterns, wherein a combination of multiple techniques must be used to achieve the best results. The common consensus among medical professionals is that only by combining multiple treatment modalities is it possible to adequately address all dimensions of facial aging. A systematic combination therapy of suspension threads, neuromodulators, and dermal fillers can create more striking and longer-lasting effects in patients. Most importantly, this combined technique is used to treat various indices of aging, such as volume loss and dynamic wrinkles depending on the age of the patient and his ethnic group, which depicts the need for a complete assessment and a customized treatment plan to attain harmonious results (Jacob et al., 2021; Moon et al., 2021). In addition, the application of dermal fillers is not limited only to facial attractiveness, with future applications extending beyond dermatologic therapies in other domains, including hand rejuvenation and scar therapy. Since technology and practitioner skills keep advancing, prospective application of dermal fillers can be expansive. In hand rejuvenation, fillers re-volumize to address the natural consequences of aging that strike the skin's plumpness and elasticity. Similarly, fillers help to cover up atrophic scars, improving the overall texture and appearance of the skin. These new applications readily illustrate the vast range of dermal fillers and how they are able to handle more of an array of aesthetic concerns. Thus, with the emergence of newer techniques and formulations, the horizon of treatable possibilities widens, reaffirming the place of dermal fillers at the fore in aesthetic treatments (Jacob et al., 2021; Moon et al., 2021).

Test Your Knowledge

1. How do dermal fillers provide immediate results, and how quickly can patients see visible improvements after the procedure?
2. What are the key advantages of dermal fillers being a minimally invasive procedure compared to more invasive treatments like surgery?

12.4. Risks and Side Effects

Learning Outcome

1. Describe common side effects
2. Explain rare but serious complications
3. Understand the importance of choosing a qualified practitioner

Use of dermal fillers, while mostly safe and effective for esthetic use, is not without risk and complications. Swelling, bruising, and redness at the site of injection have been most commonly encountered, typically resolving within a few days. More severe complications can arise, however, in the form of infection or development of granulomas—hard nodules that occur as a result of immune reactions to the filler material. These complications demand meticulous medical history and assessment prior to the treatment for the selection of suitable candidates. For instance, individuals with a history of severe allergies or specific medical conditions may be at higher risk during these treatments, indicating the importance of individualized treatment planning in evolved aesthetic clinics (Wollina & Goldman, , 2011). Beyond the obvious side effects, there are also long-term risks of dermal fillers that must be considered by practitioners and patients alike.

Vascular occlusion, where filler inadvertently enters a blood vessel, can result in tissue necrosis or even blindness if it is injected close to the region of the eyes. Technique and skill of the injector are the factors that are most critical in minimizing the risk of these; thus, selecting an experienced practitioner is most critical. Furthermore, understanding the specific properties and longevity of the filler chosen can provide for realistic patient expectations of both aesthetic outcome and possibility of side effects (Barnes et al., 2016). With the ever-evolving facial aesthetics environment constantly bringing forth new products and technologies, there is thus a constant need for ongoing education and vigilance by providers concerning safety protocols and the emergence of risks. Psychological impacts of experiencing side effects, even if they are small or extreme, should not be overlooked. The pressure to physical idealization may lead to negative self-esteem and unreasonably high expectations, particularly in younger patients who are increasingly seeking these treatments. Ethical issues regarding motivations for dermal fillers are also compounded by the huge boom in social media use, which can exacerbate body image disturbances. The control of such issues requires a combined effort through pre-procedure counseling and open discussion on the probability of side effects. Cosmetic practitioners are therefore confronted with such challenges in ensuring patient well-being and informed consent, whereby people are informed not only of the benefits of dermal fillers but also of the risks and implications involved (Wollina & Goldman, , 2011).

12.4.1. Common Side Effects

Use of dermal fillers, as increasingly popular as they are for their lack of surgery, comes with no strings attached. The most common side effects reported are localized temporary swelling, bruising, and redness at the site of injection. These symptoms resolve spontaneously within a week or a few days and thus seem most side effects to be fairly mild. However, one of the primary factors in the explanation of such overall reactions includes the injectors' technique and the nature of the filler. For instance, reactions to hyaluronic acid fillers tend to be less severe than to permanent fillers. Patients asking for fillers in delicate areas, such as the periocular region, are more at risk of complications and need to be counseled concerning potential outcomes before the treatment, with emphasis on informed consent and adequate planning (Ciesielska et al., 2025). In addition to the usual mild side effects, there are more serious complications that can occur, although less likely. Included among these are the risk of ischemic complications resulting from intra-arterial injection by mistake, for example, necrosis of the skin or loss of sight. These are disastrous outcomes that rely on proper understanding of facial anatomy and precise injection techniques. Precautionary methods have been highlighted in terms of aspirating prior to injecting and employing small, incremental volumes as a method of significantly minimizing such risks. Also, pre-treatment with imaging techniques has been proposed to decrease the incidence of serious complications. Therefore, while common side effects are primarily mild, practitioners should be prudent about the likelihood of more serious adverse results (Öztürk, 2021). Lastly, it is critical that practitioners and patients set proper expectations of dermal fillers. An informed approach can also reduce the psychological impact of first-time side effects. For instance, bruising or swelling may be problematic for patients who were not anticipating these reactions. Instructing patients regarding the typical healing time and that these effects are expected can make them more satisfied and less stressed post-procedure. Further, knowledge of the role of personal anatomy and underlying health conditions is fundamental in customizing treatment regimens and minimizing side effects. By means of open dialogue and adherence to best standards, medical practitioners can ensure that the cosmetic benefits of dermal fillers outweigh the risks involved in their application (Ciesielska et al., 2025) (Figure 12.11).

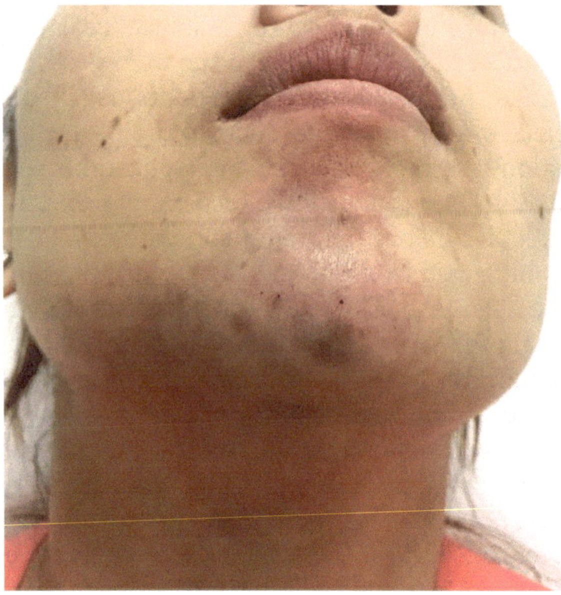

Figure 12.11. Postinjection picture taken 15 minutes after filler injection in the chin. Skin discoloration and demarcation of the ischemic area visible in the chin and neck.

Source: https://www.researchgate.net/publication/325388998/figure/fig1/AS:639994658029568@1529598025327/postinjection-picture-taken-15-minutes-after-filler-injection-in-the-chin-skin.png.

12.4.2. Rare But Serious Complications

The increasing popularity of dermal fillers has undoubtedly transformed aesthetic treatments, enabling practitioners to restore facial volume and shape with greater control. But the increasing popularity of dermal fillers has also highlighted the onset of rare but serious complications of such treatments. Ischemic complications are one such very demanding risk that arises as a result of unwanted intra-arterial injection of fillers. These conditions can lead to severe complications, including skin necrosis or total loss of sight, making it critical for practitioners to exercise careful technique and anatomical understanding in the process. As a precaution for potential occurrence of the above side effects, aesthetic medicine practitioners must invest in preventive care to avoid such occurrences as much as possible, for instance, aspirating before injecting and employing imaging techniques where necessary (Ciesielska et al., 2025). Such precautions, while seemingly cautious, can contribute significantly to procedural outcomes and patient safety. In addition to ischemic complications, inflammatory reactions are also a source of additional risk in the domain of dermal fillers. While most filler-related side effects are minor and self-limited, some patients experience prominent inflammatory reactions. A study of hyaluronic acid injection laryngoplasty revealed that 1.9% of patients experienced complications, primarily inflammatory reactions presenting as dysphonia or dyspnea following treatment (Öztürk, 2021). In such cases, systemic steroid and antibiotic administration was often required, illustrating the necessity for the identification and management of potential complications effectively. Results are such that while hyaluronic acid is largely harmless in application, it carries the risk of profound inflammatory reactions that necessitate proper patient screening and sound judgment in selection and technique. Maturity of informed consent, in which patients are informed about common and rare side effects, is still central to ethical practice. Lastly, treatment of rare yet serious complications of dermal fillers is multidisciplinary. Ongoing education and training of the practitioners are the top priority to improve the injection techniques and anatomical knowledge, thus reducing the risk of such adverse outcomes. Also, customization of treatment planning based on patient anatomy and personal requirements can reduce risks and optimize aesthetic results. Multi-disciplinary teams of dermatologists, plastic surgeons, and emergency physicians can optimize management in case complications arise by sharing expertise for delivering better patient care. Continued research and data collection on complications will continue to inform best practices, eventually leading to a safer environment in which to utilize dermal fillers (Öztürk, 2021) (Figure 12.12).

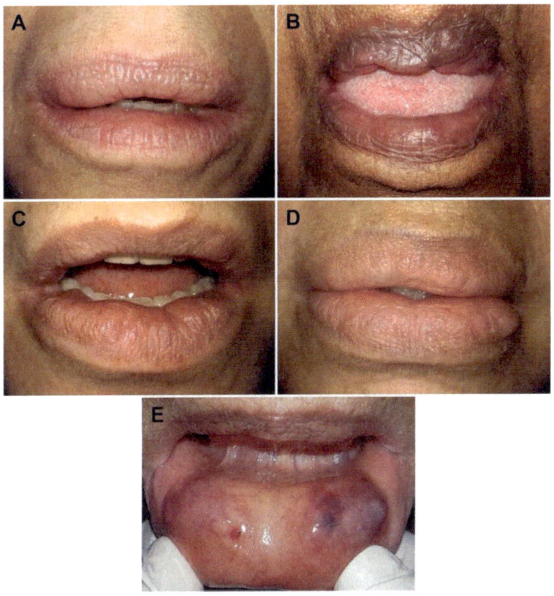

Figure 12.12. Clinical aspects of adverse reactions to dermal fillers in the oral and maxillofacial region. A–D Cases 1–4: asymptomatic and normal-colored fibrous submucosal nodules located in the upper and lower lips. E Case 5: painless bilateral nodules in the mucosa of the lower lip associated with marked redness.

Source: https://www.researchgate.net/publication/371135864/figure/fig1/AS:11431281190502934@1695348898235/Clinical-aspect-of-adverse-reactions-to-dermal-fillers-in-the-oral-and-maxillofacial.jpg

12.4.3. Importance of Choosing a Qualified Practitioner

Selection of a skilled practitioner for dermal filler procedures is essential to a patient's safety and the achievement of good aesthetic outcomes. A skilled practitioner with sufficient knowledge of the facial anatomy complexities will minimize the risk of injection-related issues leading to vascular occlusion or infection. Also, an evidence-based practitioner who is trained, as noted in Kumar (2021), can apply critical thinking and evidence-based approaches in tailoring treatments to meet the unique needs of individual patients. This sensitivity is especially critical with the abundance of dermal fillers and the range of specific indications that exist, where a trained practitioner can pick the right product and technique that aligns with a patient's desired esthetic results with safety at top priority. Aside from technical skill, the worth of selecting an experienced practitioner is also in informed consent and patient education.

A qualified practitioner should be able to describe the potential risks and benefits of various dermal fillers clearly so that patients can be well-informed before signing the consent form. Prioritizing a thorough assessment of the patient's medical history and potential contraindications is important, as outlined in leading curricula for aesthetic practitioners, including that covered in Kumar (2021). This prepares the practitioner to manage patient expectations realistically, fostering a harmonious relationship that improves overall satisfaction with the end result. The decision to choose an experienced injector therefore, has a significant impact on both procedural experience and outcome. In addition, the practitioner's adherence to ongoing education and adherence to industry standards is an important consideration in ensuring dermal filler treatment safety and effectiveness.

As the quickly evolving non-surgical aesthetic industry continues to grow, practitioners must remain constantly educated and trained and upgrade their skills in new technologies and techniques. This dedication is reinforced in works such as those compiled in, which outline comprehensive protocols for the handling of scars and wounds, emphasizing the importance of careful information in procedural applications.

Continual refinement of methods enables practitioners to utilize best practices and maximize patient safety profiles. Lastly, selecting a qualified practitioner ensures technical competence but also manifests commitment to excellence in patient treatment and aesthetic procedures.

Test Your Knowledge

1. What are the most common side effects associated with dermal fillers, and how can patients manage them during recovery?
2. Are there any rare but serious complications that could arise from dermal filler treatments, and how can these be prevented or addressed?

12.5. Injection Techniques

Learning Outcome

1. Describe different injection methods
2. Explain the importance of anatomical knowledge
3. Discuss the role of patient assessment in technique selection

Selection of injection techniques is critical for the optimization of safety and efficacy of dermal filler treatment. Proper familiarity with the anatomical landscape must be present, particularly in high-risk locations such as the periocular region, where anatomical complexity may affect the results of the injection. Practitioners must individualize their technique by first identifying the patient's individual needs and the specific facial areas to be treated. Methods such as aspiration before injection are also necessary in order to prevent unwanted intra-arterial placement of the filler, which can lead to severe complications, e.g., necrosis of the skin or even loss of vision (Ciesielska et al., 2025). In addition, employing slow injection methods in the mid or deep dermal plane allows for precise control of volume, which is crucial for minimizing side effects. These preventive actions highlight the need to fill gaps in anatomical knowledge with skilled performance to yield optimal outcomes in patients. Education and training on diverse dermal filler brands also play a significant role in the selection of appropriate injection techniques. Several different compositions, such as hyaluronic acid fillers, have certain properties that affect their utilization and handling during administration. For instance, the use of more technologically advanced fillers like VYC-25L aims to standardize technique and ensure predictability in outcome while addressing the challenges of facial remodeling in varied patient profiles (Segurado et al., 2021). The new dynamics of dermal fillers demand ongoing education and refreshing of injection skill sets to align with the latest advancements. Practitioners are encouraged to be mindful of innovations and consensus recommendations that pertain to specific techniques and complications of these products. This vigilance ensures a more successful and safer treatment process for aesthetic-challenged patients. The placement of focus on technical skill aside, another aspect that impacts the choice of injection methods involves patient evaluation as well. Each patient possesses certain characteristics that determine the best method for filler injections. Identifying all these variables, such as facial anatomy and intended aesthetic results, enables practitioners to select not only the filler but also the delivery method that will work best. For example, correction of cases such as microgenia or sagging face may require specialized techniques for optimal augmentation (Segurado et al., 2021). These are the reasons why individual treatment plans have to be developed after a proper discussion of anticipated risks and complications. Finally, open communication and a commitment to patient safety are most crucial, allowing practitioners to deliver optimal care in dermal filler treatments.

12.5.1. Different Injection Methods (E.g., Linear Threading, Bolus)

Treatment with fillers is done with a variety of injection methods, each having certain applications, advantages, and disadvantages. Linear threading is one method most often utilized to inject filler under controlled circumstances along the path of a wrinkle or fold. It allows direct placement and greater control of filler injected, resulting in a more subtle and naturally appearing outcome. Linear threading is employed by clinicians such that the product is uniformly distributed, thereby lowering the frequency of lumps or irregular texture. In addition, it is particularly handy in contouring areas of high precision that are sensitive, e.g., marionette lines and nasolabial folds. Heterogeneity of tissue response necessitates each patient having a tailored approach, and this can be maximized through efficient means like linear threading. In contrast, the bolus injection method focuses on applying large amounts of filler in specific areas to achieve immediate volume replacement. It is particularly effective in areas of extreme volume loss, such as the cheeks or the temples. By injecting the filler in favorable bolus locations, the practitioner is able to create a symmetrical lifting effect and restore the contours of youth. This method not only adds bulk but also supports underlying tissue, thus providing structural support. Complications such as swelling or bruising can be more common with bolus injections since more volume is being added at one location. Therefore, careful patient selection and optimal anatomical knowledge are important to minimize adverse results from this method of injection. The technique of injection depends commonly on the location of the treated tissue, the type of aesthetic effect, and the needs of the patient. Bolus and linear threading are effective in treating many facial manifestations of aging, including volume loss and skin laxity. Although bolus delivery might be faster, linear threading produces a more gradual effect, offering more control over the aesthetic result. Proper education about the implications of each technique, alongside comprehensive determination of personal risk profiles, enables clinicians to formulate appropriately informed decisions according to patients' expectations and goals. Some techniques, such as those for the management of infraorbital hollows, depict the importance of a personalized approach to injection techniques (Jui-Peng et al., 2020; Siperstein, 2022). This flexibility in the choice of technique finally improves patient satisfaction and outcome (Figure 12.13).

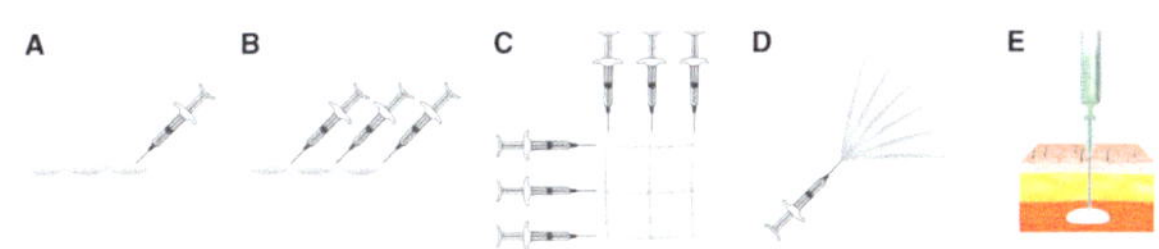

Figure 12.13. Illustration of basic injection techniques. (A) linear threading technique; (B) Serial puncture threading technique; (C) Cross-hatching technique; (D) Fan technique; and (E) Bolus techniques.

Source: https://www.researchgate.net/publication/347533970/figure/fig3/AS:983173290811405@1611418187966/Illustration-of-basic-injection-techniques-a-linear-threading-technique-B-Serial.ppm.

12.5.2. Importance of Anatomical Knowledge

A full understanding of facial anatomy is required by practitioners performing dermal filler injections. This not only assists in selecting proper filler agents and techniques but also enhances safety and outcomes during procedures. Awareness of underlying anatomy, i.e., vasculature and nerve tracts, decreases complications such as bruising, nerve damage, or vascular occlusion. Additionally, anatomical landmark familiarity allows practitioners to achieve desired aesthetic results through optimal filler placement. As highlighted in current literature, identification of morphologic diversity within ethnic groups, for instance, Asian and Caucasian patients, impacts treatment strategies and enhances patient satisfaction (Moon et al., 2021). Development of a strong anatomical knowledge base assists clinicians in tailoring interventions according to individual patient needs and, hence, maximizing the chances of favorable outcomes in aesthetic procedures. A well-defined area of anatomical knowledge in regard to facial aging and its impact on filler treatment is also of critical importance. Volume loss and tissue relocations alter the aging face profoundly, and their solution must be multidirectional in approach to aesthetic improvement. Practitioners must understand inter-relationships between facial compartments, such as superficial and deep fat layers, to restore a youthful appearance successfully. Further, understanding the patient's individual anatomic features, such as differences in skin thickness or variations of adipose distribution, allows the practitioner to customize the technique and product selection. Such individualization not only creates more esthetically pleasing outcomes but also minimizes postoperative morbidity because practitioners can anticipate the effects of aging and, accordingly, modify interventions (Moon et al., 2021). A solid background in facial anatomy is therefore essential for achieving natural outcomes, with patient safety being ensured. Last but not least, anatomical education performs an equally critical role in adopting new technologies and techniques in aesthetic surgery. The idea of ultrasound-guided injections is an advancement in the technology of injectable fillers because it allows practitioners to see the anatomy in real-time, so the placement remains precise. It keeps the basic and complex anatomy of the face more relevant. Familiarity with the physiological reactions of the skin and tissues underlying other therapies can also be useful in the choice of appropriate treatment modalities by the practitioner. As dermatologic ultrasound and other emerging technologies continue to evolve, anatomy-aware practitioners are in a position to adapt and integrate the change into their practice. Finally, the benefit of understanding anatomy transcends basic technical proficiency, warranting a general aesthetic medicine approach and long-term patient relationships based on assurance and successful outcomes.

12.5.3. Role of Patient Assessment in Technique Selection

Evaluation of patients is an important step in choosing the injection techniques for dermal fillers so that there are optimal aesthetic outcomes and fewer complications. Proper evaluation begins with patients' medical history, including the presence of any previous conditions, allergies, or cosmetic procedures done before. These factors are crucial in guiding practitioners on what type of fillers to use and how to inject them. Inadequate assessment of such factors can have undesirable effects, and these may have a considerable influence on patient safety and satisfaction. Besides facilitating the tailoring of the treatment plan, an informed assessment also facilitates the establishment of realistic expectations, a friendly setting between patient and practitioner upon which the success of treatments in aesthetic dermatology largely depends. Much more important, however, is the patient-to-patient anatomical difference to be of paramount concern at the time of patient evaluation. Different regions of the face require differing approaches due to differences in skin thickness, musculature depth, and vascular supply. As a point of reference, areas such as the periocular area, which require high fidelity, require judicious selection of technique based on in-depth knowledge of anatomy. As highlighted by research, technique misestimates may have severe complications such as ischemic injuries from inadvertent intra-arterial filler injection. Practitioners should therefore undergo comprehensive training to evaluate every patient's unique anatomical terrain for compatibility with the intended injection method. A tailored approach that incorporates both patient assessment and expert understanding of facial anatomy is needed in order to reduce risks and optimize aesthetic outcomes (Ciesielska et al., 2025). Patient assessment must also incorporate psychological considerations that entail the motivations and expectations that patients have for cosmetic interventions using dermal fillers. Understanding the patient's psychological profile allows health professionals to gauge the appropriateness of requested intervention, thereby ensuring expectations are within what can be delivered. Unrealistic patients, for instance, will be problematic in the treatment process as they will never be satisfied with what is attained.

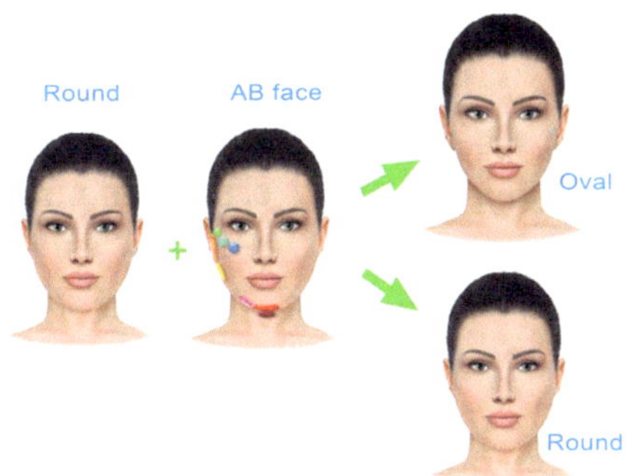

Figure 12.14. AB face technique treatment plan for the round-shaped face. The treatment with injectable fillers enhances the structure without changing the shape or may elongate the face into a more oval shape. In general, the volume of filler is distributed in the following proportion: 30% in the middle third and 70% in the lower third of the face.

Source: https://www.researchgate.net/publication/343974193/figure/fig8/AS:940739634659330@1601301215594/AB-face-technique-treatment-plan-for-the-round-shaped-face-The-treatment-with-injectable.ppm.

The integration of psychological assessment in pre-procedure evaluation increases the provider's ability to select suitable techniques and enhance communication in the treatment process. This comprehensive strategy not only addresses the technical aspects required in successful dermal filler procedures but also emphasizes the importance of all-encompassing patient care, thereby adding to the overall satisfaction and safety in aesthetic dermatology clinics (Madnani et al., 2022) (Figure 12.14).

Test Your Knowledge

1. What are the different injection methods used in dermal filler procedures, and how do they impact the outcome of the treatment?
2. How does patient assessment play a role in selecting the appropriate injection technique, and what factors are considered during this evaluation?

12.6. Post-Procedure Care

Learning Outcome

1. Understand immediate aftercare instructions
2. Focus on long-term care and maintenance
3. Discuss the signs of complications to watch for

Post-procedure care is a crucial factor in ensuring the longevity and safety of dermal filler treatments. Following the treatment, patients are most likely advised to avoid strenuous activity, excessive sun exposure, and exposure to extreme temperatures for a minimum of 24 to 48 hours. These measures are likely to minimize any potential side effects, such as swelling and bruising, that occur immediately following the treatment. Moreover, patients need to be educated about warning signs of complications, like persistent pain, skin discoloration, or vision changes, which can indicate a deeper issue related to vascular occlusion or filler migration (Ciesielska et al., 2025). The practitioner must provide complete post-treatment instructions and schedule follow-up sessions at the appropriate time to monitor and address any complications, reassuring the patient that they are not left to recover by themselves. On post-injection care, cold compresses can be utilized to reduce swelling and discomfort. Patients are advised to use a clean, cold compress at times on the first day after the procedure for the prevention of such effects. The importance of the avoidance of superficial manipulations of the injected areas cannot be overstressed, as this will lead to undesired filler migration or displacement. This must be communicated to the practitioner: proper recovery care is the solution to maintaining the early results. Post-treatment advice can also differ with the type and volume of filler used; for example, hyaluronic acid fillers can be subject to less strict aftercare compared to other materials since they can be dissolved with hyaluronidase in case of any complications (Reddy et al., 2012). Furthermore, management of post-procedure complications requires a high-level understanding of the filler used and the anatomical zone injected. In the case of fine periocular targets, there is a need for prompt identification of evidence of adverse reaction because of the risk of hazardous sequelae such as ischemia or necrosis caused by vascular compromise (Ciesielska et al., 2025). Practitioners need to be prepared to counteract immediately with appropriate interventions, which may include the administration of hyaluronidase or surgical interventions for permanent fillers. Preparedness not only enhances patient safety but also functions in a critical manner to facilitate the maintenance of aesthetic treatment outcomes. Patient education on the potential side effects and what to do if a side effect occurs reinforces the importance of post-procedure care, ultimately leading to increased satisfaction from dermal filler treatments.

12.6.1. Immediate Aftercare Instructions

Early aftercare following dermal filler injection is important to obtain optimal results and prevent complications. The patient is typically advised to avoid activities that can enhance swelling or bruising, such as strenuous exercise, sunbathing, or sauna, for 24 to 48 hours following the injection. Further, application of ice packs to the injection areas can reduce swelling and pain effectively. The application of over-the-counter painkillers like acetaminophen is also often suggested, while that of NSAIDs is to be avoided because it encourages bruising. Educating patients on the importance of following these initial aftercare procedures guarantees the best outcome and establishes their confidence in the procedure (Avelar et al., 2023). The second most important aspect of early aftercare is the monitoring for unusual responses, such as persistent swelling or aberrant discoloration. If side effects do appear, they must be instructed on the importance of contacting their physician promptly. Direct communication concerning probable potential side effects can also decrease fear and allow patients to distinguish between the usual indications of healing and complications that require attention. Furthermore, practitioners should emphasize the necessity of following up post-appointments, as follow-up sessions provide opportunities for reassessment and management of any complications that may arise after treatment. Such in-depth aftercare plans lay the groundwork for supportive ongoing care that can enhance patient satisfaction and treatment length (Alicia et al., 2017). Aside from physical welfare, psychological assistance is likewise essential during the immediate post-dermal filler injection session. Patients may be in any of several moods ranging from jubilation over their new appearance to apprehension concerning postoperative results.

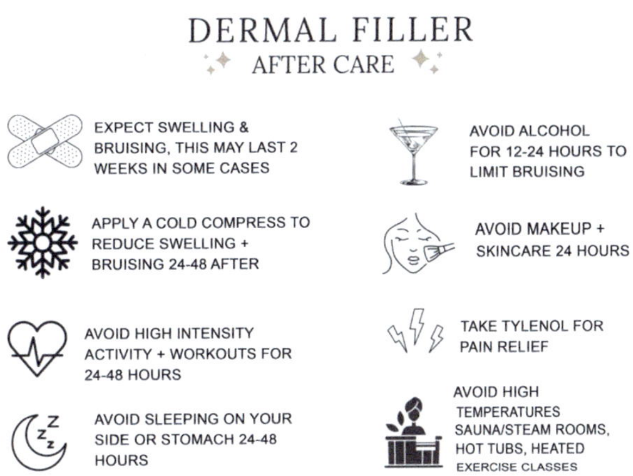

Figure 12.15. Dermal fillers: after care.

Source: https://www.newyorkliposuction.com/wp-content/uploads/2024/09/6B26B368-534D-4F5A-A72E-FF18E39EB8F8-1024x731-1.jpg.

An appropriate aftercare regimen includes not only physical healing instructions but reassurance of normality regarding these feelings. Encouraging patients to have practical expectations of the final result, particularly in the first few days when swelling can obscure the end result, helps towards better acceptance of the treatment. Connecting emotional support and practical advice, healthcare providers are able to facilitate enhanced patient experiences and outcomes, representing the complex nature of post-treatment care for aesthetic clinics (Avelar et al., 2023) (Figure 12.15).

12.6.2. Long-Term Care and Maintenance

In dermal fillers, long-term maintenance and care should be done to achieve proper results. Once the dermal filler injections are given, proper aftercare should be a priority for the patient to enhance the effects of the procedure. Regular follow-ups by a skilled practitioner allow tracking of the treatment area, verification of results, and intervention on time if necessary. In addition, proper skincare regimens, including the use of sun protection and moisturizers, can significantly affect the longevity of fillers. A daily regimen, which may include gentle cleansers and moisturizers, may improve the general well-being of the skin and consequently the long-term effects of the fillers. This active strategy for the health of the skin gives recognition to maintenance and procedural intervention with long-term dermatological treatment to achieve optimal aesthetic outcomes. Additionally, the creation of dermal fillers also plays a significant role in maintaining their effects in the long term. For instance, hyaluronic acid fillers, through their natural configuration and biocompatibility, provide compatibility with tissue integration in the skin. As has been described in recent research, newer approaches to dermal filler design have led to improved longevity and fewer side effects, and patient satisfaction has improved over the years. Advances such as cross-linking agents can dramatically enhance the stability of these fillers so that they are more durable before their effect on bulking diminishes. Similarly, the application of various types of fillers for various regions of the face underscores the need for tailored treatments based on specific requirements in order to achieve effective long-term management and a more natural result over the lifetime of the filler. Furthermore, the role of regular professional follow-ups cannot be downplayed regarding long-term maintenance. A complete awareness of personal reactions to fillers can direct modifications to treatment protocols toward achieving the best aesthetic results. Such an open discussion between the practitioner and patient allows for a cooperative strategy for managing expectations and dealing with issues that might occur after treatment. The addition of new materials, such as new biomaterials that enhance the compatibility and function of dermal fillers, also highlights the requirement for expert consultation in the maintenance stage. Research has put forward that the addition of new materials such as hydrogels would not only enhance the overall function of dermal fillers but would also introduce new functional properties (Jacob et al., 2021; Veeman et al., 2021). Lastly, long-term maintenance in the practice of dermal fillers is a multifaceted process involving patient education, follow-up, and constant developments in filler technology to attain aesthetic goals successfully.

12.6.3. Signs of Complications to Watch for

The increasing popularity of dermal fillers, particularly hyaluronic acid, necessitates awareness of potential complications that can arise during and after injection. One of the most critical signs to monitor is the onset of vascular complications, which can lead to conditions such as vascular occlusion. Patients and practitioners must be vigilant for symptoms such as sudden pain, discoloration of the skin, and changes in skin temperature, as these indications could signal compromised blood supply to the tissue. Timely recognition and intervention are essential to mitigate further damage, as outcomes can range from minor issues to significant tissue necrosis if not addressed promptly. Educating both patients and clinicians about these warning signs is crucial for maintaining safety in cosmetic procedures, allowing for early detection and appropriate management of complications related to dermal fillers (Sanders et al., 2024). In addition to vascular occlusion, clinicians should also be alert for signs of inflammation, infection, or abscess formation. Symptoms that may arise include localized swelling, redness, and the presence of pus or unusual discharge at the injection site. These issues may indicate a bacterial infection and necessitate immediate medical evaluation to prevent worsening conditions. The case of a 37-year-old patient who developed an abscess post-injection exemplifies the importance of recognizing and addressing these complications. Despite initial treatment efforts, the infection persisted, ultimately requiring surgical intervention. This underlines the need for thorough pre-procedural assessments, ensuring that patients are free from underlying periodontal conditions that could exacerbate the risk of infection (Iannitti et al., 2012).

Test Your Knowledge

1. What are the immediate aftercare instructions patients should follow after receiving dermal filler injections to ensure optimal results and minimize side effects?
2. What long-term care and maintenance practices can help prolong the effects of dermal fillers and support skin health over time?

SUMMARY

In concluding an exploration of dermal fillers, it becomes evident that these aesthetic interventions hold significant value in contemporary cosmetic medicine. The diversity of filler types, ranging from hyaluronic acid to collagen-based products, caters to a broad array of patient needs. Individuals seek dermal fillers not only for aesthetic enhancement, such as smoothing wrinkles or augmenting volume, but also for corrective measures in instances of asymmetry or post-surgical adjustments. Understanding the underlying motivations of diverse demographics, particularly younger adults in their third decade of life, emphasizes the ethical implications of aesthetic medicine as a preventive strategy, distinguishing it from mere cosmetic trends (Wollina & Goldman, 2011). This broader perspective allows practitioners to consider the psychological and social dimensions of their patients' desires, laying the groundwork for informed and responsible practice. Moreover, the administration of dermal fillers entails specific injection techniques that are vital for achieving optimal results while minimizing risks. Mastering these techniques requires thorough training and a deep understanding of facial anatomy, as well as an astute awareness of individual patient conditions. A noteworthy concern in this realm is the management of potential complications, which, although infrequent, can impact patient safety and satisfaction. For instance, studies have indicated the occurrence of inflammatory adverse reactions, particularly with hyaluronic acid injections, necessitating comprehensive strategies for monitoring and managing such incidents effectively (Öztürk, 2021). Consequently, practitioners must remain vigilant and well-informed regarding the latest techniques and approaches to mitigate these risks while delivering safe and effective treatments. Ultimately, the conclusion drawn from this examination of dermal fillers highlights not only their efficacy but also the imperative for ethical practice within aesthetic medicine. It is essential that healthcare providers balance the potential benefits of dermal fillers with a commitment to patient safety and well-being. As the field evolves, continuous education and adherence to best practices will be paramount in maintaining the integrity of the profession. The implications of aesthetic treatments as part of preventive medicine present unique challenges and opportunities, underscoring the responsibility of practitioners to deliver care that respects both the physical and emotional landscapes of their patients (Wollina & Goldman, 2011). In essence, a holistic approach that considers the diverse needs and expectations of patients will ensure the continued advancement and acceptance of dermal fillers within the broader scope of cosmetic enhancement.

In the landscape of cosmetic enhancements, dermal fillers represent a significant advancement in aesthetic medicine, offering a range of applications from volumizing to contouring the face. Various types of fillers, including hyaluronic acid, collagen-based, and APCs, cater to diverse patient needs. Hyaluronic acid fillers are highly favored due to their biocompatibility and reversibility, while collagen-based fillers typically provide longer-lasting results but may require skin testing before application. APCs, a relatively newer option, have shown promising results in facial rejuvenation and treatment of scars, underscoring the importance of interdisciplinary knowledge in choosing appropriate dermal fillers for different indications. This versatility is pivotal as practitioners strive to provide tailored treatments that align with the aesthetic goals and unique biology of each patient, ultimately enhancing satisfaction and treatment outcomes. The indications for dermal fillers extend beyond mere aesthetics, involving complex considerations that include patient safety and desired outcomes. Conditions such as volume loss due to aging, scarring from acne, and even treatment of melasma are now addressed through targeted filler applications. Recent advancements have highlighted the potential of a-PRP in combination with traditional fillers, yielding compelling results in skin rejuvenation and scar treatment (Davies & Miron, 2025). The literature suggests that such combinations may yield better aesthetic results, and additional research is needed to standardize procedures and monitor long-term effects. Having such knowledge allows clinicians to effectively balance aesthetic improvement with patient safety and satisfaction throughout the treatment journey. In terms of effectiveness, safety in dermal filler injection can be heavily reliant on the technique used. Proper technique not only influences the immediate visual outcome but also mitigates the risk of complications such as bruising, swelling, or more severe adverse effects (Téot et al., 2021). Techniques vary among practitioners and may include linear threading, bolus injection, and retrograde injection methods, each suited for different filler types and treatment areas. Training in these advanced techniques is essential, as their mastery can significantly affect patient experiences and results. Moreover, continued professional development through workshops and conferences fosters an environment of knowledge sharing, ultimately advancing the field of aesthetic medicine. As researchers and practitioners evaluate emerging technologies alongside established methods, a comprehensive understanding of injection techniques will remain fundamental to achieving optimal results in the ever-evolving domain of dermal fillers.

KEY TERMS FROM THIS CHAPTER

- Biocompatibility
- Filler treatment
- Nasolabial folds
- Safer treatment process
- Hyaluronic acid
- Poly-L-lactic acid
- Collagen fillers
- Semi-permanent fillers
- Volume restoration
- Wrinkle correction
- Calcium hydroxylapatite (CaHA)
- Heightened recognition
- Patient management
- Dermal fillers
- Calcium hydroxyapatite
- Polymethylmethacrylate (PMMA)
- Temporary fillers
- Permanent fillers
- Facial contouring
- Lip augmentation

CRITICAL THINKING QUESTIONS

1. Which of the following is the most commonly used type of dermal filler?
   a. Calcium hydroxylapatite
   b. Polymethylmethacrylate (PMMA)
   c. Hyaluronic acid
   d. Poly-L-lactic acid

2. Which area of the face is most commonly treated with dermal fillers to restore volume loss due to aging?
   a. Forehead
   b. Nasolabial folds
   c. Eyelids
   d. Chin

3. Which injection technique involves placing the filler in a linear path as the needle is withdrawn?
   a. Bolus technique
   b. Serial puncture technique
   c. Tunneling technique
   d. Fanning technique

4. Which of the following is a non-permanent dermal filler?
   a. Calcium hydroxylapatite
   b. Silicone
   c. PMMA
   d. Hyaluronic acid

5. A common complication of improper dermal filler injection into the glabella region is:
   a. Skin discoloration
   b. Infection
   c. Allergic reaction
   d. Vascular occlusion leading to tissue necrosis

Short Answer Questions

1. What are the main types of dermal fillers, and what is each type commonly composed of?
2. List three common aesthetic indications for the use of dermal fillers.
3. How does the mechanism of action differ between hyaluronic acid fillers and poly-L-lactic acid fillers?
4. What are the advantages of using hyaluronic acid fillers compared to other types?
5. What are some contraindications to dermal filler injections?
6. Describe the difference between linear threading and bolus injection techniques.
7. What are common immediate and delayed complications of dermal filler treatments?
8. How can vascular occlusion during dermal filler injections be identified and managed?

Answer to Critical Thinking Questions

1. (c); 2. (b); 3. (c); 4. (a); 5. (d)

REFERENCES

1. Alfageme, F., Wortsman, X., Catalano, O., Roustán, G., Crişan, M., Crişan, D., Gaitini, D., et al. (2020). European Federation of Societies for Ultrasound in Medicine and Biology (EFSUMB) position statement on dermatologic ultrasound. *Ultra Schall in der Medizin–European Journal of Ultrasound, 42*, 39–47. https://doi.org/10.1055/a-1161-8872.
2. Avelar, L. E. T., Ong, A. J., Ong, D. S. Y., Wai, A. C. S., Wai, A. Y. T., Sungkyu, J., Seok, L. H., et al. (2023). Consensus recommendations on the use of injectable poly-L-lactic acid in Asian patients. *Journal of Cosmetic Dermatology, 22*, 3223–3231. https://doi.org/10.1111/jocd.15969.
3. Barnes, C., Chuang, J., & Wong, B. (2016). *Overview of Facial Plastic Surgery and Current Developments*. https://core.ac.uk/download/617032104.pdf (accessed on 11th June 2025).
4. Segurado, M. A., Urdiales-Gálvez, F., Benítez, P. A., Carrasco, S., Díaz, I., Escoda, N., Farollch-Prats, L., Figueiredo, V., Ortíz, F., Sebastián, M. C., & Uva, L. (2021). An expert consensus report on the clinical use of the Vycross® hyaluronic acid VYC-25 L filler. *Journal of cosmetic dermatology, 20*(10), 3155–3164. https://doi.org/10.1111/jocd.14398 (accessed on 11th June 2025).
5. Burgess, C. M. (2006). *Principles of Soft Tissue Augmentation for The Aging Face*. https://core.ac.uk/download/pdf/8299191.pdf (accessed on 11th June 2025).
6. Catalano, C., De Rosa, M., Frezza, M. A., La Gatta, A., et al. (2016). *Biophysical and Biological Characterization of a New Line of Hyaluronan-Based Dermal Fillers: A Scientific Rationale to Specific Clinical Indications*. https://core.ac.uk/download/197708206.pdf (accessed on 11th June 2025).
7. Christen, M. O., & Vercesi, F. (2020). Polycaprolactone: How a well-known and futuristic polymer has become an innovative collagen-stimulator in esthetics. *Clinical Cosmetic and Investigational Dermatology, 13*, 31–48. https://doi.org/10.2147/ccid.s229054.
8. Ciesielska, A., Sieradzka, A., Szerej, K., Kot, A., Wojtczak, M., Myśliwiec N., ... Mawlichanów M. (2025). An Overview of Complications and Treatment Strategies in Periocular Dermal Fillers: A Literature Review. *Quality in Sport, 37*, 57034. https://doi.org/10.12775/QS.2025.37.57034(accessed on 11th June 2025).
9. Cortese, A., Chirico, F., Tartaro, G., Audino, G., Colella, G., Rugge, L., Sgaramella, N., et al. (2021). *Non-Surgical Touch-Up with Hyaluronic Acid Fillers Following Facial Reconstructive Surgery*. https://core.ac.uk/download/599516555.pdf (accessed on 11th June 2025).
10. Davies, C., & Miron, R. J. (2025). Autolougous platelet concentrates in esthetic medicine. *Periodontology 2000, 97*(1), 363–419. https://doi.org/10.1111/prd.12582(accessed on 11th June 2025).
11. Madnani, N., Vedmurthy, M., Parthasarthi, A., Dhawan, S., Kandhari, R., Pillai, R., & Nischal, K. C. (2022). Expert opinion on pre and post procedure care in aesthetic dermatology. *International Journal of Research in Medical Sciences, 10*(4), 991–1000. https://doi.org/10.18203/2320-6012.ijrms20220999(accessed on 11th June 2025).
12. Téot L, Mustoe TA, Middelkoop E, et al., editors. Textbook on Scar Management: State of the Art Management and Emerging Technologies [Internet]. Cham (CH): Springer; 2020. Available from: https://www.ncbi.nlm.nih.gov/books/NBK586066/ doi: 10.1007/978-3-030-44766-3(accessed on 11th June 2025).

13. Goldie, K., Peeters, W., Alghoul, M. S., Butterwick, K. J., Casabona, G., Chao, Y. Y. Y., Costa, J., et al. (2018). Global consensus guidelines for the injection of diluted and hyper diluted calcium hydroxyapatite for skin tightening. *Dermatologic Surgery, 44*, S32–S41. https://doi.org/10.1097/dss.0000000000001685.

14. Wollina, U., & Goldman, A. (2011). Minimally invasive aesthetic procedures in young adults. *Clinical, cosmetic and investigational dermatology*, *4*, 19–26. https://doi.org/10.2147/CCID.S17467 (accessed on 11th June 2025).

15. Iannitti, T., Marusza, W., Mlynarczyk, G., Netsvyetayeva, I., et al. (2012). *Probable Biofilm Formation in The Cheek as A Complication of Soft Tissue Filler Resulting from Improper Endodontic Treatment of Tooth 16*. https://core.ac.uk/download/pdf/8729802.pdf (accessed on 11th June 2025).

16. Jacob, S., Nair, A. B., Shah, J., Sreeharsha, N., Gupta, S., & Shinu, P. (2021). Emerging role of hydrogels in drug delivery systems, tissue engineering and wound management. *Pharmaceutics, 13*, 357. https://doi.org/10.3390/pharmaceutics13030357

17. Kumar, N. (2021). *Design, Development and Implementation Framework for A Postgraduate Non-Surgical Aesthetics Curriculum*. https://core.ac.uk/download/480391006.pdf (accessed on 11th June 2025).

18. Makvandi, P., Kirkby, M., Hutton, A. R. J., Shabani, M., Yiu, C. K. Y., Baghbantaraghdari, Z., Jamaledin, R., et al. (2021). Engineering microneedle patches for improved penetration: Analysis, skin models and factors affecting needle insertion. *Nano-Micro Letters, 13*. https://doi.org/10.1007/s40820-021-00611-9.

19. Proietti, I., Skroza, N., Mambrin, A., Marraffa, F., Tolino, E., Bernardini, N., Marchesiello, A., Rossi, G., Volpe, S., & Potenza, C. (2021). Aesthetic Treatments in Cancer Patients. *Clinical, cosmetic and investigational dermatology, 14*, 1831–1837. https://doi.org/10.2147/CCID.S342734(accessed on 11th June 2025).

20. Medeiros, C. C. G. (2013). *Estudo Experimental Em Ratos Submetidos À Injeção Intravascular De Polimetilmetacrilato: Avaliação Clínica E da Toxicidade Sistêmica*. https://core.ac.uk/download/48130605.pdf (accessed on 11th June 2025).

21. Meghe, S., Ramapure, R., Jaiswal, S., Jawade, S., & Singh, S. (2024). A comprehensive review of minimally invasive dermatosurgical procedures. *Cureus*. https://doi.org/10.7759/cureus.56152.

22. Moon, H. J., Fundaro, S. P., Goh, C. L., Hau, K. C., Paz-Lao, P., & Salti, G. (2021). A review on the combined use of soft tissue filler, suspension threads, and botulinum toxin for facial rejuvenation. *Journal of Cutaneous and Aesthetic Surgery, 14*, 147. https://doi.org/10.4103/jcas.jcas_119_20.

23. O'Connor, A., Lowe, P., Shumack, S., & Lim, A. (2017). Chemical peels: A review of current practice. *Australasian Journal of Dermatology, 59*, 171–181. https://doi.org/10.1111/ajd.12715.

24. Öztürk, K. (2021). *Inflammatory Complications of Vocal Fold Injection with Hyaluronic Acid: A Multiinstitutional Study*. https://core.ac.uk/download/630381466.pdf (accessed on 11th June 2025).

25. Peng, J. H., & Peng, H. L. P. (2020). HA filler injection and skin quality–Literature minireview and injection techniques. *Indian Journal of Plastic Surgery, 53*, 198–206. https://doi.org/10.1055/s-0040-1715545.

26. K. Rajeev Reddy, 1 K. Srinidhi Reddy, 2 V. Sridhar Reddy3. Management of Peri Implant deficiency with PRP and bone grafts – A Case Report. Effect of PRP on bone regeneration using bone substitutes RttdifPRPhhhtflllbbtitt IJCDS • MARCH, 2012 • 3(1) © 2 https://core.ac.uk/download/pdf/288292355.pdf (accessed on 11th June 2025).

27. Riggio, E. (2024). Report on the 11th National Congress AICPE (Associazione Italiana di Chirurgia Plastica Estetica) held in Rimini, Italy, 12–14 April 2024. *Surgical Techniques Development, 13*, 122–161. https://doi.org/10.3390/std13020009.

28. Sanders, G. (2024). *A Bundle of Care for Prevention, Early Recognition, And Treatment of Hyaluronic Acid Dermal Filler Associated Vascular Occlusion*. https://core.ac.uk/download/616423550.pdf (accessed on 11th June 2025).

29. Siperstein, R. (2022). Infraorbital hyaluronic acid filler: Common aesthetic side effects with treatment and prevention options. *Aesthetic Surgery Journal Open Forum, 4*. https://doi.org/10.1093/asjof/ojac001.

30. Valente, D. S., Steffen, N., & Valente, S. S. (2018). Abstract: Dermal fillers in secondary rhinoplasty. *Plastic & Reconstructive Surgery Global Open, 6*, 242–243. https://doi.org/10.1097/01.gox.0000547154.45079.71

31. Veeman, D., Sai, M., Sureshkumar, P., Jagadeesha, T., Natrayan, L., Ravichandran, M., & Mammo, W. D. (2021). Additive manufacturing of biopolymers for tissue engineering and regenerative medicine: An overview, potential applications, advancements, and trends. *International Journal of Polymer Science, 2021*, 1–20. https://doi.org/10.1155/2021/4907027.

INDEX

N

P

Q

R

S